Ways of
Living

Ways of Living

4TH EDITION

Intervention Strategies to Enable Participation

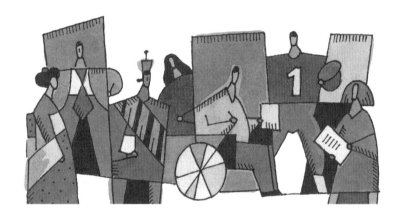

EDITED BY

CHARLES H. CHRISTIANSEN, EDD, OTR, OT(C), FAOTA

KATHLEEN M. MATUSKA, PHD, OTR/L, FAOTA

FOREWORD BY GARY KIELHOFNER, DRPH, OTR/L, FAOTA

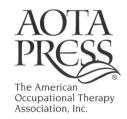

AOTA PRESS

The American Occupational Therapy Association, Inc.

AOTA Centennial Vision

We envision that occupational therapy is a powerful, widely recognized, science-driven, and evidence-based profession with a globally connected and diverse workforce meeting society's occupational needs.

Mission Statement

The American Occupational Therapy Association advances the quality, availability, use, and support of occupational therapy through standard-setting, advocacy, education, and research on behalf of its members and the public.

AOTA Staff

Frederick P. Somers, *Executive Director*
Christopher M. Bluhm, *Chief Operating Officer*

Chris Davis, *Director, AOTA Press*
Rick Ludwick, *Production Consultant*
Ashley Hofmann, *Development/Production Editor*
Victoria Davis, *Production Editor/Editorial Assistant*

Beth Ledford, *Director, Marketing*
Emily Zhang, *Technology Marketing Specialist*
Jennifer Folden, *Marketing Specialist*

American Occupational Therapy Association, Inc.
4720 Montgomery Lane
PO Box 31220
Bethesda, MD 20814
Phone: 301-652-AOTA (2682)
TDD: 800-377-8555
Fax: 301-652-7711
www.aota.org
To order: http://store.aota.org

Disclaimers

This publication is designed to provided accurate and authoritative information in regard to the subject matter covered. It is sold or distributed with the understanding that the publisher is not engaged in rendering legal, accounting, or other professional service. If legal advice or other expert assistance is required, the services of a competent professional person should be sought.
—*From the Declaration of Principles jointly adopted by the American Bar Association and a Committee of Publishers and Associations*

It is the objective of the American Occupational Therapy Association to be a forum for free expression and interchange of ideas. The opinions expressed by the contributors to this work are their own and not necessarily those of the American Occupational Therapy Association.

ISBN: 978-1-56900-298-8

Library of Congress Control Number: 2011902498

Cover Design by Debra Naylor, Debra Naylor Design, Inc., Washington, DC
Composition by Maryland Composition, Laurel, MD
Printed by AGS, White Plains, MD

Dedications

To Gary Kielhofner, DrPH, OTR/L, FAOTA, posthumously with great respect, for being friend, colleague, and inspiration; to Amy Lind, PhD, OTR, and Ruth Peterson, OTR (also posthumously), who taught me about professionalism and kindness and believed in me enough to give me a first and second chance; and to Beth A. Jones, PhD, my dear wife, who has given me an important third chance.
—*CHC*

To Tom, for 33 years as husband, father, friend, counselor, and supporter. Thanks for everything.
—*KMTM*

Contents

List of Tables, Figures, Boxes, Case Studies, and Appendixes

Chapter 8

Chapter 9

Foreword to the Fourth Edition

Occupational therapy has its origins in the observation that the way in which people live their everyday lives is a barometer of their health and well-being. The fundamental rationale for occupational therapy is grounded in the related observation that engaging clients in the tasks of everyday life has a salutary effect on their physical, psychological, and social recovery following disease, injury, and stress.

Nearly a century has passed since these observations were first codified as the cornerstones of the profession. In that time, occupational therapists have sought to translate them into knowledge about the relationship between occupation and health and into practical strategies to address the many problems that can interfere with occupation. This volume both reflects and contributes to that enterprise in important ways.

It is worth noting that the journey to realize occupational therapy's original insights concerning the reciprocal relationship between health and occupation has not been linear. The field was diverted in the last century by an alliance with medical ways of understanding and managing impairment. In the past three decades there has been a call by occupational therapy's leaders for a return to the field's original tenets and to a practice thoroughly grounded in occupation. Nonetheless, practitioners have struggled to realize the latter objective under conditions in which technical proficiency, efficiency, and productivity have become critical forces shaping the delivery of health care services.

It is in this context that *Ways of Living: Intervention Strategies to Enable Participation* makes an important contribution. The text begins with an elucidation of how engagement in the activities of daily life provides avenues of participation, identity making, and creation of a personal narrative, which are all essential to a good life. It also underscores the importance of recognizing the personal devastation that can be created when one is deprived of meaningful occupation.

These two core ideas infuse a series of chapters that discuss the occupational therapy process and that address important specifics about the services occupational therapists can provide for persons who face barriers to occupation in the form of cognitive, orthopedic, neurological, sensory, and psychiatric impairments. Other themes taken up in the book include the importance of partnerships with clients and caretakers; of environmental adaptations; and of removing social, economic, and political barriers to occupation.

To address these and other issues, this volume brings together the collective wisdom and experience of a wide range of expert practitioners who provide detailed guides as to how occupational therapists enable clients experiencing these conditions to recapture and re-engage in their lives. The authors take special care to ensure that the knowledge and know-how shared herein is in touch with contemporary conditions. This is reflected, for instance, in incorporation of the latest *Occupational Therapy Practice Framework* (American Occupational Therapy Association, 2008), an emphasis on client-centered practice, attention to the importance of evidence-based practice, and awareness of the impact of the digital age.

Readers will find in this book a wealth of information to guide practice that has been thoughtfully and thoroughly presented. Importantly, this text not only echoes and reinforces the call to occupation-oriented intervention but also provides a detailed roadmap for therapists to reach that destination.

Gary Kielhofner, DrPH, OTR/L, FAOTA
Professor, Department of Occupational Therapy
University of Illinois at Chicago

Reference

American Occupational Therapy Association. (2008). Occupational therapy practice framework: Domain and process (2nd ed.). *American Journal of Occupational Therapy, 62,* 625–683.

Preface to the Fourth Edition

If we have learned anything during the 21st century, it has been that things can change quickly in a short period. Since the third edition of this text was published in 2004, much of historical note has occurred. Hurricanes created havoc in the Gulf Coast of North America, a worldwide economic downturn occurred, the United States elected its first African American President, and the world has continued its amazing progress in the realm of digital technology. More than ever before, we are in touch and informed, with our neighbors, our communities of interest, and the world at large. Access to information has never been easier.

Because information is so easy to disseminate and access, its influence on action is more rapid, which can have both positive and negative consequences. In the world of health care, the past several years have seen a major push toward practice based on proof. A positive consequence is that evidence-based practice is becoming the norm, and although evidence can take many forms, the expected and preferred form is through controlled research. Research, of course, takes time to complete. Thus, a negative consequence is the long process of providing evidence, communicating the information, and applying it to practice. This creates a "lag" time that feels paradoxically slow in a world where so many other things seem to happen at the speed of light. At the same time, the importance of being well informed and using best evidence to guide practice has never been greater. Health care providers are being held to a higher standard of effectiveness and efficiency on all levels.

As this preface was being written, a long-awaited national debate on health care reform was taking place in the United States. This reform effort culminated in the passage of federal legislation that has major implications for the country in many ways. The legislation should expand access, create conditions that encourage the widespread implementation of digital health information systems, and assuredly increase expectations about the need for evidence as a means to control costs and improve the quality of care within the context of safety and efficacy. Occupational therapy must be able to respond to these changes in its evidence-based practice.

As occupational therapists, we hope that the benefit of occupation-oriented intervention will continue to gain recognition. There is abundant evidence that people experience and evaluate their health in terms of its impact on their lives, or their ability to participate in their worlds of meaning. Thus, meaningful occupational performance is the outcome we strive for with our clients, recognizing that physical, mental, and emotional health are enablers to that outcome. When well-focused and implemented, occupational therapy services address those qualitative aspects of care that mean the most to the client.

Since publication of the third edition of this book, the *Occupational Therapy Practice Framework* (American Occupational Therapy Association, 2008) has been updated. Although the changes are not profound, neither are they inconsequential. This fourth edition reflects those changes both in content and in terminology. It also reflects them in spirit. The subtitle has been changed to reflect a broadened application of intervention strategies beyond adaptation to ADL and IADL challenges. Content has been updated, attention to supporting evidence has been emphasized, and efforts have been made to provide information in the book as a useful resource for understanding the most practical tools to enhance occupation-oriented practice.

Several new contributors have been invited to share their expertise, and new chapter features have been added, such as a highlights box. The editors are indebted to the following individuals for their support of the project: Charles Hayden for outstanding editorial assistance, Christina Davis and Victoria Davis of AOTA Press for terrific publishing support, and Google™ for providing an outstanding search engine and facility for sharing documents online. *Google docs* is yet another digital marvel that is changing the way information is created and shared.

We are also indebted to the late Gary Kielhofner for agreeing to write the foreword. Dr. Kielhofner's work has had significant global influence over many years, and we are honored to have his words in this volume. To become a better resource in the future, *Ways of Living* will benefit from the feedback of its readers. We invite your comments and suggestions at all times, which can be made to the publisher at AOTA Press.

Charles H. Christiansen, EdD, OTR, OT(C), FAOTA
Rochester, MN

Kathleen M. Matuska, PhD, OTR/L, FAOTA
St. Paul, MN

Reference

American Occupational Therapy Association. (2008). Occupational therapy practice framework: Domain and process (2nd ed.). *American Journal of Occupational Therapy, 62,* 625–683.

About the Contributors

Beatriz C. Abreu, PhD, OTR, FAOTA, is Clinical Professor at the University of Texas Medical Branch at Galveston. She earned her undergraduate degree in occupational therapy at the University of Puerto Rico, and a doctor of philosophy in Occupational Therapy from New York University. She is an educator and master clinician honored for her contributions to brain injury rehabilitation. Dr. Abreu has significantly contributed to the neuroscience literature. She has done numerous presentations in neurorehabilitation throughout the United States, Canada, South America, Japan, China, and Italy.

Suzanne Krenek Andrews, MOT, OTR, ATP, is manager of the TIRR Memorial Hermann Out-Patient Therapy Services in Houston, Texas. She has also served as adjunct faculty at Texas Woman's University for assistive technology. She received a bachelor of science degree in Community Health at Texas A&M University and a master's degree in Occupational Therapy from Texas Woman's University in Houston, Texas. She has twelve years of experience working with persons with spinal cord injury, amputations and other neuromuscular diseases. Suzanne is an Assistive Technology Professional, specializing in advanced seating and mobility needs of clients, computer and environmental access. She has provided expert review for the Consortium for Spinal Cord Medicine Clinical Practice Guidelines for Bladder Management after spinal cord injury.

Denis Anson, MS, OTR, graduated from the University of Washington in 1980 with a bachelor's degree of occupational therapy. In 1983, he received a master's of science degree in Occupational Therapy. He worked in adult physical disabilities for 6 years, and was a lecturer in the Division of Occupational Therapy at the University of Washington, Seattle, Washington for nine years. In August, 1997, he moved to Misericordia University in Dallas, Pennsylvania, and in 2005, became the Director of Research and Development of the Assistive Technology Research Institute. Mr. Anson has been actively involved in computer and assistive technology applications for rehabilitation for almost three decades.

Diane J. Atkins, OTR, FISPO, is an occupational therapist, currently in private practice, who has specialized in upper extremity rehabilitation for the past 30 years. She is a Clinical Assistant Professor in the Department of Physical Medicine and Rehabilitation Medicine at Baylor College of Medicine in Houston. Her experience with over 1,500 amputees has enabled her to lecture and teach to professional audiences throughout the world. She is a past Board Member and Fellow in the International Society of Prosthetics and Orthotics, and Honorary Member in the American Academy of Orthotics and Prosthetics. Diane is the co-editor and author of the text *Comprehensive Management of the Upper Limb Amputee*, and a Second Edition of this text entitled *Functional Restoration for the Person With Upper Extremity Amputation*. Currently, Diane serves as a consultant to the U.S. Department of Defense.

Catherine Backman, PhD, OT(C), FCAOT, is Associate Professor, Department of Occupational Science and Occupational Therapy, The University of British Columbia, and Research Scientist, The Arthritis Research Centre of Canada, in Vancouver, BC. A graduate of the University of British Columbia, (UBC), attended graduate school at the University of Washington. She began her academic career at UBC in 1986, and interrupted her teaching to complete a doctoral degree in Health Care and Epidemiology at UBC. Catherine's research is focused on studies of intervention and participation, particularly in the area of Arthritis. She is widely published and is a Fellow of the Canadian Association of Occupational Therapists, receiving that organization's highest honour, the Muriel Driver Memorial Lectureship, in 2004.

Karin J. Barnes, PhD, OTR, is chair in the Occupational Therapy Department at The University of Texas Health Science Center at San Antonio. She teaches pediatric occupational therapy courses. Her research interest areas are children with developmental disabilities, school system occupational therapy; and activities of daily living of children with disabilities.

Alison J. Beck, PhD, OTR, is associate professor in the Department of Occupational Therapy at The University of Texas Health Science Center at San Antonio. She teaches early childhood occupational therapy courses and is in clinical practice at a local pediatric outpatient clinic. Her current research is in assessment practices of occupational therapists.

Rebecca Birkenmeier, MSOT, OTR/L, is an Instructor of Occupational Therapy and Neurology at Washington University School of Medicine. She earned her master's degree in Occupational Therapy from Washington University School of Medicine. Her research interests focus on improving arm function in order to increase participation following stroke.

Jane A. Charlton, MSEd, is a Certified Orientation and Mobility Specialist and a Certified Rehabilitation Therapist, and teaches orientation and mobility to students at the State of Wisconsin's Center for the Blind and Visually Impaired. Prior to this, she worked on an itinerant basis with adults who were visually impaired for the State of Wisconsin's Department of Health and Family Services. Before working in the field of blindness rehabilitation, Charlton held several technical writing and editing positions. She has a master's degree in Education from Northern Illinois University, and a Bachelor of Science Degree in Bacteriology and Journalism from the University of Wisconsin-Madison.

Margaret Christenson, MPH, OTR/L, FAOTA, is President of Lifease, Inc.,® developer of Home Modification and Fall Prevention software. The software customizes and prints reports with ideas and products for safety, convenience, and independence in the home setting. She is a frequent seminar leader and has spoken to several hundred consumers and professional groups on the adaptations of the living environment to compensate for age-related changes and the incorporation of universal design. She was Minnesota Occupational Therapist of the Year, chair of the Gerontology Special Interest Section of AOTA and a delegate to the White House Conference on Aging. She chaired AOTA's Home Modification Specialty Certification Committee and is co-editor of their publication *Occupational Therapy and Home Modifications: Promoting Safety and Supporting Participation.*

Charles H. Christiansen, EdD, OTR, OT(C), FAOTA, is Executive Director of the American Occupational Therapy Foundation (AOTF) and a Clinical Professor at the University of Texas Medical Branch at Galveston. Prior to his current role, he served as Vice-Provost for Health Sciences and Founding Director, Center for Allied Health Professions at the University of Minnesota, and as Dean and George T. Bryan Distinguished Professor, School of Health Professions at the University of Texas Medical Branch. He is founding editor of the journal *OTJR: Occupation, Participation and Health,* and a Fellow of the American Occupational Therapy Association [AOTA]. He has served in numerous roles as officer and board member of professional societies in occupational therapy, allied health, and occupational science, and has edited or co-authored 10 books and over 100 scientific and scholarly papers and chapters.

Penelope Moyers Cleveland, EdD, OTR/L, BCMH, FAOTA, earned a doctorate in Adult Education, with a major in Public Administration, from Ball State University, and a Master's Degree in Community Development from the University of Louisville. Her bachelor's degree in occupational therapy is from the University of Missouri. Dr. Moyers Cleveland served as President of AOTA from 2007–2010. As Dean of the Henrietta Schmoll School of Health at St. Catherine University, she draws on 29 years of experience in occupational therapy, having developed expertise in mental health practice and in upper extremity rehabilitation. Dr. Moyers Cleveland is board certified by AOTA in Mental Health. Dr. Moyers Cleveland has published extensively on the topic of substance use disorders and other topics and has worked extensively to develop evidence-based practice briefs for occupational therapy. She has served in numerous professional roles and is widely published.

Heather Schultheis Dodd, MS, OTR/L, is an occupational therapist with experience in burn and hand therapy. She is currently at the University of North Carolina (UNC) Hand Center and the North Carolina Jaycee Burn Center at UNC Healthcare in Chapel Hill.

Sandra Fletchall, OTR/L, CHT, MPA, FAOTA, occupational therapist and certified hand therapist, has specialized in catastrophic injuries of amputations, burns and complex fractures for the past 35 years. Her work experience includes providing services for catastrophic injuries in a variety of settings. For the past several years, private practice has provided the environment for continuing services to individuals with catastrophic injuries from acute care to return to work, including home and work assessments and functional assessments. Ms. Fletchall has received awards for outstanding practice and leadership from the Tennessee Occupational Therapy Association and AOTA, where she was named Fellow in 2000. She has published articles published on the topics of burns, amputations, and prosthetics.

Gelya Frank, PhD, is Professor in the Division of Occupational Science and Occupational Therapy at the School of Dentistry, University of Southern California. She is a cultural anthropologist and a founder of occupational science. Her books include: *Lives: An Anthropological Approach to Biography* (Chandler and Sharp, 1981), with L. L. Langness; *Venus on Wheels: Two Decades of Dialogue on Disability, Biography, and Being Female in America* (University of California Press, 2000); and *Defying the Odds: The Tule River Tribe's Struggle for Sovereignty in Three Centuries* (Yale University Press, 2010), with Carole Goldberg. Dr. Frank is Director of the NAPA–OT Field School in Antigua, Guatemala, an interdisciplinary project of the National Association for the Practice of Anthropology. She was honored by the Society for the Study of Occupational Science as the 2010 Ruth Zemke Lecturer in Occupational Science.

Don Golembiewski, MA, CVRT, is an instructor for the Hadley School for the Blind of Winnetka, Illinois. Previously he has served as the Coordinator of the Wisconsin Independent Living for Older Blind Individuals program and participated in the direct itinerant rehabilitation teaching services to blind adults in a nine county area in Wisconsin. Mr. Golembiewski received a master's degree in blind rehabilitation from Western Michigan University in 1977 and has held a number of leadership positions in his field. He is past president of the Madison Central Lions Club and was a Preceptor for Occupational Therapy students at the University of Wisconsin–Madison, and has worked collaboratively with Northern Colorado University, Mississippi State University, the State of Colorado Services for the Blind, Northern Illinois University, and the American Foundation for the Blind. He is a co-author of *Coping With Low Vision*.

Theresa Gregorio-Torres, MA, OTR, ATP, is a Senior Therapist for Stambush Healthcare Services providing occupational therapy services at TIRR Memorial Hermann Hospital and a PRN therapist at The University of Texas M.D. Anderson Cancer Center in Houston, Texas. She received a bachelor of science degree from University of Louisiana at Monroe, a master's degree in Occupational Therapy Education and an Occupational Therapy Ergonomics Certificate from Texas Woman's University in Houston. She has over 29 years of experience working with persons with spinal cord injury or diseases of the spine. She currently represents the AOTA on the Consortium for Spinal Cord Medicine Clinical Practice Guidelines of the Paralyzed Veterans of America. Her other interests include assistive technology evaluation and prescription.

Kristine Haertl, PhD, OTR/L, is an Associate Professor in the Department of Occupational Science and Occupational Therapy at St. Catherine University in St. Paul, Minnesota. Her clinical expertise includes areas of psychiatric, cognitive and developmental occupational therapy practice. In addition to full time faculty work, Dr. Haertl has a small private practice, is a community practitioner, serves on the executive Board for a large mental health organization in the Twin Cities, and is a former quality consultant for the Federal Head Start programs. Her research interests include the impact of environmental design, program development, and meaningful occupations on client success and quality of life. She has published and presented nationally and internationally on topics of psychiatric practice, mental health housing, and sensory processing.

Bernadette Hattjar, DrOT, MEd, OTR/L, is an Assistant Professor of Occupational Therapy at Gannon University in Erie, Pennsylvania. Dr. Hattjar has authored or co-authored a number of articles in occupational therapy publications. She has also co-authored a textbook chapter. She has been the principal investigator on a number of research projects at Gannon University. Her research focus at this time is the psychological effects of disability on life satisfaction. She is currently completing work on a user-friendly textbook on sexuality and disability for AOTA Press.

Claudia List Hilton, PhD, OTR/L, SROT, FAOTA, worked for over 25 years as an occupational therapist across the spectrum of ages and diagnostic groups, and has served on the occupational therapy faculties at Washington University and Saint Louis University in St. Louis, Missouri. She is on the editorial board for the *American Journal of Occupational Therapy*, has served as an Accreditation Council for Occupational Therapy Education reviewer, and has been a grant reviewer for several national and international granting agencies. Dr. Hilton earned her doctorate in occupational therapy and is currently completing a postdoctoral fellowship in the Department of Psychiatry at Washington University School of Medicine.

Devva Kasnitz, PhD, is a medical anthropologist, a disability studies scholar, a disability policy consultant, and the Director of Disability Studies for the NAPA–OT Field School in Antigua, Guatemala. She is a founding member of the Society for Disability Studies, the Association of Rural Programs in Independent Living, and the Disability Research group of the Society for Medical Anthropology.

Rafferty Laredo, MA, OTR, ATP, is the Occupational Therapy Clinical Coordinator for the Spinal Cord Injury Team at TIRR Memorial Hermann Hospital in the Texas Medical Center in Houston, Texas. He received his bachelor of arts degree in Psychology from Baylor University in Waco, Texas, and bachelor of science degree in Occupational Therapy from the University of Texas Health Science Center of San Antonio. He received his master's degree with specialty in Assistive Technology from Texas Woman's University in Houston, Texas. He has been invited to speak extensively on advanced spinal cord injury care, including advanced seating and mobility, assistive technology, bowel and bladder management, and innovative ADL strategies. He has provided expert review for the Consortium for Spinal Cord Medicine Clinical Practice Guidelines for Respiratory Management and Bladder Management after spinal cord injury.

Kathleen Matuska, PhD, OTR/L, FAOTA, is Associate Professor and Graduate Program Director in the Department of Occupational Therapy and Occupational Science at St. Catherine University in St. Paul, Minnesota. Dr. Matuska has done research in multiple sclerosis and has co-edited the previous two editions of *Ways of Living*. She earned a bachelor of science in Occupational Therapy, a master's degree in Public Health, and doctorate from the University of Minnesota. Her doctoral dissertation was on the topic of measuring life balance, and she has published several papers and co-edited a book on that topic, *Life Balance: Multidisciplinary Theories and Research*, which is jointly published by AOTA Press and Slack, Inc.

Kerri Morgan, MSOT, OTR/L, is an Instructor in the Program in Occupational Therapy and Neurology at Washington University Medical School, St. Louis, Missouri. Her job responsibilities include teaching an assistive technology course to first-year graduate occupational therapy students and managing several disability related grants from a variety of federal and state funding sources. Grant topics include personal assistance services, employment, outcome measures, health and wellness, community accessibility and assistive technology for people with disabilities. Ms. Morgan served as a consultant for two local independent living centers where she performed state assessments to determine the eligibility of people with disabilities for a Consumer Directed Personal Assistance Service Program.

Margaret A. Perkinson, PhD, is an Associate Professor in the Department of Occupational Science and Occupational Therapy at Saint Louis University, St. Louis, Missouri, and Director, Community-Based Gerontology, NAPA–OT Field School in Antigua, Guatemala. She received her doctoral degree in Human Development and Aging, with a concentration in medical anthropology, from the University of California, San Francisco. She serves as editor-in-chief of *Journal of Cross-Cultural Gerontology* and is on the editorial board of *Physical and Occupational Therapy in Geriatrics*. Her research interests include family care giving for older adults in the community and in nursing homes, friendship patterns and community development in continuing care retirement communities, physical activity and dementia, and aging in developing countries.

Monica Perlmutter, MA, OTR/L, is an instructor in the Program in Occupational Therapy at Washington University Medical School, St. Louis, Missouri, and the lead occupational therapist for the Program's Community Practice Low Vision Services. Academic responsibilities include teaching in the problem-based learning curriculum and in related practice courses. Her research interests currently focus on measurement of the occupational performance of older adults with vision loss and the impact of lighting on daily activities.

Janet L. Poole, PhD, OTR/L, FAOTA, is Professor and Graduate Program Coordinator, Occupational Therapy Graduate Program, Department of Pediatrics, University of New Mexico, Albuquerque, New Mexico. Dr. Pool is a Fellow of AOTA and a member of the prestigious Academy of Research of the American Occupational Therapy Foundation. She is widely published in a number of clinical areas, including arthritis and connective tissue diseases.

Mark Prochazka, OTR/L, MHA, is an occupational therapist with 7 years of trauma and burn related experience. He is currently at the North Carolina Jaycee Burn Center at the University of North Carolina Healthcare at Chapel Hill.

Sandra Rogers, PhD, OTR/L, is an Associate Professor in the School of Occupational Therapy at Pacific University in Hillsboro, Oregon. She has been teaching in occupational therapy for 10 years and is involved in research examining the relationship between neurological damage and physiological functioning and examining how occupational therapy intervention influences health. She participates in interprofessional activities with faculty and students to serve clients, including services at a high school for at-risk teens, a shelter for homeless youth and co-leads a nationally recognized camp for stroke survivors, Stroke Camp Northwest, awarded a Rosalyn and Jimmy Carter Partnership Award for University and Community Collaborations. Dr. Rogers has been recognized for teaching excellence, and has published chapters and articles and presented on occupation-based practice and physiological changes after neurological injury.

Carol Haertlein Sells, PhD, OTR, FAOTA, is a Professor of Occupational Therapy at the University of Wisconsin (UW) at Milwaukee, a Scientist with the UW–Milwaukee Center for Addiction and Behavioral Health Research, and a Major in the U.S. Army. She is a Fellow of AOTA and a past member of the AOTA Commission on Education. Her current scholarly interests include the occupational needs of wounded service members and young veterans, the reduction and prevention of college student drinking, and the examination of community success for people with serious mental illness in collaboration with Dr. Virginia Stoffel. She has been involved in several federally funded research projects, including Project ARRIVE, funded by the National Institute on Mental Health and Comparing Two Interventions for Freshmen Violators, funded by the National Institute on Alcohol Abuse and Alcoholism. She and Dr. Stoffel have also been the recipients of grant funding from AOTF, AOTA, and the Wisconsin Occupational Therapy Association's Research Fund.

Martha E. Snell, PhD, is a Professor of Education in the Curry School of Education at the University of Virginia where she directs the graduate programs in severe disabilities and early childhood special education. Believing in an interdisciplinary and collaborative teaming approach for serving children and adults with disabilities, Dr. Snell often teams with occupational therapists and other related services personnel while preparing teachers through course work and supervised field experiences. Among her research interests are instructional methods for students with severe disabilities and inclusion of students with disabilities in general education.

Virginia C. Stoffel, PhD, OT, BCMH, FAOTA, is an Associate Professor of Occupational Therapy at the University of Wisconsin – Milwaukee, coordinates the graduate program, and is a scientist and Core Leader for the Center for Addiction and Behavioral Health Research, which is also located at the University of Wisconsin – Milwaukee. She is currently Vice President of the American Occupational Therapy Association (AOTA), past chair of the AOTA Mental Health Special Interest Section, a Fellow of AOTA, and past member of the AOTA Specialties Board and Commission on Continuing Competency and Professional Development. Dr. Stoffel is Board Certified in Mental Health through AOTA's recognition program. Her clinical experiences have been in mental health and substance abuse intervention programs. She is involved in several leadership development programs, most recently the AOTA Emerging Leader Development Program, based on her doctoral emphasis.

Sydney Jane Thornton, OTR/L, is an occupational therapist with over 27 years of experience treating burn patients. She is currently the senior occupational therapist at the North Carolina Jaycee Burn Center at University of North Carolina Healthcare in Chapel Hill.

Laura K. Vogtle, PHD, OTR/L, ATP, is Professor in the Department of Occupational Therapy and the Director of the Post Professional Master's Program at the University of Alabama at Birmingham in Birmingham, Alabama. Prior to completing her Ph.D. in program evaluation, she was a pediatric clinician for 23 years. More recently, she has become involved in aging in adults with developmental disabilities. She is involved in transdisciplinary team teaching and is a strong supporter of collaborative intervention for children and adults with disabilities. Her research interests include outcomes research and the use of social context in occupational therapy treatment.

Timothy J. Wolf, OTD, MSCI, OTR/L, is an Instructor of Occupational Therapy and Neurology at Washington University School of Medicine. He earned his clinical doctorate in Occupational Therapy and master's degree in Clinical Investigation from Washington University School of Medicine. His primary research focus is work rehabilitation as it relates to individuals with cognitive deficits following stroke and other chronic neurological conditions. Currently, his work is conducted through the Cognitive Rehabilitation Research Group (CRRG) and the Occupational Performance Center (OPC) at the Rehabilitation Institute of St. Louis (TRISL).

Sybil M. Yancy, MOT, OTR, is Director of Occupational Therapy at the Transitional Learning Center in Galveston. She earned her undergraduate degree at West Texas A&M University and her Master of Occupational Therapy degree at Texas Tech University. She is a certified brain injury specialist and a Non-violent Crisis Intervention Instructor with the Crisis Prevention Institute, Inc. Additionally, she has done numerous presentations at the National level, provided OT services internationally, and has contributed to the rehabilitation literature.

About the Editors

Charles H. Christiansen, EdD, OTR, OT(C), FAOTA, is Executive Director of the American Occupational Therapy Foundation. Previously, he spent three decades in various academic leadership roles, including service at the University of Minnesota, the University of Texas Medical Branch, and the University of British Columbia. Dr. Christiansen holds degrees in educational administration, counseling psychology, and occupational therapy. His scholarly and scientific interests inhabit the domain of lifestyle and health, with a particular focus on individual patterns of activity over the life course and how these influence well-being. He is particularly interested in how the interconnections of social, psychological, and neurophysiological mechanisms explain adaptation to stressful circumstances.

Kathleen Matuska, PhD, OTR/L, FAOTA, is Professor and Master of Arts in Occupational Therapy Program Director in the Henrietta Schmoll School of Health at St. Catherine University. Dr. Matuska has extensive clinical experience in the area of physical rehabilitation, with a special interest in healthy living and life balance for all persons. Her primary areas of interest and research include life balance, fatigue management, multiple sclerosis, and healthy aging.

Chapter 1

The Importance of Participation in Everyday Activities

CHARLES H. CHRISTIANSEN, EDD, OTR, OT(C), FAOTA

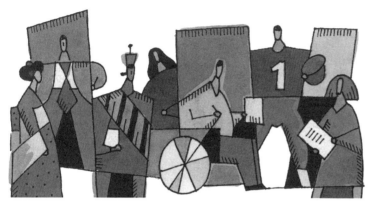

KEY WORDS

ADLs	participation
allostatic load	play
chronobiology	psychoneuroimmunology
core affect	quality of life
desynchronosis	social role
engagement	spirituality
flourishing	stigma
IADLs	work
ICF	Zeitgeber
identity	
leisure	
narrative	
occupational deprivation	
occupational disruption	

HIGHLIGHTS

- Basic and instrumental activities of daily living (IADLs) are life categories that serve as foundations for survival and participation in the community.

- IADLs include community mobility, communication, care of others (including pets), financial management, meal preparation, shopping, and care of the home.

- People understand their lives as stories consisting of activities over time that are given meaning; thus, understanding the stories of clients is an important part of clinical reasoning.

- The *International Classification of Functioning, Disability and Health (ICF)* emphasizes the importance of participation in understanding the relationships among people, their functional ability, and the environments in which they live.

- Participation in valued, meaningful activity has been shown to promote health and well-being through its psychological, neurological, endocrinological, and immunological benefits.

OBJECTIVES

After reading this material, readers will be able to

- Identify the major categories of daily activity,
- Distinguish between formal and informal ways of classifying time use,
- Explain the social importance of daily activity as identity building,
- Provide examples of how activity influences physiological processes,
- Identify common barriers to participation,
- List three examples of the relationship between daily activity and well-being, and
- Identify the major components of the *ICF* and their relationships.

This chapter is about living life or, more specifically, about the activities people do everyday, and why these activities are individually and collectively important to well-being. Being well involves more than simply feeling good. Wellness is a state of being that involves health, but it also involves the way people feel about themselves and their lives. When people can do what is important to them and feel good about what they've done, they flourish. Flourishing is a desired end-state that provides an appropriate model for understanding the link between how people feel (their core affect) and what they can do (their abilities and skills). How people feel about their health consistently and strongly predicts their mortality and their longevity more effectively than so-called "objective" measures of physical functioning (Idler & Benyamini, 1997; Lee et al., 2007). Even more importantly, participation in valued activities is strongly correlated with self-rated health (Katz et al., 2009).

In the early part of the 20th century, a small group of influential and committed people recognized that participation in daily occupations both enabled and reflected a person's state of well-being. Nearly a century later, we now know that what people are doing and how they are doing it can often provide many clues about who they are and how they are feeling, both emotionally and physically. What individuals do during a typical day often serves as a window that provides a useful view of their overall well-being.

For example, as people read this chapter, chances are they are sitting down, trying to get comfortable, and centering their mind so they can concentrate. This book is a professional text, and those reading it are most likely students studying for a professional degree. They have a goal, and completing this reading is a small step toward attaining that goal. That goal involves the reader, but it also involves others. It is likely that the importance associated with attaining the goal is influenced by an expectation that completion of a professional degree will bring respect and admiration. In reflecting on these possibilities, it is already apparent that the activities that people engage in in their lives have many dimensions beyond those that are apparent at first glance.

Yet, most people go about their daily routines without thinking too much about their activities or what they are doing at the moment. If there is a special event or person or an unusual situation that requires actions that are different from what is usually experienced, such activities gain their special attention. These events typically are accompanied by feeling states or emotions that are described in everyday language with terms such as anxiety, fear, surprise, anger, sadness, gratitude, frustration, or joy.

The feelings associated with activities can serve many purposes. They may arouse the senses and stimulate attention, motivate people to adapt to challenging or threatening circumstances, impel them to take further action, or stimulate their endocrine systems to release hormones important to their ability to respond. One theorist suggests that the feelings associated with events contribute to the interpretation of experience (Bruner, 1990) and help people learn from and remember them. That is, events may become connected in time with other experiences and through those connections help people "make sense of them." As activities are interpreted in the larger context of personal life stories, they may contribute to identity and provide a sense of continuity or overall coherence (Antonovsky, 1987b; see Box 1.1).

It is clear, then, that our everyday "occupations" are more complex than they seem. This chapter discusses the importance of participation in everyday activities to well-being and is organized in four sections. In the first section, the categories of activity that make up a typical day are discussed. In the second section, the personal and social significance of everyday activities are discussed, emphasizing the importance of daily activities to quality of life, personhood, identity, and social roles. In the third section, the way in which activities influence the body is reviewed, with emphasis on the connections between physiological changes and activity. This im-

Box 1.1. Antonovsky's Sense of Coherence

Aaron Antonovsky was an American/Israeli psychogist who was educated in the United States but emigrated to Israel. As part of his clinical practice, he became fascinated with the differences in the ability of his clients to cope with stressful conditions in life. He noticed that people who seemed to be more resilient, or less susceptible to the health consequences of their stressful episodes, seemed to have several characteristics, or orientations toward life, in common.

Resilient people had lives that were meaningful, manageable, and comprehensible. First, resilient people had *meaning* in their lives, in that they seemed to have a purpose that motivated them on a daily basis. Second, they seemed to have a belief that they could contend with the problems that came their way. Antonovsky described this using the term *manageability*. Finally, resilient people were able to make sense of their lives, even when they encountered many experiences that might otherwise make this difficult. This characteristic he described as *comprehensibility*. Altogether, Antonovsky observed that having these three characteristics helped people created a sense of coherence about their lives. A sense of coherence, Antonovky's claimed, would help people become less susceptible to conditions that would threaten their health.

Antonovsky's salotugenic theory continues to be used as a model for understanding the relationship between stress and illness. Although studies to test the validity of his theory have yielded mixed results, it is useful to note how its central features support the ideas in this chapter. Each of the features of this model correspond to themes in the chapter: meaning, life stories (comprehensibility), and having the belief that one can overcome challenging situations (manageability).

portant section describes how activities influence physiological health, how they influence the regulation of the body's internal clocks, and how reactions to participation in life's activities can influence the manner in which the body adapts to stress. In the final section, threats to participation in everyday activities are examined. These threats include limitations on participation; the section includes brief discussions of disability, disfigurement, stigma, social policy, attitudes, and environmental barriers, which

are described as forms of occupational deprivation and disruption. The chapter concludes with a review of the World Health Organization's (2001) *ICF*, a model of classifying disease and disability that reflects the multiple dimensions of people participating in activities within environments.

Defining and Describing Categories of Everyday Activities

Behavioral scientists have tried various approaches to describing or grouping activities according to their characteristics, yet no universal set of categories has been adopted. It is difficult to categorize an activity without knowing more about where it is performed, who it is performed with, when it is performed, and for what purposes (Christiansen & Townsend, 2010). For example, the game of golf can be played by professional athletes who earn a living from it or by amateurs as a type of weekly recreation. Moreover, golf is often used as a means for promoting business transactions. So, is golf a play or leisure activity, a work activity, or both? The answer depends upon the intended goals of the participants and the context or circumstances of the experience. An activity's context includes the various characteristics of the situation in which it is done.

Consider an example involving waiting, a common but unpopular activity. Now, consider two contexts in which people are waiting. In the first, a woman waits in a dentist's office to be called for a procedure that will require discomfort and possible pain. Her emotions are ambivalent. On the one hand, she wants to get the procedure over with and get on with her day. On the other hand, she dislikes sitting in the chair and having her mouth serve as the source of shrill sounds and unpleasant vibrations.

In the second example, a woman waits at the airport, and her lover is expected to land after a long absence. She can't wait to embrace and experience the joy of being together with her loved one once again. In this example, her anticipation is full of joyful expectation. The waiting period is both agonizing and pleasant because it connects previous memories of enjoyment with anticipated new experiences. In these two examples, the manners in which the participants experience waiting are vastly different because of the places, people involved, anticipated outcomes, and meanings associated with the situations. These are some of the characteristics that can influence the context in which an activity occurs and change the importance and meaning of an activity and the emotions associated with it.

Table 1.1. Time Use Categories From the International Classification of Activities for Time Use Statistics (ICATUS)

Time Use Category		Activities
01	Work for organizations	Paid work for corporations, government, nonprofits
02–05	Household work	Primary production Non-primary production Construction Services for income
06	Unpaid domestic services	Preparing and serving food Cleaning house and surroundings Clothes care Household management Shopping Travel in relation to these activities
07	Unpaid caregiving services	Care of children and adults and travel related to these activities
08	Community services	Voluntary and obligatory services for members of the community and travel related to these activities
09	Learning	Attendance of classes at all levels of instruction, including pre-primary, primary, vocational. Higher education and literacy classes; travel related to learning activities
10	Socializing and community participation	Socializing and communicating and participating in community events and related travel
11	Attending/visiting cultural, entertainment, and sports events/venues	Visiting cultural events or venues, exhibitions Watching shows, movies Visiting parks, gardens, zoos Visiting amusement centers, fairs, festivals, circuses Watching sports events Travel to and from these places
12	Hobbies, games, and other pastime activities	Active participation in arts, music, theater, dance; engaging in technical hobbies such as collecting stamps, coins, trading cards, computing, crafts Playing games Taking courses in relation to hobbies Related travel
13	Indoor and outdoor sports participation	Active participation in indoor and outdoors sports Coaching, training Looking for gym, exercise program, trainer Assembling and readying sports equipment Taking courses in relation to sports
14	Mass media	Includes reading (not related to work, learning); listening to radio or other audio devices; use of computer technology not strictly for work, learning, household management, or shopping; going to the library for leisure Travel to and from places for these purposes
15	Personal care and maintenance	Activities required by the individual in relation to meeting biological needs Performing own personal and health care and maintenance or receiving this type of care Activities in relation to spiritual/religious care Doing nothing, resting relaxing Meditating, thinking, planning

Source: Bediako and Vanek (1999).

People don't always do exactly what they want to do, because they have requirements, obligations, and expectations that influence how they use their time. One of the first researchers to create a classification system proposed that activities be classified according to whether or not they represented endeavors that were *necessary* (such as sleeping and eating), *contracted* (such as paid work or school), *committed* (such as child care, housekeeping, meal preparation, and shopping), or *free time* (activities chosen during the time remaining after attending to necessary, committed, and contracted activities) (Aas, 1980). In a similar way, time use researchers have adopted certain conventions for their research as depicted in the categories shown in Tables 1.1 and 1.2. It is important to note that these differ from categories typically used to describe everyday activities by practitioners in occupational therapy. These categorical differences are influenced by the interest of governments in measuring the economic consequences of time use rather than the social, cultural, and behavioral dimensions of how people spend their time.

Everyday Activity as Viewed Within Occupational Therapy

Occupational therapy practitioners typically divide daily living into several broad categories. These include activities done to earn a living; those related to leisure and recreation; and those related to personal care and self-maintenance, including rest and sleep. The American Occupational Therapy Association (AOTA) groups activities into categories, including activities of daily living (ADLs), instrumental activities of daily living (IADLs), rest and sleep, education, work, play, leisure, and social participation (AOTA, 2008, pp. 631–633). In Table 1.2, notice how these categories compare to those found in time diaries used in national studies of time use and depicted in Table 1.1. In the sections to follow, the specific activities and characteristics that define these categories are explained in greater detail.

Basic and Instrumental Activities of Daily Living

Activities at home and in the community designed to enable basic survival and well-being are sometimes referred to as *activities of daily living (ADLs)*. These are the duties and chores related to taking care of ourselves, including those related to basic self-care or personal care (such as toileting, bathing, grooming, and dressing), eating, using the telephone, managing medications, and sexual expression (see Figure 1.1). Sometimes, activities in this category are referred to as *personal activities of daily living*, and they are fundamental to survival and to living in a social world. This is because they are necessary for good physical and mental health and also important for group acceptance.

Although not listed in many descriptions of *basic activities of daily living (BADLs)*, sleep and its associated routines may also be considered a self-care activity. The revised *Occupational Therapy Practice Framework* (hereinafter the *Framework*; AOTA, 2008) includes rest and sleep as a separate area of human occupation. Sleep constitutes nearly one-third of each day in the lives of typical working adults (Basner et al., 2007). In addition to the time it consumes, sleep is also an obligatory occupation that is necessary for health and may have other purposes yet to be fully understood by scientists. Research has shown relationships between activity (including social involvement) and the quality and quantity of sleep (Ohayon, Zulley, Guilleminault, Smirne, & Priest, 2001; Carney, Edinger, Meyer, Lindman, & Istre, 2006).

Instrumental Activities of Daily Living

Nearly four decades ago, M. Powell Lawton, a gerontologist, recognized that living independently in the community required the ability to accomplish more than personal or basic self-care tasks (Lawton, 1971). These additional, and more complex tasks, were described by Lawton as *instrumental activities of daily living (IADLs)*. More recently, these have also been referred to as *extended activities of daily living*, or *EADLs* (Christiansen, 2004).

Activities in this category include care of others, care of pets, child rearing, communication device use (such as the telephone or TYY/TDD device for persons with deafness), *community mobility* (getting around in the community), financial management, health management and maintenance, home establishment and management, meal preparation and cleanup, safety and emergency responses, and shopping.

Together, basic self-care tasks and extended self-maintenance activities are viewed as a foundation for survival and for participation in the community. Cross-national research has shown that self-maintenance activities independent of sleep (BADLs and IADLs together) consume around 20% of the average nondisabled person's waking day (Fraire, 2006). People with disabilities and older persons may require a slightly higher proportion of time to accomplish these self-maintenance activities (Lawton, 1990; McKinnon, 1992).

Table 1.2. Terminology for ADLs From the *Occupational Therapy Practice Framework* *(cont.)*

Areas of Occupation	Specific Activities Within the Area	Definition
Various kinds of life activities in which people, populations, or organizations engage, including ADLs, IADLs, rest and sleep, education, work, play, leisure, and social participation.		
Activities of Daily Living (ADLs)—Activities that are oriented toward taking care of one's own body	Bathing, showering	Obtaining and using supplies; soaping, rinsing, and drying body parts; maintaining bathing position; and transferring to and from bathing positions.
	Bowel and bladder management	Includes complete intentional control of bowel movements and urinary bladder and, if necessary, use of equipment or agents for bladder control.
	Dressing	Selecting clothing and accessories appropriate to time of day, weather, and occasion; obtaining clothing from storage area; dressing and undressing in a sequential fashion; fastening and adjusting clothing and shoes; and applying and removing personal devices, prostheses, or orthoses.
	Eating	The ability to keep and manipulate food/fluid in the mouth and swallow it.
	Feeding	The process of setting up, arranging, and bringing food fluids from the plate or cup to the mouth.
	Functional mobility	Moving from one position or place to another (during performance of everyday activities), such as in-bed mobility, wheelchair mobility, transfers (wheelchair, bed, car, tub, toilet, tub/shower, chair, floor). Performing functional ambulation and transporting objects.
	Personal device care	Using, cleaning, and maintaining personal care items, such as hearing aids, contact lenses, glasses, orthotics, prosthetics, adaptive equipment, and contraceptive and sexual devices.
	Personal hygiene and grooming	Obtaining and using supplies; removing body hair (use of razors, tweezers, lotions, etc.); applying and removing cosmetics; washing, drying, combing, styling, brushing, and trimming hair; caring for nails (hands and feet); caring for skin, ears, eyes, and nose; applying deodorant; cleaning mouth; brushing and flossing teeth; or removing, cleaning, and reinserting dental orthotics and prosthetics.
	Sexual activity	Engagement in activities that result in sexual satisfaction.
	Toilet hygiene	Obtaining and using supplies; clothing management; maintaining toileting position; transferring to and from toileting position; cleaning body; and caring for menstrual and continence needs (including catheters, colostomies, and suppository management).

Table 1.2. Terminology for ADLs From the *Occupational Therapy Practice Framework* (cont.)

Areas of Occupation	Specific Activities Within the Area	Definition
Instrumental Activities of Daily Living (IADLs)— Activities that are oriented toward interacting with the environment and that are often complex—generally optional in nature (i.e., may be delegated to another)	Care of others (including selecting and supervising caregivers)	Arranging, supervising, or providing the care for others.
	Care of pets	Arranging, supervising, or providing the care for pets and service animals.
	Child rearing	Providing the care and supervision to support the developmental needs of a child.
	Communication device use	Using equipment or systems such as writing equipment, telephones, typewriters, computers, communication boards, call lights, emergency systems, braille writers, telecommunication devices for the deaf, and augmentative communication systems to send and receive information.
	Community mobility	Moving self in the community and using public or private transportation, such as driving, or accessing buses, taxicabs, or other public transportation systems.
	Financial management	Using fiscal resources, including alternate methods of financial transaction and planning and using finances with long-term and short-term goals.
	Health management and maintenance	Developing, managing, and maintaining routines for health and wellness promotion, such as physical fitness, nutrition, decreasing health risk behaviors, and medication routines.
	Home establishment and management	Obtaining and maintaining personal and household possessions and environment (e.g., home, yard, garden, appliances, vehicles), including maintaining and repairing personal possessions (clothing and household items) and knowing how to seek help or whom to contact.
	Meal preparation and cleanup	Planning, preparing, serving well-balanced, nutritional meals, and cleaning up food and utensils after meals.
	Safety procedures and emergency responses	Knowing and performing preventive procedures to maintain a safe environment as well as recognizing sudden, unexpected hazardous situations and initiating emergency action to reduce the threat to health and safety.
	Shopping	Preparing shopping lists (grocery and other), selecting and purchasing items, selecting method of payment, and completing money transactions.

(Continued)

Table 1.2. Terminology for ADLs From the *Occupational Therapy Practice Framework* *(cont.)*

Areas of Occupation	Specific Activities Within the Area	Definition
Rest and Sleep—Includes activities related to obtaining restorative rest and sleep that supports healthy active engagement in other areas of occupation	Rest	Quiet and effortless actions that interrupt physical and mental activity resulting in a relaxed state. Includes identifying the need to relax; reducing involvement in taxing physical, mental, or social activities; and engaging in relaxation or other endeavors that restore energy, calm, and renewed interest in engagement.
	Sleep	A series of activities resulting ingoing to sleep, staying asleep, and ensuring health and safety through participation in sleep involving engagement with the physical and social environments.
	Sleep preparation	(1) Engaging in routines that prepare the self for a comfortable rest, such as grooming and undressing, reading or listening to music to fall asleep, saying goodnight to others, and meditation or prayers; determining the time of day and length of time desired for sleeping or the time needed to wake; and establishing sleep patterns that support growth and health (patterns are often personally and culturally determined).(2) Preparing the physical environment for periods of unconsciousness, such as making the bed or space on which to sleep; ensuring warmth/coolness and protection; setting an alarm clock; securing the home, such as locking doors or closing windows or curtains; and turning off electronics or lights.
	Sleep participation	Taking care of personal need for sleep such as cessation of activities to ensure onset of sleep, napping, dreaming, sustaining a sleep state without disruption, and nighttime care of toileting needs or hydration. Negotiating the needs and requirements of others within the social environment. Interacting with those sharing the sleeping space such as children or partners, providing nighttime care giving such as breastfeeding, and monitoring the comfort and safety of others such as the family while sleeping.
Education—Includes activities needed for being a student and participating in a learning environment	Formal educational participation	Including the categories of academic (e.g., math, reading, working on a degree), nonacademic (e.g., recess, lunchroom, hallway), extracurricular (e.g., sports, band, cheerleading, dances), and vocational (prevocational and vocational) participation.
	Exploration of informal personal educational needs or interests (beyond formal education)	Identifying topics and methods for obtaining topic-related information or skills.
	Informal personal education participation	Participating in classes, programs, and activities that provide instruction/training in identified areas of interest.

Table 1.2. Terminology for ADLs From the *Occupational Therapy Practice Framework* *(cont.)*

Areas of Occupation	Specific Activities Within the Area	Definition
Work—Includes activities needed for engaging in remunerative employment or volunteer activities	Employment interests and pursuits	Identifying and selecting work opportunities based on personal assets, limitations, likes, and dislikes relative to work.
	Employment seeking and acquisition	Identifying job opportunities, completing and submitting appropriate application materials, preparing for interviews, participating in interviews and following up afterward, discussing job benefits, and finalizing negotiations. Job performance including work habits (e.g., attendance, punctuality), appropriate relationships with coworkers and supervisors, completion of assigned work, and compliance with the norms of the work setting.
	Retirement preparation and adjustment	Determining aptitudes, developing interests and skills, and selecting appropriate avocational pursuits.
	Volunteer exploration	Determining community causes, organizations, or opportunities for unpaid "work" in relationship to personal skills, interests, location, and time available.
	Volunteer participation	Performing unpaid "work" activities for the benefit of identified selected causes, organizations, or facilities.
Play—Any spontaneous or organized activity that provides enjoyment, entertainment, amusement, or diversion	Play exploration	Identifying appropriate play activities, which can include exploration play, practice play, pretend play, games with rules, constructive play, and symbolic play.
	Play participation	Participating in play; maintaining a balance of play with other areas of occupation; and obtaining, using, and maintaining, toys, equipment, and supplies appropriately.
Leisure	Leisure exploration Leisure participation	
Social Participation	Community participation Family participation Peer–friend participation	

Source. Reproduced with permission from American Occupational Therapy Association. (2008). Occupational therapy practice framework: Domain and process (2nd ed.). *American Journal of Occupational Therapy, 62,* 625–683.

Rest and Sleep

According to the *Framework* (AOTA, 2008), this category of daily occupations includes activities related to obtaining restorative rest and sleep that support healthy active engagement in other areas of occupation (see Table 1.2). The particular occupations in this category include *rest, sleep,* and *sleep preparation.* Rest includes interruptions in physical or mental activities that promote relaxation and restore energy and interest in resuming active participation. Sleep preparation includes routines related to dressing, grooming, and other practices that prepare the body and its surrounding environment for restorative sleep. Sleep itself includes falling asleep and staying asleep for sufficient duration to enable sleep quality. Sleep quality is a subjective measure but typically includes feeling a restoration of energy upon awakening.

Typically, people spend one-third of their lives sleeping, so its proportion of human time use is substantial (Roehrs & Roth, 2004). Despite this, the science underlying sleep remains in its infancy, and scientists are still not in agreement about all of the functions of sleep. Measurement of electrical activity in the brain has consistently shown that restorative sleep involves defined stages, leading to pro-

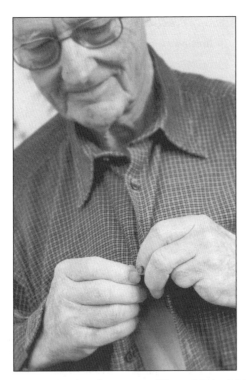

Figure 1.1. Dressing is one specific activity within the area of occupation identified as ADLs in the *Occupational Therapy Practice Framework*. This activity would be classified as personal care and maintenance in the time use categories specified by the International Classification of Activities for Time Use Statistics. Photo Credit: Image © Photos to go unlimited. Used under license.

function and other health consequences (Murphy & Delanty, 2007). The relationship between daily routines and sleep duration and quality is not fully understood, but there does appear to be useful guidance for sleep hygiene, or practices, that contribute to falling and staying asleep in a consistent manner (Atkinson & Davenne, 2007; Landis et al., 2003).

Work

Work includes activities needed for engaging in paid employment or volunteer activities (AOTA, 2008). This category includes employment and related activities (such as job seeking and acquisition), job performance, retirement-related activities, and exploration and participation in volunteerism. Time use scientists recognize that work occurs both in the home and at workplaces outside the home. When scientists want to distinguish between the work of maintaining households and that of earning a living, they refer to the latter category as *paid work*.

gressively deeper sleep and culminating in REM, or rapid eye movement sleep (Dew et al., 2003). During REM sleep the individual is dreaming, and it is widely believed that this stage of deep sleep is important for physical and mental restoration.

Research has shown that sleep deficits are related to the incidence of impaired cognition and safety issues, as well as chronic disease and life expectancy (Chaput, Després, Bouchard, & Tremblay, 2007; Dew et al., 2003). In addition to the mental and physical causes, disturbed sleep can be caused by lifestyle factors related to time use, including circadian desynchronosis, resulting from travel to other time zones, shift work, and other factors leading to temporal irregularity. The entrainment or calibration of internal physiological clocks to the external environment is an important characteristic of healthy living and is supported by regular routines. Depression, shift work, conditions that obstruct breathing, noisy environments, stress, and other circumstances can lead to sleep disturbances that, if left untreated, can lead to diminished immune

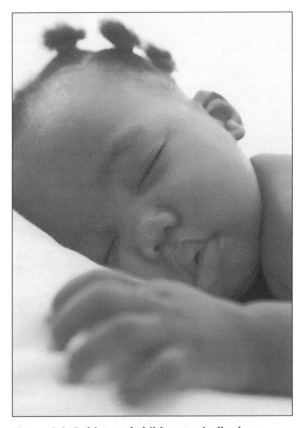

Figure 1.2. Babies and children typically sleep longer than adults, although people of all ages require adequate sleep because of its health benefits. Disturbed sleep may be a sign of circadian desynchronosis, or it can be related to disorders of breathing or mental illnesses, such as depression. Photo credit: Cathy Yeulet. Used under license from 123RF.com.

With the advent of telecommuting and the increased frequency of part-time employment arrangements, the nature of paid work is changing. However, traditional work sites and work groups provide more than income for the people employed there. Even in manufacturing jobs where wages are paid based on piecework (or each item manufactured or completed), there develops over time a set of relationships among those sharing work time that helps meet human needs for socialization and esteem. Regular work schedules also impose a temporal order on lives, so that the structure of the day and week become important parts of a person's habit patterns, routines, and lifestyle (Zerubavel, 1981). There is substantial evidence that unemployment impairs mental health (Paul & Moser, 2009).

Volunteerism consists of contributing one's time and talent toward an area of interest that benefits society or a specific group. Although it is generally accepted that public volunteerism fosters goodwill and trust in groups and in societies by promoting social capital, it also is said to offer the benefit of participation to greater numbers of people, and in so doing provides opportunities for learning and relationship building (Brudner & Kellough, 2000). Volunteerism enables an individual to contribute knowledge and skills for the benefit of others without obligation and with minimal social expectation beyond altruism and earnest effort. Recent studies have shown a relationship between volunteerism and health and longevity (Ayalon, 2008; Harris & Thoresen, 2005; Yaffe et al., 2009).

Education

Education includes activities needed for participating in a learning environment. This category of activity includes participation in both formal and informal educational pursuits and involves sensory and cognitive processing. Although education of both a formal and informal nature occurs throughout life, formal education constitutes a significant portion of time use during a typical week for children and adolescents (Hofferth & Sandberg, 2001).

Play

Play is defined by "any spontaneous or organized activity that provides enjoyment, entertainment, amusement, or diversion" (Parham & Fazio, 1997, p. 252; see Figures 1.3 and 1.4). Brian Sutton-Smith, one of the world's foremost scholars on play, notes that play is almost impossible to define because it is so ambiguous. He observes that there are many categories of play that have been named in the scholarly literature, including celebrations, rituals, contests, risky play, vicarious or audience play, mind play, solitary play, and informal social play, with each category having multiple examples of activity within it (Sutton-Smith, 2001, 2002). Play also provides an outlet for self-expression. Another scholar, Johan Huizinga, suggested that play is fundamental to culture and that it is contained within definite space and time and pursued without necessity, but with a mood of enthusiasm or rapture and absorption appropriate to the occasion or setting (Huizinga, 1950). No theory of play has yet been widely adopted, although it has been suggested that play serves important learning and adaptation functions and contributes to both variety and diversity in human activity.

Leisure

Leisure is defined as "a nonobligatory activity that is intrinsically motivated and engaged in during discretionary time; that is, time not committed to obligatory occupations such as work, self-care, or sleep" (Parham & Fazio, 1997, p. 250). As with play, leisure activities have an ambiguous nature, are freely chosen, have an attitudinal component, and are culturally defined (Thibodaux & Bundy, 1998). Stebbins identifies two broad categories of leisure, including those that involve significant personal effort or commitment, which he terms *serious leisure* (such as hobbies, volunteerism, self-development), and *casual leisure*, consisting of those activities that are pleasurable, of short duration, intrinsically rewarding, and requiring little effort (Stebbins, 1997).

Some theories suggest that leisure fulfills important psychological needs, including agency, novelty, belongingness, service, sensual enjoyment, cognitive stimulation, self-expression, creativity, competition, vicarious competition, and relaxation (Tinsley, 1995).

The potential importance of meaningful leisure activity was demonstrated in a study conducted by Waters and Moore (2002). In this interesting study, samples of employed and unemployed individuals were asked to report on their unmet needs, moods, and participation in leisure activities. Unemployed participants engaged in social leisure activities less and solitary activities more and reported higher levels of depression, lower self-esteem, and greater unmet needs. The meaning attained through social and solitary leisure activities acted to reduce perceived feelings of deprivation, and thus psychological distress, in unemployed participants. However, in the employed study participants, only social leisure had an impact on perceived deprivation and psychological health. Overall, the findings sug-

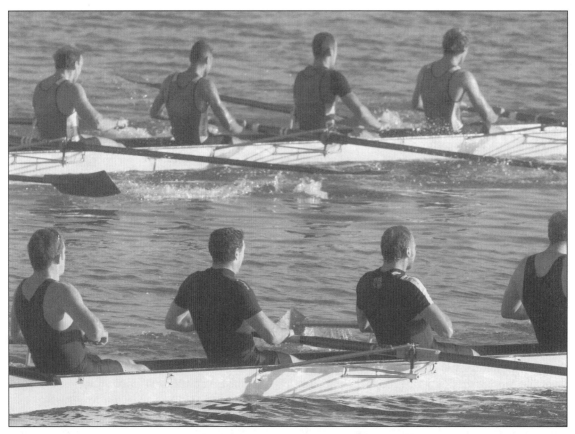

Figure 1.3. Competitive sports, such as rowing, exemplify the characteristics of play, which include enjoyment, absorption, challenge, and mastery, each meeting important human needs. Photo Credit: Image © Photos to go Unlimited. Used under license to the author.

gested that participation in leisure activities that are meaningful, rather than simply frequent, may be a constructive and readily achievable coping response during unemployment.

Social Participation

A final major area of occupation identified in the occupational therapy literature is *social participation* (see Figure 1.5). This category includes activities associated with organized patterns of behavior that are characteristic and expected of an individual or an individual interacting with others within a given social system (AOTA, 2008). Social participation includes community-based activities that result in successful interaction at the community level, as well as activities that help fulfill required or desired familial or friendship roles. This category also includes activities at different levels for intimacy, including engaging in desired sexual activity.

Psychologist Robert Hogan (Hogan, 1983; Hogan, Jones, & Cheek, 1985; Hogan & Sloan, 1991) provides an interesting and important basis for understanding the significance of social participation.

He notes that humans evolved as group-living, culture-bearing, and symbol-using animals. Being a member of a group depends on acceptance by others, and membership confers safety, access to shared resources, opportunities to learn roles through the modeling of others, and other benefits important for surviving and thriving. Once accepted, one's place in the group can confer additional advantages. Individuals vary in terms of influence within a group. We can refer to this place in the group as a person's *social standing*.

The ability to achieve and maintain standing in social groups requires a *social identity*, and Hogan notes that people spend a good deal of time developing, negotiating, repairing, enhancing, and defending who they are and would like to be. I have contended elsewhere (Christiansen, 1999) that an individual's social identity is achieved mainly through activities, and a large proportion of activities are pursued as an expression of self. This occurs through the choice of activity, with whom the activity is shared, and even where or how well the activity is conducted (McAdams, 1993).

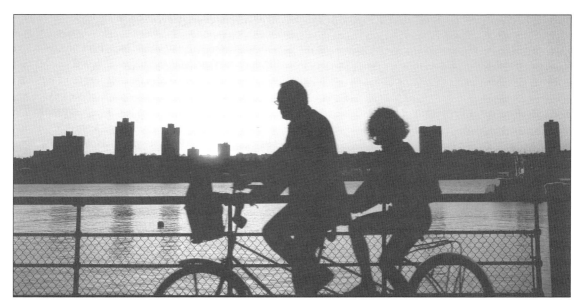

Figure 1.4. A couple bicycles along the Hudson River near New York City at dusk. Leisure and play are activity categories that share the characteristic of being freely chosen. Photo credit: Sam Aronov. Used under license to the author from 123RF.com.

It is easy to identify social activities that build relationships between people and within groups. Stroll through any park or green space on a sunny afternoon to observe people walking and enjoying nature together, jogging or cycling in groups, or playing competitive sports. What purposes do jogging and cycling serve? What are the individual or group purposes behind competitive sports or timed races?

Studies of Participation and Well-Being

The importance of engagement and full participation to well-being and a high quality of life has been demonstrated in recent research involving people with and without functional performance deficits that could limit participation in activities.

Many of the studies involving people with disabilities illustrate that functional ability is often not a significant determinant of either participation or well-being. For example, studies of persons with spinal cord injury have found that life satisfaction is most influenced by role performance and the extent of participation in everyday activities, and is not significantly influenced by degree of impairment or disability (Dijkers, 1999; Boschen, Tonack, & Gargaro, 2003; Lobello et al., 2003). A prospective study of a large group of individuals with traumatic brain injury conducted by Corrigan and colleagues (Corrigan, Bogner, Mysiw, Clinchot, & Fugate, 2001) similarly concluded that factors associated with en-gagement in valued activities in the community predicted life satisfaction.

Studies of people without disabilities have also shown that engagement in valued activities is related to higher levels of perceived well-being (happiness) and life satisfaction. For example, Menec (2003) reported on a longitudinal study of seniors living in the province of Manitoba in Canada. Findings suggested that happiness was related to a greater overall activity level. Both functional ability and mortality were also associated with activity level. Of particular interest was the finding that different activities were associated with different types of outcome. Engagement in social and productive activities predicted greater happiness, increased functional ability, and longer lifespan, whereas engagement in more solitary activities, such as hobbies requiring careful handwork, predicted only happiness. The author concluded that social and productive activities may be more active and therefore result in greater physical benefit as related to function and longer life, whereas solitary activities, such as reading, might provide important psychological benefits helping to engender a more positive sense of well-being.

These results were consistent with findings reported by Everard and colleagues (Everard, Lach, Fisher, & Baum, 2000). They found that engagement in social and high-demand leisure activities was associated with higher physical health scores, whereas engagement in low-demand leisure activities was associated with higher mental health scores. In an earlier study, Everard (1999) found that the reasons for participation also influenced well-being. Activities engaged in for social purposes predicted better well-being than activities pursued simply to pass time.

Box 1.2. Personal Projects: Explaining the Important Features of Everyday Life

Brian R. Little (1983), a Berkeley-educated Canadian psychologist who also studied at Oxford, spent an entire career studying people's personal projects. Little defined *personal projects* as the concerns, or sets of organized activity, that help people organize their lives over time. Little's research showed that most people have 15–20 "projects" that they are working on at any one time, ranging from simple and mundane endeavors like "cleaning the garage" to grander and life-changing projects such as becoming the world's best tennis player (and everything in between). Little realized that regardless of the items on an individual's project list (described as a *project system*, because projects influence each other), each project can be evaluated according to common characteristics, such as its enjoyment, difficulty, importance, perceived value, visibility, or degree of challenge, for example. Because projects vary according to these dimensions, people are able to rate each of their projects along a continuum from low to high for each dimension. These ratings can then examined in various ways to determine their relationships with other factors, such as health, well-being, perceived stress, and various other measures of psychological state.

Little's fascinating research has revealed many things about people and their engagement in activities. Perhaps most importantly, however, his work (and the work of others pursuing study of personal projects) has demonstrated the clear association between certain features of everyday activity and people's well-being. For example, people who have projects they rate more highly as important or enjoyable tend also to have higher scores on measures of well-being, and vice versa. Little's measurement approach, called *personal projects analysis*, has been used by scientists in occupational therapy and occupational science to study (and confirm) the importance of activities in promoting well-being in everyday lives.

Activities and the Self

People make sense of their lives through the activities that form their life stories (see Box 1.2). Moreover, since each person is the central figure in a life story, the activities in which they participate contribute to their personhood or sense of self (McAdams, 1993). Another word for sense of self is *identity*. It can be said that the goals and activities people choose are not only part of their life story; they also help to shape their identities, or who they are.

Many theorists agree that the formation of an acceptable identity or sense of self is central to *meaning*, or how a person understands life. It is important to realize that without the social group, activities would be devoid of shared meaning. Psychologists are in agreement that learning about the self requires social interaction, and shaping the perceptions of others occurs through the daily activities people choose. For example, I proposed (Christiansen, 1999) that activity choice and engagement are necessary parts of creating an identity that provides the personal context for creating meaning in life. By demonstrating competence and the ability to perform valued social roles responsibly, people establish themselves as accepted and valued members of groups. They also come to know who they are. Psychologist Jerome Bruner, in his well-regarded book *Acts of Meaning* (Bruner, 1990), suggests that the creation of meaning occurs through engagement in activity experiences that become part of a person's autobiography or personal story.

Narrative is a term scholars use for personal or life-related stories. The central idea behind narrative is that individuals understand themselves and their lives through storied accounts that have central figures (themselves), beginnings, middles, current situations, and future chapters. According to Mancuso and Sarbin (1985), any slice of life, when carefully considered, is interpreted and experienced as part of a story. In speaking about how narrative influences self-identity, Polkinghorne (1988) has written that

> We achieve our personal identities and self-concept...and make our existence into a whole, by understanding it as an expression of a single unfolding and developing story. We are in the middle of our stories and cannot be sure how they will end; we constantly have to revise the plot as new events are added to our lives. Self, then, is not a static thing or a substance, but a configuring of personal events into an histori-

cal unity, which includes not only what one has been but also anticipations of what one will be. (p. 150)

The possible future chapters and endings for stories involve many anticipated selves. These possible selves influence the choices people make and the behaviors they exhibit daily. People are motivated to strive to become like people they want to be (wealthy, successful, popular, and so forth) and to avoid becoming like people they do not want to be (unpopular, unattractive, unhealthy, and so on). Studies by psychologist Hazel Markus and her colleagues have shown that the images of possible selves provide important motivation to perform roles in ways that enhance people's views of self and the views others have of them (Markus & Nurius, 1986).

Psychologist Dan McAdams of Northwestern University has devoted his career to studying the identities central to life stories (McAdams, 1993, 1999). Among his many interesting findings is the observation that many stories have common overall themes and that these central themes often pertain to developing relationships with others or demonstrating one's competence through achieving important goals. McAdams's research has shown that stories in which people view themselves as overcoming adversity to achieve success are associated with perceived well-being, whereas stories where lives took an unfortunate turn for the worse and failed to realize the dreams of the individual were associated with depression and poorer overall affect (McAuley & Katula, 1998). It is important to note that these themes—developing relationships with others and demonstrating competence through the achievement of goals valued by self and/or others— occur through participation in everyday activities.

Activity Engagement and Threats to Identity

The work of occupational therapists brings them into daily contact with people whose self-identities are in transition (Mattingly & Fleming, 1993). Sometimes, because of serious illness, disease, or injury, people are not able to return to their previous living situations and are trying to make new sense of who they are now and who they will become. Their identities are changing because their ability to perform important roles as parents or spouses or workers may now be reduced.

People with spinal cord injuries offer dramatic examples of how abrupt role transitions are experi-

enced. Persons with spinal cord injuries are often young, active men in excellent physical condition who were skiing or swimming one instant and suddenly paralyzed moments later. During their rehabilitation, such individuals encounter considerable anxiety regarding their future roles as desirable marital partners, as productive members of the workforce, and as accepted members of their peer groups (Zedjlik, 1992).

However, role transitions also take place in other ways, and such changes are a normal part of life. All persons, whether disabled or not, must confront transitions during their lives because their circumstances and abilities change. For example, the process of normal aging leads to a series of role changes at predictable stages in life. Throughout life, people acquire new roles and lose old ones. As young adults, individuals may move from being students to workers, from single persons to having a partner and perhaps giving birth to or adopting children. Later, the same persons may move from being parents responsible for rearing children to becoming doting grandparents.

As life progresses, physical and sensory skills decline, and activities change. Often, as the capacity for self-reliance declines, individuals are placed in situations where choice and control are limited (such as institutions and medical facilities) and where their sense of self as competent members of society becomes diminished. During these life changes, acts that were previously viewed as ordinary or routine assume larger significance as symbols of competency. Thus, retaining or relearning the ability to perform tasks of self-maintenance (even with assistance), such as dressing without assistance, becomes a means of fostering self-identity. In many cultures, people are expected to remain self-reliant unless they are otherwise incapable of caring for themselves. On the other hand, society tends to excuse people from social obligations when they are ill or otherwise incapable of performing their roles and responsibilities on their own.

Consider the idea of the "sick role." As described by Parsons (1951, 1975), the *sick role* is a transitional state in which persons are exempted from typical role responsibilities during their recovery from an illness. Thus, for example, when we have the flu, people excuse us from our everyday obligations. We are permitted to miss work or school, and most deadlines are extended automatically. This "exemption," however, requires that we take steps to facilitate our recovery, such as limiting

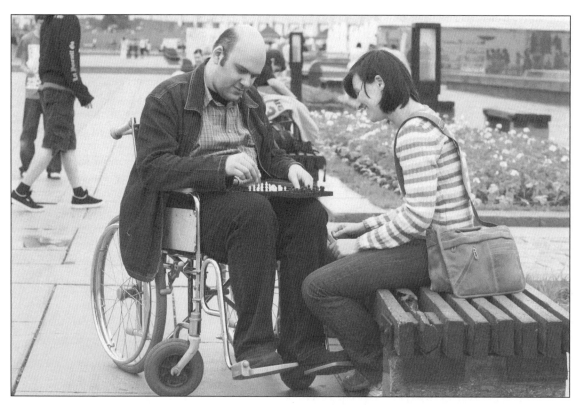

Figure 1.5. A young volunteer socializes with her companion in the park. Volunteer activities provide important opportunities for learning and building relationships, whether during young adulthood, middle age, or during the later stages of life. Social participation by persons with disabilities are important to the development of identity, or sense of self. When participation is restricted, identity is threatened. Photo credit: Tatania Belova. Used under license to the author from 123RF.com.

our social activities and seeking medical attention if appropriate.

Unfortunately, when people become old or disabled because of illness or injury, they are often viewed in a manner similar to that described in the sick role. When people are viewed in this way, they are in danger of being assigned a permanently diminished standing because they are exempted from engaging in valued social roles. In the words of noted sociologist Irving Goffman (1963), they have become the victims of stigma because they are no longer seen as people who are capable of fulfilling their roles.

Stigma

Stigma describes a social condition in which a person is devalued because he or she cannot meet expected "codes of behavior" in role performance (see Box 1.3). Goffman (1963) portrayed all interaction as consisting of crediting or discrediting role performances. A discrediting role performance can result from any number of behaviors that are different from those expected within a given social situation. For example, Goffman notes that behaviors such as yawning, stuttering, appearing nervous or self-conscious, problems with balance, losing muscular control, or losing one's temper can each diminish the "creditability" of a person during a social encounter. Because persons with physical or emotional disorders may be unable to exhibit some behaviors that would be expected in a given situation, their performances put them at risk of stigma. Thus, persons with obvious disabilities often must learn to manage the impressions they convey during social interaction to avoid the discrediting that occurs with social stigma. One advantage of the increased interaction that has occurred during the digital age is that, in general, people can become more aware and comfortable with differences, whether these differences are cultural or related to physical or social variations, or the color of one's skin.

Disfigurement

Stigma can also result from appearing to be different as a result of bodily disfigurement. *Disfigurement* refers to any physical abnormality that is sufficiently unusual as to be easily noticeable. Adolescents and young adults are frequently self-conscious about facial blemishes or acne because they believe it detracts from their appearance and places them at a disadvantage socially. In the same manner, people with severe scarring, with amputations, or with other noticeable physical conditions that mark them as atypical have concerns about how these conditions affect the manner in which they will be accepted by others. A very bad haircut can be seen as spoiling one's appearance, but this can be corrected. A permanent condition can be more problematic, and although efforts may be taken to disguise or hide disfiguration, the psychological harm of feeling stigmatized becomes a disadvantage.

Box 1.3. The Elephant Man: A Tale of Social Stigma and Identity Transformation

In the movie "Elephant Man" (Cornfeld, Sanger, & Lynch, 1980), the factual account of an Englishman, Joseph Carey Merrick (1862–1890), with a rare and severely disfiguring condition (Proteus syndrome) resulting in grotesque skin growths, is portrayed. In the 19th century, it was not unusual for persons with disfigurements to be marginalized and

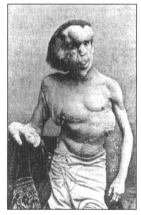

Joseph Carey Merrick ("The Elephant Man"), 1889.
Image © The Wellcome Trust. Used under license.

treated as "freaks." Befriended by a compassionate London physician, Frederick Treves, Mr. Merrick began to change his views of himself as the result of his acceptance by others. As interactions increased between Joseph Merrick and others, his disfigurement became an inconsequential personal characteristic, and people who befriended him were able to ignore it, focusing on his human characteristics of intellect and compassion.

The movie "Elephant Man" illustrates two important lessons: First, that John Merrick was himself transformed as people reacted differently to him, and, second, that an important aspect of breaking down stigma is to create pathways where initial barriers to interaction created by physical differences are overcome.

Thus, as the excerpt reveals, acceptance by others also requires maintaining expected standards of dress and appearance. People are expected to present themselves according to social norms, and the manner of their appearance and dress has been shown to influence perceptions of their status and competence. Thus, being able to manage basic self-care tasks is a fundamental prerequisite for successful social interaction for people without a disability and no less important for the person with a disability. Learning to overcome stigma and regaining an acceptable social identity may be the most significant challenge confronting someone with a disability. When others do not readily accept a person, this presents a formidable social barrier and limits participation in other activities necessary for well-being.

Important Biological Connections Between Activities and Health

In addition to their influence on social and psychological well-being through creating identity and meaning, activities also have a direct influence on physical health. When people consider relationships between activity and physical health, their first reaction is often to think about cardiovascular fitness or weight maintenance. It is true that technology and lifestyle have created sedentary behavioral patterns that are problematic for maintaining fitness and weight. Every occupational therapist should be familiar with (and model) basic concepts of fitness so that these principles can be incorporated into intervention plans.

In this section, however, the relationships between activity participation and its less obvious influences on physiological states of the body, are examined, focusing first on the important relationships between feeling states (emotions) and stress. This is followed by a discussion of the manner in which activity engagement helps keep the body attuned to the rhythms of the natural environment.

Activity and Stress

Activities influence feelings, inviting reactions that we commonly call *emotions*. When we speak of *affect* or *emotion*, we refer to how people feel at a particular moment. Behavioral scientists now increasingly understand emotion in terms of an idea called *core affect* (Russell & Feldman Barrett, 1999). The concept of core affect springs from the need to create an understandable structure to explain the very broad area of human emotion.

Although there have been many types of emotions labeled by psychologists over the years, only recently have behavioral scientists come to general agreement about the idea that people have a central disposition, or core affect. This central feeling state is based upon two dimensions or continua—*activation* and *pleasure*. People experience activation along a continuum from fatigue or listlessness to states of high alertness or excitement. Feelings at points along the activation continuum explain the level of energy with which people engage in activity. A tandem continuum is one of pleasure and displeasure. People feel happy, pleased, or positive, or they may feel sad or depressed. This dual continuum of core affect helps to explain why people with depression often feel lethargic or disinclined to act. On the other hand, it also provides a framework for understanding observed associations between energy and positive feelings.

Beyond their core affect, people may also exhibit changes in emotion based on particular events or situations. These shorter duration feelings have been described as prototypical emotional episodes and most closely resemble how activity-related emotions are described and understood by people in everyday life. These episodes have been labeled with commonly understood terms such as *surprise, fear, anger, sadness,* and *happiness*. According to current theory, however, they are labels that are more fully explained by examining how underlying levels of activation and pleasure interact with situations to produce the short-term emotional states they represent.

Regardless of the theoretical structures explaining affect, as emotional states change, the human endocrine system releases different hormones designed to ready the body for action. Through the vascular system, the body channels cells carrying nutrients or repair mechanisms to where they will be needed. In stressful circumstances, this system acts as a useful defense. If overused, this process can damage the body's immune system, much as a firefighter would get fatigued following too many false alarms. The degree of wear and tear on the human immune system is now calculated through a measurement called *allostatic load*. The entire process, from emotion to physiological changes, including the consequences of these changes over time, defines an important area of study called *psychoneuroimmunology* (McEwen, 2008). The term and process are easy to remember if the term is broken down into its component parts. Psychoneuroimmunology describes how thoughts and feelings work through the *neuro*endocrine system to influence the body's *immune* system.

Although it is important to understand how stressful circumstances can influence the immune system through the feelings or emotion-based reactions that accompany them, it is also important to recognize that a person's ability to cope with stressful circumstances involves multiple factors, many of which pertain to activities. For example, Aaron Antonovsky (1987a), who developed a widely respected theory of adaptation to stress called *salutogenesis*, identified the creation of *meaning* as an important component of resilience to the harmful affects of stress. His theory emphasizes the importance of being competent in the performance of tasks, an aspect of coping he called *manageability*, as another central feature (see Box 1.1). Manageability of life's roles requires social competence, self-confidence, and other activity-related dimensions of life.

Viewed altogether, this section emphasizes that activity-related dimensions seem to play a central role in helping people manage stress, reduce allostatic load, and thus prevent the chronic diseases that have been found to be associated with the body's physiological reactions to stress.

Activities and Internal Clocks

Another less obvious, but important, relationship between activity and health concerns *chronobiology*, or the science concerning the body's complex but important biological rhythms. In 1922, Adolf Meyer, a prominent psychiatrist now regarded as the father of American psychiatry, presented a philosophical paper to the fledgling society for the promotion of occupational therapy in which he clearly conveyed the notion of the timing and rhythm of activities as important aspects of lifestyle and health.

At the time of his remarks, chronobiology was just gaining momentum as an area of research at Johns Hopkins University, where Meyer was on the faculty. Circadian rhythms influence a wide array of behavioral and physiological events and seem to be driven by a pacemaker structure known as the *superchiasmatic nucleus*, or *SCN*, and *peripheral oscillators*. This timekeeping process influences when a person is physiologically ready for the demands of daily activity and, conversely, when he or she is in a natural period of rest or sleep. Travel across time zones results in a condition of *descynchronosis*, commonly known as "jet lag," which provides a common example of how the body is affected when its internal clocks are not entrained with the outside environment.

Scientists have discovered that certain regular activities, termed *zeitgebers*, help to entrain or synchronize the body's circadian rhythms to the external world (see Figure 1.6). These social zeitgebers include such activities as regular social interaction, routine chores such as walking the dog, the timing of meals, and when a person goes to bed. A theory proposed by Ehlers, Frank, and Kupfer (1988) claims that there is a causal relationship between the regularity of everyday activities and the stability of circadian rhythms. Consistent and predictable social contact seems to stabilize mood and circadian rhythms (Ashman, Monk, & Kupfer, 1999). Research has also shown that life events, such as the birth of a baby, can disrupt ordinary rhythms and have a harmful effect on lifestyle and relationships (Monk et al., 1996). For example, the consistency of activity routines has been shown to be related to sleep quality. These findings are part of theory called *social zeitgeber theory,* which has been supported to varying degrees by recent research (Grandin, Alloy, & Abramson, 2006; Shen, Alloy, Abramson, & Sylvia, 2008).

Social zeitgeber theory has led to intervention approaches to counteract the consequences of desynchronosis by encouraging a regimen of lifestyle regularity and balanced social interaction to help manage both unipolar and bipolar depression and anxiety (Frank et al., 2005). This approach is strikingly reminiscent of the habit-training programs for persons with mental illness used as an intervention during the era of Meyer's theory of psychobiology (Slagle, 1922).

International Classification of Functioning, Disability and Health

How can all of the various elements related to daily occupation be viewed in an overall context that allows them to be integrated or interpreted within views of health care? One global approach to doing so was developed by the World Health Organization (WHO), which published a system for classifying illness and disease, as these influence participation in the activities of everyday life. This framework is known as the *International Classification of Functioning, Disability and Health* or by its abbreviated form simply as *ICF* (WHO, 2001; see Table 1.3). This model acknowledges that *function,* or participation in valued activities, represents an interaction between a person and an environmental context recognizing that illness may or may not limit participation in activities or performance of social roles.

ICF is a classification of health and health-related domains—domains that help to describe changes in body function and structure, what persons with a health-related condition can do in a

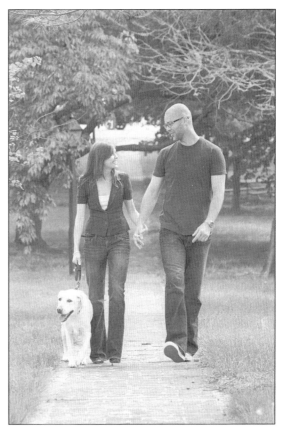

Figure 1.6. A couple strolls in the park, combining exercise with walking their dog. Regular routines, such as walking the dog, can have important functions as social zeitgebers, to help set the body's internal clocks. Photo credit: 123RF.com.

standard environment (level of capacity), as well as what persons actually do in their usual environment (level of performance). At its development, it represented a dramatic departure from traditional views of classifying illness and disability by shifting the focus of disease classification from *pathology,* or problems of structure and function in the body, to a view of illness and disability as it is revealed in the activities of everyday living. As the developers of the *ICF* note,

ICF puts the notions of "health" and "disability" in a new light. It acknowledges that every human being can experience a decrement in health and thereby experience some disability. This is not something that happens to only a minority of humanity. *ICF* thus "mainstreams" the experience of disability and recognizes it as a universal human experience. By shifting the focus from cause to impact it places all health conditions on an equal footing, allowing them to be compared using a common metric—the ruler of health and disability. (WHO, 2002, p. 3)

This description of the *ICF* emphasizes that what matters to people when they have health problems is the manner in which such problems interfere with a person's participation in valued activities. The ability to participate fully in everyday life activities is a quality-of-life issue that has a profound effect on an individual's satisfaction and well-being (Christiansen, Backman, Little, & Nguyen, 1999).

The WHO defines *quality of life* as a person's perception of his or her life as viewed in the context of goals, expectations, standards, and concerns (WHO, 1997). Quality of life is thus a broad concept influenced in a complex way by a person's physical health, psychological state, level of independence, social relationships, personal beliefs, and relationship to significant features of his or her environment. Major factors considered important to quality of life are physical function, psychological function, level of independence, environment, social relationships, and meaning (or spirituality). The

Table 1.3. Structure and Classification Definitions From the *International Classification of Functioning, Disability and Health*

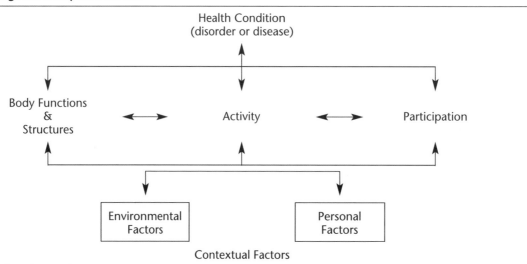

Body functions	Are the physiological functions of body systems (including psychological functions).
Body structures	Are anatomical parts of the body such as organs, limbs, and their components.
Impairments	Are problems in body function or structure, such as a significant deviation or loss.
Activity	Is the execution of a task or action by an individual.
Participation	Is involvement in a life situation.
Activity limitations	Are difficulties an individual may have in executing activities.
Contextual factors	Include personal factors and environmental factors that influence health and functioning.
Personal factors	Are internal influences on functioning and disability. These include gender, age, coping styles, social background, education, profession, past and current experience, overall behavior pattern, character, and other factors that influence how disability is experienced by the individual. These factors are not classified in *ICF* because of the wide social and cultural variation that influences these factors.
Environmental factors	Make up the physical, social, and attitudinal environment in which people live and conduct their lives. These include products and technology, the natural environment and human-made changes to the environment, support and relationships, attitudes, services.
Participation restrictions	Are problems an individual may experience in involvement in life situations.

Source: World Health Organization. (2001). *International classification of functioning, disability and health.* Geneva: Author.

first four factors are often barriers to participation in activities and therefore represent the kinds of concerns typically addressed by occupational therapy. Yet, addressing these four issues opens the door to social participation and the creation of meaning.

Illness and Disability as Participation Restrictions

People expect to be able to pursue their goals and participate in the world through their actions and activities. People seldom anticipate that these pursuits will be interrupted by unforeseen events, as they can be when individuals become isolated from opportunity, or restricted from participation by environmental circumstances, or worse yet, by illness and disability.

In 1977, Tristram Englehardt, Jr., a physician and medical philosopher, wrote a paper in which he observed "Humans are healthy or diseased in terms of the activities open to them or denied them" (Englehardt, 1977, p. 667). This quotation suggests that Dr. Englehardt has a very good understanding of what makes life meaningful. Englehardt's statement deserves further explanation in order to understand it fully. Acute illnesses, such as the flu, are nuisances because of the pain and discomfort they cause. They can be viewed as disruptions in the sense that they interfere with the normal activity routines that people experience every day. People with such illnesses may miss a day or two from their typical activities, but such inconveniences are temporary disruptions. In comparison, catastrophic illnesses and injuries, such as spinal paralysis or traumatic brain injury, result in the permanent disruption of the daily occupations that make up lives (Whiteford, 2010).

When such disastrous health problems occur, often in an instant, individuals do not understand what has happened to them. Medical diagnoses such as "cerebral infarct" or "spinal cord lesion" are not part of most people's everyday language and not readily understood. When presented with information involving such medical terminology, patients and families typically want health care professionals to provide a practical explanation related to engagement in daily activities. Thus, questions such as "Will I be able to ride my horse again?" or "Can I play the piano when I recover?" become the means for understanding medical conditions. This is because what people do every day defines their lives and who they are. People experience illness or disability not as a medical diagnosis but as an interruption or inconvenience to participating in the activities or occupations of life. When extended, such disruptions can be termed *deprivations*, in that they deprive people of participating in the activities that allow them to define who they are and gain meaning through those experiences.

Observe also that when people are first confronted with a disabling condition that will result in permanent disability, they seldom ask about whether or not they will be able to perform everyday activities, such as eating or going to the toilet, without assistance. These ordinary acts of self-maintenance were taken for granted before their disability to such an extent that their basic place in everyday life is not apparent. It is only when their performance becomes difficult or impossible that the importance of these common everyday requirements is evident. Indeed, people with disabilities who write about their own experiences typically comment about the unexpected challenges presented by their inability to perform routine daily tasks such as dressing and bathing.

In the excerpt below, from *The Body Silent,* anthropologist Robert Murphy (Murphy, 2001) provides a personal account of the effects of a spinal tumor that progressively diminished his ability to live without assistance from others:

> I was quite self-sufficient back in that stage of my disability. I could dress my upper body, though I never did master pants and shoes, and I took care of most of my personal needs. I shaved, brushed my teeth, sponge bathed most of my body, and I used the toilet without assistance. Yolanda would go off to work every day, leaving lunch in the refrigerator, and I would fend for myself. I even managed to reheat coffee. The only time that I required help was in getting dressed in the morning and undressed at night. (p. 62)

The abnormal cells that caused Murphy's tumor created gradual paralysis, which eventually cost him his life. Murphy experienced his gradual condition not as a series of biological events but rather as a progressive barrier that kept him from performing the daily tasks he had previously taken for granted. When his inability to walk and his lack of arm strength and coordination limited his ability to participate in everyday activities at home and in the community, he recognized that his very identity as a college professor, husband, and father was threatened.

Murphy was unique in the sense that he had an unusual insight into his situation and was able to continue for many years in his role as a professor despite limitations in his abilities to perform tasks. In another sense, however, his situation provides a typical example of the powerful consequences of being unable to participate in daily activities as a result of functional limitations involving thinking, feeling, or moving. These consequences included a change in his life story and a threat to his identity, which he struggled hard to maintain even when his functional skills became limited and were eventually lost.

In recent years, persons with conditions that limit their participation in society, rehabilitation professionals, and social activists have banded together to influence legislation and language in an attempt to change prejudicial attitudes and influence social policy. Recognizing that language influences thought and attitudes, they have worked hard to introduce new terminology that does not perpetuate outdated views. The term *disablement* expresses a view that an individual's ability to participate in society is based on a combination of factors. These factors include, in addition to body structure and function, people's attitudes; social policies; and physical structures in the built environment, such as buildings, vehicles, and streets.

Occupational Deprivation and Disruption

Attitudes, policies, and environmental features such as the design of objects, equipment, furniture, buildings, and even streets and parks can combine with functional deficits to interfere with engagement in valued activities. Such participation restrictions can lead to both *occupational disruption* and *deprivation*. These are terms that have been introduced into the occupational science and occupational therapy literature to describe conditions that limit activity engagement (Whiteford, 2000, 2010). *Occupational disruption* refers to a transient or temporary condition of being restricted from participation in necessary or meaningful occupations, including those caused by illness, temporary relocation, or temporary unemployment (Stone, 2003). These are conditions experienced by most people at one time or another. Although inconvenient and disruptive, most people find ways to cope with these temporary modifications of lifestyle and routine without significant lasting consequence.

In contrast, *occupational deprivation* consists of conditions where there is prolonged exclusion from engagement of occupations that are necessary or meaningful. Conditions leading to deprivation are

outside the control of the individual and include geographic isolation, incarceration, or functional disability. Occupational therapy personnel can provide valuable assistance to help ameliorate the restrictions on participation brought about by occupational deprivation.

The remaining chapters of this book focus on tools and strategies used in occupational therapy to enable individuals to participate to the maximum extent possible in the world around them. Each chapter deals with a particular condition or a category of intervention that can be employed in the service of overcoming occupational deprivation. In the years since the first edition of this book was published, great strides have been made in the development of assistive technologies to improve functional independence, mobility, and environmental access. In the years ahead, incomprehensible technological advances are likely to continue. Yet the basic aims of occupational therapy are unlikely to change. People want to live their lives fully, to participate actively in the world around them, and to enjoy their identities as part of supportive social groups. Their ability to do so will enable them to flourish and will add meaning and quality to their lives. To the extent that therapists lose sight of this ultimate goal—that of helping their clients find satisfying and meaningful ways of living—the value of their interventions will be diminished accordingly.

Summary

In this chapter, it was argued that enabling engagement in activity is an important and worthwhile goal for occupational therapy. Major categories of daily activity were identified and described in terms of their functions and characteristics as part of the daily round of human time use. It was noted that activity engagement is necessary for well-being and quality of life because humans are social and depend upon others for understanding themselves and that activity helps people construct meaning within the context of their life stories. The concept of core affect was introduced to exlain how altered feelings can lead to physiological responses that can be destructive if sustained. Relationships between activity engagement and chronobiology were also reviewed. Various threats to activity engagement and social participation were identified, including attitudinal barriers as well as other examples falling within the categories of occupational disruption and deprivation. Disability was identified as a potential cause of occupational deprivation. The chapter concluded by suggesting that the role of occupational therapists in promoting or enabling activity engagement has important benefits, including higher levels of health, life satisfaction, and well-being for people whose function is compromised as well as for those who wish to remain active and healthy during the later stages of their lives.

Study Questions

1. How do activity classifications for time use studies differ from those used by occupational therapists?
2. How do IADLs differ from BADLs?
3. What is the social importance of everyday activities?
4. How do activities contribute to identity building?
5. What are the potential threats to identity associated with illness and injury?
6. What are the differences between the concepts of occupational deprivation and occupational disruption?
7. What types of activity seem to contribute most to perceived well-being?

References

Aas, D. (1980). *Designs for large-scale time use studies of the 24-hour day.* Sofia: Institute of Sociology at the Bulgarian Academy of Science.

American Occupational Therapy Association. (2008). Occupational therapy practice framework: Domain and process (2nd ed.). *American Journal of Occupational Therapy, 62,* 625–683.

Antonovsky, A. (1987a). The salutogenic perspective: Toward a new view of health and illness. *Advances, The Journal of Mind–Body Health, 4,* 47–55.

Antonovsky, A. (1987b). *Unraveling the mystery of health: How people manage stress and stay well.* San Francisco, CA: Jossey-Bass.

Ashman, S., Monk, T., & Kupfer, D. (1999). Relationship between social rhythms and mood in patients with rapid cycling bipolar disorder. *Psychiatry Research, 86,* 1–8.

Atkinson, G., & Davenne, D. (2007). Relationships between sleep, physical activity, and human health. *Physiology and Behavior, 90*(2–3), 229–235.

Ayalon, L. (2008). Volunteering as a predictor of all-cause mortality: What aspects of volunteering really matter? *International Psychogeriatrics, 20*(5), 1000–1013.

Basner M., Fomberstein K. M., Razavi, F. M., Banks, S., William, J. H., Rosa, R. R., et al. (2007). American time use survey: Sleep time and its relationship to waking activities. *Sleep, 30*(9), 1085–1095.

Bediako, G., & Vanek, J. (1999). Trial international classification of activities for time-use statistics. In J. Merz & M. Ehling (Eds.), *Time use: Research, data, and policy* (pp.151–165). Baden-Baden, Germany: Nomos.

Boschen, K. A., Tonack, M., & Gargaro, J. (2003). Long-term adjustment and community reintegration following spinal cord injury. *International Journal of Rehabilitation Research, 26*(3), 157–162.

Brudner, J., & Kellough, K. (2000). Volunteers in state government: Involvement, management, and benefits. *Nonprofit and Voluntary Sector Quarterly, 29*(1), 111–130.

Bruner, J. (1990). *Acts of meaning.* Cambridge, MA: Harvard University Press.

Carney, C., Edinger, J., Meyer, B., Lindman, L., & Istre, T. (2006). Daily activities and sleep quality in college students. *Chronobiology International: Journal of Biological and Medical Rhythm Research, 23*(3), 623–637.

Chaput, J. P., Després, J. P., Bouchard, C., & Tremblay, A. (2007). Short sleep duration is associated with reduced leptin levels and increased adiposity: Results from the Quebec family study. *Obesity, 15*(1), 253–261.

Christiansen, C. H. (1999). Occupation as identity. Competence, coherence, and the creation of meaning. *American Journal of Occupational Therapy, 53*(6), 547–558.

Christiansen, C. H. (2004). Functional evaluation and management of self-care and other activities of daily living. In J. DeLisa et al. (Eds.), *Rehabilitation medicine: Principles and practice* (4th ed.). Philadelphia: Lippincott Williams & Wilkins.

Christiansen, C. H., Backman, C., Little, B. R., & Nguyen, A. (1999). Occupations and well-being: A study of personal projects. *American Journal of Occupational Therapy, 53*(1), 91–100.

Christiansen, C. H., & Townsend, E. (2010). *Introduction to occupation: The art and science of living* (2nd ed.). Upper Saddle River, NJ: Pearson Education.

Cornfeld, S., & Sanger, J. (Producers) & Lynch, D. (Director). (1980). *The Elephant Man* [motion picture]. London: Brooksfilms.

Corrigan, J. D., Bogner, J. A., Mysiw, W., Clinchot, D., and Fugate, L. (2001). Life satisfaction after traumatic brain injury. *Journal of Head Trauma Rehabilitation, 6,* 543–554.

Dew, M. A., Hoch, C. C., Buysse, D. J., Monk, T. H., Begley, A. E., Houck, et al. (2003). Healthy older adults' sleep predicts all-cause mortality at 4 to 19 years of follow-up. *Psychosomatic Medicine, 65*(1), 63–73.

Dijkers, M. (1999). Correlates of life satisfaction among persons with spinal cord injury. *Archives of Physical Medicine and Rehabilitation, 80*(8), 867–876.

Ehlers, C., Frank, E., & Kupfer, D. (1988). Social zeitgebers and biological rhythms. *Archives of General Psychiatry, 45,* 948–952.

Englehardt, Jr. H. T. (1977). Defining occupational therapy: The meaning of therapy and the virtues of occupation. *American Journal of Occupational Therapy, 31*(10), 666–672.

Everard, K. (1999). The relationship between reasons for activity and older adult well-being. *Journal of Applied Gerontology, 18*(3), 325–340.

Everard, K., Lach, H. W., Fisher, E. B., & Baum, M. C. (2000). Relationship of activity and social support to the functional health of older adults. *Journal of Gerontology: Psychological Sciences, 55,* S208–S212.

Fraire, M. (2006). Multiway data analysis for comparing time use in different countries. *International Journal of Time Use Research, 3*(1), 88–109.

Frank, E., Kupfer, D. J., Thase, M. E., Mallinger, A. G., Swartz, H. A., Fagiolini, et al. (2005). Two-year outcomes for interpersonal and social rhythm therapy in individuals with bipolar I disorder. *Archives of General Psychiatry, 62*(9), 996–1004.

Goffman, I. (1963). *Stigma: Notes on the management of a spoiled identity.* Englewood Cliffs, NJ: Prentice-Hall.

Grandin, L. D., Alloy, L. B., & Abramson, L. Y. (2006). The social zeitgeber theory, circadian rhythms, and mood disorders: Review and evaluation. *Clinical Psychology Review, 26*(6), 679–694.

Harris, A., & Thoresen, C. (2005). Volunteering is associated with delayed mortality in older people: Analysis of the longitudinal study of aging. *Journal of Health Psychology, 10*(6), 739–752.

Hofferth, S. L., & Sandberg, J. F. (2001). How American children spend their time. *Journal of Marriage and the Family, 63*(2), 295–308.

Hogan, R. (1983). A socioanalytic theory of personality. *Nebraska Symposium on Motivation* (pp. 55–90). Lincoln: University of Nebraska Press.

Hogan, R., Jones, W. H., & Cheek, J. M. (1985). Socioanalytic theory: An alternative to armadillo psychology. In B. R. Schlenker (Ed.), *The self and social life* (pp. 175–201). New York: McGraw-Hill.

Hogan, R., & Sloan, T. (1991). Socioanalytic foundations for personality psychology. *Perspectives in Personality, 3*(Part B), 1–15.

Huizinga, J. (1950). Homo ludens: *A study of the play element in culture.* Boston: Beacon Press.

Idler, E., & Benyamini, Y. (1997). Self-rated health and mortality: A review of twenty-seven community studies. *Journal of Health and Social Behavior, 38,* 21–37.

Katz, P., Morris, A., Gregorich, S., Yazdany, J., Eizner, M., Yelin, E., et al. (2009). Valued life activity disability played a significant role in self-rated health among adults with chronic health conditions. *Journal of Clinical Epidemiology, 62*(2), 158–166.

Landis, C. A., Frey, C. A., Lentz, M. J., Rothermel, J., Buchwald, D., & Shaver, J. L. (2003). Self-reported sleep quality and fatigue correlates with actigraphy in midlife women with fibromyalgia. *Nursing Research, 52,* 140–147.

Lawton, M. P. (1971). The functional assessment of elderly people. *Journal of the American Geriatric Society, 19*(6), 465–481.

Lawton, M. P. (1990). Age and the performance of home tasks. *Human Factors, 32*(5), 527–536.

Lee, S., Moody-Ayers, S., Landefeld, C., Walter, L., Lindquist, K., Segal, M., et al. (2007). The relationship between self-rated health and mortality in older black and white Americans. *Journal of the American Geriatric Society, 55,* 1624–1629.

Little, B. R. (1983). Personal projects: A rationale and method for investigation. *Environment and Behaviour, 15*(3), 273–309.

Lobello, S. G., Underhil, A. T., Valentine, P. V., Stroud, T. P., Bartolucci, A. A., & Fine, P. R. (2003). Social integration and life and family satisfaction in survivors of injury at 5 years post injury. *Journal of Rehabilitation Research and Development, 40*(4), 293–300.

Mancuso, J. C., & Sarbin, T. R. (1985). The self narrative in the enactment of roles. In T. R. Sarbin & K. E. Schiebe (Eds.), *Studies in social identity* (pp. 233–253). New York: Praeger.

Markus, H., & Nurius, P. (1986). Possible selves. *American Psychologist, 41,* 954–969.

Mattingly, C., & Fleming, M. (1993). *Clinical reasoning: Forms of inquiry in a therapeutic practice.* Philadelphia: F. A. Davis.

McAdams, D. P. (1993). *The stories we live by: Personal myths and the making of the self.* New York: Guilford Press.

McAdams, D. P. (1999). Personal narratives and the life story. In L. A. Pervin & O. P. John (Eds.), *Handbook of personality: Theory and research* (pp. 478–500). New York: Guilford Press.

McAuley, J., & Katula, J. (1998). Physical activity interventions in the elderly: Influence on physical health and psychological function. In G. Schulz, G. Maddox, & P. Lawton (Eds.), *Interventions research with older adults: Annual review of gerontology and geriatrics* (pp. 18, 111–155). New York: Springer.

McEwen, B. S. (2008). Central effects of stress hormones in health and disease: Understanding the protective and damaging effects of stress and stress mediators. *European Journal of Pharmacology, 583*(2–3), 174–185.

McKinnon, A. L. (1992). Time use for self-care, productivity, and leisure among elderly Canadians. *Canadian Journal of Occupational Therapy, 59*(2), 102–110.

Menec, V. H. (2003). The relation between everyday activities and successful aging: A 6-year longitudinal study. *Journal of Gerontology, 58*(2), S74–S82.

Meyer, A. (1922). The philosophy of occupational therapy. *Archives of Occupational Therapy 1*(1). Reprinted: *American Journal of Occupational Therapy, 31,* 639–642.

Monk, T., Essex, M., Smider, N., Klein, M., Lowe, K., & Kupfer, D. (1996). The impact of the birth of a baby on the time structure and social mixture of a couple's life and its consequences for well being. *Journal of Applied Social Psychology,* **26**(14), 1237–1258.

Murphy, K., & Delanty, N. (2007). Sleep deprivation: A clinical perspective. *Sleep and Biological Rhythms, 5*(1), 2–14.

Murphy, R. (2001). *The body silent.* New York: W. W. Norton.

Ohayon, M. M., Zulley, J., Guilleminault, C., Smirne, S., & Priest, R. G. (2001). How age and daytime activities are related to insomnia in the general population: Consequences for older people. *Journal of Gerontology, 49*(4), 360–366.

Parham, L. D., & Fazio, L. S. (1997). *Play in occupational therapy for children.* Philadelphia: Mosby.

Parsons, T. (1951). *The social system.* London: Routledge & Kegan Paul.

Parsons, T. (1975). The sick role and the role of the physician reconsidered. *Milbank Memorial Fund Quarterly: Health and Society, 53*(3), 257–278.

Paul, K., & Moser, K. (2009). Unemployment impairs mental health: Meta analyses. *Journal of Vocational Behavior, 74*(3), 264–282.

Polkinghorne, D. (1988). *Narrative knowing and the human sciences.* Albany: State University of New York Press.

Roehrs, T., & Roth, T. (2004). Sleep disorders: An overview. *Clinical Cornerstone, 6*(Suppl 1C), S6–S16.

Russell, J. A., & Feldman Barrett, L. (1999). Core affect, prototypical emotional episodes, and other things called emotion: Dissecting the elephant. *Journal of Personality and Social Psychology, 76,* 805–819.

Shen, G. H., Alloy, L. B., Abramson, L. Y., & Sylvia, L. G. (2008). Social rhythm regularity and the onset of affective episodes in bipolar spectrum individuals. *Bipolar Disorders, 10*(4), 520–529.

Slagle, E. C. (1922). Training aids for mental patients. *Archives of Occupational Therapy, 1,* 11–17.

Stebbins, R. A. (1997). Casual leisure: A conceptual statement. *Leisure Studies, 16,* 17–25.

Stone, S. (2003). Workers without work: Injured workers and well-being. *Journal of Occupational Science, 10*(1), 7–13.

Sutton-Smith, B. (2001). *The ambiguity of play.* Cambridge, MA: Harvard University Press.

Sutton-Smith, B. (2002). Recapitulation redressed. In J. Roopnarine (Ed.), *Play and culture studies* (Vol. 4, pp. 3–21). Westport, CT: Ablex.

Thibodaux, L. R., & Bundy, A. C. (1998). Leisure. In D. Jones, S. Blair, T. Hartery, & R. Jones (Eds.), *Sociology and occupational therapy: An integrated approach* (pp. 157–169). London: Churchill Livingstone.

Tinsley, H. (1995). Psychological benefits of leisure participation: A taxonomy of leisure activities based on their need-gratifying properties. *Journal of Counseling Psychology, 42*(2), 123–132.

Waters, L., & Moore, K. (2002). Reducing latent deprivation during unemployment: The role of meaningful leisure activity. *Journal of Occupational and Organizational Psychology, 75*(1), 15–32.

Whiteford, G. (2000). Occupational deprivation: Global challenge in the new millennium. *British Journal of Occupational Therapy, 64*(5), 200–210.

Whiteford, G. (2010). When people cannot participate: Occupational deprivation. In C. Christiansen & E. Townsend (Eds.), *Introduction to occupation: The art and science of living* (pp. 221–242). Upper Saddle River, NJ: Prentice-Hall.

World Health Organization. (1997). *WHOQOL: Measuring quality of life.* Geneva: Author.

World Health Organization. (2001). *International classification of functioning, disability and health.* Geneva: Author.

World Health Organization. (2002). *Towards a common language for functioning, disability and health.* Geneva: Author.

Yaffe, K., Fiocco, A. J., Lindquist, K. Vittinghoff, E., Simonsick, E. M., Newman, A. B., et al. (2009). Predictors of maintaining cognitive function in older adults: The Health ABC Study. *Neurology, 72*(23), 2029–2035.

Zedjlik, C. P. (1992). *Management of spinal cord injury.* Boston: Jones & Bartlett.

Zerubavel, E. (1981). *Hidden rhythms: Schedules and calendars in social life.* Berkeley: University of California Press.

Chapter 2

The Meaning of Self-Care Occupations

Gelya Frank, PhD, and Devva Kasnitz, PhD

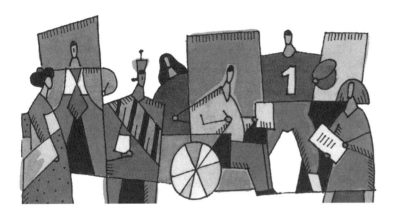

KEY WORDS

activity limitation	impairment
ADLS	impairment effects
biological citizenship	participation
biopower	personal assistance services
disability	self-care
disease	sick role
embodiment	social suffering
empathic witnessing	stigma
ICF	
illness	

HIGHLIGHTS

- The overarching goal of occupational therapy is social participation.
- Discrimination and oppression have historically been part of the social experience of living with a disability.
- Terminology and language relating to disability are important because they communicate messages that influence social perceptions and policy.
- Knowing the *techniques* for teaching a person self-care skills is not sufficient; knowing the *meaning* of the activity, as understood by the client, might be the most important therapeutic knowledge of all.
- Because the meanings attached to activities are important, occupational therapists should approach interventions with flexibility and with options in mind so the optimal approach for a given situation can be offered.
- Cultural stereotypes of beauty and ability create social conditions that marginalize and stigmatize people with differences.
- Independence is defined by decision making and self-determination, not by independent performance.

OBJECTIVES

After reading this material, readers will be able to

- Define and discuss meaningful distinctions among the terms *illness, disease, impairment, activity limitation,* and *disability;*

- View self-care activities from the standpoint of social participation;

- Draw examples from interdisciplinary perspectives to illustrate the personal, social, and cultural meanings of ADLs;

- Explain how the ability to do self-care ADLs independently or with a consumer-directed personal assistant can influence a person's self-concept;

- Describe how some institutional personal care solutions can lead to the alienating feeling of being an object rather than a person;

- Discuss how occupational therapists can support clients to discover better ways to accomplish personal care ADLs; and

- Understand how independent living and disability rights activists and disability studies can provide resources on the services that people with disabilities might prefer.

Perspectives from occupational science, anthropology, and disability studies can deepen our appreciation of the situations, tasks, settings, and challenges that face occupational therapists as they begin their practice. Knowing how to help people eat, bathe, use the toilet, dress, and groom themselves requires more than mastery of clinical techniques. Interdisciplinary perspectives can teach occupational therapists to recognize the diverse meanings that people attach to these self-care activities. Such perspectives also help prepare occupational therapists for the various ways that people may prefer to accomplish self-care.

An interdisciplinary approach is important for occupational therapy to remain vital, dynamic, competitive, and relevant as a 21st-century profession (Frank, Block, & Zemke, 2008). The American Occupational Therapy Association's (AOTA's) *Centennial Vision* states "We envision that occupational therapy is a powerful, widely recognized, science-driven, and evidence-based profession with a globally connected and diverse workforce meeting society's occupational needs" (AOTA, 2007, p. 613).

With this broad vision in mind, this chapter introduces some information, concepts, terms, and theories and accounts concerning the experiences of self-care among people with chronic illness and disability. We look at the meanings of self-care activities as they relate to two themes, embodiment and participation. *Embodiment* views the body as the instrument with which people perceive the world and the site where the world engages them. *Participation* looks at individuals and their daily activities in terms of social participation—in families, households, employment, community settings, and as citizens with rights and duties.

A focus on *embodiment* and *participation* can help occupational therapists work with patients, clients, and consumers to achieve more satisfying self-care strategies and solutions. Later, the chapter will examine narrative accounts by people with chronic illness and disability—and their caregivers—that illustrate some of the varied meanings of self-care activities. But first, we will discuss foundational concepts and definitions and explain where the chapter's key terms come from, how they have been changing, and why these changes matter.

Embodied Meanings

The concept of *embodiment* offers a way to think about the experiences of mind and body taken for granted as we engage in our usual routines and occupations. For example, we don't think about the fact that our entire body scheme, such as the upright position in which we sit and walk, is oriented with respect to gravity. We would become aware of this fact of our embodiment if we were to enter a zero-gravity environment or have an injury to the ear or the brain that affects our balance and orientation in space. This view of embodiment comes from the work of Maurice Merleau-Ponty (1907–1961), a contributor to the phenomenological movement in philosophy (see Merleau-Ponty, 1962; Spiegelberg, 1976). The concept of embodiment has been applied by anthropologists and other social scientists to better understand how disability and other atypical conditions are experienced (Csordas, 1994; Frank, 2000).

Another view of embodiment is that of Michel Foucault (1926–1984), a prolific thinker whose work has had widespread influence in medical anthropology (Scheper-Hughes & Lock, 1987). Foucault's concept of "biopower," which appeared in his later lectures and books, addresses how social institutions such as schools, hospitals, and the prison system discipline bodies in ways that mark how specific classes or groups are to be treated (Foucault, 1984, 2003). An example is the federal government boarding schools of the late 19th and early 20th centuries, where Native American children were punished for speaking their languages and were forced to dress and groom themselves to emulate the appearance of non-Indians (Lomawaima, 1995). Just as biopower is now recognized in political theory as a way to regulate and control populations (Hardt & Negri, 2001), it is also now seen as the basis of "biological citizenship" (Rose, 2007). *Biological citizenship* refers to the identities, associations, and political movements among people with specific genetic makeup and other forms of difference (Das & Addlakha, 2001; Rapp & Ginsburg, 2001).

The experience, however, of chronic illness and disability cannot be predicted from diagnoses alone, such as blindness, multiple sclerosis, spinal cord injury, or amputation. There must be some knowledge of the patient's or population's life history and life context (Ingstad & Whyte, 1995, 2007). Evidence of this need to understand appears in studies by anthropologists of spinal cord injury in the (then) People's Republic of China since the late 1960s (Kohrman, 2005), of Alzheimer's disease in postcolonial India (Cohen, 1998), and of impairments caused by genetic defects resulting from the 1986 Chernobyl radiation spill in Ukraine (Petryna, 2002).

Some meanings of embodiment are nearly universally shared by people with and without disabilities alike. Others may be specific to people with certain impairments that lend a sense of biological citizenship. Still other meanings will be unique to each individual, based on his or her experiences. With regard to self-care, "toileting," "feeding," and "grooming" should be understood as more than mere functions—they are meaningful activities that can support or disrupt embodied identities and the ability to participate in a full and rewarding life. It is essential that occupational therapists ask questions, listen, and be observant in order to understand what is at stake for each individual.

Defining *Disease, Illness, Impairment, Disability,* and *Participation*

The goal of occupational therapy is not simply to improve function but to maximize a person's social participation. Careful use of terminology can help us to appreciate the meanings attached to self-care in this regard. Many scholars and practitioners now find it useful, for example, to distinguish between *disease* and *illness*. *Disease* refers to a biologically defined disorder; *illness* refers to an individual's experience of the disorder (Eisenberg, 1977). People may have a disease without feeling ill or feel ill without having a disease.

Arthur Kleinman (1988), a psychiatrist and medical anthropologist, offers examples of illness experiences in terms of activity limitations:

> We may be unable to walk up our stairs to our bedroom. Or we may experience distracting low back pain while we sit at work. Headaches may make it impossible to focus on homework assignments or housework, leading to failure and frustration. Or there may be impotence that leads to divorce. (p. 4)

Kleinman has proposed that before offering practical interventions, the health care professional should first strive to be an "empathic witness to the experience of suffering." Empathic witnessing comes from recognizing feelings of distress and their causes.

Kleinman and colleagues, therefore, also note dimensions of *social suffering,* given that so many of the mental and physical illnesses seen in clinics are associated with poverty, natural disasters, accidents, wars, epidemics, labor migration, street violence, and other social precursors (Das, Kleinman, Lock, Ramphele, & Reynolds, 2001; Kleinman, Das, & Lock, 1997). Many challenges and frustrations faced by people with chronic illness and disability might have been prevented or alleviated by prudent social policies, such as access to primary health care, safer communities, cleaner environments, better education, occupational safety laws, and more generous and comprehensive income supplements (CSDH, 2008). Many occupational therapists worldwide are taking into account these social determinants of health (Kronenberg, Pollard, & Simó Algado, 2005; Pollard, Sakellariou, & Kronenberg, 2008; Watson & Swartz, 2004). Social participation should be the goal that underlies public policy in just societies.

In the mid–1990s, the World Health Organization (WHO) engaged scientists, scholars, professionals, and disability activists to redefine its *International Classification of Functioning, Disability and Health (ICF),* which defines the terms used internationally to gather statistics and frame policies related to disability (WHO, 2002; also see www.who.int/classifications/icf/en/). The *ICF,* which was established in 1980, was based initially on medical diagnoses relating to body structures and functions. In 2001, the 191 members states of WHO voted to make a paradigmatic shift in this underlying conceptual basis. The most fundamental change was to add the factor of environmental context to the phenomena of disability. Disability, then, occurs when impairment, in the social and environmental context, causes inequity in access to social participation. Thus, the *ICF* now focuses on the individual's level of participation in life situations, not solely on the presence or absence of impairment but on the individual's ability to engage in his or her world as influenced by both biological and social factors. The *ICF* also retired the term "handicap" (WHO, 2001), replacing it with "activity limitation."

Occupational therapist Beth Ann Wright (2004), who also is a lawyer and disability studies scholar, explains the shift in the *ICF* approach:

> The World Health Organization includes participation as a core component of assessing health and disability within the new *ICF* instrument. WHO defines participation as involvement in a life situation. In *ICF*, participation is categorized under the following domains: learning and applying knowledge; general tasks and demands; communication; mobility; self-care; domestic life; interpersonal interactions and relationships; major life areas such as work or school; and community, social, and civic life.

Occupational therapists who participated in the *ICF* revision process helped to argue for the new focus on participation (Frank, Baum, & Law, 2010). As Mary Law (2002) notes, occupational therapy research has consistently shown that participation in meaningful everyday occupations, including formal and informal activities, has a positive influence on health and well-being: "Participation is a vital part of the human condition and experience—it leads to life satisfaction and a sense of competence and is essential for psychological, emotional, and skill development" (Law, 2002). The new field of disability studies, which emerged in the mid–1980s, also helped to spur the WHO to revise the *ICF*.

The Society for Disability Studies, an interdisciplinary forum, was established in 1982. Since then, disability studies programs and courses have been added to university and college campuses at an impressive rate (Cushing & Smith 2009; Kasnitz, Pfeiffer, Bonney, & Aftendelian, 2000; Pfeiffer & Yoshida, 1995). Susan Magasi (2008a), an occupational therapist and disability studies scholar, explains,

> Disability studies is a field of critical study that emerged from the disability rights movement as a challenge to the medicalization of the lives of people with disabilities. Disability studies, while often critical of medicine and rehabilitation, has the potential to inform and improve practice by mak-

ing it more responsive and relevant to the long-term needs and desires of people with disabilities. (p. 283)

The perspectives of the profession of occupational therapy and the interdisciplinary field of disability studies can be complementary, especially with regard to giving occupational therapists better access to evidence and rationales for the preferences of disabled people (Kasnitz, 2008; Magasi, 2008a, 2008b; Mulhorn, 2004; Wright, 2004). But the perspectives also sometimes clash when, for example, occupational therapists tend to think of people with disabilities only as their "patients" and do not see beyond the impairment (Padilla, 2003). Conversely, disabled activists and disability studies scholars are often wary of the "helping" professions, which tend to view people with disabilities as patients needing to be "fixed" through the application of expert knowledge rather than as consumers exercising the right to evaluate, choose, and even reject or modify prescribed health care services. Conflicting perspectives may exist even with regard to the use of "people-first language." Magasi (2008a) writes,

> "People with disabilities" has been adopted by many governmental, advocacy, and service organizations. The use of people-first language is seen as giving primacy to the person, with the disability as a secondary trait. The term "disabled people" is, however, preferred by many in disability studies and the disability rights movement who see disability not as a characteristic of the individual but as a form of social oppression imposed on people with impairments. (p. 284)

Increased collaboration and continued exchanges between occupational therapy and disability studies can result in a disabled people, as pointed out by Magasi (2008a, 2008b; see also Frank et al., 2008; Kasnitz, 2008).

Looking at how terms change lends insight into how to focus our energies as professionals seeking to support positive social change (DePoy & Gilson, 2004). Disability studies scholars do not view *disability* as synonymous with *impairment, disease,* or *illness*. Instead, they define *disability* as the disadvantage that results when people are excluded from social participation because of their differences (Crewe & Zola, 1983; Linton, 1998). Such exclusion tends to have two dimensions: (1) cultural beliefs, prejudices, and assumptions about associating with persons who are devalued because of their differences (Goffman, 1963; Hahn, 1988) and (2) physical and social environments that impose limitations because of beliefs, rules, and laws governing how activities should be performed (Crewe & Zola, 1983).

Although disability studies have focused greatly on challenging the medical definitions of disability that tend to reinforce views of disability as deficits, the pendulum is swinging back to center as disability scholars turn their attention once again to the experience and the effects of bodily impairments. Carol Thomas (2007) has suggested the term *impairment effects* to describe the actual experiences and consequences of impairments. Disability scholar Tom Shakespeare (2006), for his part, believes that focusing on impairments can result in knowledge specific to certain diagnoses that can decrease distress or discomfort and increase function and participation. Occupational therapists and disability scholars can help create useful solutions by understanding not only disability but also a sociology of impairment (Paterson & Hughes, 1999). This includes how symptoms and impairment effects interact with the environment in order to equalize access for specific groups of people with roughly the same kinds of impairments and activity limitations—as, for example, in Project Shake It Up, a camp for children with multiple sclerosis (Block, Vanner, Keys, Rimmer, & Skeels). Occupational therapists can often also serve their patients and clients indirectly by connecting them with advocates working to remove barriers (Kasnitz, 2008).

Embodiment and Participation in Self-Care

We turn now to some first-person accounts of illness experiences in which self-care has been affected. Occupational science teaches occupational therapists to view self-care activities as part of repertoires and routines of purposeful, meaningful activities (Clark et al., 1991; Yerxa et al., 1990). Starting from childhood, we expect most self-care activities to become habitual and easier to perform with practice over time; self-care comprises a common denominator of skills and routines. When an individual has a stroke or spinal cord injury or becomes the parent of a child with an impairment that affects self-care activities, the profound embodied meaning of self-care activities is revealed.

Agnes de Mille, dancer and choreographer, first noticed symptoms of the stroke she suffered in 1975, in her 70s, when her hand didn't work to sign a contract. de Mille saw this activity limitation as a threat to her lifetime identity: "Please do something fast," she told her doctor, "because I've got to be on the stage in one hour delivering a very difficult lecture, and I've never been late for anything in the theater in my life" (1981, pp. 21–22). People who become impaired often say that their bodies or some body parts become alien to them. Sometimes parts of their bodies even seem dead. Describing the weeks imme-

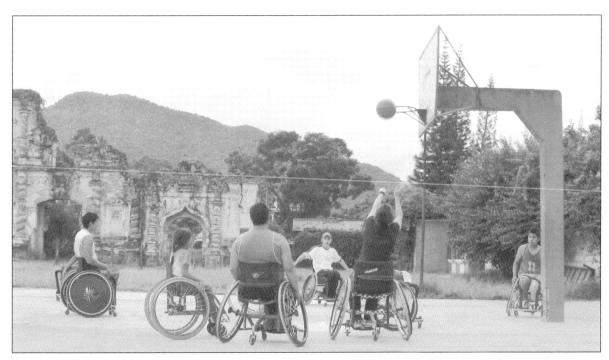

Figure 2.1. Basket! The Transitions Team, Antigua, Guatemala, second rated in Central America, is part of an innovative independent living center. Photo credit: Devva Kasnitz.

diately after her stroke, de Mille wrote, "Half of me was imprisoned in the other half" (p. 57). Six months later, she felt as if her whole self were split in two: "My right arm, my right leg, that whole side of my body gone. I was to be two bodies, one of them not my friend, alien" (p. 219).

The ability to engage in customary daily occupations remains crucial over time. Poet Audre Lorde, 9 months after a modified radical mastectomy for breast cancer, longed for a past self who could perform daily activities effortlessly. "I can never accept this, like I can't accept that turning my life around is so hard, eating differently, sleeping differently, moving differently, being differently. . . . I want the old me" (1980, pp. 11–12). A professor of anthropology who suffered a neurological tumor, Robert F. Murphy (1987) wrote that his life was "divided radically into two parts: pre-wheelchair and post-wheelchair." But his return to the lecture halls of Columbia University and the ability to engage in his customary occupations, even in a wheelchair, meant a return to his former self: "Hey, it's the same old me inside this body!" (p. 81).

It is rarely possible to recover the "same old me" without reevaluating one's identity. Social psychologists working in rehabilitation say that "adjustment" to disability requires accentuating the positive—one's remaining assets—and turning away from the negatives—what is missing (Wright, 1983). The process of reconstructing one's personal identity after chronic illness and disability has been called "biographical work" (Corbin & Strauss, 1988). Disability rights activists use the same strategy when they say that negative illness experiences and impairment effects are not part of the disabled person. Doing self-care differently, or with help, should not bar people from social participation.

Toileting

Excretion in many cultures is supposed to be among the most private and unseen activities. Agnes de Mille (1981), who finally managed to get to the toilet at night by using a three-pronged cane to keep from falling or bumping herself, wrote, "My trip to the bathroom in privacy and decency meant more to me than a rave notice in the [*New York*] *Times*" (p. 167). Irish author Christopher Nolan (1987) writes about his "agony" as a 15-year-old schoolboy trying to sit through a science lesson and control his bowels after a dose of laxative. Born with cerebral palsy, he was used to asking for help, except in going to the bathroom. "He knew he cast roles of responsibility on his fresh-faced friends, but bringing him to the toilet was a chore he would never ask them to do

for him" (p. 117). Activity limitations in using the toilet may disgust not only strangers but also our friends and relatives, resulting in personal shame. As has been noted by disability scholars (see, for example, Campbell, 2009), shame can result in *internalized oppression*, under the weight of which people with impairments devalue themselves.

The problems involved in going to the toilet are closely entwined with our identities, including our gender identities. Irving Kenneth Zola (1982), a sociologist and spokesperson for the Independent Living Movement, lived for a week as a participant observer at the village of Het Dorp, a planned independent living community in the Netherlands for people with physical impairments. During his stay, Zola decided to use a wheelchair to report how, from this new vantage point, he handled what he described as the usually "unspeakable" practices of urinating and defecating. It was an experience that led him to reevaluate the part disability played in his masculinity and identity as a disabled person. Getting off the wheelchair and onto the toilet, sitting on the toilet, and getting back onto the wheelchair, Zola realized that the bathroom's barrier-free, or universal, design made using the toilet easier than he remembered it. Using the grab bar, he was able to raise himself from the toilet despite his weak stomach muscles and legs. He became aware of how unnecessary his previous difficulties in going to the bathroom had been. But Zola also felt uncomfortable using the toilet from a seated position because he felt that a man of his age ought to urinate standing up:

> As a Western man I had been trained to urinate standing with both feet firmly planted on the ground. Thus, to sit and urinate took some getting used to. This did, however, provide a side benefit. Standing I had always needed one hand free to steady myself. Sitting at least made it a more relaxed activity. (pp. 65–66)

Before leaving the bathroom, Zola continued,

> I tried to think if I had "to go" again. Once more I was reduced to the status of a child as I recalled parental admonitions to the effect, "We are starting on a trip, so you better use the toilet now." I did the same thing with my own children. What were the toilet facilities like elsewhere in the Village? Would they be as easy to negotiate as the one in my room?

Zola's remembered association of using the toilet with childlike dependency and infantalization has been echoed in the next generation of disabled activists.

Alana Theriault (2008), now a national expert in disability benefits and personal assistance policies, contributed her memoir to a treasure trove of oral histories titled *The Disability Rights and Independent Living Movement*, housed at the Bancroft Library of the University of California, Berkeley (http://bancroft.berkeley.edu/collections/drilm/). Theriault relates an early experience that made her anxious about asking for help in the bathroom:

> Fumbling around in the bathroom, and my best friend and the mom were trying to do an untrained pivot transfer onto the toilet and trying to get my pants down at the same time. I mean, I didn't get hurt. I was a pretty resilient crawl-on-the-floor-or-whatever kind of kid, I wasn't fragile. But it was just a fumbling mess. I remember realizing, "Wow, Alana, that was kind of stupid to demand the bathroom when you really didn't need to pee that bad." But it was just sort of—I look back, and it was really the final nail in the coffin of my sense of entitlement about basic bodily functions. . . "Oh well. You don't need to pee out in public, because it's too hard" . . . I mean, my whole mode was, "Just don't be a burden. Don't be a hassle. Make it easy for you; make it easy for other people." I didn't even get the concept of entitlement until I was sixteen and moved out on my own, and that's a whole other chapter in my life, post-nursing home. But I was finally able to hire people. (p. 15)

Zola's and Theriault's stories show how the ability and willingness to adapt behavior—even in the most private situations—may hinge on unspoken cultural rules defining social identity. Zola was helped to adapt by his ability to step back and reflect on his reactions. Theriault was inspired by reading work like Zola's and by meeting pioneers of the disability studies movement and other role models like him. Such critical thinking can also help other people with disability experience make choices about what works for them and what options occupational therapists should promote for universal design and individual accommodation.

Eating

Unlike toileting, which involves cultural rules about privacy, eating is the most social of activities. Ideally, meals are shared. The breaking of bread together reflects trust, reciprocity, and membership in recognized family and community life. The phrase *making a mess,* appears frequently in the accounts of people with impairment effects when they talk about their frustration, disgust, and fears—to borrow another metaphor—of losing their place at the table. Murphy's (1987) inability to feed himself resulted in frustration and anger, not because he

would go hungry but because he had lost an essential mark of his human identity:

> A paralytic may struggle to walk and become enraged when he cannot move his leg. Or a quadriplegic may pick up a cup of coffee with stiffened hands and drop it on his lap, precipitating an angry outburst. I had to give up spaghetti because I could no longer twirl it on my fork, and dinner would end for me in a sloppy mess. This would so upset me that I would lose my appetite. (pp. 106–107)

Disabled people may experience shame about not being able to eat in a typical manner when in public. Diane DeVries, a woman born in 1950 without legs and with short arm stumps, imposed strict standards of table behavior upon herself and others with impairments similar to her own (Frank, 1986, 2000). DeVries remarked that despite having no forearms or hands,

> whatever I did, like feed myself, drink, I was able to do it without any sloppiness. You know, I've even seen a girl at camp with no arms that bent down and lapped her food up like a dog. . .And I knew her. And I went up to her and said, "Why in the hell do you do that?" And I said, "They asked if you wanted a feeder or your arms on. You could have done either one, but you had to do that." She said, "Well, it was easy for me." To me that was gross. She finally started wearing arms, and she started feeding herself. But that to me was just stupid, because people wouldn't even want to eat at the same table as her. (as cited in Frank, 1986, p. 209)

Providing, preparing, and sharing food are important blocks in the foundation of social life, yet people with chronic illness and disability may have less freedom and choice in defining themselves with food because they lack the mobility and income to dine in public places, among other factors. A Louis Harris and Associates (1986) survey indicated that Americans who experienced disability shopped and ate out much less often than other Americans and were three times more likely never to eat in restaurants than their peers without disabilities. As many as to 13% of them never shopped for groceries, compared to only 2% of the population without disabilities.

"The dining room is concerned, of course, with food" writes de Mille (1981) "and therefore had been the focal point of my life as a child. It was the place of family interchanges" (p. 197). For de Mille's 32nd wedding anniversary, one month after her stroke, her husband Walter arranged a party at the hospital.

The celebration was topped by the hospital's present, a great big beautiful wedding cake, very rich and delicious. (The wedding cake Walter and Jonathan had brought was later given to the nurses.) And I knew that my friends and Walter were glad that I was alive, glad for me, glad for Walter. Glad for what I was beginning to be able to do. And there was happiness there because I was going to live. And we had toasts, many of them. They did. I had only a thimbleful of the champagne. (p. 79)

The celebration strengthened de Mille's determination to recover. "I'm going to live," she told her husband. "I'm going to make it. I'll be out of here soon" (p. 80).

Family needs can sometimes challenge the goal of independent self-feeding that occupational therapists encourage in their clients. The mother of a small child who is blind continued to spoon-feed her child to preserve the quality of life for her family.

Rosalyn Gibson. . .told the group that she still spoon-fed her blind three-year-old because the alternatives created such chaos. Meanwhile, the teachers encouraged Nancy to feed herself at school and urged Rosalyn to follow their lead. . . .they spoke of time saved in the long run. Rosalyn thought about the family meals ruined by flying food and recrimination, and the long hours of clean-up. (Featherstone, 1980, p. 29)

Similarly, if occupational therapist Esther Huecker was to succeed in getting Timmy, who was totally dependent on intravenous feeding, to eat, she had to engage him in a social relationship. Her task was to get Timmy to enjoy food despite his unfamiliarity with hunger and reluctance to put objects in his mouth. Her lure was her own participation in the experience of getting to know food. After months of treatment, a successful meal became like a "dance" between them:

We began our usual rituals. He brushed his teeth, washed his face, opened all of the containers, and began to smell and name what was on his plate. Timmy picked up a green bean and dipped it into the gravy to lick. I talked about putting gravy on his potatoes, but there was no hole to keep it from spilling. He gingerly poked a hole with his finger and licked the potatoes. He helped to mince some chicken in a grinder and then took small tastes from a spoon. The meal felt like a well-choreographed dance. I could anticipate his needs and prepare him for his risk-taking actions. His success generated more risk-taking.

After exploring and tasting everything on his tray several times, Timmy announced he was "all done." Picking him up from the high chair, I felt exhilarated that the experience had been so satisfying. Timmy put his arms around my neck and gave me a kiss, something that had never occurred in a spontaneous moment. (Frank, Huecker, Segal, Forwell, & Bagatell, 1991, p. 258)

Murphy (1987) writes that when people cannot reciprocate, cannot help those who help them get and eat food, or perform other tasks, they feel less valuable than others; they lose self-respect. He describes two young women living together in a wheelchair-adapted apartment in a retirement housing project, whose creative solution to feeding problems challenged that potential devaluation:

One is a spinal cord-damaged quadriplegic with good upper body strength, although she has considerable atrophy of the hands. The other has cerebral palsy; she has moderate speech impairment and very limited arm and hand use. Both women use wheelchairs. Nevertheless, they both completed college, where they lived in dorms, and now were sharing an apartment. Each had a van, and the two did their own cooking and shopping, taking care of all their needs. The woman with cerebral palsy was unable to hold and use eating implements, so she was hand-fed by the other. (pp. 201–202)

In the mutual relationship of these two women, one helping the other, takes place within a larger context of give and take. Together, they appear to transform one's "feeding" the other into dining together. This reciprocal help is not uncommon in the disability rights community: It is not uncommon, for example, for a person with paraplegia to hire a blind person as an attendant and to then help them read their mail. In occupational therapy, even when the immediate (short-term) treatment goal is focused narrowly on helping a person get food to his or her mouth with built-up utensils, eating remains an expression of social membership, cultural values, and personal preferences. The ultimate goal of treatment is to enable the patient to participate in all of these. In some situations, participation may trump self-feeding. The occupational therapist should always consider flexibility and multimodal solutions a viable choice.

Grooming and Dressing

Grooming, including bathing and dressing, is often affected by chronic health conditions or disability. Yet clothing, hairstyle, figure, jewelry, and cosmetics are important markers of a person's social identity, tending to display a person's gender, age, occupation, status, ethnicity, and class (Storm, 1987). Changes in personal appearance often send a message that the person's place in society has changed. Hospital gowns or pajamas, nightgown and slippers worn as regular daytime attire, wheelchairs and other adaptive equipment announce "Here is a sick person!" Uncombed hair and strong body odors, at least in mainstream North American culture, mark a person as an outsider, someone on the margins of society. They are examples of "stigma symbols" (Goffman, 1963) that suggest the individual is not competent to participate in society.

Chronic illness and disability are likely to stigmatize a person only when they become obvious to others. Individuals with such illnesses or disability may often hide or cover up aspects of their appearance that could be discredited and try to "pass" as normal. The United States once had "ugly laws" that kept those with observable physical difference off the streets and protected the "delicate sensibilities" of "normal" people (Schweik, 2009). Profound discrimination and oppression historically have accompanied disability and still affect disabled people in some parts of the country and regions of the world (Pernick, 1996). Though grooming and dressing reveal information that can improve one's social identity, they can equally conceal or reveal information that would be socially damaging. Gaining control over and maintaining one's appearance can help avoid the stigma of being labeled as disabled or change attitudes that lead to devaluing those with disability or impairment.

Being put in the "sick role" can be particularly distressing for people with chronic illness and disability, who live with conditions that are never going to be cured (Crewe & Zola, 1983; Parsons, 1951). Being sick temporarily excuses them from work—but the cost is loss of social status and control of their situations until declared well by a medical authority. Some members of the independent living and disability rights movement resist this identification by "claiming disability" rather than rejecting it; they work at the experience and display "disability pride," sometimes as a result of becoming activists (Linton, 1998). They make a point of showing their "stigma symbols" to protest stereotypes of social inferiority and to combat discrimination, and have achieved changes in laws, policies, and social awareness and helped create support for disability arts, disability studies, and other forms of disability culture (Berkowitz, 1987; Charlton, 1998; Longmore, 2003).

Like others, disabled people use clothing and cosmetics to conceal a defect, distract attention away from it, or compensate for it (Kaiser, Freeman, & Wingate, 1990). Agnes de Mille (1981) used all three of these strategies after her stroke, without, however, dressing to comply with mass market styles.

> I bought Chinese suits with long coats and the brace was hidden in my pants [concealment] and I was told I looked very smart. . . . indulging myself with the loveliest tunics and Indian Benares silk pants of contrasting or complementary tones and little colored slippers [deflecting attention]. The more decrepit my body, the more dashing my dress [compensation]—plain but très gai, très daring. Another flag went up the mast to signal my recovering and making my new life a happy one. (p. 223)

Rosemarie Garland-Thomson, who herself shortens one sleeve of her elegant suits to accommodate a congenital partial arm amputation, in *Staring: How We Look* (2009), speaks to how both the viewer and the disabled being viewed manipulate and represent *looks*. Not all people are able or want to invest themselves or their resources in grooming and dress. But grooming and dress, or their absence, serve expressive functions in any event (Mairs, 1987, 1989). Dress made it possible for his family to recognize Billy, born with multiple impairments, dependent on a ventilator, and fed through a gastrostomy tube, as a person (Pierce & Frank, 1992). Occupational therapist Doris Pierce writes, "When Billy was dressed in his first baby outfit, his oldest brother, who had refused to see Billy since his first visit, stayed with him all day" (p. 974). In her field notes, Pierce recorded the brother's comment, "He looks like a real baby!"

Finally, there are circumstances in which the display of stigmatizing behaviors may be either self-protective or involuntary. Anthropologist Paul Koegel (1987) writes about homeless mentally ill women in Los Angeles: "Were they chronically mentally ill, or were they simply reacting very sanely to the enormous stress of an insane situation? Was the fact that they wore four pairs of pants during the summer a reflection of an inability to properly identify weather-appropriate clothing, or was it a highly conscious strategy aimed at frustrating potential rapists? Was their poor hygiene the result of poor self-management skills or their restricted access to sinks and showers?" (p. 30).

Occupational therapist Sandra Greene (1992), who studied a day shelter for women in the Los Angeles area, found a wide range of strategies related to grooming and dress among its homeless clients. A few were able to maintain a normal appearance, taking pride in their personal cleanliness and dress. Some rented storage spaces to protect their clothing from theft. They were aware that carrying suitcases or bundles of possessions marked them as homeless. For others, just taking a shower was important, even when they made no attempt in their dress to conceal their homelessness.

> For women who value passing as a non-homeless woman, the availability of a place to keep clean is extremely important so that they don't "look like one of these filthy women." For some women who do not seem to take steps to pass as a non-homeless woman, this service is still considered important and is often mentioned as one of the services they like to use at the shelter. (p. 168)

Writers in the disability rights movement are challenging mainstream stereotypes of beauty and sexuality in society. Research shows that people tend to attribute positive personal characteristics to those who are physically attractive and negative characteristics to those who are seen as abnormal or different (Kaiser et al., 1990). Negative stereotypes of men and women deemed disabled have been perpetuated in television and films, fiction, and drama (Garland-Thomson, 2009; Kent, 1987; Longmore, 1987).

Political scientist Harlan Hahn (1988), a polio survivor, poses the question "Can disability be beautiful?" Hahn suggests that, when confronted with disability, people without a disability tend to experience an "existential" anxiety (the projected threat of the loss of physical capabilities) and an "aesthetic" anxiety (fear of others whose traits are perceived as disturbing or unpleasant). His historical research indicates, however, that Western cultures have eroticized as well as stigmatized people with physical differences. Although it is rarely openly acknowledged, Hahn argues, disabled people in art and literature often have been portrayed with a certain sexual appeal. Campbell (2009) concurs and analyzes people who are "devotees" of people with amputations and other impairments.

Hahn urges disabled people to speak out as cultural critics of rigid, conformist ideals of the body beautiful. The culturally shared "language" of grooming and dress provides a vocabulary to do so. Some students with disability, for example, wear T-shirts with disability rights mottos and humorous slogans that display their social uniqueness and suggest a desire for more reexamination of their representation in society. Examples include "I'm no quad; I'm just tired of walking," "High-level quads do it with a joy stick," "I'm accessible," and "If I prove I'm better, will you admit I'm equal?" (Kaiser et al., 1990, p. 42).

Growing up without legs and arms except for above-elbow stumps, Diane DeVries has made choices since childhood about her grooming and

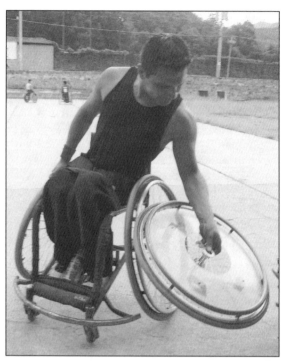

Figure 2.2. Edwin, changing a wheel, Antigua, Guatemala, where he is making chairs for a women's team. Photo credit: Devva Kasnitz.

dress (Frank, 2000). She accepted cultural ideals of attractiveness yet also challenged negative stereotypes about the "handicapped." As a child, Diane wore shift dresses over a three-wheeled "scooter" used with a crutch. During puberty, she decided that the scooter looked strange and decided to use an electric wheelchair instead. While any piece of adaptive equipment may be a "stigma symbol," Diane came to feel that a wheelchair was more appropriate for than her three-wheeled scooter, especially at the county rehabilitation facility where she then lived among other disabled teenagers and young adults. There, as a member of a culture of disability, Diane modeled herself after a young woman with a spinal cord injury who encouraged her to use her female assets.

> To go around in whatever you're in, your wheelchair, or your braces, or whatever, and not look clumsy. . .I mean, people are already looking at you. You know, any crip's going to be looked at. But at least if they look at you, at least they'll say, "Wow, look at that person in the wheelchair. Hey, but you know, not too bad!" (Frank, 1986, p. 208)

Diane DeVries prefers to wear close-fitting clothes that accentuate her assets instead of attempting to conceal her multiple limb deficiencies. "Like when I was a kid, I hated wearing skirts and dresses, because with a skirt you could notice even more that there are legs missing than when you wore shorts and a top. Shorts and a top fitted your body, made the fact that no legs were there not look so bad" (Frank, 1986, p. 209). But another woman with amputations chooses to wear long sleeves or full skirts to cover their missing limbs:

> I get a different response from people when I wear short sleeves so I very seldom wear short sleeves. It camouflages my disability (missing arm) when I wear long sleeves. Because of my amputation at the hip, I prefer dresses without a waist or gathering at the bodice of the dress. Dresses that flare out more at the tail are more attractive. (Kaiser et al., 1990, p. 39)

The bottom line is that disabled people wish to choose how to present themselves socially but often are unable. For Alana Theriault (2008), issues with grooming presented a barrier to her social participation:

> I mean, junior high—another memory is dirty hair, being embarrassed about it. Being able to wash your hair only once a week when you're in junior high is not cool, I mean, especially with all those hormones going, and your body's gross, and changing. I mean, I felt really embarrassed about who I was, I felt ugly, I felt dirty, and at the same time, my sister was starting to do the big feathered hair thing, and the makeup. And I wasn't able to do all that grooming stuff. I was a tomboy anyway, so I was kind of—I really held onto that as, "Well, this is the reason why I don't do all these things." (p. 15)

Alana later realized that being a tomboy was only a rationale that she had adopted to help her cope with the lack of adequate support for her self-care:

> But in reality—I borrowed my sister's razor and tried to shave my legs. I played with the makeup. I wanted to do the girly things, but they were extra. They weren't part of what my mother or sister would be willing to do to get me up in the morning. I mean, bathing is not even happening, and I could no longer sit on a toilet, so my bowel program was a major ordeal, too, because having a bowel movement on a bedpan requires a laxative, requires two hours of putzing around. So already, I felt like I was too much of a burden. (p. 10)

Not uncommonly, the choices that disabled people make in grooming and dress may conflict with preferences and expectations held by helpers or assistants—whether family members, occupational therapists, other professionals, or paid attendants. When disabled people depend on others, there is often a fine line between help and control. When she was a young teenager, Diane DeVries liked dresses with narrow straps that she could slip into by herself and that allowed her the greatest freedom of movement. Some members of her rehabilitation team, however, challenged her right to determine what was appropriate dress (Frank, 1986, p. 207). Diane suggests that people with impairments learn to say "no" and to stay in control of their grooming and dress when helped by another.

> Like me, I would never wear a skirt, a long skirt, like they used to. I've even seen some people with no arms wearing long sleeves pinned up or rolled clumsily so they're *this* fat. You can find a lot of clothes that fit you. It's not hard. If they have someone take care of them, they won't tell them: "No. I want my hair this way." They'll just let them do it. That's dumb. It's your body. They're helping you out. (Frank, 1986, p. 210)

At conventions of Little People of America (LPA), a self-help organization for people of profound short stature, one of the best-attended events is the annual fashion show (Ablon, 1984). Although most little people can wear children's clothing with minor alterations and children's shoes, children's styles are inappropriate for mature people. The fashion show displays clothing made by the models themselves or made for them and adult-size clothing with major alterations. Women model elegant suits, dresses, and sports clothes, while men usually model formal suits. LPA members also attend sewing workshops and patronize representatives of tailoring firms who fit them and take custom orders. Women sometimes order shoes from Hong Kong, where average sizes are smaller than in the United States. Several people have also started firms making clothing for people who never stand—that won't ride up or catch in the mechanism of a wheelchair.

Ernestine Amani Patterson (1985) had an intense desire to wear her hair braided in cornrows, African-style, but her blindness prevented her from doing them herself, and beauticians and others discouraged her. A beautician from Liberia finally satisfied her insistence on having her hair done in cornrows with colorful beads and tinkling bells. She helped Patterson reject the isolating stigma of blindness and claimed her identity as a Black sister:

> Of course, people are still the same—inevitable and specific in their cruelty. "Your hair is pretty," or "Your dress is pretty." The lines between womanhood and blindness are

never supposed to meet. And with Blackness on top of that, what must people be seeing! And although I seldom hear, "You are looking nice," I am not the same, even if they are. Since that Saturday in the shop with the wooden floor and squeaky steps, where the heater had to be turned on against the chilly morning, I have always looked forward to the bus ride and short walk there. Mrs. Younger [her Liberian beautician] has not only increased her clientele, other girlfriends of hers from Africa help out with the hair. So it's lovely talking to all of them. And since most of these women are used to me now, we relate as Black sisters. And though this was not a first step in my growth, mine is actually a case wherein the style of my hair altered the shape of my head within. (p. 243)

Self-Care and Assisted Care

The disability studies and independent living movements have focused on the most essential of ADL tasks as a litmus test for self-determination. The focus is on choice and the availability of all options, from occupational therapy and assistive technology, that may allow someone to do self-care alone, to access to paid, consumer-controlled personal assistant services, referred to as *personal care assistance* or *attendant care* when ADLs are involved. The Research and Training Center on Personal Assistance Services (http://www.pascenter .org/home/index.php) provides rich information for consumers, providers, and others and tracks changes in public programs and regulations by state as program improvements are made. The work includes models for personal assistance in the workplace, a key service for many people who otherwise could not work (Stoddard, 2006).

Whether we think about toileting, eating, grooming, or other self-care, such as going to and getting up from bed, the physical and social environment is always a deciding factor to access. Physical barriers are relatively simple to understand, if not to prevent. In Zola's case, barriers that he had experienced before when manipulating a wheelchair were not present in a bathroom at Het Dorp. In her full oral history, Theriault (2008) describes how she brought a table into a bathroom at her workplace so she could lie down to urinate.

In the best of cases, disabled people are able to build accessible physical and human environments that give them the best balance of independence and assistance in accomplishing ADLs. The issue is often not what someone can do alone but what is the cost

in energy and time of doing it alone. The independent living movement is clear that independence is about decision making, self-determination, choice, and control, not about doing things alone. Some people take great pleasure in slowly cooking a meal but prefer to have help dressing because it takes longer to do alone than they feel is warranted. The same person may then do schoolwork alone, with an elaborate system of computer hardware and software, instead of dictating to an assistant. These choices between low- or high-tech and human assistance with ADLs are exemplified by the video "A Day in the Life of Richard Devylder," produced by the California Department of Rehabilitation (2005). Devylder, the deparment's former deputy director, takes us through the combination of solutions he uses as a congenital quadrilateral amputee, like Diane DeVries, to accomplish basic self-care. Resources such as this are enormously helpful in giving a consumer perspective and demystifying disability.

When people do need and want help with ADLs, they are usually dependent on family and local community charity. Paid assistance is of critical importance but still covers only the tip of the iceberg of need. Institutionalization because of an inability to perform self-care was once common and is still feared. In 1999, the U.S. Supreme Court upheld a provision that states that people have the right to personal care in the "least restrictive environment" (Center for an Accessible Society, 1999). For many, this has meant an opportunity to have home and community-based services where they may even be allowed to pay family members as caregivers from public funding streams. However, these options are still underfunded; vary enormously by state, county, and even city; and are controversial.

Caregiving

When people need or prefer help, a caregiver or assistant often ascribes a different meaning to self-care from that of the person he or she is assisting. Consequently, how the recipient of care experiences eating, dressing, bathing, and going to the bathroom will be colored by the experiences of the caregiver.

Most ADL assistance happens within the family and is unpaid. Couples typically work together to manage activity limitations (Corbin & Strauss, 1988). When a spouse or children take care of another family member's basic needs, the division of labor in the family often becomes unbalanced. Newman (2002) examines the assumption that children suffer when they become caregivers for their disabled parents, an assumption his research questions—though in family-based care feelings of exhaustion, depression, anxiety about money, self-pity, and resentment are common.

Caregivers often feel guilty about having these reactions. In a study of couples managing chronic illness at home, one woman described her exhaustion over the physical work she did to help her husband.

> All night long he would say, "Get me water, put me on the commode." I would tell K., "Let me sleep; let me rest. I don't mind waiting on you hand and foot during the day, but at night let me sleep". . . . He got out of bed one night and urinated all over the floor. I had to get up and clean him up and put him back to bed. I didn't realize he was taking up so much of my energy. That twenty-four hour stuff was getting to me. (Corbin & Strauss, 1988, pp. 293–294)

Too much responsibility on her shoulders as a parent caused Helen Featherstone's (1980) outrage when a practitioner suggested a small addition to her son Jody's home program. It was recommended that she brush Jody's teeth three times a day, for 5 minutes, with an electric toothbrush to counteract gum overgrowth caused by his antiseizure medication. Featherstone, mother of three children, was handling so many demands already that she exploded.

> "Jody," I thought, "is blind, cerebral-palsied, and retarded. We do his physical therapy daily and work with him on sounds and communication. We feed him each meal on our laps, bottle him, change him, bathe him, dry him, put him in a body cast to sleep, launder his bed linens daily, and go through a variety of routines designed to minimize his miseries and enhance his joys and his development. (All this in addition to trying to care for and enjoy our other young children and making time for each other and our careers.)" Now you tell me that I should spend fifteen minutes every day on something that Jody will hate; an activity that will not help him to walk or even defecate, but one that is directed at the health of his gums. (pp. 77–78)

People who receive their care from family often are acutely aware of the sacrifices necessary and try to avoid demanding too much. Disabled children are aware of the burden they place on their parents. Shaw's (2001) study of teenagers shows that they would prefer a formal arrangement for help with ADLs from their age-mates rather than their parents.

The recipient and caregiver shape the meaning of care; so, in an important sense, does public policy

(Fisher & Tronto, 1990; Strauss & Corbin, 1988). Access to health insurance; insurance coverage for rehabilitation services; the availability and quality of nursing homes; community-based personal assistant services, including personal attendant care at school and work; and respite care all contribute to the meaning of self-care in relationships among providers and the clients, friends, or family members they care for, with or without training, supervision, or payment.

Hospital policy also shapes the experience of self-care for patients and their families. Patients depend on strangers for their care and routines dictate not only when to eat, when to comb hair and wash, but even on occasion when to go to the bathroom.

> If dinner is scheduled for 4:30 p.m., as it was on a floor in which I once spent two months, then that's when you eat. And if your bowels don't move often enough to suit the nursing staff, laxatives are the answer. The infamous routine that demands that all temperatures be taken at 6:00 a.m. is well known to all who have been patients. I even spent five weeks on one floor where I was bathed at 5:30 every morning because the daytime nurses were too busy to do it. (Murphy, 1987, pp. 20–21)

Arnold Beisser (1989) was hospitalized for 3 years beginning in 1950 after becoming paralyzed by polio. His alienation from his own failed body grew worse because of depersonalized care. Beisser spent every moment of the first year and a half on his back in an iron lung. He was a young man in his mid-20s, who had been a national tennis champion and was a medical school graduate.

> Intermittently people would open one or another of the portholes of my new metal skin and invade my private space. They would enter the most personal and private parts of me as they reached inside to move a leg or arm, or insert a needle or a bedpan. There was not even the pretense that my new space belonged to me, and entry beneath my new metal skin was at the discretion of others. (p. 18)

People who must depend on others for help with bowel and bladder functions are sometimes infantilized. Beisser realized that he was seen as a baby. Some of his caregivers were concerned with controlling an unruly child, others with nurturing a helpless infant. In Alana Theriault's life, the experience of institutionalization was galvanizing.

> Nursing home was never something I even conceived of. I think me dying was more the expected scenario. This was pre-ventilator, and I always had a respiratory infection every year. The muscular dystrophy clinic was al-

ways saying, "Well, it will be a very amazing thing if Alana lives through this next winter." Everybody was expecting me to die of a respiratory infection, and I think my family was part of that, and my internal little monologue was, "Fuck that shit! I'm not going to die. I'll show you!" and I just became a fighter then. (2008, p. 9)

The group ADAPT is an ardent promoter of the availability of community-based, consumer-directed personal assistance services as an alternative to institutional care:

ADAPT is a national grass-roots community that organizes disability rights activists to engage in nonviolent direct action, including civil disobedience, to assure the civil and human rights of people with disabilities to live in freedom. There's no place like home; and we mean real homes, not nursing homes. We are fighting so people with disabilities can live in the community with real supports instead of being locked away in nursing homes and other institutions. (http://www.adapt.org/)

Largely with ADAPT's urging, independent living centers have taken on the task of emancipating people from nursing homes, with some success (RTC–RURAL, 2008). Researchers have studied the safety, quality, and efficacy of consumer-directed personal assistance services models (e.g., Benjamin, Matthias, & Franke, 2000); the model is now well established, and a second wave of work has begun on setting training and working standards (although Medicare funding for this as part of home care is currently in question). Together with adequate, affordable, general health care, nothing can make more of a difference in the lives of people with ADL-affecting impairments than access to assistive technology and personal assistance services.

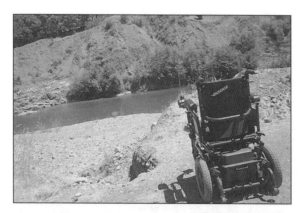

Figure 2.3. Stopping for a swim, outside of Garberville. Photo credit: Neil Marcus.

Conclusion

Bringing us back to our themes of embodiment and participation, self-care is not simply an objective routine. While impairment challenges the body, every experience of disability oppression also challenges the embodied human being who interrelates with family, friends, helpers, and who wants to participate meaningfully in the society of which he or she is a part. The narratives of people with chronic illness, impairment, and disability show that their experience is *occupational*. That is to say, performance differences of their bodies or "activity limitations" in an inaccessible environment that provides no assistance, can cause *occupational injustice* and prevent people from engaging in the customary activities that enrich their lives and give them meaning. Personal identity and social relations are at stake in even the simplest activities of self-care, however accomplished, alone or with assistance, resulting in either self-esteem or profound shame.

Occupational therapists can help people with disability experience by recognizing that self-care occupations are deeply meaningful—and about power. People must cope with feelings of frustration when their ability to perform daily activities breaks down, when they encounter environmental barriers, or when needed assistance or assistive tools are absent. They experience anger and depression over the lack of control and choice. They experience negative feelings about being helpless or dependent on others or when they are perceived to be so. They feel distress and guilt about the necessary reorganization of family and other relationships or their inability to participate in routine reciprocal roles. These feelings are normal and often justified.

Fortunately, attitudes can and do change as people grow and develop new skills and understand the accommodation choices to which they have access. People adapt to new impairments over time. Their attitudes toward their impairments and occupational changes—the meanings they attach to them—depend partly on where they stand on the developmental or rehabilitation path.

Professional, community, and family assistants' attitudes can change, too. The ability to reevaluate cultural rules about "the right way" to do things and the meaning of doing them can make impairments less disabling and less stigmatizing. Occupational therapists can make a tremendous contribution to their clients by helping them and their families gain the occupational skills needed to implement their personal care choices. With experience and over time, a concerned occupational therapist can learn to guide clients in ways that take basic embodied meaning into consideration and enhance rather than limit personal and social identity, choice, and participation.

People with chronic illness or disability, in order to exercise their right to full social participation, need access to basic health care and functional assistance through adequate insurance, rehabilitation services, attendant care, respite care, adaptive equipment, employment opportunities, and income supports. These resources must be provided by enlightened social policy. In each of these areas, compassionate assistance that emphasizes participation and choice can make an important difference in the quality of life of the disabled person and their significant others.

Acknowledgment

The authors thank Carol Stein, MA, OTR/L, for her contributions as coauthor of a previously published version of this chapter. Carol Stein retired in 2009 as Chief of Occupational Therapy of the Veterans Administration Healthcare System facilities of Greater Los Angeles. A founding member of the discipline of occupational science at the University of Southern California, she has had 30 years of experience as an occupational therapist.

Study Questions

1. Describe the importance of embodiment and participation in thinking about solutions to problems around essential ADLs.
2. Explain the differences among *illness, impairment,* and *disability* as used by WHO and disability studies scholars.
3. How does the body affect a person's sense of self? Identify some of the meanings associated with toileting, eating, and grooming. How does the setting in which an activity or occupation occurs influence its meaning?
4. Consider potential strategies for helping people express their sense of control and selfhood over basic ADLs and problems often encountered in families and community settings around these issues.
5. Describe possible occupational therapy activities, and what you need to know about someone's life, to help a person maximize participation and make choices about self-care and assisted care for essential ADLs.

References

Ablon, J. (1984). *Little people in America: Social dimensions of dwarfism.* New York: Praeger.

American Occupational Therapy Association. (2007). *Centennial Vision,* and executive summary. *American Journal of Occupational Therapy, 61,* 613–614.

Beisser, A. R. (1989). *Flying without wings: Personal reflections on being disabled.* New York: Doubleday.

Benjamin, A. E., Matthias, R., & Franke, T. (2000). Comparing consumer-directed and agency models for providing supportive services at home. *Health Services Research, 35*(1), Part II, 351–366.

Berkowitz, E. D. (1987). *Disabled policy: America's programs for the handicapped.* New York: Cambridge University Press.

Block, P., Vanner, E., Keys, C. B., Rimmer, J., & Skeels, S. (in press). Project Shake-It-Up! A disability studies framework of empowerment for capacity building and health promotion. *Disability and Rehabilitation.*

California Department of Rehabilitation. (2005). *A day in the life of Richard Devylder* [Video]. Retrieved May 4, 2009, from http://www.rehab.cahwnet.gov/rd_video.htm

Campbell, F. K. (2009). *Contours of ableism: The production of disability and abledness.* New York: Macmillan.

Center for an Accessible Society. (1999). *Supreme Court upholds ADA "Integrati Mandate" in Olmstead decision.* Retrieved November 1, 2009, from http:// www.accessible society.org/topics/ada/olmstead overview.htm

Charlton, J. (1998). *Nothing about us without us: Disability oppression and empowerment.* Berkeley: University of California Press.

Clark, F. A., Parham, D., Carlson, M. E., Frank, G., Jackson, J., Pierce, et al. (1991). Occupational science: Academic innovation in the service of occupational therapy's future. *American Journal of Occupational Therapy, 45*(4) 300–310.

Cohen, L. (1998). *No aging in India: Alzheimer's, the bad family, and other modern things.* Berkeley: University of California Press.

Corbin, J. M., & Strauss, A. (1988). *Unending work and care: Managing chronic illness at home.* San Francisco, CA: Jossey-Bass.

Crewe, N., & Zola, I. K. (1983). *Independent living for physically disabled people.* San Francisco, CA: Jossey-Bass.

CSDH. (2008). *Closing the gap in a generation: Health equity through action on the social determinants of health.* Final Report of the Commission on Social Determinants of Health. Geneva: World Health Organization. Retrieved May 1, 2009, from http://www.who.int/social_determinants/en/

Csordas, T.J. (1994). The body as representation and being in the world. In T.J. Csordas (Ed.), *Embodiment and experience: The existential ground of culture and self* (pp. 1–23). London: Cambridge University Press.

Cushing, P., & Smith, T. (2009). Multinational review of English language disability studies degrees and courses. *Disability Studies Quarterly, 29*(3).

Das, V., & Addlakha, R. (2001). Disability and domestic citizenship: Voice, gender and the making of the subject. *Public Culture, 13*(3), 511–531.

Das, V., Kleinman, A., Lock, M., Ramphele, M., & Reynolds, P. (Eds.). (2001). *Remaking a world: Violence, social suffering, and recovery.* Berkeley: University of California Press.

de Mille, A. (1981). *Reprieve: A memoir.* New York: Doubleday.

DePoy, E., & Gilson, S. (2004). *Rethinking disability: Principles for professional and social change.* Pacific Grove, CA: Wadsworth.

Eisenberg, L. (1977). Disease and illness: Distinctions between professional and popular ideas of sickness. *Culture, Medicine, and Psychiatry, 1,* 9–23.

Featherstone, H. (1980). *A difference in the family: Living with a disabled child.* New York: Penguin.

Fisher, B., & Tronto, J. (1990). Toward a feminist theory of caring. In E. K. Abel & M. K. Nelson (Eds.), *Circles of care: Work and identity in women's lives* (pp. 35–62). Albany: State University of New York Press.

Foucault, M. (1984). *The Foucault reader.* New York: Pantheon Books.

Foucault, M. (2003). *The essential Foucault.* New York: New Press.

Frank, G. (1986). On embodiment: A case study of congenital limb deficiency in American culture. *Culture, Medicine, and Psychiatry, 10,* 189–219.

Frank, G. (2000). *Venus on wheels: Two decades of dialogue on disability, biography, and being female in America.* Berkeley: University of California Press.

Frank, G., Baum, C., & Law, M. (2010). Chronic conditions, health, and well-being in global contexts: Occupational therapy in conversation with critical medical anthropology. In L. Manderson & C. Smith-Morris (Eds.), *Chronic conditions, fluid states: Globalization and the anthropology of illness.* New Brunswick, NJ: Rutgers University Press.

Frank, G., Block, P., & Zemke, R. (2008). Introduction, special theme issue, anthropology, occupational therapy and disability studies: Collaborations and prospects. *Practicing Anthropology, 30*(3).

Frank, G., Huecker, E., Segal, R., Forwell, S., & Bagatell, N. (1991). Assessment and treatment of a pediatric patient in chronic care: Ethnographic methods applied to occupational therapy practice. *American Journal of Occupational Therapy, 45,* 252–263.

Garland-Thomson, R. (2009). *Staring: How we look.* New York: Oxford.

Goffman, E. (1963). *Stigma: Notes on the management of spoiled identity.* Englewood Cliffs, NJ: Prentice Hall.

Greene, S. L. (1992). *An ethnographic study of homeless mentally ill women: Adaptive strategies, needs, and services.* Unpublished master's thesis, University of Southern California, Los Angeles.

Hahn, H. (1988). Can disability be beautiful? *Social Policy, 18,* 26–32.

Hardt, M., & Negri, A. (2001). *Empire.* Cambridge, MA: Harvard University Press.

Harris, L., & Associates. (1986). *The ICD survey of disabled Americans: Bringing disabled Americans into the mainstream.* New York: International Center for the Disabled.

Ingstad, B., & Whyte, S. R. (Eds.). (1995). *Disability and culture.* Berkeley: University of California Press.

Ingstad, B., & Whyte, S. (Eds.). (2007). *Disability in local and global worlds.* Berkeley: University of California Press.

Kaiser, S. B., Freeman, C. M., & Wingate, S. B. (1990). Stigmata and negotiated outcomes: Management of appearance by persons with physical disabilities. In M. Nagler (Ed.), *Perspectives on disability* (pp. 33–45). Palo Alto, CA: Health Markets Research. Reprinted from *Deviant Behavior, 6,* 205–224.

Kasnitz, D. (2008). Collaborations from anthropology, occupational therapy and disability studies, special theme issue anthropology, occupational therapy and disability studies: Collaborations and prospects. *Practicing Anthropology, 30*(3).

Kasnitz, D., Pfeiffer, D., Bonney, S., & Aftendelian, R. (2000). The Development of Disability Studies Curricula. *Disability Studies Quarterly, 20*(2), 5–18.

Kent, D. (1987). Disabled women: Portraits in fiction and drama. In A. Gartner & T. Joe (Eds.), *Images of the disabled, disabling images* (pp. 47–63). New York: Praeger.

Kleinman, A. (1988). *The illness narratives: Suffering, healing, and the human condition.* New York: Basic Books.

Kleinman, A., Das, V., & Lock, M. (Eds.). (1997). *Social suffering.* Berkeley: University of California Press.

Koegel, P. (1987). Ethnographic perspectives on homeless and homeless mentally ill women. In P. Koegel (Ed.), *Proceedings of a two-day workshop sponsored by the Division of Education and Service Systems Liaison.* Bethesda, MD: National Institute of Mental Health.

Kohrman, M. (2005). *Bodies of difference: Experiences of disability and institutional advocacy in the making of Modern China.* Berkeley: University of California Press.

Kronenberg, F., Pollard, N., & Simó Algado, S. (2005). *Occupational therapy without borders: Learning from the spirit of survivors.* Edinburgh, Scotland: Elsevier.

Law, M. (2002). Participation in the occupations of everyday life. *American Journal of Occupational Therapy, 56*(6), 640–649.

Linton, S. (1998). *Claiming disability: Knowledge and identity.* New York: New York University Press.

Lomawaima, K. T. (1995). Domesticity in the Federal Indian schools: The power of authority over mind and body. In J. Terry & J. Urla (Eds.), *Deviant bodies* (pp. 197–218). Bloomington: Indiana University Press.

Longmore, P. K. (1987). Screening stereotypes: Images of disabled people in television and motion pictures. In A. Gartner & T. Joe (Eds.), *Images of the disabled, disabling images* (pp. 65–78). New York: Praeger.

Lorde, A. (1980). *The cancer journals.* San Francisco: Spinsters Ink.

Magasi, S. (2008a). Infusing disability studies into the rehabilitation sciences. *Topics in Stroke Rehabilitation, 15*(3), 283–287.

Magasi, S. (2008b). Disability studies in practice: A work in progress. *Topics in Stroke Rehabilitation, 15*(6), 611–617.

Mairs, N. (1987). On being a cripple. In M. Saxton & F. Howe (Eds.), *With wings: An anthology of literature by and about women with disabilities* (pp. 118–127). New York: Feminist Press.

Mairs, N. (1989). *Remembering the bone house: An erotics of place and space.* New York: Harper & Row.

Merleau-Ponty, M. (1962). *Phenomenology of perception.* New York: Humanities Press. (Original work published 1945)

Mulhorn, K. A. (Ed.). (2004). Disability studies in public health and health professions, Special Theme Issue. *Disability Studies Quarterly 24*(4). Retrieved 11/22/2009 from http://www.dsq-sds.org/article/view/882/1057

Murphy, R. F. (1987). *The body silent.* New York: Henry Holt.

Newman, T. (2002). 'Young carers' and disabled parents: Time for a change of direction? *Disability and Society, 1*(6), 613–625.

Nolan, C. (1987). *Under the eye of the clock: The life story of Christopher Nolan.* New York: St. Martin's.

Padilla, R. (2003). Clara—A phenomenology of disability. *American Journal of Occupational Therapy, 57*, 413–423.

Parsons, T. (1951). Illness and the role of the physician: A sociological perspective. *American Journal of Orthopsychiatry, 21*, 452–460.

Paterson, K., & Hughes, B. (1999). Disability studies and phenomenology: The carnal politics of everyday life. *Disability and Society, 14*(5), 597–610.

Patterson, E. A. (1985). Glimpse into transformation. In S. E. Browne, D. Connors, & N. Stern (Eds.), *With the power of each breath: A disabled women's anthology* (pp. 240–243). Pittsburgh, PA: Cleis Press.

Pernick, M. S. (1996). *The black stork: Eugenics and the death of "defective" babies in American medicine and motion pictures since 1915*. New York: Oxford University Press.

Petryna, A. (2002). *Life exposed: Biological citizens after Chernobyl*. Princeton, NJ: Princeton University Press.

Pierce, D., & Frank, G. (1992). A mother's work: Feminist perspectives on family-centered care. *American Journal of Occupational Therapy, 46*, 972–980.

Pfeiffer, D., & Yoshida, K. (1995). Teaching disability studies in Canada and the USA. *Disability and Society, 10*, 475–499.

Pollard, N., Sakellariou, D., & Kronenberg, F. (Eds.). (2008). *A political practice of occupational therapy*. Edinburgh, Scotland: Elsevier.

Rapp, R., & Ginsburg, F. (2001). Enabling disability: Rewriting kinship, reimagining citizenship. *Public Culture, 13*(3), 533–556.

Rose, N. (2007). *The politics of life itself: Biomedicine, power, and subjectivity in the twenty-first century*. Princeton, NJ: Princeton University Press.

RTC–RURAL. (2008, March). *Nursing home emancipation: Accomplishments of urban and rural centers for independent living, rural disability, and rehabilitation*. Research Progress Report 39. Research and Training Center on Disability in Rural Communities, University of Montana Rural Institute. Retrieved December 2, 2009, from http://rtc.ruralinstitute.umt.edu/IL/Nursing HomeEmancipationUrbanRural.html

Scheper-Hughes, N., & Lock, M. (1987). *Medical Anthropology Quarterly, 1*, 6–41. Retrieved November 24, 2009, from www.anthrosource.net/doi/abs/10.1525/maq.1987.1.1 .02a00020

Shakespeare, T. (2006). *Disability rights and wrongs*. New York: Routledge.

Shaw, M. (2001). Personal assistance services and youth in transition. In L. J. Rogers & B. B. Swadener (Eds.), *The semiotics of dis/ability: Interrogating categories of difference* (pp. 165–187). Buffalo: State University of New York Press.

Schweik, S. (2009). *The ugly laws: Disability in public*. New York: New York University Press.

Spiegelberg, H. (1976). *The phenomenological movement: A historical introduction* (2nd ed.). The Hague, Netherlands: Martinus Nijhoff.

Stoddard, S. (2006). Personal assistance services as a workplace accommodation. *Work: A Journal of Prevention, Assessment, and Rehabilitation, 27*(4), 363–369.

Storm, P. (1987). *Functions of dress: Tool of culture and the individual*. Englewood Cliffs, NJ: Prentice Hall.

Strauss, A., & Corbin, J. M. (1988). *Shaping a new health care system: The explosion of chronic illness as a catalyst for change*. San Francisco: Jossey-Bass.

Theriault, A. (2008). *"Crafting a life of independence and advocacy," conducted by Laura Hershey in 2007*. Berkeley: Regional Oral History Office, Bancroft Library, University of California.

Thomas C. J. (Ed.). (1994). *Embodiment and experience: The existential ground of culture and self*. New York: Cambridge University Press.

Thomas, C. (2007). *Sociologies of disability and illness: Contested ideas in disability studies and medical sociology*. London: Palgrave Macmillan.

Watson, R., & Swartz, L. (Eds.). (2004). *Transformation through occupation*. London: Whurr.

World Health Organization. (2001). *International classification of functioning, disability and health (ICF)*. Geneva: Author.

World Health Organization. (2002). *Towards a common language for functioning, disability and health (ICF)*. Geneva: Author.

Wright, B. A. (1983). *Physical disability: A psychosocial approach* (2nd ed.). New York: Harper & Row.

Wright, B. A. (2004). Redefining disability to promote equality: The role of disability studies in educating occupational therapists. *Disability Studies Quarterly 24*(4). Retrieved December 11, 2009, from http://www.dsq-sds.org/article/view/885/1060

Yerxa, E. J., Clark, F., Frank, G., Jackson, J., Parham, D., Pierce, D., et al. (1990). A foundation for occupational therapy in the 21st century. *Occupational Therapy in Health Care 6*(4), 1–18.

Zola, I. K. (1982). *Missing pieces: A chronicle of living with a disability*. Philadelphia: Temple University Press.

Chapter 3

Evaluation to Plan Intervention

CHARLES H. CHRISTIANSEN, EDD, OTR, OT(C), FAOTA;
KRISTINE HAERTL, PHD, OTR/L; AND SANDRA ROGERS, PHD, OTR/L

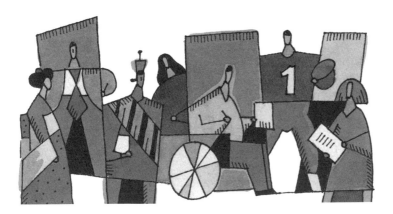

KEY TERMS

analysis of
    occupational
    performance
assessment
correlation
evaluation
norms

occupational profile
Rasch analysis
reliability
stability

HIGHLIGHTS

- *Evaluation* consists of formal and informal collection of useful information about the client.
- Occupational therapy evaluation consists of an occupational profile and an analysis of occupational performance.
- The suitability of a measure depends on the nature of the client, the purpose of evaluation, and the setting in which evaluation is performed.
- Evaluation instuments should be practical, reliable, and valid for their intended purposes.

OBJECTIVES

After reading this material, readers will be able to

- Describe the basic purposes of evaluation and assessment;
- List questions appropriate to the development of an occupational profile;
- Understand the meaning of "performance contexts";
- Identify important characteristics of assessment instruments;
- Appreciate the relationship between target outcomes and assessment selection;
- Describe the purposes and characteristics of selected assessment instruments suitable for measuring occupational performance in ADLs, IADLs, play, leisure, work and education, environmental contexts, and social participation; and
- Understand how informal and formal assessment methods are used in combination during the analysis of occupational performance.

The evaluation process consists of the formal and informal collection of useful information (sometimes called *data*) from multiple sources. Informal data collection includes casual observation, interactions with clients and/or people in the client's life, and general knowledge of communities and situations. Formal data collection usually involves assessment tools. These, too, incorporate observation and interaction by occupational therapy personnel or by other professionals.

Occupational therapy evaluation is a dynamic, two-part process. It relies on informal and and formal observation methods to develop an occupational profile of the client and assess his or her occupational performance (Figure 3.1).

Ideally, the evaluation process emphasizes data reflecting the client's performance of activities in natural contexts (that is, the settings in which they typically live). Doing so provides a more representative indication of strengths and weaknesses of contextual (situational) factors, person-related factors, and activity-related factors. A complete evaluation attends to performance issues in all areas that affect the person's ability to engage in occupations and in activities. The evaluation process gathers information on performance skills, performance patterns, and the contextual or situational factors that influence performance, as well as activity demands and client factors.

When the occupational therapist gathers information on performance skills, his or her attention is directed to specific features of doing (such as bending or choosing) rather than the underlying body functions or capacities that support those acts, such as joint range of motion, or motivation. A client demonstrates a performance skill when the demands of an activity (which include such aspects as necessary objects, space, sequencing, required actions, required body functions, and structures) and the contexts of the activity (the cultural, physical location, social, personal, spiritual, temporal, and virtual factors) come together during the performance of that activity. The client, the demands of an activity, and the contexts of the activity combine as factors that influence occupational performance.

Development of the Occupational Profile

As a first step in the evaluation process, the client must be understood through development of an occupational profile (American Occupational Therapy Association, 2008). The occupational profile provides a summary of the client's identity and occupational history and his or her priorities, interests, values, and needs. The intent is to understand the client as an occupational being from his or her perspective in order to provide client-centered care.

The occupational profile helps the therapist formulate an "occupational" view of the client, which in turn enables the development of a working hypothesis concerning identified problem areas. The therapist forms a preliminary understanding of the client's strengths and weaknesses and the causes of the client's occupational performance problems. The therapist's impressions must be tested through the use of assessment tools and strategies: the analysis of occupational performance.

Analysis of Occupational Performance

The analysis of occupational performance involves determining a client's ability to carry out the activities of daily life in the various areas of occupation. This analysis requires the identification of performance skills and patterns used in performance and other aspects of occupational engagement that affect performance skills and patterns. The process enables the identification of facilitators as well as barriers to performance and requires an appreciation of the complex nature of occupational performance. That is, therapists must recognize that occupational performance involves a dynamic interaction among

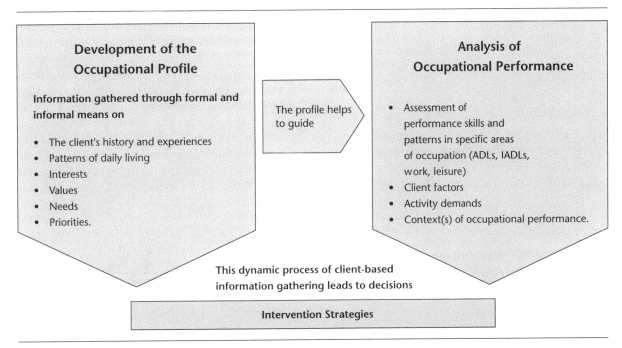

Figure 3.1. Summary of the evaluation process.

skills, activity demands, client factors, and contexts. Information from the occupational profile guides the therapist in identifying specific areas needing evaluation and for selecting specific assessment tools. Typically, particular conceptual frames of reference will also direct attention toward specific and theoretically consistent tools or approaches.

The therapist can use several factors to determine the suitability of a particular scale. These include basing the assessment on the client's needs and circumstances, understanding the relationship between performance of everyday activities and the elements of skill, and appreciating the important difference between assessments based on self-report versus those based on observation of the individual's actual performance (Finlayson, Havens, Holm, & Van Denend, 2003; Rogers et al., 2003).

Evaluation often is biased toward using standardized assessment tools. A *standardized tool* is one that has well-defined procedures for administration and scoring. Some tools are based on normative data gathered from sample populations. A limitation of standardized instruments is that one set of items and procedures must be used for all clients and situations. Standardized instruments do not have items that represent all situations. Additionally, instruments that provide normative data may have little meaning within specific contexts because the norm provides information on a statistically derived "typical situation and client,"

which may resemble but does not accurately describe any specific situation or client. Moreover, a long list of every possible task would be impractical and would make it difficult to compare the efficacy of treatment approaches across large numbers of clients.

The therapist can gain valuable information that contributes to a client's evaluation during informal observation and interactions, as well as during more structured interviews. The development of the occupational profile informs both the selection of assessment instruments and provides information that helps to validate findings from standardized assessment tools. Both standardized and nonstandardized approaches have a place in assessing occupational performance.

Some assessment approaches are based on the reports of clients or family members, often when they are used to follow up on client status following discharge or termination of care. Studies of self-report instruments have shown that what clients or those living with them say a client can do may not always match the individual's actual day-to-day performance. A client may be capable of doing a defined task under certain circumstances or occasionally but is unable to do it regularly. It is important to determine an individual's consistent level of function. This can be done reliably and validly only in the environment in which people experience their day-to-day living (Christiansen, 2004).

A client's ability to perform daily occupations is influenced by the demands of the activity, the context(s) of action, and client factors. The client's general health and physical abilities, mental and emotional states, living environment, and relationships with others can influence the performance of tasks in any occupational area. Understanding the relative influence of these various factors on a given client's performance helps the therapist to consider all the barriers to function during intervention planning. Ideally, clients should be assessed in environ- ments that represent their everyday living situations (Moore, Palmer, Patterson, & Jeste, 2007; Rogers & Holm, 1994; see Box 3.1). Effective evaluations are always individualized and capture the uniqueness of the client. This book includes a case study (see Box 3.2) that illustrates how the various components of the evaluation process, including the development of the occupational profile, the analysis of occupa- tional performance, and the assessment of contexts, provide the basis for identifying intervention needs formulating goals for intervention. This case study

---

Box 3.1. Selecting Assessment Instruments

Researchers consider numerous characteristics when developing an instrument to measure any aspect of occupational performance. These include the

- Scope of tasks addressed by the instrument,
- Instrument's sensitivity to changes in the client,
- Reliability of the assessment procedures,
- Validity of the instrument,
- Nature of resulting data, and
- Feasibility of the assessment instrument.

Some instruments cover a broad range of func- tional tasks; others limit themselves to a few self-care tasks. The extent to which instruments address each self-care task or assess the client's level of function also varies. For example, one instrument may evalu- ate the task of dressing using a single item that refers to the complete task, and another instrument may use several items to address the task's component parts, such as putting on socks, fastening shirt but- tons, and so forth.

An instrument's sensitivity reflects the degree to which it detects small changes in the client. Sensitiv- ity is particularly important in measuring the effects of intervention. An instrument that lacks sensitivity will fail to indicate small gains in the client's ability to perform self-care tasks.

The procedures for administering and scoring the instrument must be stated clearly in the test manual or protocol. Reliable procedures will yield consistent scores or descriptors from one assessment period to another and among assessments given by different individuals.

Validity relates to what behaviors the assess- ment instrument measures and how well it does so. A test that is valid in one situation may not be valid in different or changed circumstances. For example, a test of mobility that was developed for ambula- tory subjects may be unsuitable for assessing mobil- ity in wheelchair users. In this example, the content validity is not precisely determined by a statistical calculation; rather, it is a judgment call made by the potential test user. How well a test measures what it purports to measure may be more precisely mea- sured by comparing performance on the test with the results of another instrument already consid- ered to be an accurate indicator of the behavior of interest. If two tests measure the same thing, a per- son's performance using the first measure should relate to his or her performance on the second. The comparison often is expressed as a correlation coef- ficient, indicating the extent of relationship be- tween two instruments.

A completed assessment instrument may pro- vide a detailed profile that describes the client's self- care ability, or it may result in a single code or nu- merical value that represents a measure of overall function. Instruments may be descriptive or evalua- tive, and the purpose of the assessment directs the type of data collected. Useful evaluative instruments quantify function, the assumption being that the nu- merical score will change as the subject's perfor- mance changes. A single overall score for something as complex as self-care is misleading, however, so caution is advised when interpreting a global score that represents the sum of several subtests. Most as- sessment instruments for adults are designed to yield scores that allow practitioners to measure change or compare performance to normative data. Some tests have a developmental focus so that the resulting data indicate the subject's performance in relation to a developmental continuum.

The training, equipment, and time required to administer the assessment all influence the useful- ness of the instrument in any given setting.

Assessment instruments that are suitable for program evaluation and research purposes will have similar desirable characteristics. Comprehensiveness, accuracy, sensitivity to change, and feasibility are just some of the characteristics to be considered before making a choice.

Box 3.2. Case Study of Irene: Information Gathered for an Occupational Therapy Evaluation

Occupational Profile
(Gathered from interview)

Irene is a 52-year-old divorced woman who was diagnosed with multiple sclerosis 20 years ago. Until a recent exacerbation of her symptoms, Irene lived alone in an apartment and was independent in all areas of self-care, including driving. Disabling fatigue forced her to quit her job several years ago. Irene has been very active in her church, attending weekly services and the women's club. She loves to go to movies and restaurants and has averaged about two social outings per week, accompanying either her daughter or a friend. She loves to read.

Irene's usual pattern has been to sleep until about 8:00 a.m. She does most of her housework and errands on rising in the morning, when she has the most energy and feels the best. After the work is done, she either goes to a church activity or takes a half-mile walk before lunch. Typically she feels exhausted by the afternoon and naps for 2 or 3 hours. She generally spends evenings reading or watching TV, with occasional outings.

Irene recently experienced an exacerbation of her symptoms, including double vision, left-sided weakness and numbness, and cognitive problems. All of Irene's symptoms worsen with fatigue.

Analysis of Occupational Performance
(Gathered from the Canadian Occupational Performance Measure and Activity Card Sort and from observation during the interview)

1. Irene now struggles more with dressing and bathing because these tasks take her longer and are more fatiguing. Although she can complete the tasks, she finds it easier to bathe less frequently and to wear the same clothes for several days without removing them at night.
2. She has not been cooking. Instead, she depends on eating the food her daughter brings over. She reports that she can cook, but it takes too much effort.
3. Irene's daughter has been doing the laundry.
4. She has not been driving because of her double vision. Therefore, she depends on her daughter for delivering groceries and doing her banking.
5. She has stopped going to the church group meetings and is too fatigued for outings in the evening.
6. Reading has become difficult, especially in the evening.
7. Irene spends most of her day listening to the TV, sleeping, and talking with friends on the telephone.

Assessment of Client Factors
(Gathered from manual muscle testing, sensory testing, and interview)

1. Irene's left arm and hand are weak. She has grade 3/5 muscle strength throughout, and her maximal grip was 10 pounds.
2. She can discriminate sensations on her arm and hand but reports a feeling of tingling in the fingers and forearm.
3. Irene's vision is best in the morning; her vision worsens as the day progresses. At times she can see the TV well enough to watch it, but later in the day she cannot see well enough to read.
4. She has short-term memory problems that worsen with fatigue.
5. She reports her level of fatigue as severe.
6. She admits to feeling depressed.

Assessment of Performance Contexts
(Gathered from observation in her home and interviews with Irene and her daughter)

1. Irene's apartment is small, and she keeps it clutter-free and minimally furnished. The building's laundry room is three doors down on the same, first-story level as the apartment. She has a wheeled laundry cart.
2. Irene's bathroom has a combination tub and shower. She had grab bars installed several years ago as a precaution against falling.
3. She wears knit, stretchy clothes for ease and comfort.
4. Irene's apartment is well lit for reading and other tasks.
5. Her daughter works during the day but has been coming over two or three nights a week to take care of miscellaneous housework and to bring several meals.
6. Her friends at the church have been calling her on the telephone, and some have volunteered to pick her up to attend group meetings, but she has declined their offers.
7. Irene's daughter is very concerned about her mother's apparent lack of interest in bathing, dressing, hygiene, and household tasks. She believes Irene is forgetting things more often and that she sleeps too much. The daughter is unable to take her mother to her church groups during the day, and she is very concerned about Irene's limited social activity. She has a family of her own and finds it very difficult to attend to all her mother's needs.

Note: This case study continues in Chapter 4 with a discussion of Irene's goals and the intervention planning her therapist completes in collaboration with her.

continues in Chapter 4 to illustrate how evaluation leads to the planning of interventions that are described for various conditions reviewed in this book.

In the remainder of this chapter, we identify and discuss specific assessment tools for analysis of occupational performance. An exhaustive review of all available tools in each occupational area is not possible here. The intent here is to provide examples of scales that are broadly used (by occupational therapists or other professionals) in each occupational area. Note that not all occupational areas have measures that can be applied to individual clients, groups, and populations. Before using any instrument, it is important for professionals to gather as much information as possible on the measure's procedures, strengths, limitations, and evidence of reliability and validity. This information can be gained from the professional literature and (for published tests) by consulting recent editions of the *Mental Measurements Yearbook* (Geisinger, Spies, Carlson, & Plake, 2007), or *Tests in Print*, available in printed form or online through the Buros Institute, Lincoln, NE. For tools listed, only summary information on characteristics and reliability and validity studies is provided. Additional details and citations can be found in Table 3.6 at the end of the chapter.

Assessment of Activities of Daily Living

The literature provides many instruments and recommendations for evaluating the performance of ADLs Christiansen, 2004). The challenge for occupational therapists is to develop effective strategies for determining clients' basic ADL performance by selecting the most appropriate instruments. In the past, rehabilitation experienced an era where instruments proliferated, and few were well standardized, validated, or based in theory (McDowell & Newell, 1996). Fortunately, greater attention has been given to the consistent use of fewer, higher-quality tools, and therapists have come to appreciate that it is important to use only instruments with documented reliability and evidence of validity.

When a therapist evaluates a client, he or she makes several important decisions based on the person's ability to perform ADL safely and independently. It is important to remember that independent performance does not always equate with safe performance (Rogers, Holm, Beach, Schulz, & Starz, 2001). When an individual cannot eat, bathe, or dress independently, some type of personal assistance usually is required. The person's occupational roles and social and physical environments may change. Evaluation of ADLs may lead to determinations about whether care or assistance may be necessary and the degree of care or assistance required. These determinations contribute to decisions regarding discharge from care settings into long-term care, skilled nursing, or supported home care environments (Hoogerduijn, Schuurmans, Duijnstee, de Rooij, & Grypdonck, 2007).

Selected Measures of Basic Activities of Daily Living

Several specific instruments evaluate everyday tasks that are sometimes called *basic activities of daily living (BADLs)*. BADLs typically include bathing or showering, bowel and bladder management, dressing, eating, feeding, functional mobility, personal device care, personal hygiene and grooming, sexual activity, sleep and rest, and toilet hygiene. Instruments that assess other types of ADLs and combined or global instruments are discussed in separate sections later in the chapter. Instruments in this section are presented in the order of their development and appearance in the literature. An attempt has been made to include those scales most widely used in the United States and in the international community.

Barthel Index

In 1965, Mahoney and Barthel published a weighted scale for measuring BADLs with chronically disabled patients (Mahoney & Barthel, 1965). The Barthel Index includes 10 items, including feeding, transfers, personal grooming and hygiene, bathing, toileting, walking, negotiating stairs, and controlling bowel and bladder. Items are scored differentially according to a weighted scoring system that assigns points based on independent or assisted performance. For example, a person who needs assistance in eating would receive 5 points, whereas independence in eating would be awarded 10 points. A patient with a maximum score of 100 points is defined as continent, able to eat and dress independently, walk at least a block, and climb and descend stairs. The authors were careful to note that a maximum score did not necessarily signify independence, because instrumental activities of daily living (IADLs) such as cooking, housekeeping, and socialization are not assessed.

The Barthel Index may be the most widely studied and used self-care scale globally. Several studies have shown that the scale has acceptable psychometric properties, including that it is sensitive to change over time, that it is a significant predictor of rehabilitation outcome, and that it relates significantly with other measures of client status.

Shortened versions of the Barthel Index (BI–3 and BI–5) have also been developed, and these have shown evidence of satisfactory psychometric characteristics and predictive validity acceptable for outcome use (Ellul, Watkins, & Barer, 1998; Hsueh, Huang, Chen, Just, & Hsieh, 2000). A mailed self-report version has also been reported (Gompertz, Pound, & Ebrahim, 1994). The Extended Barthel Index (EBI; Prosiegel et al., 1996) was developed to address perceived limitations by adding items for comprehension, expression, social interaction, problem solving, memory, learning, orientation, and vision/neglect.

Katz Index of Independence in Activities of Daily Living

The Katz Index of Independence in ADL was originally developed to study results of treatment and prognosis in elderly persons and individuals with chronic illness (Katz, Ford, Moskowitz, Jackson, & Jaffe, 1963). Development of the index was based on observations of a large number of activities performed by a patients following hip fracture (Katz, Downs, Cash, & Grotz, 1970).

The index is based on an evaluation of the functional independence of patients in bathing, dressing, going to the toilet, transfers, continence, and feeding. Using three descriptors for rating independence in each of six subscales, the rater is able to derive an overall grade of independence with the aid of specific rating criteria. Depending on the determined level of independence, a patient is graded as A, B, C, D, E, F, G, or other. According to the scale, a patient graded as A would be functioning independently in all six functions, whereas a patient graded as G would be dependent in all rated functions. Patients graded as other are dependent in at least two functions but not classifiable as C, D, E, or F. Over a defined period of time, the observer determines whether the patient is assisted or whether the patient functions on his or her own when performing the six activities. Assistance is graded as active personal assistance, directive assistance, or supervision. A video demonstrating the use of the Katz Index is available for free online at http://links.lww.com/A241.

Studies have demonstrated that the scoring reflects an ordered pattern, meaning that someone who was able to perform a given activity independently at higher levels would be able to perform all activities performed by persons graded at lower levels. This hierarchical structure correctly classifies the

functional ability of patients 86% of the time and reflects a desirable property of scalability (Guttman, 1950). The Katz Index of Independence in ADL has been used as a tool to accumulate information about clients with many types of conditions, including stroke, amputation, hip fracture, dementia, and age-related disability (Christiansen, Rogers, & Haertl, in press). The Katz Index seems to have good inter-rater reliability (Brorsson & Asberg, 1984) and has been used successfully across various cultural groups.

Combined ADL/IADL Measures for Adults

A few global measures are available that combine basic ADL with items that measure IADLs. Scales described in this section include the Functional Independence Measure (now the FIM™), the Kohlman Evaluation of Living Skills, the Performance Assessment of Self-Care Skills, and the Canadian Occupational Performance Measure.

The FIM™

The FIM™ evolved from a Task Force of the American Congress of Rehabilitation Medicine and the American Academy of Physical Medicine and Rehabilitation, which met to develop a reliable and valid instrument that could be used to document the severity of disability as well as the outcomes of rehabilitation treatment as part of a uniform data system (Hamilton, Granger, Sherwin, Zielezny, & Tashman, 1987).

The FIM™ consists of 18 items organized under 6 categories, including self-care (eating, grooming, bathing, upper body dressing, lower body dressing, and toileting); sphincter control (bowel and bladder management); mobility (transfers for toilet, tub, or shower, and bed, chair, wheelchair); locomotion (walking, wheelchair, and stairs); communication, including comprehension and expression; and social cognition (social interaction, problem solving, and memory). Using the FIM™, patients are assessed on each item with a seven-point scale, ranging from 1 = *total assistance required* to 7 = *complete independence* (see Figure 3.2).

The FIM™ has been widely studied with a wide range of conditions and across multiple settings, demonstrating good reliability and strong evidence of predictive and concurrent validity (Ottenbacher, Hsu, Granger & Fiedler, 1996). It has also been studied using different formats of administration, with good results. Ceiling effects using the FIM™ have been reported (Hall et al., 1996). A ceiling effect is created when scores on a scale tend to cluster at the

Motor Items	Cognitive Items	Levels of Scoring
Self-Care	*Communication*	*Independence*
A. Eating	N. Comprehension	7 = Complete independence (timely, safely)
B. Grooming	O. Expression	6 = Modified independence (device)
C. Bathing	*Social Cognition*	*Modified Independence*
D. Dressing upper body	P. Social interaction	5 = Supervision
E. Dressing lower body	Q. Problem solving	4 = Minimal assistance (subject 75%+)
F. Toileting	R. Memory	3 = Moderate assistance (subject 50%+)
Sphincter Control		*Complete Dependence*
G. Bladder management		2 = Maximal assistance (subject 25%+)
H. Bowel management		1 = Total assistance (subject 0%+)
Transfer		
I. Bed, chair, wheelchair		
J. Toilet		
K. Tub, shower		
Locomotion		
L. Walk, wheelchair		
M. Stairs		

Legend: An administration protocol is used for guidance in evaluating a patient's performance in completing the tasks or movements required under each item category. Based on observed performance, the patient is assigned a score of 1–7, and the scores on each item are summed to yield a total score. This score represents the patients' level of independence in the activities of daily living evaluated at the time of scale administration.

Figure 3.2. Components of The FIM.™

high end. This characteristic may limit the scale's usefulness in measuring change within groups. In 1995, the U.S. Centers for Medicare and Medicaid Services (CMS) contracted to use the FIM™ system as the basis for prospective payment in rehabilitation and to use the FIM™ instrument as part of a patient assessment instrument known as the Inpatient Rehabilitation Facility-Patient Admission and Information Report (IRF–PAI). The IRF–PAI is discussed later in this chapter.

Kohlman Evaluation of Living Skills (KELS)

The Kohlman Evaluation of Living Skills (KELS; Thomson, 1992) was designed to evaluate ADLs and IADLs in adult populations. Although originally intended for inpatient psychiatric clients, the evaluation has since been used in long-term settings, and populations have been broadened to geriatrics as well as those with cognitive conditions. The KELS assesses 17 different living skills categorized under (a) self-care, (b) safety and health, (c) money management, (d) transportation and telephone, and (e) work and leisure. Criterion-based scoring results in either "independent" or "needs assistance" within each area. A cumulative score of 5½ or less suggests a person may be capable of living independently. As with any ADL/IADL measure, additional information should be taken into account before making recommendations for level of independence. According to Thomson

(1999), limitations of the evaluation include the fact that some of the items are knowledge based versus performance based, and clients may answer only part of individual questions, thus complicating the scoring. The quality of the client safety photographs for assessment is an additional limitation some practitioners report.

Research has demonstrated the reliability and validity of the KELS (Pickens et al., 2007; Thomson 1992, 1999). It has also been validated for use with elderly populations in Israel (Zimnavoda, Weinblatt, & Katz, 2002). The evaluation has been used in research to assess skills of homeless women (Davis & Kutter, 1998), to identify elders at risk for self-neglect (Naik, Burnett, Pickens-Pace, & Dyer, 2008; Pickens et al., 2007), and to measure the effectiveness of goal attainment scaling for persons with cognitive disorders (Rockwood, Joyce, & Stolee, 1997).

Performance Assessment of Self-Care Skills (PASS)

The Performance Assessment of Self-Care Skills (PASS; version 3.1) is a criterion-referenced instrument designed to evaluate independent living capacity in adults. It has been used with healthy adults as well as those with disabilities (Holm & Rogers, 1999). The PASS has been used for planning intervention as well as for documenting change over time.

The 26 items in the PASS scale address functional mobility, personal care, and home management.

Tasks in three performance areas—independence, safety, and outcome—receive independent scores on a four-point scale that ranges from 0 = *dysfunction* to 3 = *function*. Each task is broken down into subtasks, which allows the evaluator to pinpoint the specific aspects of performance that may be problematic. The scale also documents the amount of assistance needed to complete tasks, thus providing a guide for quantifying the caregiving support necessary for the client.

The PASS is based on four established functional assessment tools for seniors. Its reliability as measured through estimates of internal consistency, test–retest, and inter-rater consistency has been reported at .80 and above (Rogers, Holm, Goldstein, McCue, & Nussbaum, 1994). The PASS has been used with a wide range of clients, including people without health problems and people with many types of diagnoses having functional sequelae, such as traumatic brain injury, multiple sclerosis, spinal cord injury, arthritis, CVA, macular degeneration, and depression (Rogers & Holm, 2000; Rogers et al., 2001, 2003). The scale can discriminate among clients on the basis of their ability to perform complex tasks and by the severity of their conditions, and studies have shown additional evidence of its convergent validity (Rogers et al., 1994; Rogers & Holm, 2000).

Canadian Occupational Performance Measure (COPM)

The Canadian Occupational Performance Measure (COPM) is an outcome measure that was developed in consultation with the Department of National Health and Welfare and the Canadian Association of Occupational Therapy (Law et al., 1994; Law et al., 2005). The COPM uses a client-centered approach in order to detect client perception of occupational performance over time (Baptiste, 2008; Law et al., 2005). The therapist and client collaborate within the administration of the measure to identify goal areas, plan intervention, and provide a baseline for reassessment. The COPM includes roles and role expectations from within the client's living environment using a semistructured, individualized interview approach that takes approximately 15 to 30 minutes to perform (Law et al., 2005). The measure was originally developed based on the Canadian Model of Occupational Performance, which identifies occupations under the categories of self-care (occupations that one performs in the care of self such as personal care, functional mobility, and leisure management); productivity (paid or unpaid work, household management,

school, and play); and leisure (quiet recreation, active recreation, and socialization) (McColl et al., 2003). Based on this model, the COPM focuses primarily on activities related to self-care, productivity, and leisure but may also be used to assess a client's strengths and limitations. The COPM was developed to help therapists establish functional performance goals based on a client's perceptions of need and to provide an objective measure of change in specific problem areas.

The COPM can be used to measure outcomes across a broad range of situations and clients. A caretaker may complete the scale if the client is unable to do so. The COPM considers the client's views of the importance of each activity and client's satisfaction with his or her performance. The instrument takes into account client roles and role expectations and, in focusing on the client's own environments and priorities, ensures that contextual factors are considered in the assessment process. Administration requires a five-step process using a semistructured interview conducted by the therapist together with the client or caregiver. These steps include

- Problem identification/definition,
- Initial assessment,
- Occupational therapy intervention,
- Reassessment, and
- Calculation of change scores.

During administration, problems are identified and defined jointly by the therapist, the client, and appropriate caregivers. After activities of concern are identified, the client is asked to rate the importance of each activity on a scale of 1 to 10. These ratings are for information and not considered in the determination of client change. The client or caregiver must then rate the client's ability to perform the specified activities and his or her satisfaction with performance on the same scale of 1 to 10. These scores are then compared over time. The scale yields two scores, one for performance and the other for satisfaction. Weaknesses of the COPM may include the time required for administration and reported difficulties by some clients in self-ratings (Bodiam, 1999). Strengths include its holistic, client-centered approach and its flexibility, as reported use has gone beyond different types of clients from multiple cultures and age groups to include systems, communities, and external stakeholders (Baptiste, 2008). Overall, the COPM appears to provide useful and important information regarding ADL and IADL performance from the perspective of the recipient of care.

Measuring ADLs/IADLs in Children

In this section, measures of ADLs and IADLs specifically designed for children are described. These include the WeeFIM II© and the Pediatric Evaluation of Development Inventory.

Functional Independence Measure for Children (WeeFIM II©)

In 1987, the FIM™ was adapted to meet the need for a reliable and valid functional assessment tool that would be useful in measuring the severity of disability in children. The resulting Functional Independence Measure for Children (WeeFIM) (Uniform Data System, 1990) was designed to measure functional ability in a developmental context. In 2005, the WeeFIM II System Clinical Guide was developed and added a zero–three module in addition to an Internet-based software program to the existing WeeFIM system (Uniform Data System, 2005). The WeeFIM II is designed for children ages 3 to 7 (or those falling below a developmental age of 7) and includes a minimal data set of 18 items that measure performance in the areas of self-care, mobility, and cognition. The scale uses the same seven-point ordinal scale to assess level of function (graded from dependence to independence) as the parent tool, the FIM. The WeeFIM II 0–3 module is designed for children ages 0 to 3 and measures developmental performance in motor, cognitive, and behavioral performance using a three-level rating system (3 = *usually*; 2 = *sometimes*; 1 = *never*). The 0–3 module is designed to measure early functional performance and serve as a measurement for functional outcomes over time.

In conjunction with the development of the WeeFIM II, clinicians may now subscribe to the WeeFIM II system through the Uniform data System for Medical Rehabilitation. Subscription to the system includes specific modules and the 0–3 assessment tool. In addition, subscribers also receive quarterly benchmark reports, clinical and technical support, software for reporting and submitting online data, and a variety of other services.

Pediatric Evaluation of Development Inventory (PEDI)

The Pediatric Evaluation of Development Inventory (PEDI) is a comprehensive assessment that samples key functional capabilities and performance in children from the ages of 6 months to 7.5 years (Haley, Coster, Ludlow, Haltiwanger, & Andrellos, 1992). The scale was developed for use with children having a variety of disabling conditions for the purposes of measuring functional deficit and developmental delay or monitoring progress. Professionals may administer the PEDI through structured interview or by parental report (Haley et al., 1992). During development of the PEDI, content validity was determined through use of a multidisciplinary panel of experts (Haley et al., 1992). Items were derived from a wide array of functional performance and development scales. Normative data were collected from 412 children and families from the northeastern United States, with a sample stratified to represent national population demographics. A detailed manual with scale development data, administration instructions, and scoring are available, as are published scoring forms and software. The PEDI's six domain scores enable the tester to develop a profile of the client's relative strengths.

The PEDI six domains address both capability and performance in the areas of self-care, mobility, and social function (see Table 3.1). The three functional domains are further divided into subunits that make up each task. Capability is determined by identifying the functional skills for which a child has demonstrated mastery, with scores reflected on the Functional Skills Scales. Two other subscales are provided. One is the Caregiver Assistance Scale, which measures the extent of help provided the child during typical daily situations, and the other is the Modifications Scale, a measure of environmental modifications and equipment used routinely in daily activities. The PEDI has 197 functional skill items and 20 items that measure caregiver assistance and environmental modifications. The PEDI was designed to determine functional capabilities and deficits, to monitor progress, and to evaluate therapeutic outcomes.

Six domain scores are provided that enable a profile of relative strengths and weaknesses in both functional skills and caregiver assistance across the domains tested. No composite summary score is provided, with the rationale that this would obscure meaningful differences in functional performance within specific domains. Scaled scores can be computed to provide an indication of where a child's performance falls relative to the possible maximum. Item difficulty for the PEDI was determined through Rasch analysis, which was also used to estimate goodness of fit between individual subject profiles and the overall hierarchy, intended for each subscale. Because each scale is self-contained, it can be used individually or in combination with other scales. The average time for administration is 45 to 60 minutes.

The PEDI has wide range applicability across diagnostic groups, but further research is needed to explore its reliability and validity in various cultures. Overall, the PEDI can be described as an instrument that is useful for measuring basic and extended functional ADL status and change in children with disabilities from ages 6 months to 7.5 years.

Assessment Tools to Evaluate IADLs

IADLs are complex activities that support life in the home and community; examples include meal preparation, home management, shopping, and community mobility (AOTA, 2008; Bookman, Harrington, Pass, & Reisner, 2007). Wade (1992) has suggested that these types of ADLs be described as *extended activities of daily living (EADLs)*. Other terms in use for similar scale items are *social ADLs* and *advanced ADLs* (Chong, 1995). In this section, several scales that focus specifically on IADL performance are reviewed, including the Assessment of Motor and Process Skills, the Nottingham Extended Activities of Daily Living Scale, and the Frenchay Activities Index.

Assessment of Motor and Process Skills (AMPS)

The Assessment of Motor and Process Skills (AMPS) is a standardized, criterion-referenced observational evaluation system for persons ages 3 or older that simultaneously examines a client's ability to perform IADLs and the underlying motor and process capacities necessary for successful performance (AMPS Project International, 2009; Fisher, 2006). The AMPS requires a trained clinician to observe a person performing IADLs as he or she would normally perform them. The client selects two or three familiar tasks among more than 50 possibilities offered in the manual. After the tasks are performed, the clinician rates the person's performance in two skill areas: IADL motor and IADL process (Table 3.2). These tasks are analogous to classifications under Activities and Participation domains of the *International Classification of Functioning* and the World Health Organization (AMPS Project International, 2009); thus, the instrument is widely used internationally. Following completion and scoring of the performance of the tasks, scores received in each component area are processed by computerized software calibrated to the item difficulty, task challenge, and the therapist's pre-established observation style.

The AMPS defines motor skills as observable actions that are supported by underlying abilities, including postural control, mobility, coordination,

Table 3.1. Performance Items in the Pediatric Evaluation of Disability Inventory

Functional Skills Content (197 Items)

Self-Care	Mobility	Social Function
Fasteners	Ability to negotiate outdoor surfaces	Community function
Hairbrushing	Bed mobility/transfers	Complexity of expressive communication
Handwashing	Car transfers	Comprehension of sentence complexity
Management of bladder	Chair/wheelchair transfers	Comprehension of word meanings
Management of bowel	Distance traveled and speed indoors	Functional use of expressive
Nose care	Distance traveled and speed outdoors	communication
Pants	Going down stairs	Household chores
Pullover/front-opening	Going up stairs	Peer interactions
garments	Method of indoor locomotion	Problem resolution
Shoes/socks	Method of outdoor locomotion	Self-protection
Toileting tasks	Pulls or carries objects	Self-information
Toothbrushing	Toilet transfers	Social interactive play
Types of food textures	Tub transfers	Time orientation
Use of drinking containers	Bed mobility/transfers	Functional comprehension
Use of utensils	Car transfers	Functional expression
Washing body and face	Chair/toilet transfers	Joint problem solving
Bathing	Indoor locomotion	Play with peers
Bladder management	Outdoor locomotion	Safety
Bowel management	Stairs	
Dressing lower body	Tub transfers	
Dressing upper body		
Eating		
Grooming		
Toileting		

Note. Adapted from "Functional Evaluation and Management of Self-Care and Other Activities of Daily Living," by C. H. Christiansen, in *Rehabilitation Medicine: Principles and Practice* (4th ed.), by J. Delisa et al. (Eds.), 2004, Philadelphia: Lippincott Williams & Wilkins. Copyright © 2004 by Lippincott, Williams & Wilkins. Adapted with permission.

Table 3.2. Skills Measured Through Task Performance Using the Assessment of Motor and Process Skills

Motor Skills

Paces	Inquires	Searches/Locates
Attends	Initiates	Gathers
Chooses	Continues	Organizes
Uses	Sequences	Restores
Handles	Terminates	Navigates
Heeds		

Process Skills

Stabilizes	Coordinates	Lifts
Aligns	Manipulates	Calibrates
Positions	Flows	Grips
Walks	Moves	Paces
Reaches	Transports	Endures
Bends		

Process Skills—Adaptation

Notices/Responds	Adjusts
Accommodates	Benefits

and strength. The AMPS motor items represent an observable taxonomy of actions used to move the body and objects during actual performance. In comparison, process skills include actions that demonstrate the organization and execution of a series of actions over time in order to complete a specified task. Thus, process skills may be related to a person's underlying attention, conceptual, organizational, and adaptive capabilities. The AMPS process and motor skill items are designed to represent a universal taxonomy of actions that can be observed during any task performance.

During each task performed for the assessment and for each of the 16 motor and 20 process skills (see Table 3.2), the person is rated on a four-point scale: 1 = *deficit*, 2 = *ineffective*, 3 = *questionable*, and 4 = *competent*. The raw ordinal scores are analyzed using a probability model known as many-faceted Rasch analysis. This approach rests on a mathematical model of likelihood that the person will receive a given score on each of the motor and process skill items. The AMPS motor and process scales represent continua of increasing instrumental ADL motor or process skill ability, and the person's estimated position on the AMPS motor and process scales, expressed in logits, represents his or her instrumental ADL motor and process skill ability (Fisher, 1993). The ability measure produced by the Rasch analysis is the estimated person ability plotted on a linear scale and is defined by the skill item easiness and task simplicity but adjusted for the rater who scored the task performance (Kinnman, Andersson,

Wetterquist, Kinnman, & Andersson, 2000; McNulty & Fisher, 2000; Waehrens & Fisher, 2007).

Because the AMPS adjusts the person ability measures for task simplicity, the therapist can use the measures to predict whether a client will have the motor and process skills necessary to perform tasks that are more difficult than those performed in the assessment. Additionally, since the AMPS includes a wide variety of possible instrumental ADL tasks, and each person is observed performing only two or three, there are many possible alternative task combinations. Regardless of how many different tasks the individual performs, however, the ability measure is always adjusted to account for the ease and simplicity of those particular tasks. Therefore, direct comparisons can be made, even among people who performed completely different tasks.

Nottingham Extended Activities of Daily Living Index (NEADL)

The Nottingham Extended Activities of Daily Living Index (NEADL) was developed by Nouri and Lincoln (1987). This self-report index organizes 22 items into four sections: mobility, kitchen tasks, domestic tasks, and leisure activities. Scoring is along a four-item range of discrete categories, ranging from not done not at all to done alone easily. Unfortunately, there are currently no guidelines for assigning scores. Because of the range of extended ADL tasks reported, the scale has intuitive appeal as an outcome measure of rehabilitation and social participation (Table 3.3). Existing literature suggests that it is a suitable instrument for evaluating extended ADL function in the community.

Frenchay Activities Index (FAI)

The Frenchay Activities Index (FAI) (Holbrook & Skibeck, 1983) was initially developed for use in clinical social work for stroke survivors and has emerged as a frequently used measure of IADLs (Buck, Jacoby, Massey, & Ford, 2000). The Frenchay Activities Index consists of 15 items divided into two sections. Its purpose is to record changes in patterns of activity pre- and post-stroke and to reflect quality of life (Woodson, 2008). The first section records activities performed within the 3 months preceding completion of the scale and includes standard mobility, household maintenance, and meal preparation items. The second section consists of items performed in the 6 months prior to scale completion and reports on work, leisure, travel, and household/car maintenance. Items are scored on a four-point scale from 0 to 3 according to well-defined guidelines. The index is designed as a mailed questionnaire

Table 3.3. Nottingham Extended Activities of Daily Living Index

Questions	Answers			
	Not At All	With Help	Alone With Difficulty	Alone Easily
Mobility—Do you:				
Walk around outside?				
Climb stairs?				
Get in and out of the car?				
Walk over uneven ground?				
Cross roads?				
Travel on public transport?				
Kitchen tasks—Do you:				
Manage to feed yourself?				
Manage to make yourself a hot drink?				
Take hot drinks from one room to another?				
Do the washing up?				
Make yourself a hot snack?				
Domestic tasks—Do you:				
Manage your own money when you are out?				
Wash small items of clothing?				
Do your own shopping?				
Do a full clothes wash?				
Leisure activities—Do you:				
Read newspapers or books?				
Use the telephone?				
Go out socially?				
Manage your own garden?				
Drive a car?				

Note. Based on Nouri, F., & Lincoln, N. (1987). An extended activities of daily living scale for survivors of stroke. *Clinical Rehabilitation, 1,* 301–305.

to be completed by self-report. Although most of the studies using the FAI have been related to outcomes following stroke, other populations have also been studied. In general, these studies support the reliability and validity of the FAI.

Assessment Tools to Evaluate Leisure Activity

The term *leisure* typically denotes a choice in time use for personal satisfaction that may or may not be structured (for example, a hobby or specific craft). Stebbins (1997) characterized two types of leisure: casual and serious leisure, the latter often requiring more structure and at times a specific skill set, such as in a hobby. Stebbins challenged the concept of freedom to choose one's leisure given the fact that there are various sociocultural and leisure constraints that inhibit an individual's choice of leisure (for example, socioeconomic and geographical constraints might limit the choice to participate in the leisure pursuit of surfing). Given inherent barriers to complete choice of leisure pursuits, Stebbin identified leisure as "uncoerced activity undertaken during free time where such activity is something people want to do, and, at a personally satisfying level using their abilities and resources they succeed in doing" (Stebbins, 2005, p. 350). Historically, developments in leisure theory and measurement have occurred largely outside the field of occupational therapy, principally in leisure science, therapeutic recreation, exercise science, and related fields. Measures in this area of occupation have concerned themselves with leisure awareness or knowledge, leisure attitudes and interests, skills, leisure satisfaction, and participation. In this section, three measures of leisure will be described: the Leisure Satisfaction Scale, the Leisure Competence Measure, and the Leisure Diagnostic Battery.

Leisure Satisfaction Scale

The Leisure Satisfaction Scale is a self-report measure developed by Beard and Ragheb in 1980. The scale consists of 51 items scored on a five-point scale and provides information on six aspects of leisure engagement: psychological, educational, social, relaxation, physiological, and aesthetic domains. It takes approximately 30 minutes to complete (Beard & Ragheb, 1980). Studies have validated the content validity of the Leisure Satisfaction Scale, and the reliability estimates range from .82 to .86 (Beard & Ragheb, 1980). Unfortunately, few studies have been done to test the scale's validity. Additional studies have used the scale to measure health, stress, and

quality of life as related to leisure satisfaction. A study by Kanters (1995) failed to support a hypothesis that increased leisure satisfaction would be associated with reduced stress. Lloyd and Auld (2002) found that leisure satisfaction, as measured by the Leisure Satisfaction Scale, was the best predictor of quality of life in the sample of those studied. Pearson (1998) showed that leisure satisfaction and job satisfaction were positive and significant predictors of psychological health in a sample of employed people. More recent studies have used the Leisure Satisfaction Scale in studies of adolescents using online games (Wang, Chen, Lin, & Wang, 2008), the leisure satisfaction of elders (Broughton & Beggs, 2006), the influence of family environment on leisure participation (Garton, Harvey, & Price, 2004), and leisure satisfaction as compared to mental health for people with spinal cord injuries (Raj, Manigandan, & Jacob, 2006). Given the continued use of the Leisure Satisfaction Scale in both practice and research, additional studies on reliability and validity are recommended.

Leisure Competence Measure

The Leisure Competence Measure is a measure of adult leisure functioning developed by Kloseck and Crilly (1997). The scale was originally designed for therapeutic recreation as a measure of adult leisure functioning and as way to document change over time. Kloseck and Crilly selected items based on leisure science theory using information provided by 25 content experts. Items in the scale are organized into nine categories: leisure awareness, leisure attitude, leisure skills, cultural behaviors, social behaviors, interpersonal skills, community integration, social contact, and community participation, with each item rated on a seven-point rating scale. The rater assigns points to each item based on observation, the client's record, an interview, and reports from other people who are aware of the client's behavior.

The Leisure Competence Measure requires about 1 hour for administration and additional time for scoring. No normative data are available, but reliability estimates for internal consistency and stability over time are .89 (Kloseck, Crilly, & Hutchinson-Troyer, 2001). The scale has been reported as sensitive to changes in leisure participation over time (Strain, Grabusic, Searle, & Dunn, 2002), and construct validity studies have shown that it correlates significantly with mental state, life satisfaction, and depression. Additionally, the Leisure Competence Measure has shown sensitivity to measuring change following leisure education (Searle, Mahon, Iso-Ahola, & Sdrolias, 1998). Strengths of the Leisure Competence Measure are that it is easily incorporated into practice and may be used to measure change in leisure practices over time.

Leisure Diagnostic Battery (LDB)

The Leisure Diagnostic Battery (LDB) was originally developed in 1986 as a self-reporting measure to determine an individual's perceptions of personal leisure competence. The LDB (Witt & Ellis, 1989) includes self-report instruments that may be used with adolescents and adults of all ages and abilities. Version A of the battery is for adolescents and includes 95 items related to competence, control, needs depth, and playfulness; 24 items related to perceived barriers to leisure participation; and 28 items related to knowledge of leisure activities. Items are rated on a three-point scale on which subjects are asked to determine the extent to which a statement about leisure is applicable to them. Version B is for use with adults. A 25-item short form of the LDB is also available for both A and B versions of the battery. Administration of the long and short forms requires approximately 40 minutes and 15 minutes, respectively. An administration manual is available, and an automated scoring and report writing system is available on the Internet for use with desktop computers. Several studies have validated the LDB, including a study that confirmed by factor analysis the independence of the battery's separate scales (Dunn, 1987; Ellis & Witt, 1986). The scale has been shown to have internal consistency, with alpha coefficients of .83 to .94 for the long form and .89 to .94 for the short form (Chang & Card, 1994).

The number of studies used to examine the psychometric properties suggests the appropriateness of its use in both clinical and research settings (Witt, 1990). Correlational studies have validated the LDB with other measures of leisure, including knowledge of leisure activities and barriers. Scores on the battery are sensitive to change on the basis of clients' participation in recreation programs. Although many of the studies conducted on this tool occurred in the late 1980s and 1990s, the tool is fairly widely used in recreation/leisure settings and recently was used in a study to examine the efficacy of a family-centered leisure approach (Ryan, Stiell, Gailey, & Makinen, 2008). The study asserted the need for a comprehensive team and family-centered approach in enhancing client participation.

Assessment Tools to Evaluate Play Activity (Children)

Through play and spontaneous engagement in the environment, children develop social, emotional, physical, and cognitive skills essential for development (Haertl, 2010). Play is a major means by which children develop competence and mastery (Rodger & Ziviani, 1999) and an area used in occupational therapy evaluation and intervention. Two commonly used assessments of play are the Preschool Play Scale Revised and the Test of Playfulness.

Preschool Play Scale–Revised (PPS–R)

In 1974, Knox developed the Preschool Play Scale, a structured observational scale that could be used to determine a child's developmental play age and provide a profile of play behaviors of children (Knox, 1974). The original scale measured four dimensions: space management, material management, imitation, and participation. Revised by Bledsoe and Shepherd in 1982, the scale was renamed the Preschool Play Scale, or PPS (Bledsoe & Shepherd, 1982). Study of the revised scale's reliability and validity suggested that it provided consistent and valid information on childhood play (Harrison & Kielhofner, 1986) but recommended that the PPS be revised to include a dimension that measured the degree of a child's engagement in play. Other studies showed that the PPS could not measure differences in play between age groups or in children with conditions affecting their development (Bledsoe & Shepherd, 1982; Morrison, Bundy, & Fisher, 1991).

In 1997, Knox further revised the Preschool Play Scale and renamed it the Preschool Play Scale–Revised (PPS–R) (Knox, 1997). Changes included revisions to the definitions of the dimensions and the renaming of the imitation dimension. The PPS–R now focuses on the child's capacity to play and is suitable for use for children from birth to 6 years of age. The scale is designed to function both as a diagnostic tool and as an outcome measure to determine the effectiveness of intervention. The PPS–R remains an observational assessment of four play dimensions that are now defined as space management, material management, imitation, and participation. While observing the child at play in familiar environments (both outside and indoors), the examiner scores the child's behaviors on items associated with each dimension. Dimension scores are determined by averaging the item scores, and a total score is determined by averaging the scores on individual dimensions. The PPS–R takes about 1 hour to administer.

Early reliability data showed that the pre-revised version of the scale had good inter-rater reliability (Bledsoe & Shepherd, 1982). Because the PPS has evolved based on thorough reviews of the literature, its content validity can be described as good.

Recent research further demonstrated the tool's construct validity and inter-rater reliability (Jankovich, Mullen, Rinear, Tanta, & Deitz, 2008). Additional studies have shown that the PPS correlates significantly with measures of social play development and chronological age, yet should be used with additional data such as parent interviews and would benefit from more research on its psychometric properties (Jankovich et al., 2008; Knox, 1997). The PPS has been used in a number of recent studies (Messier, Ferland, & Majnemer, 2008; Ziviani, Rodger, & Peters, 2005) and continues to have broad utility in both research and clinical settings.

Test of Playfulness (TOP)

The Test of Playfulness (TOP) is an observational instrument developed by Bundy to measure four elements of playfulness in children: intrinsic motivation, internal control, freedom from some constraints of reality, and the ability to give and read cues (Bundy, 1997). The scale was updated in 2000 and again in 2003 (Bundy, 2000, 2003) and may be used with all ages of children, from infancy through adolescence (Bundy, 2000). Administration of the scale involves observing a child during 15 to 20 minutes of free play in an environment familiar to the child. The TOP consists of 24 items, with each item scored on a four-point scale to reflect extent of play, intensity, and skill. Studies have generally demonstrated that the TOP has good psychometric properties, can be reliably administered with 15 minutes of observation, and shows evidence of concurrent validity.

Assessment Tools for Evaluating School and Work Occupational Performance

Tools for measuring school- and work-related occupational performance include the School Function Assessment, the VALPAR Component Work Samples, the Career Ability Placement Survey, and the Employee Aptitude Survey. Note that these tests measure functional performance of cognitive and motor skills necessary for productive engagement in activities necessary for school or work.

School Function Assessment (SFA)

The School Function Assessment (SFA) measures the functional skills necessary for children to perform the required education-based and social tasks for elementary school (Coster, Deeney, Haltiwanger, & Haley, 1998). The purpose of the scale is to facilitate collaborative program planning for children with disabilities. The SFA is made up of three parts: participation, which examines the student's participation level in six major school activity settings; task supports, which assesses the supports provided for the student to perform daily functional tasks; and activity performance, which examines the student's performance on school-related activities (for example, moving through the classroom, using materials, following rules, and interacting with others). Scores are obtained from observations of a child's performance in the school setting using 26 scales, with each scale scored using either a four- or six-level rating. The items are completed as a team or coordinated by a leader who collects scores from those school professionals who have observed the performance of the child in the academic setting and completes the scale. Items for the development of the SFA were selected from a review of the literature that identified those tasks that were related to successful school performance. The items for the scale were developed through an iterative statistical process that involved a broad sample of children with and without disabilities from across the United States and Puerto Rico. Published in 1998 (Coster et al., 1998), the original research on the tool yielded excellent reliability estimates for internal consistency at .92 to .98 and test–retest at a range of .82 to .98. The developers report that the scale has excellent predictive validity and is capable of discriminating between students who are at risk and those who are more likely to succeed in the academic environment. The scales with the lowest reliability are those associated with task support (Coster, 1998).

VALPAR Component Work Samples

The VALPAR consists of 23 simulated work sample performance tests that are designed to assess the ability of an individual to successfully engage in various work-related tasks. Each sample task has been standardized and can be evaluated according to job requirements identified by the U.S. Department of Labor taxonomy. The VALPAR is suitable for use by adolescents and adults. Completion of each work component takes from 10 to 30 minutes. The VALPAR compares client scores to two main types of criterion-referenced standards: the U.S. Department of Labor's work-related factor system as described in the *Revised Handbook for Analyzing Jobs* (U.S. Department of Labor, 1991) and Methods–Time Measurement (MTM) standards. MTM standards may be used in two ways. They may be interpreted directly, and they may be used to help determine whether the client has demonstrated the U.S. Department of Labor factors at the levels needed for success in specific jobs and occupations. VALPAR Component Work Samples 1, 2, 4, 8, 9, and 10 can be modified for use by persons with blindness and visual impairments using a special modification (B–Kit) available from the publisher.

The VALPAR has an examiner's manual with detailed instructions. Stability for the VALPAR is reported as good to excellent for Work Samples 14 through 16, using test–retest correlations. Criterion validity as reported in the manual is good for most samples. As of September 2007, manufacturing of the work samples was transferred to a new company and are undergoing change; the first new wave of samples are available at http://www.basesofva.com/.

Career Ability Placement Survey (CAPS)

The Career Ability Placement Survey (CAPS) is a timed and standardized paper-and-pencil test battery consisting of eight subtests. The battery measures a person's abilities in the conceptual skills required for entry-level performance in the majority of jobs found in 14 occupational clusters listed in the *Dictionary of Occupational Titles* maintained by the U.S. Department of Labor (Knapp, Knapp, & Knapp-Lee, 1992). The subtests measure abilities in mechanical reasoning, spatial relations, verbal reasoning, numerical ability, language usage, word knowledge, perceptual speed and accuracy, and manual speed and dexterity. The CAPS is suitable for clients who are in junior high or older and takes approximately 50 minutes to administer and score. Examiners may score the CAPS subtests manually or by machine. The CAPS is part of the COPSystem (Career Occupational Preference System), a battery of work ability, interest, and value tests that is widely used in Canada. Extensive research on the CAPS has demonstrated strong evidence of reliability and validity. Internal consistency, stability, and inter-rater coefficients have been reported as satisfactory to excellent (Knapp, Knapp, & Michael, 1977).

Employee Aptitude Survey (EAS)

The Employee Aptitude Survey (EAS) is a battery of standardized and timed multiple-choice subtests designed to measure the cognitive, perceptual, and psychomotor abilities that are required for successful job performance in a wide variety of occupations. Each of the EAS tests can be used individually or as part of a battery. The 10 subtests measure verbal comprehension, numerical ability, visual pursuit, visual speed and accuracy, space visualization, numerical reasoning, verbal reasoning, verbal fluency, manual speed and accuracy, and symbolic reasoning (Ruch & Stang, 1994). The EAS is suitable for a client population from ages 12 and older and takes approximately 5 to 10 minutes per subtest to administer.

The EAS has shown satisfactory reliability (Ruch & Stang, 1994). Content-related evidence of validity for the EAS was gathered during the test construction process by representatively sampling defined content domains. Test developers first identified 10 abilities as important for a wide variety of jobs, then selected item types that had been shown to evaluate the ability. Criterion-related evidence of validity for the EAS has been gathered for more than 40 years (Table 3.4). Summaries of the 725 validity coefficients from 160 studies appear in the technical manual for the survey (Grimsley, Ruch, Ruch, Warren, & Ford, 1983). The EAS has been found to be statistically predictive of both training success and job performance. Construct validity evidence for the EAS, provided by factor analyses and correlations with other measures of identified constructs, shows that common, general mental abilities are associated with certain job categories (Table 3.4). Factor analysis has identified eight primary factors across the eight subtests. Percentile norms are available for close to 100 occupational and educational classifications based on more than 200,000 test scores. Computer-based, Web-based and paper-and-pencil versions of the tests are available.

Measures of the Environment

All human activities take place within an environmental context. For assessments conducted outside a rehabilitation center, hospital, or skilled-care facility, it is appropriate and relevant to determine the safety and adequacy of the setting and the extent to which it supports the performance of activities and occupations in the home, community, school, or workplace. Given the broad variety of contexts, any one instrument is limited in its ability to measure the many factors in an environmental situation that can influence engagement in occupations. Cooper, Letts Rigby, Stewart, and Strong (2001) suggested that because occupational engagement represents a transaction between an individual and the environment in which occupation takes place, the best measures are those that incorporate the dynamic nature of that transaction.

In this section scales that measure the attributes of environments to support performance are

Table 3.4. Correlation Coefficients for Studies of the Employment Aptitude Survey and Criterion Variables

Performance Dimensions	Occupational Grouping									
	Professional, Managerial, and Supervisory		Clerical		Light Industry, Production, Mechanical		Technical		All Jobs	
	Job Performance	Training Success	Job Performance	Training Success	Job Performance	Training Success	Job Performance	Training Success	Job Performance	Training Success
Verbal comprehension	.53	.42	.38	—	.35	.63	.17	.45	.35	.53
Numerical ability	.55	.60	.46	—	.38	.69	.53	.76	.41	.66
Visual pursuit	—	.27	—	—	.35	—	—	.41	.37	.39
Visual speed and accuracy	—	.28	.46	—	.32	.31	.31	.40	.39	.37
Space visualization	—	.34	.50	—	.38	.48	.38	.47	.38	.45
Numerical reasoning	.53	.31	.29	—	—	.31	.52	.61	.10	.51
Verbal reasoning	.53	.29	.46	—	.13	—	.33	.48	.33	.47
Word fluency	—	.40	—	—	—	—	—	.22	.47	.41
Manual speed and accuracy	—	.27	.27	—	.29	—	—	.30	.22	.34
Symbolic reasoning	—	.48	—	—	—	—	.57	.53	.44	.59

Note: Dashes are shown where correlations were not computed.

reviewed. These include those suitable for examination of factors in the home, such as the SAFER, HOEA, and HOME tools, as well as those focusing on the work environment, including the Work Environment Scale and the Work Environment Impact Scale. The final scale described in this section is the Environmental Independence Interaction Scale.

Safety Assessment of Function and the Environment for Rehabilitation Tool (SAFER)

The Safety Assessment of Function and the Environment for Rehabilitation Tool (SAFER) was designed to identify risk factors in the living setting that can result in injury and to permit recommendations regarding safety (Letts & Marshall, 1995; Oliver, Blathwayt, Brackley, & Tamaki, 1993). The SAFER tool uses items grouped into 14 domains: living situation, mobility, kitchen, fire hazards, eating, household, dressing, grooming, bathroom, medication, communication, wandering, memory aids, and general. The SAFER was developed by occupational therapists to address the need for an "acceptable, standardized instrument focusing on safety and function within the home environment" (Letts & Marshall, 1995, p. 53; Oliver et al., 1993). The original SAFER tool predated the development of the SAFER HOME and included

evaluations based on an environmental checklist that rated Addressed, Not Applicable, and Problem. The new SAFER HOME version expanded the checklist to increase sensitivity to change over time and now includes No Identified Concern, Mild Problem, Moderate Problem, and Severe Problem (Chiu, Oliver, Faibish, & Cawley, 2002). The SAFER HOME is designed as an outcome measure to facilitate plans for intervention and is based on the original SAFER instrument (Chiu & Tickle-Degnan, 2002). An interesting attribute of the SAFER tool is the choice of items that reflect a transactional relationship between the individual and the environment. The items were selected systematically by a panel of clinicians and seniors, and some items were discarded after analysis of content and construct validity. The item selection process also provided a basis for developing guidelines to assist clinicians in using the tool. These guidelines have been organized in the form of questions to consider when completing an environmental assessment.

The SAFER tool is a descriptive environmental assessment that demonstrates acceptable reliability and validity in measuring a person's ability to function safely within a home environment. The newest version (SAFER HOME–3) consists of 75 questions divided into 12 categories (Chiu et al., 2006). A study found that the original SAFER tool demonstrated that environments with greater safety risk correlated with cognitive impairment, suggesting that a relationship exists between level of independence and safety (Letts, Scott, Burtney, Marshall, & McKean, 1998). A study of the most recent version of the SAFER HOME instrument established initial positive results on the reliability and validity of the revised version but asserted the need for continued studies in the tool's long-term development (Chiu & Oliver, 2006).

Home Occupation Environment Assessment (HOEA)

The Home Occupation Environment Assessment (HOEA) (Baum, Edwards, Bradford, & Lane, 1995) is an assessment developed specifically for clients with dementia. The assessment addresses behavioral and environmental items that suggest the client's ability to live safely in a given environment. Items on the scale were initially developed based on expert opinion and then factor-analyzed to determine those item clusters that correlate with high risk. A checklist allows the therapist to indicate whether or not a given item was assessed and to provide a score on a four-point scale (*no problem observed, requires monitoring, requires attention,* or *high-risk situation*).

Behavioral items include impaired judgment, disheveled appearance, possible abuse/neglect, depressed mood, difficulties with finance, difficulties with managing medications, awareness of surroundings, understands questions, slurred speech, slow response, difficult to understand, hearing problem, smell, and vision. Environmental items include the following categories: accessibility within the home, sanitation, food storage, and general safety issues. Because the HOEA is a new scale, it has not yet been validated or studied extensively, and research continues. Further study is needed with this instrument aimed at persons with cognitive deficits.

Home Observation for Measurement of the Environment (HOME Revised)

The Home Observation for Measurement of the Environment (HOME) is a standardized screening instrument designed to identify attributes of the home environment that contribute to cognitive, social, and emotional development for children (Caldwell & Bradley, 1984). The focus is on the child as a recipient of environmental inputs, including objects, events, and transactions occurring in connection with the family and caregivers in the surroundings (Bradley, 1993). The tool is intended for clinicians and researchers and is administered through semistructured interview and observation. Four versions of the HOME inventory include the Infant/Toddler, Early Childhood, Middle Childhood, and Early Adolescent. The original Infant/Toddler version was developed by Caldwell and colleagues in the 1960s to examine relationships between a child's home environment, day care, and effects on developments (Elardo, Bradley, & Caldwell, 1975). Subsequent versions were developed using exploratory factor analysis resulting in the widely used HOME tools (Caldwell & Bradley, 1984).

The full version of the HOME takes approximately an hour to administer for each age group and includes a combination of interview and observation. Each version of the inventory includes subscales of measurement (for example, parental responsivity, organization of the environment, learning materials, and emotional environment). Although the current items within the HOME scales are identical to the original, they have been re-ordered in the latest Administration and Scoring Manual published in 2001 (Caldwell & Bradley, 2001). Practitioners may also elect to use the short form (HOME–SF), which replicates content in all four versions, yet is condensed for efficiency of time. Similar to the HOME, the short version of the measure includes interview and observation and may be used for individual assessment or within research as independent variables to measure childhood developmental outcomes, or may be used as measures themselves to understand relationships among environment, familial characteristics, and childhood development (Mainieri, 2006).

Work Environment Scale (WES)

The Work Environment Scale (WES) was designed to evaluate productivity, assess employee satisfaction, and clarify employee work expectations to ensure a healthy work environment (Moos, 1993, 1994). The WES consists of 90 items organized in 10 subscales with 9 items in each. A 40-item short form is also available. The scale allows workers to report perceptions of both their real and ideal work settings and uses a two-point true–false question format (Kotzner, 2008). The subscales include assessment of the following work environment factors: involvement, coworker cohesion, supervisory support, autonomy, task orientation, work pressure, clarity, managerial control, innovation, and physical comfort. The WES is designed for completion by adult workers but may be performed by service providers as well. The assessment may be completed through a structured interview or in a naturalistic context by observing the work setting. The scale takes approximately 30 minutes to complete. Scoring is complex, so examiner training is recommended. The WES may be administered to individuals or groups. The manual provides normative data and information on clinical, consulting, and program evaluation uses. It also has updated and expanded research information. Normative data for the WES have been collected from more than 8,000 workers in a variety of work settings (Moos, 1981). The user's guide assists with the interpretation of results and provides scale assessment information. The WES comes in a self-score format with an interpretive report form that can be used to explain the results.

Reliability of the WES is considered to be excellent (Abraham & Foley, 1984; Moos, 1981). Studies have demonstrated that the WES has good content, construct, and criterion-related validity (Moos, 1994; Moos & Moos, 1998). Although often used internally as an evaluation of employee satisfaction and perceived work environment, the tool was recently used to research nursing staff perceptions of their real and ideal work environmenta (Kotzer, 2008; Kotzer, Koepping, & LeDuc, 2006) and burnout in teachers (Goddard, O'Brien, & Goddard, 2006). The scale appears to have properties useful for assessment of the perceptions of the work environment and utility in research studies.

Environment Independence Interaction Scale (EIIS)

The Environmental Independence Interaction Scale (EIIS) was developed to measure contextual factors that are significantly related to independent performance among people receiving rehabilitation services (Teel, Dunn, Jackson, & Duncan, 1997). The EIIS identifies four domains as contextual factors: physical factors (including nonhuman aspects, such as objects and devices that enhance or inhibit performance); social factors (including the availability and actions of significant people in the client's environment); cultural factors (including customs, beliefs, and expectations); and temporal factors (including timing of interventions and time available for practicing skills).

The content of the EIIS was developed in concert with the construction of a conceptual model known as the Ecology of Human Performance (EHP). The EIIS and EHP were based on an extensive review of the literature that identified environmental factors related to success (Dunn, Brown, & Mc-Cuigan, 1994). Different groups of caregivers were

used to test the original version of the scale, including family members of people receiving rehabilitation at home, clients receiving care in facilities, and professionals providing care in facilities.

The EIIS consists of 20 items; 5 items rate factors in each of the physical and social environment areas, 6 items rate the cultural environment, and 4 items assess temporal factors. Using a five-point rating scale with values representing ranges between *not at all* to *a great deal*, informants express their opinions regarding attitudes, care practices, and features of the home- or facility-based rehabilitation program in which the client is receiving care. Reliability of the tool has been reported as good to excellent (Teel et al., 1997).

Studies of the scale's validity have been limited. Content validity can be judged as excellent based on the manner in which items were chosen. Evidence of construct and criterion validity is being gathered. The score provided by the EIIS is intended to show the extent to which a rehabilitation environment supports or interferes with a client's independence (Teel et al., 1997).

Assessment Tools to Evaluate Social Participation

The final area appropriate for use in developing an occupational profile is social participation. The evidence for the importance of the social environment for health is indisputable. Aspects of the social environment include social networks, social structures, social cohesion, social support, and community integration or reintegration. Many of these aspects of the social environment are multidimensional constructs, with components ranging from the more quantitative (number of social encounters per day) to the more qualitative (feeling cared for, loved, and valued). Social participation is a dimension of participation with the framework of the World Health Organization's (WHO's) *International Classification of Functioning, Disability and Health* (ICF; WHO, 2001). The scales included in this section were chosen because they appreciate and record the personal nature of social participation and recognize the contribution of social participation to health. Additionally, scales have been selected for their widespread use and utility in clinical practice or research. The scales include the Activity Card Sort, the Assessment of Communication and Interaction Skills, the Craig Handicap Assessment and Reporting Technique, the Children's Assessment of Participation and Enjoyment/the Preferences for Activities of Children, the Interview Schedule for Social Interaction, the Reintegration to

Normal Living Scale, the Community Integration Questionnaire, and the Short Form–36 Health Measure. Other scales exist in the literature that may be suitable for assessment in this domain. The scales presented here are intended to be representative of the larger domain of available instruments.

Activity Card Sort (ACS)

The Activity Card Sort (ACS), a broad assessment of life activity developed by Baum and Edwards (2001), was recently revised (Baum & Edwards, 2008). It was designed to determine an individual's level of participation in instrumental, leisure, and social activities. The ACS captures differences in activity patterns that have clinical usefulness and gives the practitioner an immediate impression of the person's activities to use in treatment planning. The scale uses a Q-Sort methodology that can be used with clients or others familiar with an individual's life activities (Figure 3.3). Although it was originally designed for the assessment of individuals with cognitive deficits, it can be used with adult populations with or without conditions that limit function (Katz, Karpin, Lak, Furman, & Hartman-Maeir, 2003). It includes 20 instrumental activities, 35 low-physical-demand leisure activities, 17 high-physical-demand leisure activities, and 17 social activities and allows for the calculation of the percentage of activity retained.

The Q-Sort methodology uses cards that are sorted into categories by the client or proxy (person completing the assessment on behalf of the client). The ACS uses 89 photographs of individuals performing activities. There are three versions of the instrument (Institutional, Recovering, and Community Living); the versions differ with respect to the categories used for sorting the cards. An institutional version and a recovering version have been developed. For example, the institutional version uses the activity cards sorted into two groups (done prior to illness and not done). This approach allows the therapist to identify premorbid activity data that are useful for planning intervention. The cards with photographs of activities that are sorted into five categories for the healthy older adult version (never done, not done, do now, do less, given up); two groups for the institutional version (done prior to illness, not done), and four in the recovering version (not done in the past 5 years, gave up due to illness, beginning to do again, do now). These categories can be modified according to the questions of interest to the evaluator.

Administration takes approximately 20 minutes. If the provider wishes to interview the client about details associated with sorting results, this

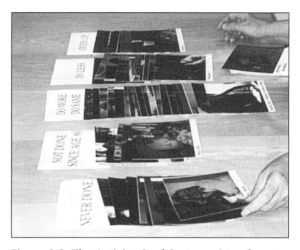

Figure 3.3. The Activity Card Sort consists of a set of labeled cards with photographs of common household and leisure tasks. The client, using a Q-Sort method, places the cards into defined categories depicting current functional status. Photo credit: M. C. Baum.

lengthens the time of administration. Because the ACS is a method for gathering data rather than a scale, it is flexible and can be adjusted to client groups and cultures with the addition of cards depicting photographs of activities.

Assessment of Communication and Interaction Skills (ACIS)

The Assessment of Communication and Interaction Skills (ACIS) is a structured observational rating scale designed to measure a client's social interaction abilities (Forsyth, Lai, & Kielhofner, 1999; Simon, 1989). Based on the conceptual framework of the model of human occupation, the ACIS is intended to capture characteristics of social interaction during participation in ordinary everyday activities. The ACIS is structured around the assumption that communication and interaction during activity have two important outcomes: goal accomplishment and social impact (effect on others). The current version (version 4.0) of the scale reflects several revisions from the original designed to use behavioral criteria precisely to identify the demonstration of skills used in social interaction.

The ACIS consists of 20 verbs that describe performance, with items grouped into the following three domains: physicality, information exchange, and relations. The professional provider rates each skill item after observing the client in a social situation using a four-point rating scale. The scoring of individual items permits the identification of strengths and weaknesses useful for social skills intervention. Items are scored after observation in four types of situations, including an unstructured situation, a parallel task group, a cooperative group situation, and dyadic or one-to-one situations. Skills related to each domain are rated on a four-point scale as *competent, questionable, ineffective,* or *deficient.*

Studies with earlier versions of the ACIS resulted in refinement of the skill item definitions. One study used Rasch analysis and found evidence of construct validity but shortcomings in the scale's ability to distinguish among clients with known social deficits (Salamy, 1993). A more recent study using 52 trained raters established the construct validity of the scale through comparison of the calibrated and ranked statistics using Rasch analysis (Forsyth et al., 1999). In this study, the scale was able to discriminate between clients with different diagnostic profiles and demonstrated unidimensionality as well as satisfactory inter-rater reliability. The ACIS has not yet been well researched and therefore must be viewed as an emerging but promising measure of skill in social participation. In another study, a Swedish version of the ACIS investigated whether ratings according to the ACIS–S are related to the settings in which the skills are assessed and whether the clients' comprehension of the setting is related to the ACIS–S rating scores (Haglund & Thorell, 2004). Additionally, a Chinese version of the ACIS (ACIS–C) demonstrated validity and sensitivity with Chinese clients and suggested that an understanding of communication and interaction as conceptualized in the model of human occupation is generalizable to an Eastern population (Hsu, Pan, & Chen, 2008).

Children's Assessment of Participation and Enjoyment (CAPE) and Preferences for Activities of Children (PAC)

The Children's Assessment of Participation and Enjoyment (CAPE) and the Preferences for Activities of Children (PAC) are two companion measures of children's participation. Both are self-report measures of children's participation in recreation and leisure activities outside of mandated school activities. The CAPE is designed to document how children with or without disabilities participate in everyday activities outside of their mandated school activities and measures the children's diversity and intensity of participation in activities in their usual context and their enjoyment of these activities. The PAC determines activity preferences and addresses the child's preferences for those activities. Given together these assessments can investigate a child's participation in several dimensions of activity: diversity of activities, intensity of participation, social engagement/with whom, location, and enjoyment.

The CAPE and PAC are designed to be used with children 6 to 21 years of age and can be either interviewer administered using the Activity Cards and Visual Response pages or completed independently by the child as a questionnaire. Both the CAPE and PAC can be administered using the same record form. There are 55 items on the questionnaire for the CAPE/PAC. The CAPE takes 30 to 45 minutes to complete and the PAC takes 15 to 20 minutes to complete. Reliability is very good for both internal consistency and test–retest, as well as inter-rater. Validity is excellent for providing information about activity patterns and preferences. Scores on these instrumens should be interpreted jointly to accurately reflect the child's participation/enjoyment patterns (Imms, 2008; King et al., 2004).

Community Integration Measure

The Community Integration measure (CIM) is a brief client–centered measure of community integration. This instrument has been designed to assess community integration from the client's perspective of belonging and participating. Designed to be used with adults with disabilities who are community dwelling, it may be administered in person or via the telephone. It consists of a 10-item checklist that has been written at a basic comprehension level and can be completed within 5 minutes. The developers used an empirically derived definition and model of community integration. The four categories that contribute to community integration include: general assimilation (conformity, orientation, acceptance), social support (close and diffuse relationships), occupation (leisure, productivity) and independent living (personal independence, satisfaction with living arrangement) (McColl, Davies, Carlson, Johnston, & Minnes, 2001).

Unlike some other measures of community integration, the focus of the CIM is subjective experiences rather than objective or observable aspects of integration. For example, the measure does not assume that independent participation in a community activity is any better than being supported by a career, family member, or partner.

It has been tested primarily on adults with brain injury; however, it can be used with community-dwelling adults with disabilities. Test items should be read to clients with cognitive difficulties. For each of the 10 items on the checklist, there are 5 response options (5 = *always agree*, 1 = *always disagree*). Item scores are summed, giving a total score of 10–50, with higher scores indicating greater community integration. The CIM possesses good internal reliability; Cronbach's alpha = .87, or .72–.83 reported by others (Reistetter, Spencer, Trujillo, & Abreu, 2005) and has low criterion validity through its correlation with the Community Integration Questionnaire (Reistetter et al., 2005). Although the CIM was not intended to be a multidimensional scale, testing suggests that the operationalizing of community integration as independent living, occupation, and social support is valid (Reistetter et al., 2005).

Community Integration Questionnaire (CIQ)

The Community Integration Questionnaire (CIQ) was developed to measure social disadvantage as an aspect of outcome following rehabilitation after brain injury (Willer, Rosenthal, Kreutzer, Gordon, & Rempel, 1993). Although the scale was developed for a specific population (those sustaining brain injuries), it has been used more broadly. The CIQ consists of 15 items that are contained in three subscales pertaining to home integration, social integration, and engagement in productive activities. Scale items assess behavioral indications of integration rather than self-perceived emotional status or feelings and are presented in a multiple-choice format. Response options are graded to reflect either the frequency of the activity in question or in what manner the individual performs the activity (alone, with someone else, or dependent on someone else). Item scores are summed to provide subscale scores, which can then be tallied to provide a total CIQ score out of a possible 29 points. Higher scores represent greater levels of community integration. The CIQ can be administered as a telephone interview or directly with clients. Administration time is approximately 10 minutes.

The CIQ has become one of the most broadly used and evaluated tools with a population of those with brain injury. An extensive review of all aspects of the CIQ was completed by Salter and colleagues and represents the accumulation of information regarding the CIQ in brain injury (Salter, Foley, Jutai, Bayley, & Teasell, 2008). In general, the reliability for the CIQ is satisfactory, with total score internal consistency estimated at .76.

Craig Handicap Assessment and Reporting Technique (CHART)

The Craig Handicap Assessment and Reporting Technique (CHART) is designed as an objective measure of the degree to which impairments and disabilities limit social and community integration (Whiteneck, Charlifue, Gerhart, Overholser, & Richardson, 1992). The CHART is based on the *International Classification of Impairments, Disabilities and Handicaps* (WHO, 1997) the precursor to the *ICF*, and was developed to provide a simple, objective measure of the degree to which impairments and disabilities result in handicaps after initial rehabilitation. It was initially designed for clients with spinal cord injuries, it has also been used with clients who have traumatic brain injury, cerebrovascular accident, multiple sclerosis, burns, and amputations. Still, it remains the most widely used quantitative measure for individuals with spinal cord injury in determining community participation (Magasi, Heinemann, & Whiteneck, 2008). A 32-item questionnaire addresses specific areas of function in six domains: Physical Independence, Mobility, Occupation, Social Integration, Economic Self-Sufficiency, and Orientation. Points are assigned to responses, with a maximum of 100 points for each domain. It is given in an interview format that can be used as a self-report or by a caregiver as a proxy. CHART Short Form (CHART–SF) is also available to serve as a screening tool with 19 items. A maximum score of 100 is considered typical performance in each domain by a person without disabilities.

Normative data have been established on 1,998 cases in the National Spinal Cord Injury Statistical Center database that provides the basis for norms by neurologic category (Hall, Dijkers, Whiteneck, Brooks, & Krause, 1998). High domain scores indicate greater social and community participation, and low domain scores indicate less social and community participation. Test–retest reliability was demonstrated by subscale coefficients ranging from $r = 0.80$ to 0.95 and total score at $r = 0.93$. Rasch analysis supported construct validity of CHART as a valid measure of social and community participation (Hall et al., 1998). The comparison of total CHART score to FIM score for clients who had a stroke was 0.70 when the domain of Economic Self-Sufficiency was removed (Segal & Schall, 1995). Studies affirmed that the CHART is a valid measure of social and community participation (Magasi et al., 2008).

Interview Schedule for Social Interaction (ISSI)

The Interview Schedule for Social Interaction (ISSI) is a well-validated structured interview that contains 52 items providing scores in the following four subscales: availability of attachments or close relationships, adequacy of attachments, availability of social interaction or more distant relationships, and adequacy of social interaction (Henderson, Duncan-Jones, Byrne, & Scott, 1980). The interview schedule has 52 items, with varying response formats available. On average, the interview requires about 45 minutes to administer (Henderson, 1980). It is a widely used scale, accepted by clinicians and patients as well as researchers to identify and assess the availability and adequacy of social relationships. Its use has been documented with individuals with cancer, those with multiple mental health issues, and the general population with no stated impairments as a measure of social support (Bengtsson-Tops et al., 2005; Hansson & Bjorkman 2007; Hansson, Rundberg, Zetterlind, Johnsson, & Berglund, 2007).

Overall, the scale has been well accepted by professionals and seems suitable for use in measuring behaviors related to social interaction and thus a client's tendencies and resources that would affect social participation. The ISSI demonstrated both construct and discriminant validity differentiating among three populations of individuals with mental illness; it also demonstrated similar results in varying samples of individuals with mental health, despite varying prerequisites for social interaction, strongly supporting the validity of the ISSI (Eklund, Bengtsson-Tops, & Lindstedt, 2007).

Reintegration to Normal Living Index (RNL)

The Reintegration to Normal Living Index (RNL) was developed with input from health care consumers, family members, and professionals concerning the factors that explain community reintegration following functional disruption related to injury or illness (Wood-Dauphinee, Opzoomer, Williams, Marchand, & Spitzer, 1988). The RNL is made up of 11 declarative statements. A visual analogue scale accompanies each statement (VAS 0–10). The scale is anchored by the statements "does not describe my situation" and "fully describes my situation" (Finch, Brooks, Stratford, & Mayo, 2002).

The total score is obtained by summing the individual scores for each statement, with 0 designating *no reintegration* to 10 that equates to *complete integration*, for each statement. This index has a possible range of 11 to 110 (Tooth, McKenna, Smith, & O'Rourke, 2003). Higher scores denote better reintegration. For ease of interpretation, the total score is then proportionally converted to a score out of 100 (Wood-Dauphinee et al., 1988). The scale is typically used with rehabilitation clients having sudden-onset disability (Wood-Dauphinee & Willliams, 1987).

The RNL requires approximately 10 minutes to complete and can be administered through interview or completed by the client. Reliability for the measure is excellent, with internal consistency estimates (using Cronbach's alpha) of .90–.95 (Wood-Dauphinee & Willliams, 1987). Factor analysis supports a one-factor solution that explains 49% of the variation in client scores. Content validity of the RNL is good, based on the iterative three-stage process employed in its development. The scale has also evidenced criterion and construct validity, with scores on the RNL correlating significantly with work and disease status but not living situation. The RNL also correlates with measures of quality of life and affect. The RNL is available from Finch and colleagues (Finch et al., 2002).

Short Form–36 Health Measure

The SF–36 is a multipurpose, short-form health survey with 36 questions (Ware & Sherbourne, 1992). It yields an eight-scale profile of functional health and well-being scores as well as psychometrically based physical and mental health summary measures and a preference-based health utility index. It is a generic measure, as opposed to one that targets a specific age, disease, or treatment group. Accordingly, the SF–36 has proven useful in surveys of general and specific populations, comparing the relative burden of diseases, and in differentiating the health benefits produced by a wide range of different treatments. Initially it was developed for the RAND Corporation's Health Insurance Experiment as a general health measure. It was refined and later used in the Medical Outcomes Study, intended for a variety of health conditions (Ware & Sherbourne, 1992). It is a practical, reliable, and valid measure of physical and mental health that can be completed in 5 to 10 minutes.

Although many studies appear to be relying on the SF–36 as the principal measure of health outcome, among the most useful studies are those that use it as a core of assessments to evaluate a particular population (Jenkinson, Wright, & Coulter, 1994). As a generic measure, the SF–36 makes it possible to compare results across studies and populations and accelerates the accumulation of interpretation guidelines that are essential to determining the clinical, economic, and social relevance of differences in health status and outcomes. Because it is short, the SF–36 can be reproduced in a questionnaire with ample room for other more precise general and specific measures (McDowell, 2006).

This instrument incorporates questions regarding physical and mental health as well as functional limitations resulting from ill health. Respondents select ratings on various topics, such as activities they might do on a typical day or whether they experienced limitations due to physical or emotional health problems. Eight-scale scores are reported, as are summary scores for physical health and mental health. The eight-scale scores relate to physical functioning, role limitations resulting from physical health problems, bodily pain, social functioning, general mental health, role limitations due to emotional problems, vitality, and general health perceptions. Scoring the instrument requires detailed guidance to calculate raw scores and *t* scores.

The SF–36 is a psychometrically sound instrument demonstrating internal consistency (alpha coefficients of all scales exceeded 0.80, except for the Social Functioning scale [0.76]), test–retest reliability (mean alpha was 0.84). Extensive validity testing on criterion validity, predictive validity, discriminant validity, and convergent validity gives the clinician confidence in using this tool to compare populations and predict health status in the short term. Clinically, it is a useful tool as it has demonstrated sensitivity to change in health status and has considerable information about norms and benchmarks useful in comparing well and sick populations and for estimating the burden of specific condition. Normative information by age group and gender is included for all subscales, allowing easy comparison of client scores to national norms. Although the questionnaire alone is available through Quality Metrics for no cost (http://www.qualitymetric.com/default.aspx), this measure can be scored electronically, and other scoring forms are also available.

Reimbursement-Related Assessment Tools to Measure Functional Status and Outcomes in Postacute Care

Various assessment tools have been developed in the United States to measure functional status and outcomes in care facilities receiving payment under federal programs for elderly and disadvantaged persons. In this section, current tools of this nature are described briefly because occupational therapy personnel working in rehabilitation encounter them in intermediate care, skilled-nursing, and long-term-care facilities. These include the Care Tool, the AMPAC, the OASIS, and the IRF–PAI. These instruments are developed under the auspices of the Centers for Medicare and Medicaid Services (CMS). Brief individual descriptions of the instruments are provided below. Readers should be alert to ongoing changes in government policy that may change the characteristics or use of these instruments.

CMS Continuity Assessment Record Evaluation Tool (CARE)

The CMS initiated an effort in 2006 to develop an assessment instrument for postacute care intended for use in skilled-nursing, long-term-care, inpatient rehabilitation facilities, and home health agencies. Using the acronym CARE, for *Continuity Assessment Record Evaluation*, the instrument is being developed to measure the health and functional status of patients at discharge and to measure changes in severity and other outcomes for patients covered under Medicare. The purpose of the CARE tool is to improve the quality and safety of patient transitions from one facility or setting to another.

The CARE tool has been designed to use the latest digital and Internet technologies to measure intervention outcomes while controlling for factors that can affect such outcomes, such as cognitive impairments and social and environmental factors. The Web-based technology will allow for future changes in data sets to incorporate advances in evidence-based medicine. The system is also designed to reduce the burden on caregivers by enabling item subsets to be used when appropriate for measuring each domain, based on the patient's characteristics.

The tool is designed with four primary domains: medical, functional, cognitive impairments, and social/environmental factors. These domains either measure case mix severity differences within medical conditions or predict outcomes such as discharge to home or community, rehospitalization, and changes in functional or medical status. The development of the CARE tool builds on existing research and extensive provider feedback. It is comprehensive; includes both ADL and IADL performance information; includes environmental, temporal, cognitive, and medical information; and requires and reports information gained through patient interaction, including orientation and mood. As this chapter is being written, the CARE tool remains under development, being tested and refined in facilities throughout the United States. The final version will be implemented by 2011. Readers are encouraged to consult the CMS Web site for the most up-to-date information on development of this instrument at http://www.cfmc.org/caretransitions/care.htm.

Activity Measure for Postacute Care (AMPAC)

The AMPAC was developed at Boston University. A comprehensive list of functional items was developed from the *ICF* and reviewed by clinical experts. The resulting items were then used to measure the function of patients with varying diagnoses in different settings. The test is now computerized and uses a process known as computer-adaptive testing to select the most appropriate items for each patient. This increases the precision of the measure while reducing the need for caregivers to respond to unnecessary items (Haley et al., 2004). Both paper and computerized versions are available.

The AMPAC has basic mobility, daily activity, and applied cognitive domains. Using computer-adaptive testing, a subsample of items is chosen for each individual based on the patient's level of function and diagnosis. Research has shown that this approach enables a patient's functional status to be measured accurately with fewer items, resulting in less time required of professional staff to document functional status (Coster, Haley, & Jette, 2006).

Outcomes and Assessment Information Set (OASIS)

The OASIS is a key Medicare assessment instrument developed for use by the home care industry to encourage and monitor outcomes. The CMS have proposed the use of OASIS as a necessary and integral part of qualification by home health agencies for federal reimbursement under Medicare. Most data items in the OASIS were developed over a decade-long national research program. The core data items were refined through several iterations of clinical and empirical research. Other items were added later by a workgroup of home care experts to augment the outcome data set with selected items viewed as essential for patient assessment.

OASIS data items encompass sociodemographic, environmental, support system, health status, and functional status attributes of adult patients. CMS provides an online training course to learn how to administer and complete OASIS according to current reimbursement policies at http://www.oasistraining.org/upfront/u1.asp. Additional information on OASIS can be found at http://www.cms.hhs.gov/oasis/.

Inpatient Rehab Facility Patient Assessment Instrument (IRF–PAI)

The IRF–PAI has served as the assessment instrument required of inpatient rehabilitation facilities in the United States since the CMS inaugurated prospective payment reimbursement for those types of facilities in 2002. IRF–PAI will most likely continue to be used by inpatient rehabilitation facilities until the CARE tool, currently under development, is implemented as planned in 2011.

The IRF–PAI is a patient status and outcome instrument that includes information on the patient's identity, demographic, and condition at admission, and at points postadmission. In addition to identity-related information, the IRF–PAI includes sections

on preadmission living setting characteristics; insurance payer information; diagnosis or impairment-related information, including comorbidities; and functional information, which consists of functional modifiers and FIM items. Functional modifiers include information on mobility independence, including transfers, and bowel and bladder control. The focus is on providing a description of the amount of assistance required by the patient in performing basic ADLs. A final section pertains to medical and safety needs and includes the patient's level of alertness, pain, ability to swallow, dehydration, respiratory status, the presence of pressure ulcers, balance, and risk for falls.

Data are entered on admission, at defined points during the stay, and at discharge. Discharge information also includes characteristics of the discharge facility. These data are gathered to determine outcomes of the admission as well as the factors that might influence changes in patient status during the inpatient rehabilitation stay, including the intensity of care of services required.

Conclusion

In this chapter, the process of developing a client's occupational profile using observations and instruments from several domains was described. Examples of useful instruments from the areas of ADLs, IADLs, leisure, play, school, and work were presented. Additional instruments for measuring the performance environment and social participation were reviewed. Table 3.5 presents a summary of the characteristics of these assessment instruments, Table 3.6 presents additional information on validity studies.

Effective assessment of occupational performance is essential to planning and modifying intervention strategies and making informed choices about safe and satisfying performance options for clients. The choice of an instrument for assessing a client will depend on the characteristics of the setting, the characteristics of the client, and the purpose of the assessment. No one "gold standard" for occupational assessment is ideally suited for each of the purposes outlined at the beginning of this chapter. Ultimately, the choice of assessments must be geared toward the development of a useful occupational profile.

There is a great need for more studies of how existing scales perform in varied settings and with different populations. Are they sensitive to change? Do they predict future occupational performance at home or in the natural living environment? Can ex-

Table 3.5. Characteristics of Instruments Reviewed

Instrument	Area(s) Measured	Reliability	Validity	Measurement Method(s)
Activity Card Sort (ACS)	IADLs/leisure/social	Internal consistency = .61–.82	Evidence of content and criterion validity	Q-sort
Assessment of Communication and Interaction Skills (ACIS)	Social interaction skills (physicality, information exchange, and relations)	$r = .96$	Evidence of content, criterion, and construct validity (few studies)	Observation of performance
Assessment of Motor and Process Skills (AMPS)	IADLs/education tasks	95% inter-rater reliability using Rasch analysis	Validity testing ongoing; concurrent validity established	Observation of performance
Barthel Index (BI)	Basic ADLs (extended version measures additional functional items)	Stability = .89 Inter-rater = .95	Criterion = .89 Detects change in parallel with Katz	Interview Observation Chart review
Canadian Occupational Performance Measure (COPM)	ADLs/IADLs/leisure	Stability = .63–.84 ICC = .90 and above	Evidence of content and criterion validity	Interview
Career Ability Placement Survey (CAPS)	Work-related conceptual skills and perceptual/ manual speed and dexterity	Split-half = .70–.95	Evidence of content, concurrent, criterion, and construct validity	Written performance test
Community Integration Questionnaire (CIQ)	Social participation (engagement in productive activities in the home and community)	Internal consistency = .76 Test–retest = .90	Evidence of content, concurrent, and criterion validity	Interview
Employee Aptitude Survey (EAS)	Work-related cognitive, perceptual, and psychomotor abilities	Alternate forms = .76–.91 Test–retest = .75	Evidence of content, concurrent, criterion, and construct validity	Written performance test
Environmental Independence Interaction Scale (EIIS)	Living context (physical, social, and temporal factors that influence independence)	Internal consistency = .92–.96; individual areas have alpha coefficients of .68–.90	Evidence of content validity, but other validity studies are under way	Report based on observation
Frenchay Activities Index (FAI)	IADLs/work/ leisure/social	Kappa = .60 Inter-rater = .93	Evidence of concurrent, construct, and criterion validity	Report/interview (mailed version)
Functional Independence Measure (The FIM™)	ADLs/IADLs	Inter-rater = .95 Test–retest = .95 Equivalence = .92 Subttests = .78–.95	Large number of studies showing concurrent, predictive, and construct validity	Interview Telephone report Direct observation
Functional Independence Measure for Children (WeeFIM)	ADLs/social cognition	Inter-rater = .98 Stability = .83–.99 ICC = .95 total score ICC = .73–.99 for subscales	Scores predict amount of caregiver assistance needed; correlates with measures of developmental status; has criterion validity	Interview Observation

(Continued)

Table 3.5. Characteristics of Instruments Reviewed *(cont.)*

Instrument	Area(s) Measured	Reliability	Validity	Measurement Method(s)
Home Observation for Measurement of the Environment (HOME)	Performance context (home); attributes that influence cognitive, social, and emotional development of children	Internal consistency = .89 or greater Inter-rater ≥ .90 Stability = .64	Evidence of content, criterion, and construct validity	Interview/survey
Home Occupation Environment Assessment (HOEA)	Performance context (home)	Inter-rater = .95	Content through expert opinion; factor analysis	Observation
Interview Schedule for Social Interaction (ISSI)	Social interaction	Internal consistency = .67–.81 Test–retest = .75–.79	Evidence of content, concurrent, criterion, and construct validity	Interview
Katz Index of Independence in ADL	Basic ADLs	Scalability = .74–.88	Criterion = discharge score; predicts need for personal assistance	Observation
Leisure Competence Measure	Leisure behaviors	Internal consistency and stability > .90	Evidence of content, concurrent, and criterion validity	Report Interview/survey
Leisure Diagnostic Battery (LDB)	Leisure knowledge, needs, and attitudes	Internal consistency = .83–.94 for long version and .89–.94 for short form	Evidence of concurrent, criterion, and construct validity (including confirmatory factory analysis)	Interview/survey
Leisure Satisfaction Questionnaire	Leisure satisfaction	Internal consistency = .82–.86	Evidence of content and predictive validity	Interview/survey
Nottingham Extended Activities of Daily Living Scale (NEADL)	IADLs/leisure	Internal consistency = .72–.94 Inter-rater reliability = .81–.90	Evidence of construct and concurrent validity	Report
Pediatric Evaluation of Disability Index (PEDI)	ADLs/cognition	Inter-rater reliability = .96–.99 Internal consistency = .95–.99	Expert panel content: scores correlate with age and with WeeFIM and Battelle Scores (.62–.97)	Interview Observation
Performance Assessment of Self Care Skills (PASS)	ADLs/IADLs	Inter-rater agreement = 96%–99% Internal consistency and test–retest > .80	Evidence of content, concurrent, criterion, and construct validity	Observation
Preschool Play Scale Revised (PPS–R)	Play behaviors (underlying capacity to play)	Inter-rater = .88–.99 Test–retest = .91–.97	Evidence of content, concurrent, and criterion validity	Report/survey
Reintegration to Normal Living Index (RNL)	Activity participation following rehabilitation	Internal consistency = .90–.95	Evidence of content, criterion, and construct validity	Interview/ self-report
Safety Assessment of Function and the Environment for Rehabilitation (SAFER) Tool	Features (safety) of living context	Inter-rater = .80 Internal consistency = .83	Evidence of content and concurrent validity	Observation

Table 3.5. Characteristics of Instruments Reviewed *(cont.)*

Instrument	Area(s) Measured	Reliability	Validity	Measurement Method(s)
School Functional Assessment (SFA)	Learning and social skills	Internal consistency = .92–.98 ICC = .80–.99	Evidence of concurrent and criterion validity	Observation
Test of Playfulness (TOP)	Play behaviors	Inter-rater ≥ .90	Evidence of concurrent, construct, and criterion validity	Observation
VALPAR Component Work Samples	Work performance	Stability = .70–.99	Evidence of criterion validity for all samples	Observation of performance
Work Environment Scale (WES)	Work context (productivity, satisfaction, expectations)	Internal consistency ≥ .69–.86 Test–retest = .69–.83 Stability = .51–.63	Evidence of content, construct, and criterion validity	Interview/survey

Note. ADLs = activities of daily living; IADLs = instrumental activities of daily living; ICC = intraclass correlation coefficient.

isting interview and self-report instruments be modified to include observation of performance in addition to reported performance? Studies that support the development and validation of existing scales are needed. The use of ad hoc or "homemade" evaluations is no longer acceptable. Because occupational therapists have extensive expertise in the assessment of function and in interventions that help adapt tasks, tools, and environments so that occupations can be pursued, they should be at the forefront of the development of performance-based assessments related to the important need to engage in activities and, in so doing, participate in the social world.

Acknowledgment

Catherine Backman, PhD, OT(C), made valuable contributions to earlier versions of this chapter. We are grateful for her past and continuing support of this book.

Study Questions

1. Describe the occupational therapy evaluation process.
2. What is an occupational profile, and how does it contribute to the occupational therapy evaluation?
3. Describe an analysis of occupational performance.

(Text continues on p. 78)

Table 3.6. Supplementary Notes on Validity Studies for Selected Measures

Instrument	Research and Citations Relating to the Instrument
Assessment of Motor and Process Skills (AMPS)	Several investigations using the AMPS with persons who have psychiatric, orthopedic, neurological (Mercier, Audet, Hebert, Rochette, & Dubois, 2001), cognitive (Lange, Spagnolo & Fowler, 2009; Liu et al., 2007; Waehrens & Fisher, 2007), and developmental disabilities (Hallgren & Kottorp, 2005; Kottorp, 2008, McNulty & Fisher, 2000) have been reported. The AMPS's ability to analyze the separate contributions of motor and process variables has provided knowledge about the specific variables contributing to task limitations in various conditions. Validity studies have suggested that the AMPS can help predict home safety (McNulty & Fisher, 2000), level of support needed in the community (Kottorp, 2008), and measure improvements following intervention for multiple sclerosis (Kinnman et al., 2000) and stroke (Tham, Ginsburg, Fisher, & Tegner, 2001). The AMPS has demonstrated consistency across different cultural groups (Fisher & Duran, 2000; Fisher, Liu, Velozo, & Pan, 1992). These, along with other studies (e.g., Douglas, Letts, & Liu, 2007), have also established the reliability and validity of the AMPS.
	In addition to the original AMPS, a school-based version is available to measure school based performance in typical classroom settings (Fisher, Bryze, Hume, & Griswold, 2005). The test measures quality of school performance, the impact of the child's process skills, and change in performance over time. The School AMPS has been used

(Continued)

Table 3.6. Supplementary Notes on Validity Studies for Selected Measures *(cont.)*

Instrument	Research and Citations Relating to the Instrument
	in a number of studies to compare children with various diagnoses to normally developing children (e.g., Granberg, Rydberg, & Fisher, 2008; Munkholm & Fisher, 2008). The School AMPS has been shown a valid instrument for measuring school performance in a naturalistic setting in the measurement of school-based motor and process skills (Fingerhut, Madill, Darrah, Hodge, & Warren, 2002).
Barthel Index (BI)	The initial BI score was found to be the most reliable predictor of final rehabilitation outcome in study of stroke patients (Hertanu, Demopoulos, Yang, Calhoun, & Fenigstein, 1984). It also correlates significantly with type of discharge and shorter length of stay for patients with stroke (Granger, Hamilton, Gresham, & Kramer, 1989; Wylie & White, 1964) and independent living outcome for patients with spinal cord injury (DeJong, Branch, & Corcoran, 1996) as well as participation of young adults with disabilities (Bent, Jones, Molloy, Chamberlain, & Tennant, 2001). The Extended Barthel Index (EBI; Prosiegel et al., 1996) was developed to address perceived limitations by adding items for comprehension, expression, social interaction, problem solving, memory, learning, orientation, and vision/neglect. One study showed that the EBI is a reliable, valid, and practical instrument that is sensitive to changes over time (Jansa, Pogacnik, & Gompertz, 2004).
Career Ability Placement Survey (CAPS)	Validity has been demonstrated through studies of the association of CAPS test scores with scores of clients on comparable tests, such as the Employee Aptitude Scale (EAS), General Aptitude Test Battery, and others (Katz, Beers, Geckle, & Goldstein, 1989; Knapp, Knapp, Strand, & Michael, 1978; Knap-Lee, 1995). Factor analysis of the CAPS has identified three primary factors, including Verbal Comprehension, Perceptual Skill, and Response Speed (Knapp et al., 1992). The CAPS has been used to study the effectiveness of retraining programs for airline workers (Deis & Scott, 2002) and may be useful in clinical and research settings related to the efficacy of specific training programs.
Community Integration Questionnaire (CIQ)	Coefficients for the subscales show greater variability: home subscale = .84, social subscale = .73, and productivity subscale = .35. Test–retest reliability has been reported at over .90 (Willer, Linn, & Allen, 1993). Content for the CIQ was derived from the literature and a panel of consumers, professionals, and researchers (Willer et al., 1993). Subscale and total scores differentiated between subjects with and without traumatic brain injury (TBI) and between subjects with TBI living in different settings (independent, supported community, and institution) (Willer, Ottenbacher, & Coad, 1994). Convergent validity was established using the Craig Handicap Assessment and Reporting Technique (0.62 for subjects with TBI; 0.70 for family members) (Corrigan & Deming, 1995; Zhang et al., 2002). The CIQ is available free of charge. The scale along with rating forms and information regarding administration may be downloaded from the Center for Outcome Measurement in Brain Injury.
Canadian Occupational Performance Measure (COPM)	Three phases of studies established the psychometric properties of the COPM (Carswell et al., 2004; Law et al., 1993; Law et al., 1994). Additional studies have reported high reliability for both performance and satisfaction scores (Sewell & Singh, 2001). Cusick, Lannin, and Lowe (2007) studied the internal reliability and validity of an adapted version of the COPM with young children. The study concluded the adapted version was psychometrically robust and appropriate to pediatric populations. Adult validity studies have been equally encouraging. Trombly and colleagues studied goal achievement by adults with TBI and found that client perceptions of progress as measured by the COPM were accompanied by improved scores on scales of independent living and social participation (Trombly, Radomski, & Davis, 1998). A comparative study of rehabilitation settings for survivors of stroke using the COPM showed that participant satisfaction with goal achievement was independent of setting and consistent with the results of performance measured by IADLs and health outcome scales (Law, Wishart, & Guyatt, 2000). A study by Simmons and colleagues found that using the COPM in combination with The FIM enhanced accuracy in prediction of outcomes for rehabilitative services for people in adult physical disabilities settings (Simmons, Crepeau, & White, 2000). These and several other studies have demonstrated that the COPM correlates well with other measures of ADL outcome, motivates active participation and adherence to rehabilitation regimens, and improves

Table 3.6. Supplementary Notes on Validity Studies for Selected Measures *(cont.)*

Instrument	Research and Citations Relating to the Instrument
	client satisfaction with services for a variety of diagnostic groups and ages (Carpenter, Baker, & Tyldesley, 2001; Gilbertson & Langhorne, 2000; Law et al., 1997; Ripat, Etcheverry, Cooper, & Tate, 2001; Rochman, Ray, Kulich, Mehta, & Driscoll, 2008; Verkerk, Wolf, Louwers, Meester-Delver, & Nollet, 2006; Wressle, Eeg-Olofsson, Marcusson, & Henricksson, 2002). Cross-cultural studies of the COPM include the following: (Eyssen, Beelen, Dedding, Cardol, & Dekker, 2005; Pan, Chung, & Hsin-Hwei, 2003), Diagnostic category studies include the following: (Case-Smith, 2003; Cresswell & Rugg, 2003; Eyssen et al., 2005; Harper, Stalker, & Templeton, 2006). Age groups studies include the following: (Cusick et al., 2007; Verkerk et al., 2006).
	During initial development, the authors reported findings on an extensive pilot study of the COPM that involved administration in several countries, including New Zealand, Greece, and Great Britain (Law et al., 1994). The scale has since been translated and used in several additional countries. Early findings indicated that the average change scores for performance and satisfaction were approximately 1.5 times the standard deviation of the scores, indicating sensitivity of the instrument to perceived changes in occupational performance by clients. The COPM is seen as a flexible instrument and appeals to clinicians who value the client-centered philosophy underlying its development (Toomy, Nicholson, & Carswell, 1995). Some reports have indicated that clients occasionally experience difficulty with the process of self-rating of performance (Bodiam, 1999), and the suitability of the measure for use with clients demonstrating cognitive or affective difficulties has been questioned. Some studies have shown these concerns to be overstated (Chesworth, Duffy, Hodnett, & Knight, 2002). Additional concerns have been raised regarding the length of time it takes to administer the measure, although familiarity with the instrument and model seem to facilitate ease of use (Baptiste, 2008).
The FIM™	Validity has been demonstrated with foreign (translated) versions of The FIM™ (Lundgren-Nilsson et al., 2005). The FIM does have limitations, however. The FIM was found to have acceptable scalability only when broken down into two parts that treat the 13 motor and 5 cognitive items as separate subscales. Recent studies of the Self-Reported Functional Measure show that the instrument predicts inpatient hospitalization but not outpatient health care use (Hoenig, Hoff, McIntyre, & Branch, 2001) and that it can also predict caregiver hours (Samsa, Hoenig, & Branch, 2001). A study of elderly patients with hip fracture by Young, Fan, Hebel, and Boult (2009) demonstrated that The FIM had concurrent validity when administered by trained interviewers (Hoenig et al., 2001).
Frenchay Activities Index (FAI)	Although most of the studies using the FAI have been related to outcomes following stroke (Chen, Hsieh, Mao, & Huang, 2007; Combs, Winchell, & Forsyth, 2007; Johansson, Mishina, Ivanov, & Bjorklund, 2007; Kwakkel, Kollen, & Wagenaar, 2002; Young, Bogle, & Forster, 2001), the index has also been used for other populations, including those with complex disabilities (Haig, Nagy, Lebreck, & Stein, 1995), limb amputations (Miller, Deathe, & Harris, 2004), brain injury (Middelkamp et al., 2007; Van Baalen et al., 2007), cardiac conditions (Lennon, Carey, Gaffney, & Stephenson, 2007; Middelkamp et al., 2007), and caregivers (Baalen et al., 2007; Mant, Carter, Wade, & Winner, 2000). The scale has also been translated for and used to study rehabilitation outcomes in Japan (Hachisuka et al., 1999), China (Hsieh & Hsueh, 1999), Denmark, and Spain (Carod-Artal, Egido, Gonzalez, & de Seijas, 2000).
	Studies demonstrate the reliability and validity of the FAI with some moderate limitations. Turnbull et al. (2000) studied 1,280 people to construct preliminary norms and to determine evidence of reliability and validity. They concluded that the FAI is reliable and shows good evidence of validity with the elderly population but would benefit from adding items relating to sport, physical exercise, and caring for children. This would make it a tool more useful for a broader segment of the population. One study showed that the FAI has excellent inter-rater reliability (Piercy, Carter, Mant, & Wade, 2000). However, Schuling and others suggested that the instrument's reliability could be improved by deleting two items and creating two subscale scores, one for

(Continued)

Table 3.6. Supplementary Notes on Validity Studies for Selected Measures *(cont.)*

Instrument	Research and Citations Relating to the Instrument
	domestic activities and the other for outdoor activities (Schuling, Dehaan, Limburg, & Groenier, 1993). Studies using the FAI and measure of BADLs, particularly the BI, demonstrated that the scales measure different factors and may be useful in combination (Hsieh & Hsueh, 1999). Green and colleagues studied the test–retest reliability of the FAI and other scales of stroke outcome. Their study found that the FAI had only moderate reliability and higher random error when stroke survivors were measured twice within a one-week interval (Green, Forster, & Young, 2001). Shepers and colleagues (2006) examined various functional measures for survivors of stroke suggested the BI as the measure of choice in acute phases of stroke and the FAI as more appropriate in chronic phases. Miller and colleagues (2004) studied the psychometric properties of the FAI for persons with lower limb amputations. This study concluded the FAI has acceptable reliability and validity for this population, with higher sensitivity in detection of group vs. individual differences.
Interview Schedule for Social Interaction (ISSI)	The ISSI has satisfactory internal, consistency (Cronbach's alpha coefficients range from .67–.81 for the four subscales), and test–retest reliability for the subscale ranges from .75–.79, Factor analysis has confirmed validity of the four subscales as measuring distinct facets of social interaction (Duncan-Jones, 1981a, 1981b). Studies have shown evidence of construct validity. ISSI scores are associated with marital status and age and correlate significantly in expected directions with measures of neuroticism, depression, and extraversion (Morris, Robinson, Raphael, & Bishop, 1991; Thomas, Garry, Goodwin, & Goodwin, 1985). The scale does not seem to be influenced by social desirability response tendency. Norms are also available for defined populations (Henderson, Byrne, & Duncan-Jones, 1981).
Katz Index of Independence in ADL	In addition to its high coefficients scalability, the Katz Index also has demonstrated good inter-rater reliability (Brorsson & Asberg, 1984). Reijneveld and colleagues (2007) have reported successful use of the Katz scale with Dutch, Turkish, and Moroccan populations. A culturally equivalent Portuguese version of the Katz index is also available (Lino, Pereira, Camacho, Ribeiro, & Buksman, 2008).
Pediatric Evaluation of Disability Index (PEDI)	The psychometric properties of the PEDI are reported in the administration manual. Reliability data (internal consistency) for the six scale scores were computed using Cronbach's alpha, with coefficients ranging from .95–.99 (Haley et al., 1992). Initial data collected on the normative sample reflected an expected progression of functional skills according to age. Initial concurrent validity was established through comparison of scores on the PEDI with scores on the Battelle Developmental Inventory Screening Test and the WeeFIM.™ These correlations were generally high for self-care and mobility but lower for social function. In early studies of the PEDI's ability to detect change, results were mixed, with one clinical sample of children with mild to moderate traumatic injuries demonstrating positive changes on the PEDI in all domains. Another clinical sample involving children with multiple significant disabilities showed positive change after 8 months only on the mobility scale. Some scores for this group decreased, indicating that the children were falling behind their peers in age-expected functional levels. Ludlow and Haley (1996) studied the influence of setting (context) on rating of mobility activities and found that parents in the home setting tend to use stricter criteria in their ratings than rehabilitation professionals in the school setting, although both can be trained to attain a satisfactory level of consistency. Numerous clinical studies using the PEDI have been reported. These have related to measuring the developmental status of very-low-birthweight children and for various rehabilitation or surgical interventions with children in various diagnostic categories, including TBI (Thomas-Stonell et al., 2006), spinal bifida (Schoenmakers et al., 2005), cerebral palsy (Novack, Cusick, & Lowe, 2007), and osteogenesis imperfecta (Engelbert et al., 1999). In addition, several reports have been published where the PEDI has been used to measure outcomes following targeted medical and surgical interventions for

Table 3.6. Supplementary Notes on Validity Studies for Selected Measures *(cont.)*

Instrument	Research and Citations Relating to the Instrument
	cerebral palsy. Ketelaar and colleagues (1998) studied the properties of 17 scales assessing the functional motor abilities of children with cerebral palsy and concluded that the PEDI was one of only two measures that demonstrated acceptable psychometric properties while having the capability to document changes in function over time. Studies of children from outside the United States have been reported to ascertain the suitability of using the PEDI with other cultural groups. For example, a study of the applicability of the PEDI in Slovenia found statistically significant differences in functional skills and caregiver assistance scores between Slovene children and the American normative group (Srsen et al., 2005) but concluded that the American normative data are not fully appropriate for reference with the Slovene population. In Norway, a study of the applicability of the PEDI recommended further research from which Norwegian reference values can be derived (Berg et al., 2003).
Safely Assessment of Function and the Environment for Rehabilitation (SAFER) Tool	The original SAFER tool predated the development of the SAFER HOME and included evaluations based on an environmental checklist rated "Addressed," "Not Applicable," and "Problem". The new SAFER HOME version expanded the checklist to increase sensitivity to change over time and now includes "No Identified Concern," "Mild Problem," "Moderate Problem," and "Severe Problem" (Chiu et al., 2002). The SAFER HOME is designed as an outcome measure and to facilitate plans for intervention and is based on the original SAFER instrument (Chiu & Tickle-Degnan, 2002). An interesting attribute of the SAFER tool is the choice of items that reflect a transactional relationship between the individual and the environment. The items were selected systematically by a panel of clinicians and seniors, and some items were discarded after analysis of content and construct validity. The item selection process also provided a basis for developing guidelines to assist clinicians in using the tool. These guidelines have been organized in the form of questions to consider when completing an environmental assessment.
School Functional Assessment (SFA)	The SFA has also been used in a variety of outcomes and comparison studies. Examples of research include use of the SFA in measuring differences in children with and without cerebral palsy (Schenker, Coster, & Parush, 2006), differences in children with and without congenital hemiplegia (Burtner, Dukeminier, Ben, Qualls, & Scott, 2006), as a standardized measure related to inter-rater reliability of assigning children *ICF* codes (Ogonowski, Kronk, Rice, & Feldman, 2004), to examine factors that facilitate or hinder children with disabilities in school performance (Eglison & Traustadottir, 2009), and to identify the responsiveness of outcome measures related to school based programs (Wright, Boschen, & Jutai, 2005). In addition to its utility in research, the SFA is useful in educational and practice settings to facilitate evaluation and intervention planning, measure change in performance, and collect administrative date to meet state and federal guidelines (Pearson Education, 2008).
Test of Playfulness (TOP)	Rasch analysis revealed evidence that 100% of the raters scored the TOP reliably, and data for 88% of the children with disabilities conformed to the pattern of playfulness typical of most of the children represented in the test's normative data set. Four TOP items accounted for most of the unexpected ratings. In another study, children diagnosed with attention deficit hyperactivity disorder (ADHD) were found to have lower mean scores on the TOP than children without ADHD. A study by Harkness and Bundy (2001) showed no significant differences between comparison groups of children with and without disabilities and also demonstrated acceptable reliability for administration. The TOP has been found to be significantly correlated with its companion instrument, the Test of Environmental Supportiveness (Bronson & Bundy, 2001), and has been found to measure similar constructs of play to the Pediatric Volitional Questionnaire (Reid, 2005) and the Children's Playfulness Scale (Muys, Rodger, & Bundy, 2006). Additional studies have demonstrated the psychometric properties of the TOP (Brentnall, Bundy, & Kay, 2008; Hamm, 2006). In response to clinical and research questions related to the optimal time for observation when administering the TOP,

(Continued)

Table 3.6. Supplementary Notes on Validity Studies for Selected Measures *(cont.)*

Instrument	Research and Citations Relating to the Instrument
	Brentnall et al. (2008) found the use of 15-minute observations superior to 30-minute sessions and similar to previous studies and the test–retest reliability at a significant level however, they recommended additional studies to substantiate the reliability and validity of the test. This parallels Skard and Bundy's (2008) assertion that a single 15-minute observation is sufficient to score the TOP.
The WeeFIM II	Comparisons of the WeeFIM with the Pediatric Quality of Life Inventory appear to be fair to moderately correlated in areas of physical health, but significant differences were not found in areas of psychosocial function suggesting the tools may measure different constructs within the psychosocial area (Grilli et al., 2006).
	Comparisons of WeeFIM scores with other developmental tests, including the Vineland Adaptive Behaviors Scales and the Battelle Developmental Inventory Screening Test, found subscale correlations of 0.42 to 0.92 and total score correlations of 0.72 to 0.94 (Ottenbacher, Taylor, et al., 1996). Additional research comparing the WeeFIM to two standardized language tests, the Symbolic Play Test and the Reynell Language Development Scale, demonstrated high correlations in a Hong Kong pediatric population, and the authors concluded from their pilot study that the WeeFIM appears to be an easy-to-use functional assessment of language in children with developmental delays (Wong, Trevor, & Law, 2005).
	Several studies have been conducted on the validity of the WeeFIM. The WeeFIM has been used to assess the developmental and functional status of children with and without disability (Ottenbacher, Hsu, Granger & Fielder, 1996) and across cultures (e.g., Wong & Wong, 2007). The scale has also been used to assess the functional status and rehabilitative progress in those with various types of congenital problems, including both common (Hogan & Park, 2000) and rare genetic disorders (Colvin et al., 2003). The WeeFIM has also been used to measure rehabilitation outcomes in larger populations across diagnostic, age, and rehabilitation cohorts (Chen et al., 2004).
	Although continued research is needed on the WeeFIM II and the use of the 0–3 module, there is sufficient data to warrant the use of the WeeFIM in a variety of pediatric populations. Studies of the WeeFIM have shown a strong correlation between the scale scores and age, with the subscale scores involving gross and fine motor skill demonstrating the highest correlations (Ottenbacher et al., 1999). Data showed that tasks on the WeeFIM demonstrate a developmental sequence, with an observed positive relationship between the complexity of tasks and the age at which children achieve independence in their performance (Braun & Granger, 1991). Repeated evaluations of the scale and comparisons of personal and telephone interview ratings have demonstrated that the scale has excellent reliability (Ottenbacher, Hsu et al., 1996; Ottenbacher et al., 1997). Additional research is warranted to continue to validate psychometric properties in the newer version, including the 0–3 module and the WeeFIM's application to other cultures.

4. Discuss some of the differences between scales that measure ADL skills and those that measure IADL skills.
5. Identify and briefly describe 2 instruments for each of the following categories of occupational performance: ADLs, IADLs, leisure, play, education, work, and social participation.
6. If you had a 65-year-old client with a recent stroke who wished to return to independent living at home, which of the instruments discussed may be appropriate to use during evaluation, and why?
7. What are some important considerations in evaluating environmental context? Describe 2 instruments you could use and the utility of each.
8. What is social participation, and how does it relate to occupational performance? Describe 2 instruments you could use to evaluate social participation and the utility of each.

References

Abraham, I., & Foley, T. (1984). The work environment scale and the ward atmosphere scale (short forms): Psychometric data. *Perceptual and Motor Skills, 58,* 319–322.

American Occupational Therapy Association. (2008). Occupational therapy practice framework: Domain and process (2nd ed.). *American Journal of Occupational Therapy, 62,* 625–683.

AMPS Project International. (2009). *Assessment of Motor and Process Skills (AMPS).* Retrieved September 17, 2009, from http://www.ampsintl.com/AMPS/index.php

Baalen, B. V., Ribbers, G. M., Medema-Meulepas, D., Odding, M. S., & Stam, H. J. (2007). Being restricted in participation after a traumatic brain injury is negatively associated by passive coping style of the caregiver. *Brain Injury, 21,* 925–931.

Baptiste, S. (2008). Client–centered assessment: The Canadian Occupational Performance Measure. In B. J. Hemphill-Pearson (Ed.), *Assessment in occupational therapy mental health: An integrative approach* (2nd ed.; pp. 35–47). Thorofare, NJ: Slack.

Baum, C. M., & Edwards, D. F. (2001). *The Washington University Activity Card Sort.* St. Louis, MO: Washington University.

Baum, C. M., & Edwards, D. F. (2008). *Activity Card Sort* (2nd ed.). Bethesda, MD: AOTA Press.

Baum, C., Edwards, D. F., Bradford, T., & Lane, R. (1995). *Home–Occupation–Environment Assessment (HOEA).* St. Louis, MO: Occupational Therapy Program, Washington University.

Beard, J., & Ragheb, M. (1980). Measuring leisure satisfaction. *Journal of Leisure Research*, 20–33.

Bengtsson-Tops, A., Hansson, L., Sandlund, M., Bjarnason, O., Korkeila, J., Merinder, L., et al. (2005). Subjective versus interviewer assessment of global quality of life among persons with schizophrenia living in the community: A Nordic multicentre study. *Quality of Life Research, 14*(1), 221–229.

Bent, N., Jones, A., Molloy, I., Chamberlain, M., & Tennant, A. (2001). Factors determining participation in young adults with a physical disability: A pilot study. *Clinical Rehabilitation, 15,* 552–561.

Berg, M., Jahnsen, R., Holm, I., & Hussain, A. (2003). Translation of a multi-disciplinary assessment. Procedures to achieve functional equivalence. *Advances in Physiotherapy, 5,* 57–66.

Bledsoe, N., & Shepherd, J. (1982). A study of the reliability and validity of a preschool play scale. *American Journal of Occupational Therapy, 36,* 783–788.

Bodiam, C. (1999). The use of the Canadian Occupational Performance Measure for the assessment of outcome on a neurorehabilitation unit. *British Journal of Occupational Therapy, 2,* 123–126.

Bookman, A., Harrington, M., Pass, L., & Reisner, E. (2007). *Family caregiver handbook: Finding elder care resources in Massachussetts.* Cambridge: Massachussetts Institute of Technology.

Bradley, R. H. (1993). Children's home envionments, health, behavior, and intervention efforts: A review using the HOME inventory as a marker measure. *Genetic, Social, and General Psychology Monographs, 119,* 437–490.

Braun, S., & Granger, C. (1991). A practical approach to functional assessment in pediatrics. *Occupational Therapy Practice, 2,* 46–51.

Brentnall, J., Bundy, A. C., & Kay, F. C. (2008). The effect of the length of observation on Test of Playfulness Scores. *OTJR: Occupation, Participation and Health, 28,* 133–140.

Bronson, M., & Bundy, A. C. (2001). A correlational study of a test of a playfulness and a test of environmental supportiveness for play. *OTJR: Occupation, Participation and Health, 21,* 242–259.

Brorsson, B., & Asberg, K. (1984). Katz Index of Independence in ADL: Reliability and validity in short-term care. *Scandinavian Journal of Rehabilitation Medicine, 16,* 125–132.

Broughton, K., & Beggs, B. A. (2006). Leisure Satisfaction of Older Adults. *Activities, Adaptation, and Aging, 31,* 1–18.

Buck, D., Jacoby, A., Massey, A., & Ford, G. S. (2000). Evaluation of measures used to assess quality of life after stroke. *Stroke, 31,* 2004–2010.

Bundy, A. C. (1997). Play and playfulness: What to look for. In L. Parham & L. Fazio (Eds.), *Play in occupational therapy for children* (pp. 52–66). St. Louis, MO: Mosby.

Bundy, A. C. (2000). *Test of Playfulness manual* (ver. 3). Ft. Collins, CO: Colorado State University.

Bundy, A. C. (2003). *Test of Playfulness manual* (ver. 4). Sydney, Australia: University of Sydney.

Burtner, P. A., Dukeminier, A., Ben, L., Qualls, C., & Scott, K. (2006). Visual perceptional skills and related school functions in children with hemiplegic cerebral palsy. *New Zealand Journal of Occupational Therapy, 53,* 24–29.

Caldwell, B., & Bradley, R. H. (1984). Home *Observation for Measure of the Environment* (rev. ed.). Little Rock: University of Arkansas.

Caldwell, B., & Bradley, R. H. (2001). *Home Inventory and Administration Manual* (3rd ed.). Little Rock: University of Arkansas.

Carod-Artal, J., Egido, J. A., Gonzalez, J. L., & de Seijas, E. V. (2000). Quality of life among stroke survivors evaluated 1 year after stroke—Experience of a stroke unit. *Stroke, 31,* 2995–3000.

Carpenter, L., Baker, G., & Tyldesley, B. (2001). The use of the Canadian Occupational Performance Measure as an outcome of a pain management program. *Canadian Journal of Occupational Therapy, 68,* 16–22.

Carswell, A., McColl, M., Baptiste, S., Law, M., Polatajko, H., & Pollock, N. (2004). The Canadian Occupational Performance Measure: A research and clinical update. *Canadian Journal of Occupational Therapy, 71,* 16–22.

Case-Smith, J. (2003). Outcomes in hand rehabilitation using occupational therapy services. *American Journal of Occupational Therapy, 57,* 499–506.

Chang, Y., & Card, J. (1994). The reliability of the leisure diagnostic battery short form Version AB in assessing healthy, older individuals. A preliminary study. *Therapeutic Recreation Journal, 28,* 163–167.

Chen, C. C., Heinemann, A. W., Bode, R. K., Granger, C. V., & Mallinson, T. (2004). Impact of pediatric rehabilitation services on children's functional outcomes. *American Journal of Occupational Therapy, 58,* 44–53.

Chen, M. H., Hsieh, C. L., Mao, H.-F., & Huang, S. L. (2007). Differences between patient an proxy reports in the assessment of disability after stroke. *Clinical Rehabilitation, 21,* 351–356.

Chesworth, C., Duffy, R., Hodnett, J., & Knight, A. (2002). Measuring clinical effectiveness in mental health: Is the Canadian Occupational Performance an appropriate measure? *British Journal of Occupational Therapy, 65,* 30–34.

Chiu, T., & Oliver, R. (2006). Factor analysis and construct validity of the SAFER-HOME. *OTJR: Occupation, Participation and Health, 26,* 132–142.

Chiu, T., Oliver, R., Ascott, P., Choo, L. C., Davis, T., Gaya, A., et al. (2006). *Safety Assessment of Function and the Environment for Rehabilitation (SAFER) Health Outcome Measurement and Evaluation (HOME),* version 3. Toronto, Ontario: COTA Health.

Chiu, T., Oliver, R., Faibish, S., & Cawley, B. (2002). *Addendum: Introduction of the SAFER-HOME.* Toronto, Ontario: COTA Comprehensive Rehabilitation and Mental Health Services.

Chiu, T., & Tickle-Degnan, L. (2002). Learning from evidence: Service outcomes and client satsifaction with occupational therapy home-based services. *American Journal of Occupational Therapy, 56,* 217–220.

Chong, D. S. (1995). Measurement of instrumental activities of daily living in stroke. *Stroke, 26,* 1119–1122.

Christiansen, C. H. (2004). Functional evaluation and management of self-care and other activities of daily living. In J. DeLisa (Ed.), *Rehabilitation medicine: Principles and practice* (pp. 975–1004). Philadelphia: Lippincott Williams & Wilkins.

Christiansen, C. H., Rogers, S. L., & Haertl, K. L. (in press). Functional evaluation and management of self-care and other activities of daily living. In J. A. DeLisa et al. (Eds.), *Rehabilitation medicine: Principles and practice* (5th ed.). Philadelphia: Lippincott Williams & Wilkins.

Colvin, L., Fyfe, S., Leonard, S., Schiavello, T., Ellaway, C., De Klerk, N., et al. (2003). Describing the phenotype in Rett syndrome using a population database. *Archives of Disability in Childhood, 88*(1), 38–43.

Combs, S., Winchell, E., & Forsyth, E. (2007). Motor and functional outcomes of a patient post-stroke following combined activity and impairment level training. *Physiotherapy Theory and Practice, 23,* 219–229.

Cooper, B., Letts, L., Rigby, P., Stewart, D., & Strong, S. (2001). Measuring environmental factors. In M. Law, W. W. Dunn, & C. M. Baum (Eds.), *Measuring occupational performance* (pp. 229–232). Thorofare, NJ: Slack.

Corrigan, J. D., & Deming, R. (1995). Psychometric characteristics of the Community Integration Questionnaire: Replication and extension. *Journal of Head Trauma Rehabilitation, 10*(4), 41–53.

Coster, W. (1998). Occupation centered assessment for children. *American Journal of Occupational Therapy, 52,* 337–354.

Coster, W., Deeney, T., Haltiwanger, J., & Haley, S. (1998). *Manual for the School Function Assessment.* San Antonio, TX: Psychological Corporation.

Coster, W., Haley, S., & Jette, A. (2006). Measuring patient-reported outcomes after discharge from inpatient rehabilitation settings. *Journal of Rehabilitation Medicine, 38,* 237–242.

Cresswell, M. K., & Rugg, S. A. (2003). The Canadian Occupational Performance Measure: Its use with clients with schizophrenia. *International Journal of Therapy and Rehabilitation, 10,* 544–553.

Cusick, A., Lannin, N., & Lowe, K. (2007). Adapting the Canadian Occupational Performance Measure for use in a paediatric clinical trial. *Disability and Rehabilitation, 10,* 761–766.

Davis, J., & Kutter, C. J. (1998). Independent living skills and posttraumatic stress disorder in women who are homeless: Implications for future practice. *American Journal of Occupational Therapy, 52,* 39–44.

Deis, M. H., & Scott, J. S. (2002, Spring). An evaluation of retraining programs for dislocated workers in the airline industry. *SAM Advanced Management Journal,* pp. 15–22.

DeJong, G., Branch, L., & Corcoran, P. (1996). Independent living outcomes in spinal cord injury: Multivariate analyses. *Archives of Physical Medicine and Rehabilitation, 77,* 883–888.

Douglas, A., Letts, L., & Liu, L. (2007). Review of cognitive assessment for older adults. *Physical and Occupational Therapy in Geriatrics, 26,* 13–43.

Duncan-Jones, P. (1981a). The structure of social relationships: Analysis of a survey instrument, Part 1. *Social Psychiatry, 16,* 55–61.

Duncan-Jones, P. (1981b). The structure of social relationships: Analysis of a survey instrument, Part 2. *Social Psychiatry, 16,* 143–149.

Dunn, J. (1987). *Generalizability of the leisure diagnostic battery.* Unpublished doctoral dissertation, University of Illinois, Champagne.

Dunn, W. W., Brown, C., & McCuigan, A. (1994). The ecology of human performance: A framework for considering the effect of context. *American Journal of Occupational Therapy, 48,* 595–607.

Eglison, S. T., & Traustadottir, R. (2009). Participation of students with physical disabilities in the school environment. *American Journal of Occupational Therapy, 63,* 264–272.

Eklund, M., Bengtsson-Tops, B., & Lindstedt, H. (2007). Construct and discriminant validity and dimensionality of the Interview Schedule for Social Interaction (ISSI) in three psychiatric samples. *Nordic Journal of Psychiatry, 61,* 182–188.

Elardo, R., Bradley, R. H., & Caldwell, B. M. (1975). The relation of infants' home environments to mental test performance from six to thirty-six months. A longitudinal analysis. *Child Development, 46,* 71–76.

Ellis, G. D., & Witt, P. A. (1986). The leisure diagnostic battery: Past, present, and future. *Therapeutic Recreation Journal, 19,* 31–47.

Ellul, J., Watkins, C., & Barer, D. (1998). Estimating total Barthel scores from just three items: The European Stroke Database "minimum dataset" for assessing functional status at discharge from hospital. *Age and Ageing, 27*(2), 115–122.

Engelbert, R. H., Beemer, F. A., van der Graaf, Y., & Helders, P. J. (1999). Osteogenesis imperfecta in childhood: Impairment and disability—A follow-up study. *Archives of Physical Medicine and Rehabilitation, 80,* 896–903.

Eyssen, I. C., Beelen, A., Dedding, C., Cardol, M., & Dekker, J. (2005). The reproducibility of the Canadian Occupational Performance Measure. *Clinical Rehabilitation, 19,* 888–894.

Finch, E., Brooks, D., Stratford, P. W., & Mayo, E. N. (2002). Reintegration to normal living (RNL) index. In E. Finch, D. Brooks, P. W. Stratford, & E. N. Mayo (Eds.), *Physical rehabilitation outcome measures* (2nd ed., pp. 201–203). Philadelphia: Lippincott Williams & Wilkins.

Fingerhut, P., Madill, H., Darrah, J., Hodge, M., & Warren, S. (2002). Classroom-based assessment: Validation for the School AMPS. *American Journal of Occupational Therapy, 56,* 210–213.

Finlayson, M., Havens, B., Holm, M., & Van Denend, T. (2003). Integrating a performance-based observation measure of functional status into a population-based longitudinal study of aging. *Canadian Journal on Aging, 22,* 185–195.

Fisher, A. (1993). The assessment of IADL motor skill: An application of the many-faceted Rasch analysis. *American Journal of Occupational Therapy, 47,* 319–329.

Fisher, A. G. (2006). *Assessment of Motor and Process Skills: Volume 1: Development standardization and administration manual* (6th ed.). Fort Collins, CO: Three Star.

Fisher, A. G., Bryze, K., Hume, V., & Griswold, L. A. (2005). *School AMPS: School version of the assessment of motor and process skills.* Fort Collins, CO: Three Star.

Fisher, A., & Duran, L. (2000). ADL performance of black Americans and white Americans on the assessment of motor and process skills. *American Journal of Occupational Therapy, 54,* 607–613.

Fisher, A., Liu, Y., Velozo, C., & Pan, A. (1992). Cross-cultural assessment of process skills. *American Journal of Occupational Therapy, 46,* 876–885.

Forsyth, K., Lai, J., & Kielhofner, G. (1999). The assessment of communication and interaction skills (ACIS): A measurement profile. *British Journal of Occupational Therapy, 62*(2), 69–74.

Garton, A. F., Harvey, R., & Price, C. (2004). Influence of perceived family environment on adolescent leisure participation. *Australian Journal of Psychology, 56,* 18–24.

Geisinger, K. F., Spies, R. A., Carlson, J. F., & Plake, B. S. (Eds.). (2007). *The Seventeenth Mental Measurements Yearbook.* Lincoln, NE: Buros Institute of Mental Measurements.

Gilbertson, L., & Langhorne, P. (2000). Home-based occupational therapy: Stroke patients' satisfaction with occupational performance and service provision. *British Journal of Occupational Therapy, 63,* 464–468.

Goddard, R., O'Brien, P., & Goddard, M. (2006). Work environment predictors of beginning teacher burnout. *British Educational Research Journal, 32,* 857–874.

Gompertz, P., Pound, P., & Ebrahim, S. (1994). A postal version of the Barthel Index. *Clinical Rehabilitation, 8*(3), 233–239.

Granberg, M., Rydberg, A., & Fisher, A. (2008). Activities in daily living and schoolwork task performance in children with complex congenital heart disease. *Acta Paediatrica, 97,* 1270–1274.

Granger, C., Hamilton, B., Gresham, G., & Kramer, A. (1989). The stroke rehabilitation outcome study: Part II. Relative merits of the total Barthel Index score and a four-item sub score in predicting patient outcomes. *Archives of Physical Medicine and Rehabilitation, 70,* 100–103.

Green, J., Forster, A., & Young, J. D. (2001). A test–retest reliability study of the Barthel Index, the Rivermead Mobility Index, the Nottingham Extended Activities of Daily Living Scale, and the Frenchay Activities Index in stroke patients. *Disability and Rehabilitation, 23,* 670–676.

Grilli, L., Feldman, D. E., Majnemer, A., Couture, M., Azoulay, L., & Swaine, B. (2006). Associations between a functional independence measure (WeeFIM) and the pediatric quality of life inventory (PedsQL4.0) in young children with physical disabilities. *Quality of Life Research, 15*(6), 1023–1031.

Grimsley, G., Ruch, F., L., Ruch, W., Warren, N. D., & Ford, J. S. (1983). *Employee Aptitude Survey Technical Manual.* Glendale, CA: Psychological Services.

Guttman, L. E. (1950). The basis for scalogram analysis. In S. Stouffer, L. Guttman, E. Suchman, P. Lazarsfield, S. Star, & J. Clausen (Eds.), *Measurement and prediction* (pp. 60–90). Princeton, NJ: Princeton University Press.

Hachisuka, K., Saeki, S., Tsutsui, Y., Chisaka, H., Ogata, H., Iwata, N., et al. (1999). Gender-related differences in scores of the Barthel Index and Frenchay Activities Index in randomly sampled elderly persons living at home in Japan. *Journal of Clinical Epidemiology, 52,* 1089–1094.

Haertl, K. L. (2010). A frame of reference to enhance childhood occupations: Scope-IT. In P. Kramer & J. Hinojosa (Eds.), *Frames of reference for pediatric occupational therapy* (3rd ed., 266–305). Baltimore: Lippincott Williams & Wilkins.

Haglund, L., & Thorell, L. (2004). Clinical perspective on the Swedish version of the assessment of communication and interaction skills: Stability of assessments. *Scandinavian Journal of Caring Sciences, 18,* 417–423.

Haig, A., Nagy, A., Lebreck, D., & Stein, G. (1995). Outpatient planning for persons with physical disabilities: A randomized prospective trial of physiatrist alone versus a multidisciplinary team. *Archives of Physical Medicine and Rehabilitation, 76,* 341–348.

Haley, S. M., Coster, W. J., Andres, P. L., Ludlow, L. H., Ni, P., Bond, T. L., et al. (2004). Activity outcome measurement for postacute care. *Medical Care, 42*(1 Suppl.), I49–I61.

Haley, S., Coster, W., Ludlow, L., Haltiwanger, J., & Andrellos, P. (1992). *Pediatric Evaluation of Disability Inventory—Development, standardization and administration Manual.* Boston: PEDI Research Group.

Hall, K. M., Dijkers, M., Whiteneck, G., Brooks, C. A., & Krause, J. S. (1998). The Craig Handicap Assessment and Reporting Technique (CHART): Metric properties and scoring. *Topics in Spinal Cord Injury Rehabilitation, 4*(1), 16–30.

Hall, K., Mann, N., High, W., Wright, J., Kreutzer, J., & Wood, D. (1996). Functional measures after traumatic brain injury: Ceiling effects of FIM, FIM+FAM, DRS, and CIQ. *Journal of Head Trauma Rehabilitation, 11*(5), 27–39.

Hallgren, M., & Kottorp, A. (2005). Effects of occupational therapy intervention on activities of daily living and awareness of disability in persons with intellectual disabilities. *Australian Occupational Therapy Journal, 52,* 350–359.

Hamilton, B., Granger, C., Sherwin, F., Zielezny, M., & Tashman, M. (1987). A uniform national data system for medical rehabilitation. In M. Fuhrer (Ed.), *Rehabilitation outcomes: Analysis and measurement* (pp. 137–147). Baltimore: Paul H. Brookes.

Hamm, E. M. (2006). Playfulness and the environmental support of play in children with and without disabilities. *OTJR: Occupation, Participation and Health, 26*, 88–96.

Hansson, L., & Bjorkman, T. (2007). Are factors associated with subjective quality of life in people with severe mental illness consistent over time? A 6-year follow-up study. *Quality of Life Research, 16*(1), 9–16.

Hansson, H., Rundberg, J., Zetterlind, U., Johnsson, K. O., & Berglund, M. (2007). Two-year outcome of an intervention program for university students who have parents with alcohol problems: A randomized controlled trial. *Alcoholism: Clinical and Experimental Research, 31*(11), 1927–1933.

Harkness, L., & Bundy, A. C. (2001). The test of playfulness and children with physical disabilities. *OTJR: Occupation, Participation and Health, 21*, 73–89.

Harper, K., Stalker, C. A., & Templeton, G. (2006). The use and validity of the Canadian Occupational Performance Measure in a posttraumatic stress program. *OTJR: Occupation, Participation and Health, 26*, 45–55.

Harrison, H., & Kielhofner, G. (1986). Examining reliability and validity of the Preschool Play Scale with handicapped children. *American Journal of Occupational Therapy, 40*, 167–173.

Henderson, S. (1980). A development in social psychiatry: The systematic study of social bonds. *Journal of Nervous and Mental Diseases, 168*, 63–69.

Henderson, S., Byrne, D., & Duncan-Jones, P. (1981). *Neurosis and the social environment*. New York: Academic Press.

Henderson, S., Duncan-Jones, P., Byrne, D., & Scott, R. (1980). Measuring social relationships: The Interview Schedule for Social Interaction. *Psychological Medicine, 10*, 723–734.

Hertanu, J., Demopoulos, J., Yang, W., Calhoun, W., & Fenigstein, H. (1984). Stroke rehabilitation: Correlation and prognostic value of computerized tomography and sequential functional assessments. *Archives of Physical Medicine and Rehabilitation, 65*, 505–508.

Hoenig, H., Hoff, J., McIntyre, L., & Branch, L. (2001). The Self-Reported Functional Measure: Predictive validity for health utilization in multiple sclerosis and spinal cord injury. *Archives of Physical Medicine and Rehabilitation, 82*(5), 613–618.

Hogan, K., & Park, J. (2000). Family factors and social support in the developmental outcomes of very low-birth weight children. *Clinics in Perinatology, 27*(2), 433–459.

Holbrook, M., & Skilbeck, C. (1983). An activities index for use with stroke. *Age and Ageing, 12*, 166–170.

Holm, M., & Rogers, J. (1999). Performance assessment of self-care skills. In B. Hemphill-Pearson (Ed.), *Assessments in occupational therapy mental health: An integrated approach*. Thorofare, NJ: Slack.

Hoogerduijn, J. G., Schuurmans, M. J., Duijnstee, M. S. H., de Rooij, S. E., & Grypdonck, M. F. H. (2007). A systematic review of predictors and screening instruments to identify older hospitalized clients at risk for functional decline. *Journal of Clinical Nursing, 16*(1), 46–57.

Hsieh, C., & Hsueh, I. (1999). A cross validation of the comprehensive assessment of activities of daily living after stroke. *Scandinavian Journal of Rehabilitation Medicine, 31*, 83–88.

Hsu, W. L., Pan, A. W., & Chen, T. J. (2008). A psychometric study of the Chinese version of the Assessment of Communication and Interaction Skills. *Occupational Therapy in Health Care, 22*(2–3), 177–185.

Hsueh, I. P., Huang, S. L., Chen, M. H., Jush, S. D., & Hsieh, C. L. (2000). Evaluation of survivors of stroke with the extended activities of daily living scale in Taiwan. *Disability and Rehabilitation, 22*, 495–500.

Hwang, J. L. (2005). The reliability and validity of the School Function Assessment–Chinese version. *OTJR: Occupation, Participation and Health, 25*, 44–54.

Imms, C. (2008). Review of the Children's Assessment of Participation and Enjoyment (CAPE) and the Preferences of Activity of Children (PAC). *Physical and Occupational Therapy in Pediatrics, 28*(4), 389–404.

Jankovich, M., Mullen, J., Rinear, E., Tanta, K., & Deitz, J. (2008). Revised Knox Preschool Play Scale: Interrater agreement and construct validity. *American Journal of Occupational Therapy, 62*, 221–227.

Jansa, J., Pogacnik, T., & Gompertz, P. (2004). An evaluation of the extended Barthel Index with acute ischemic stroke patients. *Neurorehabilitation and Neural Repair, 18*, 37–41.

Jenkinson, C., Wright, L., & Coulter, A. (1994). Criterion validity and reliability of the SF-36 in a population sample. *Quality of Life Research, 3*(1), 7–12.

Johansson, A., Mishina, E., Ivanov, A., & Bjorklund, A. (2007). Activities of daily living among St. Petersburg women after mild stroke. *Occupational Therapy International, 13*, 170–182.

Kanters, M. (1995, October). *Leisure satisfaction, stress, and health*. Unpublished paper presented at the Leisure Research Symposium.

Katz, L., Beers, S., Geckle, M., & Goldstein, G. (1989). The clinical use of the Career Ability Placement Survey versus the GATB for persons having psychiatric disabilities. *Journal of Applied Rehabilitation Counseling, 20*(1), 13–19.

Katz, N., Karpin, H., Lak A., Furman, T., & Hartman-Maeir, A. (2003). Participation in occupational performance: Reliability and validity of the Activity Card Sort. *OTJR: Occupation, Participation and Health, 23*(1), 10–17.

Katz, S., Downs, T., Cash, H., & Grotz, R. (1970). Progress in development of an Index of ADL. *Gerontologist, 10*, 20–30.

Katz, S., Ford, A. B., Moskowitz, M., Jackson, B. A., & Jaffe, M. W. (1963). Studies of illness in the aged. The index of ADL: A standardized measure of biological and psychosocial function. *Journal of the American Medical Association, 185*, 914–919.

Ketelaar, M., Vermeer, A., & Helders, P. (1998). Functional motor abilities of children with cerebral palsy: A systematic literature review of assessment measures. *Clinical Rehabilitation, 12*, 369–380.

King, G. A., Law, M., King, S., Hurley, P., Rosenbaum, P., Hanna, S., et al. (2004). *Children's assessment of participation and enjoyment and preferences for activities of kids.* San Antonio, TX: Pearson/Psych-Corp.

Kinnman, J., Andersson, U., Wetterquist, L., Kinnman, Y., & Andersson, U. (2000). Cooling suit for multiple sclerosis: Functional improvement in daily living? *Scandinavian Journal of Rehabilitation Medicine, 32,* 20–24.

Kloseck, M., & Crilly, R. (1997). *Leisure competence measure: Adult version.* London, Ontario: Data System.

Kloseck, M., Crilly, R., & Hutchinson-Troyer, L. (2001). Measuring outcomes in rehabilitation: Further reliability and validity testing of the Leisure Competence Measure. *Therapeutic Recreation Journal, 1,* 31–42.

Knapp, L., Knapp, R., & Knapp-Lee, L. (1992). *Career Ability Placement Survey manual.* San Diego: Educational and Industrial Testing Service.

Knapp, L., Knapp, R., & Michael, W. (1977). Stability and concurrent validity of the Career Ability Placement Survey (CAPS) against the DAP and GATB. *Educational and Psychological Measurement, 37,* 1081–1085.

Knapp, L., Knapp, R., Strand, L. I., & Michael, W. (1978). Comparative validity of the Career Ability Placement Survey and the GATB for predicting high school course marks. *Educational and Psychological Measurement, 38,* 1053–1056.

Knapp-Lee, L. (1995). Use of the COP System in career assessment. *Journal of Career Assessment, 3*(4), 411–428.

Knox, S. (1974). A play scale. In M. Reilly (Ed.), *Play as exploratory learning* (pp. 247–266). Beverly Hills, CA: Sage.

Knox, S. (1997). Development and current use of the Knox Preschool Play Scale. In L. D. Parham & L. S. Fazio (Eds.), *Play in occupational therapy for children* (pp. 35–51). St. Louis, MO: Mosby.

Kottorp, A. (2008). The use of Assessment and Motor Process Skills (AMPS) in predicting need assistance for adults with mental retardation. *OTJR: Occupation, Participation and Health, 28,* 72–80.

Kotzer, A. M. (2008). Defining an evidenced-based work environment for nursing in the USA. *Journal of Clinical Nursing, 17,* 1652–1659.

Kotzer, A. M., Koepping, D. M., & LeDuc, K. (2006). Perceived nursing work environment of acute care pediatric nurses. *Pediatric Nursing, 32,* 327–332.

Kwakkel, G., Kollen, B., & Wagenaar, R. J. (2002). Long-term effects of intensity of upper and lower limb training after stroke: A randomized trial. *Journal of Neurology, Neurosurgery, and Psychiatry, 72,* 473–479.

Lange, B., Spagnolo, K., & Fowler, B. (2009). Using the Assessment of Motor and Process Skills to measure functional change in adults with severe traumatic brain injury: A pilot study. *Australian Occupational Therapy Journal, 56,* 89–96.

Law, M., Baptiste, S., Carswell, A., McColl, M. A., Polatajko, H., & Pollock, N. (1993). *COPM user survey.* Unpublished manuscript, McMaster University, School of Rehabilitation Science, Hamilton. Ontario.

Law, M., Baptiste, S., Carswell, A., McColl, M. A., Polatajko, H., & Pollock, N. (2005). *Canadian Occupational Performance Measure* (4th ed.). Ottawa, Ontario: CAOT Publications.

Law, M., Baptiste, S., McColl, M. A., Opzoomer, A., Polatajko, H., & Pollock, N. (1994). The Canadian Occupational Performance Measure: An outcome measure for occupational therapy. *Canadian Journal of Occupational Therapy, 57,* 82–87.

Law, M., Polotajko, H., Pollock, N., McColl, M., Carswell, A., & Baptiste, S. (1994). Pilot testing of the Canadian Occupational Performance Measure: Clinical and measurement issues. *Canadian Journal of Occupational Therapy, 61,* 191–197.

Law, M., Russell, D., Pollock, N., Rosenbaum, P., Walter, S., & G., K. (1997). A comparison of intensive neurodevelopmental therapy plus casting and a regular occupational therapy program for children with cerebral palsy. *Developmental Medicine and Child Neurology, 39,* 664–670.

Law, M., Wishart, L., & Guyatt, G. J, (2000). The use of a simulated environment (Easy Street) to retrain independent living skills in elderly persons: A randomized controlled trial. *Journal of Gerontology (Medical Sciences), 55,* M578–M584.

Lennon, O., Carey, A., Gaffney, N., & Stephenson, J. (2008). A pilot randomized controlled trial to evaluate the benefit of the cardiac rehabilitation paradigm for the non-acute ischaemic stroke population. *Clinical Rehabilitation, 22,* 125–133.

Letts, L., & Marshall, L. (1995). Evaluating the validity and consistency of the SAFER tool. *Physical and Occupational Therapy in Geriatrics, 13,* 49–66.

Letts, L., Scott, S., Burtney, J., Marshall, L., & McKean, M. (1998). The reliability and validity of the Safety Assessment of Function and the Environment for Rehabilitation (SAFER) Tool. *British Journal of Occupational Therapy, 61,* 127–132.

Lino, V. T. S., Pereira, S. R. M., Camacho, L. A., Ribeiro, S. T., & Buksman, S. (2008). Cross-cultural adaptation of the Independence in activities of daily living index (Katz index). *Cadernos De Saude Publica, 24*(1), 103–112.

Liu, K. P, Chan, C. C., Chu, M. M. Chu, L. W., Hui, F. S., Yuen, H. K., et al. (2007). Activities of daily living performance in dementia. *Acta Neurologica Scandinavica, 116,* 91–95.

Lloyd, K., & Auld, C. (2002). The role of leisure in determining quality of life: Issues of content and measurement. *Social Indicators Research, 57,* 43–71.

Ludlow, L., & Haley, S. (1996). Effect of context in rating of mobility activities in children with disabilities: An assessment using the Pediatric Evaluation of Disability Inventory. *Education and Psychological Measurement, 56*(1), 122–129.

Lundgren-Nilsson, A., Grimby, G., Ring, H., Tesio, L., Lawton, G., & Slade, A., (2005). Cross-cultural validity of Functional Independence Measure items in stroke: A study using Rasch analysis. *Journal of Rehabilitation Medicine, 37*(1), 23–31.

Magasi, S. R., Heinemann, A. W., & Whiteneck, G. G. (2008). Participation following traumatic spinal cord injury: An evidenced-based review for research. *Journal of Spinal Cord Medicine, 31,* 145–156.

Mahoney, F., & Barthel, D. (1965). Functional evaluation: The Barthel Index. *Maryland State Medical Journal, 14,* 56–61.

Mainieri, T. (2006). *The panel study of income dynamics: Child development supplement—User Guide for CDS II.* Ann Arbor: Institute for Social Research, University of Michigan.

Mant, J., Carter, J., Wade. D. T., & Winner, S. (2000). Family support for stroke: A randomized controlled trial. *Lancet, 356,* 808–813.

McColl, M., Davies, D., Carlson, P., Johnston, J., & Minnes, P. (2001). The community integration measures: Development and preliminary validation. *Archives of Physical Medicine and Rehabilitation, 82,* 429–434.

McColl, M., Law, M., Stewart, D., Doubt, L., Pollock, N., & Krupa, T. (2003). *Theoretical basis of occupational therapy* (2nd ed.). Thorofare, NJ: Slack.

McDowell, I. (2006). *Measuring health: A guide to rating scales and questionnaires.* New York: Oxford University Press.

McDowell, I., & Newell, C. (1996). *Measuring health: A guide to rating scales and questionnares.* New York: Oxford University Press.

McNulty, M., & Fisher, A. (2000). Validity of using the assessment of motor and process skills to estimate overall home safety in persons with psychiatric conditions. *American Journal of Occupational Therapy, 55,* 649–655.

Mercier, L., Audet, T., Hebert, R., Rochette, A., & Dubois, M. F. (2001). Impact of motor, cognitive, and perceptual disorders on ability to perform activities of daily living after stroke. *Stroke, 32,* 2602–2608.

Messier, J., Ferland, F., & Majnemer, A. (2008). Play behavior of school age children with intellectual disability: Their capacities, interests, and attitude. *Journal of Developmental and Physical Disabilities, 20,* 193–207.

Middelkamp, W., Moulaert, V. R., Verbunt, J. A., van Heugten, C. M., Bakx, W. B., & Wade, D. T. (2007). Life after survival: Long-term daily life functioning and quality of life of patients with hypoxic brain injury as a result of a cardiac arrest. *Clinical Rehabilitation, 21,* 425–431.

Miller, W. C., Deathe, A. B., & Harris, J. (2004). Measurement properties of the Frenchay Activities Index among individuals with lower limb amputation. *Clinical Rehabilitation, 18,* 414–422.

Moore, D. J., Palmer, B. W., Patterson, T. L., & Jeste, D. V. (2007). A review of performance-based measures of functional living skills. *Journal of Psychiatric Research, 41,* 97–118.

Moos, R. (1981). *A social climate scale: Work Environment Scale manual.* Palo Alto, CA: Consulting Psychologists Press.

Moos, R. (1993). *Work Environment Scale: An annotated bibliography.* Palo Alto, CA: Stanford University Medical Center.

Moos, R. (1994). Work as a human context. In M. Pallack & R. Perloff (Eds.), *Psychology and work—Productivity, change, and employment* (Vol. 5, pp. 9–52). Washington, DC: American Psychological Association.

Moos, R., & Moos, B. (1998). The staff workplace and the quality and outcome of substance abuse treatment. *Journal of Studies on Alcohol, 59,* 43–51.

Morris, P. L. P., Robinson, R. G., Raphael, B., & Bishop, D. P. (1991). The relationship between the perception of social support and post-stroke depression in hospitalized patients. *Psychiatry, 54,* 306–316.

Morrison, C., Bundy, A., & Fisher, A. G. (1991). The contribution of motor skills and playfulness to play performance of preschool aged children. *American Journal of Occupational Therapy, 45,* 687–694.

Munkholm, M., & Fisher, A. (2008). Students with mild disabilities demonstrate lower quality of schoolwork performance as measured by School AMPS compared to typically developing students. *Australian Occupational Therapy Journal, 56,* 293–296.

Muys, V., Rodger, S., & Bundy, A. C. (2006). Assessment of playfulness in children with autistic disorder: A comparison of the Children's Playfulness Scale and the Test of Playfulness. *OTJR: Occupation, Participation and Health, 26,* 159–170.

Naik, A. D., Burnett, J., Pickens-Pace, S., & Dyer, C. B. (2008). Impairment of instrumental activities of daily living and the geriatric syndrome of self-neglect. *The Gerontologist, 48,* 388–393.

Nouri, F., & Lincoln, N. (1987). An extended activities of daily living scale for survivors of stroke. *Clinical Rehabilitation, 1,* 301–305.

Novak, I., Cusick, A., & Lowe, K. (2007). A pilot study on the impact of occupational therapy home programming for young children with cerebral palsy. *American Journal of Occupational Therapy, 61,* 463–468.

Ogonowski, J. A., Kronk, R. A., Rice, C. N., & Feldman, H. M. (2004). Inter-rater reliability in assigning *ICF* codes to children with disabilities. *Disability and Rehabilitation, 26,* 353–361.

Oliver, R., Blathwayt, J., Brackley, C., & Tamaki, T. (1993). Development of the Safety Assessment of Function and Environment for Rehabilitation (SAFER) Tool. *Canadian Journal of Occupational Therapy, 60,* 78–82.

Ottenbacher, K., Hsu, Y., Granger, C., & Fiedler, R. (1996). The reliability of the Functional Independence Measure: A quantitative review. *Archives of Physical Medicine and Rehabilitation, 77,* 1226–1232.

Ottenbacher, K., Taylor, E., Msall, M., Braun, S., Lane, S., Granger, C., et al. (1996). The stability and equivalence reliability of the functional independence measure for children (WeeFIM)®. *Developmental Medicine and Child Neurology, 38*(10), 907–916.

Ottenbacher, K., Msall, M., Lyon, N., Duffy, L., Granger, C. V., & Braun, S. (1997). Interrater agreement and stability of the functional independence measure for children (WeeFIM™): Use in children with developmental disabilities. *Archives of Physical Medicine and Rehabilitation, 78*(12), 1309–1315.

Ottenbacher, K., Msall, M., Lyon, N., Duffy, L., Granger, C., & Braun, S. (1999). Measuring developmental and functional status in children with disabilities. *Developmental Medicine and Child Neurology, 41*(3), 186–194.

Pan, A. W., Chung, L., & Hsin-Hwei, G. (2003). Reliability and validity of the Canadian Occupational Performance Measure for clients with psychiatric disorders in Taiwan. *Occupational Therapy International, 10,* 269–277.

Pearson Education. (2008). *Technical Report: School Function Assessment.* Old Tappan, NJ: Author.

Pickens, S., Naik, A. D., Burnett, J., Kelly, P. A., Gleason, M., & Dyer C. B. (2007). The utility of the KELS test in substantiated cases of elder self-neglect. *Journal of the American Academy of Nurse Practitioners, 19,* 137–142.

Piercy, M., Carter, J., Mant, J., & Wade, D. T. (2000). Inter-rater reliability of the Frenchay Activities Index in patients with stroke and their carers. *Clinical Rehabilitation, 14,* 433–440.

Prosiegel, M., Boettger, S., Give, T., Koenig, N., Marolf, M., Vaney, C., et al., (1996). The Extended Barthel Index—A new scale for the assessment of disability in neurological patients. *Neurorehabilitation, 1,* 7–13.

Raj, J. T., Manigandan, C., & Jacob, K. S. (2006). Leisure satisfaction and psychiatric morbidity among informal carers of people with spinal cord injury. *Spinal Cord, 44,* 676–679.

Reid, D. (2005). Correlation of the Pediatric Volitional Questionnaire with the Test of Playfulness in a virtual environment: The power of engagement. *Early Child Development and Care, 175,* 153–164.

Reijneveld, S. A., Spijker, J., & Dijkshoorn, H. (2007). Katz' ADL index assessed functional performance of Turkish, Moroccan, and Dutch elderly. *Journal of Clinical Epidemiology, 60*(4), 382–388.

Reistetter, T. A., Spencer, J. C., Trujillo, L., & Abreu, B. C. (2002). Examining the Community Integration Measure (CIM): A replication study with life satisfaction. *NeuroRehabilitation, 20*(2), 139–148.

Ripat, J., Etcheverry, E., Cooper, J., & Tate, R. (2001). A comparison of the Canadian Occupational Performance Measure and the Health Assessment Questionnaire. *Canadian Journal of Occupational Therapy, 68,* 247–253.

Rochman, D. L., Ray, S. A., Kulich, R. J., Mehta, N. R., & Driscoll, S. (2008). Validity and utility of the Canadian occupational performance measure as an outcome measure in a craniofacial pain center. *OTJR: Occupation, Participation and Health, 28,* 4–11.

Rockwood, K., Joyce, B., & Stolee, P. (1997). Use of goal attainment scaling in measuring clinically important change in cognitive rehabilitation patients. *Journal of Clinical Epidemiology, 50,* 581–588.

Rodger, S., & Ziviani, J. (1999). Play-based occupational therapy. *International Journal of Disability, Development and Education, 46,* 337–365.

Rogers, J., & Holm, M. (1994). *Performance Assessment of Self Care Skills (PASS).* Pittsburgh: University of Pittsburgh.

Rogers, J. C., & Holm, M. B. (2000). Daily-living skills and habits of older women with depression. *Occupational Therapy Journal of Research, 20,* 68S–85S.

Rogers, J., Holm, M., Beach, S., Schulz, R., Cipriani, J., Fox, A., et al. (2003). Concordance of four methods of disability assessment using performance in the home as the criterion method. *Arthritis and Rheumatism— Arthritis Care and Research, 49*(5), 640–647.

Rogers, J., Holm, M., Beach, S., Schulz, R., & Starz, T. (2001). Task independence, safety, and adequacy among nondisabled and osteoarthritis—Disabled older women. *Arthritis and Rheumatism, 45*(5), 410–418.

Rogers, J., Holm, M., Goldstein, G., McCue, M., & Nussbaum, P. (1994). Stability and change in functional assessment of patients with geropsychiatric disorders. *American Journal of Occupational Therapy, 48*(10), 914–918.

Ruch, W., & Stang, S. (1994). *Employee Aptitude Survey examiner's manual* (2nd ed.). Glendale, CA: Psychological Services.

Ryan, C. A., Stiell, K. M., Gailey, G. F. & Makinen, J. A. (2008). Evaluating a family-centered approach to leisure education and community reintegration following a stroke. *Therapeutic Recreation Journal, 2,* 119–131.

Salamy, M. (1993). *Construct validity of the assessment for communication and interaction skills.* Unpublished master's thesis, University of Illinois, Chicago.

Salter, K., Foley, N., Jutai, J. Bayley, M., & Teasell, R. (2008). Assessment of community integration following traumatic brain injury. *Brain Injury, 22*(11), 820–835.

Samsa, G., Hoenig, H., & Branch, L. (2001). Relationship between self-reported disability and caregiver hours. *Archives of Physical Medicine and Rehabilitation, 80*(9), 674–684.

Schenker, R., Coster, W., & Parush, S. (2006). Personal assistance, adaptations, and participation in students with cerebral palsy mainstreamed in elementary schools. *Disability and Rehabilitation, 28,* 1061–1069.

Schoenmakers, M. A., Uiterwaal, C. S., Gulmans, V. A., Gooskens, R. H., & Helders, P. J. (2005). Determinants of functional independence and quality of life in children with spina bifida. *Clinical Rehabilitation, 19,* 677–85.

Schuling, J., Dehaan, R., Limburg, M., & Groenier, K. (1993). The Frenchay Activities Index: Assessment of functional status in stroke patients. *Stroke, 24,* 1173–1177.

Searle, M., Mahon, M., Iso-Ahola, S., & Sdrolias, H. (1998). Examining the long-term effects of leisure education on a sense of independence and psychological well-being among the elderly. *Journal of Leisure Research, 30*(3), 331–340.

Segal, M. E., & Schall, R. R. (1995). Assessing handicap of stroke survivors. A validation study of the Craig Handicap Assessment and Reporting Technique. *American Journal of Physical Medicine and Rehabilitation, 74,* 276–286.

Sewell, L., & Singh, S. (2001). The Canadian Occupational Performance Measure: Is it a reliable measure in clients with chronic obstructive pulmonary disease? *British Journal of Occupational Therapy, 64*(6), 305–310.

Shepers, V. P., Ketelaar, M., Visser-Meily, J. M., Dekker, J., & Lindeman, E. (2006). Responsiveness of functional health status measures frequently used in stroke research. *Disability and Rehabilitation, 28,* 1038–1040.

Silverman, M. K., & Smith, R. O. (2006). Consequential validity of an assistive technology supplement for the School Function Assessment. *Assistive Technology, 18,* 155–165.

Simmons, D., Crepeau, E., & White, B. (2000). The predictive power of narrative data in occupational therapy evaluation. *American Journal of Occupational Therapy, 54,* 471–476.

Simon, S. (1989). *The development of an assessment for communication and interaction skills.* Unpublished master's thesis, University of Illinois, Chicago.

Skard, G., & Bundy, A. C. (2008). Play and playfulness. In L. D. Parham & L. S. Fazio (Eds.), *Play in occupational therapy for children* (2nd ed., pp. 71–93). St. Louis, MO: Mosby.

Srsen, K. G., Vidmar, G., & Zupan, A. (2005). Applicability of the pediatric evaluation of disability inventory in Slovenia. *Journal of Child Neurology, 20*(5), 411–416.

Stebbins, R. A. (1997). Casual leisure: A conceptual statement. *Leisure Studies, 16,* 17–25.

Stebbins, R. A. (2005). Research reflections: Choice and experiential definitions of leisure. *Leisure Studies, 27,* 349–352.

Strain, L., Grabusic, C., Searle, M., & Dunn, N. (2002). Continuing and ceasing leisure activities in later life: A longitudinal study. *Gerontologist, 42,* 217–223.

Teel, C., Dunn, W. W., Jackson, S., & Duncan, P. (1997). The role of the environment in fostering independence: Conceptual and methodological issues in developing an instrument. *Topics in Stroke Rehabilitation, 4*(1), 28–40.

Tham, K., Ginsburg, E., Fisher, A. G., & Tegner, R. (2001). Training to improve awareness of disabilities in clients with unilateral neglect. *American Journal of Occupational Therapy, 55,* 46–54.

Thomas, P. D., Garry, P. J., Goodwin, J. M., & Goodwin, J. S. (1985). Social bonds in a healthy elderly sample: Characteristics and associated variables. *Social Science and Medicine, 20,* 365–369.

Thomas-Stonell, N., Johnson, P., Rumney, P., Wright, V., & Oddson, B. (2006). An evaluation of the responsiveness of a comprehensive set of outcome measures for children and adolescents with traumatic brain injuries. *Pediatric Rehabilitation, 9,* 14–2.

Thomson, L. K. (1992). *Kohlman Evaluation of Living Skills* (3rd ed.). Bethesda, MD: American Occupational Therapy Association.

Thomson, L. K. (1999). The Kohlman Evaluation of Living Skills. In B. Hemphill (Ed.), *Assessments in occupational therapy mental health: An integrative approach* (pp. 231–242). Thorofare, NJ: Slack.

Toomey, M., Nicholson, D., & Carswell, A. (1995). The clinical utility of the Canadian Occupational Performance Measure. *Canadian Journal of Occupational Therapy, 62,* 242–249.

Tooth, L. R., McKenna, K. T., Smith, M., & O'Rourke, P. K. (2003). Reliability of scores between stroke patients and significant others on the Reintegration to Normal Living (RNL) Index. *Disability and Rehabilitation, 25,* 433–440.

Trombly, C., Radomski, M., & Davis, E. (1998). Achievement of self-identified goals by adults with traumatic brain injury: Phase I. *American Journal of Occupational Therapy, 52,* 810–818.

Turnbull, J., Kersten, P., Habib, M., McLellan, D., Mullee, M., & George, S. (2000). Validation of the Frenchay Activities Index in a general population aged 16 and over. *Archives of Physical Medicine and Rehabilitation, 81,* 1034–1038.

Uniform Data System for Medical Rehabilitation. (1990). *Guide for the use of the pediatric functional independence measure.* Buffalo: Research Foundation—State University of New York.

Uniform Data System for Medical Rehabilitation. (2005). *The WeeFIM II™ System Clinical Guide, version 6.0.* Buffalo, NY: Author.

U.S. Department of Labor. (1991). *Revised handbook for analyzing jobs.* Washington, DC: U.S. Government Printing Office.

Van Baalen, B., Ribbers, G. M., Medema-Meulepas, D., Pas, M. S., Odding, E., & Stam, H. J. (2007). Being restricted in participation after a traumatic brain injury is negatively associated by passive coping style with the caregiver. *Brain Injury, 21,* 925–931.

Verkerk, G. J., Wolf, M. J., Louwers, A. M., Meester-Delver, A., & Nollet, F. (2006). The reproducibility and validity of the Canadian Occupational Performance Measure in parents of children with disabilities. *Clinical Rehabilitation, 20,* 980–988.

Wade, D. (1992). *Measurement in neurological rehabilitation.* Oxford, England: Oxford University Press.

Waehrens, E. E., & Fisher, A. G. (2007). Improving quality of ADL performance after rehabilitation among people with acquired brain injury. *Scandinavian Journal of Occupational Therapy, 14,* 250–257.

Wang, E. S., Chen, L. S., Lin, J. Y., & Wang, M. C. (2008). The relationship between leisure satisfaction and the satisfaction of adolescents concerning online games. *Adolescence, 43,* 177–184.

Ware, J. E., & Sherbourne, C. D. (1992). The MOS 36-item Short Form Health Survey: Conceptual framework and item selection. *Medical Care, 30*(6), 473–483.

Whiteneck, G. G., Charlifue, S. W., Gerhart, K. A., Overholser, J. D., & Richardson, G. N. (1992). Quantifying handicap: A new measure of long-term rehabilitation outcomes. *Archives of Physical Medicine and Rehabilitation, 73,* 519–526.

Willer, B., Linn, R., & Allen, K. (1993). Community integration and barriers to integration for individuals with brain injury. In M. Finlayson & S. Garner (Eds.), *Brain injury rehabilitation: Clinical considerations.* Baltimore: Williams & Wilkins.

Willer, B. S., Ottenbacher, K. J., & Coad, M. L. (1994). The Community Integration Questionnaire: A comparative examination. *American Journal of Physical Medicine and Rehabilitation, 73*(2), 103–111.

Willer, B., Rosenthal, M., Kreutzer, J., Gordon, W., & Rempel, R. (1993). Assessment of community integration following rehabilitation for traumatic brain injury. *Journal of Head Trauma Rehabilitation, 8,* 75–87.

Witt, P. A. (1990, May). *Overview and conclusions based on recent studies using the Leisure Diagnostic Battery.* Proceedings of the Sixth Canadian Congress on Leisure Research, Waterloo, Ontario.

Witt, P. A., & Ellis, G. (1989). *The Leisure Diagnostic Battery: User's manual.* State College, PA: Venture.

Wong, S. S. N., & Wong, V. C. N. (2007). Functional Independence Measure for Children: A comparison of Chinese and Japanese children. *Neurorehabilitation and Neural Repair, 21,* 91–96.

Wong, V., Trevor, Y. C., & Law, P. K. (2005). Correlation of Functional Independence Measure for Children (WeeFIM) with developmental language tests in children with developmental delay. *Journal of Child Neurology, 7,* 613–616.

Wood-Dauphinee, S., Opzoomer, A., Williams, J., Marchand, B., & Spitzer, W. (1988). Assessment of global function: The reintegration to normal living index. *Archives of Physical Medicine and Rehabilitation, 69,* 583–590.

Wood-Dauphinee, S., & Willliams, J. (1987). Reintegration to normal living as proxy to quality of life. *Journal of Chronic Diseases, 40,* 491–499.

Woodson, A. M. (2008). Stroke. In M. V. Radomski & C. A. Latham (Eds.), *Occupational therapy for physical dysfunction* (6th ed., pp. 1002–1041). Philadelphia: Lippincott Williams & Wilkins.

World Health Organization. (1997). *International classification of impairments, disabilities and handicaps.* Geneva: Author.

World Health Organization. (2001). *International classification of functioning, disability and health.* Geneva: Author.

Wressle, E., Eeg-Olofsson, A., Marcusson, J., & Henriksson, C. (2002). Improved client participation in the rehabilitation process using a client-centered goal formulation structure. *Journal of Rehabilitation Medicine, 34,* 5–11.

Wright, F. V., Boschen, K., & Jutai, J. (2005). Exploring the comparative responsiveness of a core set of outcome measures in a school-based conductive education programme. *Childcare, Health, and Development, 31,* 291–302.

Wylie, C., & White, B. (1964). A measure of disability. *Archives of Environmental Health, 8,* 834–839.

Young, J., Bogle, S., & Forster, A. (2001). Determinants of social outcome measured by the Frenchay Activities Index at one year after stroke onset. *Cerebrovascular Diseases, 12,* 114–120.

Young, Y., Fan, M. Y., Hebel, J. R., & Boult, C. (2009). Concurrent validity of administering the Functional Independence Measure (FIM) instrument by interview. *American Journal of Physical Medicine and Rehabilitation, 9,* 766–770.

Zhang, L., Abreu, B. C., Gonzales, V., Seale, G., Masel, B., & Ottenbacher, K. J. (2002). Comparison of the community integration questionnaire, the Craig Handicap Assessment and Reporting Technique and the Disability Rating Scale in traumatic head injury. *Journal of Head Trauma Rehabilitation, 17,* 497–509.

Zimnavoda, T., Weinblatt, N., & Katz, N., (2002). Validity of the Kohlman Evaluation of Living Skills (KELS) with Israeli elderly individuals living in the community. *Occupational Therapy International, 9,* 312–325.

Ziviani, J., Rodger, S., & Peters, S. (2005). The play behavior of children with and without autistic disorder in a clinical environment. *New Zealand Journal of Occupational Therapy, 52,* 22–30.

Chapter 4

Planning Intervention

PENELOPE A. MOYERS CLEVELAND, EdD, OTR/L, BCMH, FAOTA

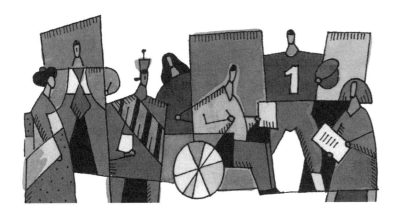

KEY TERMS

electronic documentation

ICF

intervention approach

intervention plan

intervention type

occupational performance

outcome

problem statement

professional reasoning

HIGHLIGHTS

- The intervention process is divided into three parts: (1) creating the intervention plan, (2) implementing the intervention, and (3) intervention review.

- In planning intervention, therapists should avoid oversimplification and seek to use digital documentation systems that support decision making.

- The occupational performance problem statement should identify intervention needs and priorities identified by the client.

- A careful consideration of how the client's context influences health, performance, and participation should guide intervention goal setting.

- The intervention plan normally includes objective and measurable goals that can be accomplished in a given timeframe, the occupational therapy intervention approach and types of intervention, the mechanism of service delivery, the discharge plan, the chosen outcome measures, and recommendations or referrals to others as needed.

- Main approaches in an intervention plan typically include create and promote (health promotion), establish and restore (remediation and restoration), maintain and modify (compensation and adaptation), and prevent (disability prevention).
- Careful selection of outcome measures is key to documenting goal attainment and can influence payment for services.

OBJECTIVES

After reading this material, readers will be able to

- Appreciate the difference between independence and interdependence;
- Understand that intervention planning requires careful professional reasoning;
- List the elements of the intervention plan;
- Understand the difference between intervention approaches and types of intervention;
- Identify and understand the distinctions among the various intervention approaches—create and promote, establish and restore, maintain, modify, and prevent;
- Appreciate the need for client and caregiver collaboration throughout the intervention planning process;
- Write appropriate intervention goals, including all the necessary elements;
- Delineate the criteria for selecting outcome measures; and
- Understand the importance of theory and use of evidence-based information in selecting intervention approaches and types of intervention.

This chapter describes the client-centered and evidence-based occupational therapy processes that are integral to intervention planning. The *Occupational Therapy Practice Framework: Domain and Process* (2nd ed., American Occupational Therapy Association [AOTA], 2008), hereinafter referred to as the *Framework*, provides the terminology that guides intervention planning. The World Health Organization's (2001) *International Classification of Functioning, Disability and Health (ICF)* prompts the occupational therapist to focus intervention planning on the client's need to sustain health through engagement in activity and participation in various contexts (see Table 4.1).

Also in this chapter, the occupational areas of activities of daily living (ADLs), rest and sleep, and instrumental activities of daily living (IADLs) are highlighted in the discussion of intervention planning. There is also discussion of new electronic documentation systems and innovative knowledge-based systems and how they may affect occupational therapists' professional reasoning. The focus is on improving the efficiency and effectiveness of intervention planning so client outcomes are more likely to be achieved.

Support of Professional Reasoning

There are considerable differences in the ways occupational therapists use professional reasoning strategies to guide the intervention planning process. Tomlin (2008) suggests that experienced therapists may be subject to some bias in their judgments because they rely on past cases that seem similar to their client's situation and on traditional intervention methods—and may be subject to a very human tendency to oversimplify. Using cognitive shortcuts or heuristics to process potential overload is particularly attractive to a therapist who has large caseloads and limited time. Data-entry methods that reduce the therapist's reliance on past interactions may be a solution, for example, handheld devices that allow immediate data entry instead of paper evaluation forms. Such electronic documentation systems, however, can lead in their own way to oversimplification if their standardized checklists limit the therapist's ability to attack individual problems with customized interventions.

There is a growing number of requirements that occupational therapists be more accountable by using evidence to support their choices of assessment instruments, outcome instruments, and intervention methods (Von Krogh & Naden, 2008). To address the simultaneous need for efficiency and effectiveness, any electronic documentation process should include a knowledge-based system that supports reasoning (Falvey, Bray, & Hebert, 2005; Vess, 2001; Wang, Cheung, Lee, & Kwok, 2007). Such a system would help the therapist understand underlying factors and how they affect occupational performance, ensuring that the most appropriate intervention plans are consistent with client data.

Decision-making aids should be readily available that show the therapist the relationships among outcomes of specific interventions in given populations. Although this type of system is in its

Table 4.1. World Health Organization (2001) *International Classification of Functioning, Disability and Health*

Parts	Components (Definition)	Positive Aspect	Negative Aspect
Functioning and Disability	Body functions and structures (Physiology and anatomy)	Functional and structural integrity	Impairment
	Activities and participation (Task execution and involvement)	Activities and participation	Activity limitation or participation restriction
Contextual Factors	Environmental factors (Physical, social, attitudinal environments)	Facilitators	Barriers
	Personal factors (Attributes)	Not applicable	Not applicable

early days, AOTA is devising templates that gather data that will become part of a national outcomes database and that inform choices for occupation-based interventions that are consistent with recommended occupational performance outcome measures (Strzelecki, 2009).

Prerequisite to Planning

The goal of occupational therapy is to focus on the occupations and activities that clients have determined they need and want to do (Pierce, 2001). Good intervention planning depends on the therapist having worked through the process of *evaluation*. This involves completing an occupational profile and an in-depth analysis of the occupational performances that the client or client's caregivers indicate are important for improved health and participation in the community (AOTA, 2008). The occupational profile helps the occupational therapist understand the "client's occupational history and experiences, patterns of daily living, interests, values, and needs" (AOTA, 2008, p. 649). It also helps the occupational therapist determine the client's current concerns about performing these important activities, especially inasmuch as engagement in occupation is a key factor in quality of life, health, well-being, and life satisfaction.

During the occupational performance analysis, the occupational therapist observes the client's current performance in a variety of situations, in one or more occupations and activities of concern. He or she notes how the interaction among the person, the activity, and the environment influences performance, community participation, and health (Law, Baum, & Dunn, 2005). The goal is to determine whether the client can engage in occupations in a way that supports health over time and participation in his or her usual living environments, or *contexts* (AOTA, 2008). During the analysis, the therapist notes how the selected activities, when performed in specific environments, make demands on the client's body functions and structures, performance skills, and current habits and routines. Ultimately, the occupational therapist highlights assets and barriers to performance, participation, and health within contexts and social roles.

Identifying Occupational Performance Problems

Based on the evaluation and the reason for the referral to therapy, the therapist formulates an occupational performance problem statement. It succinctly describes the occupational status of a person amenable to intervention—or any health risks related to occupational performance and participation that require prevention or health promotion strategies. The statement involves several elements (Table 4.2). It is imperative to work with the client and caregivers to prioritize the occupations and activities that will guide the intervention (Rogers & Holm, 2009). This list of priorities is perhaps the most significant aspect of the occupational performance problem statement because it is heavily influenced by the social roles that the client values.

For example, the client might demonstrate problems in many ADL areas but prefers to concentrate first on feeding and functional mobility, even though dressing and bathing are also problems. The client might indicate that he or she wants to be able to dine out with family members because that social interaction would provide the motivation to keep working

Table 4.2. Elements of the Occupational Performance Problem Statement

1. Intervention focus or the prioritized occupations and activities, with a descriptor of the problem or potential health issue
   - Loss of independence
   - More assistance needed
   - Loss of safety
   - Decreased efficiency
   - Changed effectiveness.

2. Explanation of the underlying factors contributing to the performance problem or potential health issue and those that may assist in improving performance and health
   - Performance patterns
     - Habits
     - Routines
     - Roles
     - Rituals
   - Performance skills
     - Sensory–perceptual skills
     - Motor and praxis skills
     - Emotional regulation skills
     - Cognitive skills
     - Communication and social skills
   - Client factors
     - Values, beliefs, and spirituality
     - Body functions
     - Body structures
   - Activity demands
     - Objects used and their properties
     - Space and social demands
     - Sequencing and timing
     - Required actions/performance skills
     - Required body functions/body structures.

3. Impact of context on performance in terms of barriers and supports and in terms of standards or criteria for measuring performance and health. Contexts include
   - Cultural
   - Personal
   - Temporal
   - Virtual
   - Physical
   - Social.

on other problem areas later. The client might, therefore, initially need total assistance with dressing and bathing in order to focus on the activities necessary for social participation as a family member.

Given the prioritized list of activities targeted for improvement, the occupational therapist must delineate the skills and patterns needed for performance, the factors contributing to performance or health risk, and the influence of context on performance, participation, and health. Issues of skill and habit, along with underlying factors, often can be anticipated in light of the diagnostic information or potential health concerns provided by the physician or other health care practitioners. Such information would be pertinent, for example, when people have experienced a cerebral vascular accident (CVA), or stroke. Depression is common after a stroke—which can influence motivation to engage in intervention activities. There may also be specific perceptual problems and problem-solving limitations that limit some activities or suggest others. CVAs occur in people with other medical or potential health risks, such as obesity, hypertension, macular degeneration, prescription drug abuse, or smoking. These medical and health risk factors also influence intervention planning.

Using the *Framework* (AOTA, 2008) as a guide, the evaluation helps the occupational therapist determine whether the client has deficits in—or is at risk for problems in—motor and praxis capabilities, sensory–perceptual capabilities, emotional regulation, cognition, or communication and social skills.

The performance problem statement also indicates any performance pattern issues that might interfere with occupational performance. These performance patterns include habits, performing routines and rituals, or meeting role obligations.

The factors influencing the client's occupational performance range from body function and body impairments to activity demands to his or her values, beliefs, and spirituality. The body function impairments most likely amenable to interventions include mental or cognitive functions, sensory disorders and pain, neuromusculoskeletal and movement-related dysfunction, cardiovascular and respiratory disorders, and skin problems that require special adaptive precautions or procedures (AOTA, 2008).

The client's values, beliefs, and spirituality often influence her or his choice of prioritized occupations and activities. Their influence sometimes can be seen in the way an activity is performed—using a kitchen utensil passed down through generations, for example, to cook a meal associated with a religious holiday. The therapist analyzes the activities important to the client to understand how such objects are used, the space needed and social demands, the sequencing and timing, and any required actions that make physical demands on the client. The therapist also notes how these demands may impact health in the future. This analysis helps prioritize the impairments or risks of impairment in body and other functions that need intervention and indicates how each activity may need modification.

Finally, the occupational therapist analyzes the context—How does it support or inhibit health, performance, and participation in the community? Understanding context helps identify any modifications needed and delineates how performance can be judged in terms of standards or norms. According to the *Framework* (AOTA, 2008), cultural, physical, social, personal, temporal, and virtual contexts could need modification to facilitate health and occupational performance and participation. For instance, the physical context could be modified for a person with a CVA to facilitate wheelchair access, (e.g., by building ramps into or in the home, replacing carpeting with wood or linoleum flooring, and widening doors). The personal context—age, gender, and socioeconomic and educational status—helps the therapist understand performance expectations and priorities, potential health issues, social roles, and resources needed.

Formulation of the occupational performance problem statement is a complex process involving professional reasoning. As indicated previously, experienced occupational therapists can and do tap their previous experiences to analyze current information and discern similarities. This can help them quickly develop tentative hypotheses about the most important occupational performance problems and their underlying factors and health risks (Tomlin, 2008). However, because past experience cannot be the sole determinant, they must generate several alternative hypotheses explaining the occupational performance and participation problems—and withhold final judgment until robust data are collected. In the end, identification of occupational performance problems and their health risks is the result of a client-centered approach based on careful attention to health, medical, and occupational therapy profile information; observation data and assessment results that confirm hypotheses about the relationships among underlying factors, occupational performance, and contexts; and the therapist's previous experiences with similar client situations.

Intervention Process

According to the *Framework* (AOTA, 2008), the intervention process is divided into three parts: (1) creating the intervention plan, (2) implementing the intervention, and (3) intervention review. This chapter focuses on only the intervention plan (Table 4.3).

The principles of client-centered care require that intervention planning be a collaborative process among the client, the caregiver, and the occupational therapist (Law & Mills, 1998). Occupational therapy assistants may contribute to the planning process within their competency and under supervision, but responsibility for the final development of the plan is within the scope of only the occupational therapist (AOTA, 2009).

The content of the intervention plan is based on the results of the occupational profile and analyses and on the occupational performance problem statement. The plan is formulated to guide intervention so that the performance of specific activities in a variety of contexts improves, or the risk of health problems, activity limitations, or participation restrictions diminishes. The intervention plan normally includes objective and measurable goals that can be accomplished within a given timeframe,

Table 4.3. Intervention Plan Components

Intervention Goals	Definitions
• Time frame	Days, weeks, or months
• Underlying factors	Client factors, performance skills, performance patterns
• Activity method change	Steps, techniques, procedures, equipment, context modification
• Focus of intervention	Occupational area
• Measurement parameter	Independence/assistance levels, safety, quality/adequacy
Outcome Measures	**Examples**
	Occupational performance, role competence, adaptation, health and wellness, participation, prevention, quality of life, self-advocacy, occupational justice
Intervention Approaches	**Match Intervention Focus**
• Remediate,	Impairments
restore,	Performance skills and patterns
establish	Habilitation of skills and patterns
• Maintain	Protection of current performance
• Modify	Activities, contexts, caregivers
• Prevent	Risk reduction
• Create/Promote	Lifestyle change
Types of Intervention	**Definitions**
• Therapeutic use of self	Planned use of personality, insights, perceptions, and judgments
• Therapeutic use of occupations/activities	Occupation-based activities in client's own context; purposeful activities occur in therapeutically designed context; preparatory methods prepare for occupational performance
• Consultation process	Therapist not directly responsible for intervention
• Education process	Imparting knowledge and information
• Advocacy	Empowering clients to seek and obtain resources
Mechanisms of Service Delivery	**Definitions**
• Frequency	Number of times per week, per month
• Duration	Total number of visits or total time period
• Personnel involved	Occupational therapist, occupational therapy assistant, caregivers
• Location of intervention	Clinical sites, occupational performance contexts, community settings
Discharge Plan	**Examples**
• Discharge plan	Context support, social capital, self-management, maintenance plans
• Referrals	Expert occupational therapists, other health care professionals
• Recommendations	Community resources

the occupational therapy intervention approach and types of intervention, the mechanism of service delivery, the discharge plan, the chosen outcome measures, and recommendations or referrals to others as needed (AOTA, 2008).

Intervention Goals

Intervention goals should reflect the client's priorities for improvement in occupational performance and participation or reduction in health risks (Wressle, Lindstrand, Neher, Marcusson, & Henriksson, 2003). Box 4.1 illustrates how the occupational

therapist works with Irene to verbalize her goals for therapy (see Chapter 3). Goals focus the intervention on occupational areas, performance skills, and performance patterns. They are client-centered when they are written in collaboration with the client and caregivers in order to achieve significant changes in social participation and health risk reduction. Goals may be classified as *long-term*, reflecting the outcome expected by the time therapy is discontiued, or *short-term*, consisting of the various steps needed to reach the final outcome. When the intervention timeframe is of short duration, however, the therapist may not need to separate goals in this manner.

Box 4.1. Goal Setting for Irene

[See evaluation results from Chapter 3.]

Irene is lonely and unhappy about her life and wants to go back to doing things she enjoys. She feels worthless and guilty about the burden she is placing on her daughter but does not know how to get out of it. She knows she cannot drive unless her vision improves, so she will need to readjust how she does things. Her fatigue makes it difficult for her to even want to try. The therapist helped her focus on actions by asking her to identify goals she would like to achieve within the next 2 months.

Irene's goal areas are as follows:

- Complete bathing and dressing tasks daily in a timely manner without fatigue
- Prepare a light meal daily without fatigue
- Complete one housekeeping task each day without fatigue
- Resume walking for pleasure at least twice per week
- Attend a church group meeting or social activity at least once per week
- Spend time reading or enjoying a leisure activity instead of sleeping excessively.

The therapist then uses these prioritized goal areas to create specific, measurable goals for tracking Irene's progress.

Whatever the duration, goals must indicate the change in underlying factors that will lead to an improvement in occupational performance, community participation, and health. Goals must specify the timeframe in which goal achievement is expected. They also indicate any change in context and activity method that will support performance and health risk reduction. For example, a measurable goal might be written as follows:

> Within 4 weeks [timeframe], client will demonstrate the upper extremity strength and endurance [underlying factors] to use assistive devices and a modified task procedure [activity method change or context modification] to dress [occupational area or focus of intervention] independently within 30 minutes [measurement parameters of independence level and societal standard].

Note that the parameters of goal achievement can vary among therapists and settings delivering services (Table 4.3). Goals can be written in terms of the level of independence the person can be expected to achieve (Box 4.2) or of the level of assistance needed in the performance of the valued occupations and activities (Table 4.4). Other measures of change could be the client's ability to perform occupations and activities in a safe manner or the addition of daily occupations and activities that reduce health risks. The quality or adequacy of performance may improve (Rogers & Holm, 2009): Parameters such as levels of difficulty, pain, fatigue and dyspnea, and satisfaction may change; duration may increase; societal standards may be achieved; fewer resources may be used or existing resources used more effectively; and aberrant performance and unhealthy behaviors may cease.

Outcome Measures

Prioritized goals are really statements indicating the outcomes expected as the result of occupational therapy intervention. However, the occupational therapist, the client, and the caregivers will not know whether therapy is successful unless the therapist selects outcome measures that indicate progress (or lack of it). A variety of measures are needed, depending on the outcomes in the intervention goals; these typically directly or indirectly address one or more of the following: occupational performance, participation, role competence, adaptation, health and wellness, prevention, quality of life, self-advocacy, and occupational justice (AOTA, 2008).

Emphasis on holding occupational therapy practitioners accountable for the results of their intervention is growing, as major governmental payers implement "pay for performance"—meaning payment depends upon effectiveness (Sautter et al., 2007). Choosing outcome measurement early in the intervention planning process is additionally important in guiding the occupational therapist to select the most effective intervention approaches (Prvu Bettger, Coster, Latham, & Keysor, 2008). Evidence helps determine which intervention methods are most likely to produce the results targeted in the goals and in the outcome measures (Coster, Haley, Jette, Tao, & Siebens, 2007).

Occupational therapists may work in settings where the outcome measures are interdisciplinary. Often the administration or a facility-wide committee chooses the outcome measurement tool. It remains important, however—because of the growing emphasis on accountability—that the therapist contribute to the selection of the instrument(s) or discuss concerns if the measures will not adequately as-

---

Box 4.2. Independence or Interdependence?

What does *independence* mean? Certainly, it means more that simply doing something on one's own. A person can be considered independent while performing tasks that require the use of adapted devices or environments or while overseeing others to meet various needs. In truth, few people in the modern world can claim that they are entirely self-reliant. Most of us depend on others extensively as we manage the affairs of our daily lives. The dependence is practical—we depend on those who transport goods to the market; on those who manufacture and sell goods; and on those who work in service occupations, such as police officers, hair stylists, butchers, mechanics, bus drivers, and employees of public utilities.

We also depend on other people for emotional support and behavioral models and expectations that guide and influence our behavior. Our understanding of the events in our daily lives is derived from shared interpretations of the world around us.

Therefore, it can be said that we are dependent on others for providing the structure that gives us our sense that the reality of daily life has stability and continuity. We are not independent, but interdependent.

Many people have argued that making independence a principal goal in occupational therapy is a misleading and a potentially damaging concept. Instead, adopting a recovery model that recognizes and values *interdependence* will improve therapy and more accurately reflect the realities of our social existence. A focus on interdependence can provide a broader, more socially appropriate set of options for the therapist in planning intervention than can placing an emphasis on independence. The primary objective may thus involve helping the client learn how to take advantage of the view that we are all interdependent by nature, thereby defining performance outcome success as effectively creating and managing this web of interdependence.

---

sess the goals usually developed in collaboration with clients. It may be that the therapist should add additional measures to ensure appropriate outcome measurement (Andresen, 2000). Adding measures is particularly important when the program-wide outcome measures are restricted to activity and do not address participation or health risk reduction, or when cognition and emotional and regulation skills and their impact on occupational performance and participation are not included (Coster, Haley, Ludlow, Andres, & Ni , 2004).

To select the best outcome measure, the occupational therapist must ensure that the instrument focuses on the construct most affected by the intervention plan and intervention process, is least affected by outside influences, is relevant in terms of the client's age or other personal characteristics, and is easily interpreted (Finch, Brooks, Stratford, & Mayo, 2002). In measuring occupational performance, the occupational therapist should select the outcome instrument according to the occupational area of interest and the specific activities involved,

Table 4.4. Levels of Performance Assistance and Levels of Independence

Assistance Levels (Independence Levels)	Definition
Total assistance (Dependent)	The need for 100% physical and cognitive assistance to perform functional activities
Maximum assistance (25% Independent)	The need for 75% physical and cognitive assistance to perform functional activities
Moderate assistance (50% Independent)	The need for 50% physical and cognitive assistance to perform functional activities
Minimum assistance (75% Independent)	The need for 25% physical and cognitive assistance to perform functional activities
Standby assistance	The need for supervision to perform new activity procedures without error and with anticipation of the need for using appropriate safety precautions
Independent status (100% Independent)	No physical or cognitive assistance required to safely perform functional activities

such as using an ADL outcome instrument that emphasizes dressing, bathing, toileting, feeding, and personal device use (Cohen & Marino, 2000; Salter et al., 2005). The instrument must always be able to measure improvement, especially when only small gains are expected rather than gross changes (Coster, Haley, & Jette, 2006).

When a performance deficit is not present, but there is a need to prevent problems or risks in daily life occupation, the instrument should be able to measure enhancements (AOTA, 2008). Outcome measures may need to focus upon IADLs (e.g., home management and finances) and participation in the community (Jette Keysor, Coster, Ni, & Haley, 2005), such as the outcome referred to as role competence in the *Framework* (AOTA, 2008). Instruments that measure adaptation will provide outcome data on changes in client response to an occupational challenge, such as ability to use relapse-specific coping or emotional regulation skills to avoid using addictive substances during occupational performance

To better meet the outcome measurement needs of occupational therapy services post-acute care, AOTA (Strzelecki, 2009) has endorsed the Boston University Activity Measure for Post-Acute Care (AMPAC; Haley et al., 2004) for the purpose of creating a national occupational therapy database where users may benchmark their intervention outcomes across facilities and against national averages. The AMPAC assesses a client's functional status across three domains: basic mobility, daily activities, and applied cognition.

Health-related quality-of-life outcome measures might be useful in measuring various aspects of health and wellness, prevention, and life satisfaction. These measures assess various domains such as physical, emotional, cognitive, and social role functioning, and perceptions of health and well-being (Finch et al., 2002). Such measures can be generic (Haywood, Garratt, & Fitzpatrick, 2005) in that they can be used with a broad population, or they can be disease-specific (e.g., arthritis; Valderas & Alonso, 2008). Often, disease-specific quality-of-life measures enable the person to compare himself or herself with others who have similar health conditions.

Intervention Approaches

In collaboration with the client and caregivers, the occupational therapist selects the therapy approaches best suited to the focus of intervention and the expected outcomes; the client's values and capacity for learning; the prognosis for the impairments; the time available for intervention; the prob-

able discharge environment; and the expected client follow-through, with recommendations (Rogers & Holm, 2009). According to the *Framework* (AOTA, 2008), the main intervention approaches will

- Create and promote (health promotion),
- Establish and restore (remediation and restoration),
- Maintain and modify (compensation and adaptation), and
- Prevent (disability prevention).

These categories are summarized below. Throughout the following discussion, refer to Table 4.5 to see how the occupational therapist may address Irene's goals through the use of a combination of approaches.

Create and Promote (Health Promotion)

Health promotion approaches are not based on the assumption that a disability is present or that any factors are present that would interfere with performance (AOTA, 2008). Instead, the focus is on reduction of health risks. For instance, by learning how to structure one's daily routine, unnecessary stress and its physical consequences can be avoided. Health promotion also involves strategies to improve the client's sense of life satisfaction and well-being. Lifestyles that include goal-directed occupations that reflect competence, that are viewed as less stressful, and that lead to meaning and the adequate expression of personal identity are likely to result in greater levels of life satisfaction (Wilcock, 2006).

Establish and Restore (Remediation and Restoration)

Remediation approaches focus on changes in client variables, including body functions and body structures; values, beliefs, and spirituality; performance skills; performance patterns; and occupational performance. Restoring body functions and body structures, such as range of motion and strength, attempts to influence biological, physiological, or neurological processes. Restoration approaches are also used to reestablish the client's occupational performance, performance skills, and habits and routines. If skills, habits, and occupational performance procedures have never been learned, then establishing the necessary motor and praxis skills, sensory–perceptual skills, emotional regulation skills, cognitive skills, and communication and social skills is necessary, as is organizing those skills into new and healthy occupational performance processes, habit patterns, and routines. Typically,

Table 4.5. Example of an Intervention Approach for Each of Irene's Goals

Goal	Intervention Approaches				
	Establish/Restore	Modify	Maintain	Prevent	Create/Promote
Complete bathing and dressing tasks daily in a timely manner without fatigue	Use or complete a strengthening program to improve grip for ease in bathing and dressing	Bathe and dress at a time with higher energy or before bed	Irene and her daughter will learn energy conservation principles and remediation techniques	Use nonskid flooring on the tub and make sure grab bars are positioned properly and secured	Recall the importance of bathing and proper dressing as fundamental to social interactions and sense of well-being
Prepare a light meal daily without fatigue	Complete a strengthening program to improve arm strength for ease in meal preparation	Sit to cook (use a stool) and use energy-saving devices (e.g., electric mixer)	Use daily planners and organizational strategies for meal planning	Irene's daughter arranges supplies to eliminate need for risky reaching or bending	Irene's daughter finds healthy foods that come in convenient sizes and packaging
Complete one housekeeping task each day without fatigue	Build endurance through an exercise program	Modify routines and habits to incorporate energy conservation principles (e.g., spread the task throughout the day)	Irene's daughter organizes cleaning supplies and equipment to be easily accessible	Rest before getting tired	Use a method of prioritizing activities such that energy is saved for the most valued activities
Resume walking for pleasure at least twice per week	Develop a progressive walking schedule that gradually builds endurance	Bring an adapted cane that opens to a stool for needed rests	Interpret and implement a written walking program	Use comfortable clothing and sturdy walking shoes	Join or create a peer group of walkers for support and socialization, and walk in stimulating places such as a mall or sports center
Attend a church group meeting or social activity at least once per week	Complete memory and cognitive retraining	Irene's daughter arranges rides from the group members	Irene's daughter develops a car-pool list and has Irene swap rides for other services such as bringing treats	Plan day to allow rest before attending the group	Learn about the importance of meaningful activity to health and quality of life
Spend time reading or enjoying a leisure activity instead of sleeping excessively	Complete visual exercises	Use books on tape, magnifiers, or both when vision is poor	Irene's daughter has supplies readily available for games and crafts that interest her and sensory changes	Understand precautions related to her weak grip	Participate in a book club or activity group for social and mental stimulation

restoring or establishing ADL and IADL occupational performance takes place over extended periods and involves careful structuring of activities and tasks, frequent monitoring to identify problems, and feedback to correct performance errors.

Maintain

Maintenance involves strategies to ensure that the client does not lose current levels of functioning or that improvements in occupational performance continue once therapy ends. Maintainance approaches can also focus on slowing the anticipated loss of functioning associated with a progressive condition such as Alzheimer's disease. Maintenance can also involve training caregivers to ensure that clients follow therapeutic recommendations; training the client to use exercise routines or splinting schedules; and incorporating therapy "booster" sessions to briefly retrain the client in the face of gradual degradation of client factors, occupational performance, and performance skills and patterns.

Modify (Compensation and Adaptation)

The objective of modification is to identify new ways to accomplish the required activities or tasks so that occupational performance occurs. The idea is that the client use the remaining performance capabilities or client factors and performance skills during occupational performance. Often, the context can be modified to enable successful occupational performance. Thus, modification approaches may focus on modifying the activity, the context, or both.

Many strategies can be used to modify an activity and the context to enable a client to meet ADL and IADL goals. First, the client can be taught to perform the activity within his or her capabilities. Doing so often involves a change in task method, for example, putting on pants while seated instead of standing. Second, the context can be modified to permit accomplishment of the task despite limitations in ability or skill, such as by installing grab bars in the shower stall. Third, systems or devices can be designed or acquired to enable performance despite limited cognition, strength, or sensory ability, such as using a transfer board to enable car–wheelchair transfer.

Another modification approach involves having an agent or caregiver assist with the parts of the task that overly tax the client's capabilities. For example, the caregiver could carry the client's lunch tray from the cafeteria line to the table. Each category of modification approach is described in more detail in the sections that follow.

Use of Adaptive Systems and Devices

Occupational therapy practitioners often use the broad term *assistive technology* to refer to systems and devices that help clients compensate for lost or diminished functions. Devices range from those described as *low-technology,* such as special utensils with built-up handles or elastic shoelaces that need not be tied, to *high-technology,* such as robots that vacuum the floor, remote-control devices that activate appliances, and speech synthesizers that store and speak words and sentences. Clients may need equipment at one phase of their intervention but not after remediation or restoration approaches have improved capacity in body function and body structure. The prescription of adaptive systems and devices should be made carefully after fully understanding the client's capabilities, financial situation, and psychological reaction to the equipment; the equipment's impact on safety in occupational performance and the ease of incorporating it into habit patterns and routines; the context for its use; and the patterns of the client's energy and time availability.

Environmental Modifications

Environmental modifications can vary from rearranging furniture to major alterations in the design of rooms or dwellings. Common examples include widening doorways, building ramps, and converting family rooms into bedrooms because of the lack of wheelchair access to bedrooms located on a second storey of the house. Within bathrooms, the addition of grab bars, special toilet seats, and other safety equipment can dramatically improve ADL completion.

In the United States, the Americans with Disabilities Act (ADA) of 1990, efforts by advocacy groups, and the universal design movement have made apparent the need to design environments that are accessible without requiring special accommodations. The ADA has also been instrumental in promoting the modification of environments created prior to the emphasis on universal access. Without universal access, people with impairments may experience activity limitations and participation restrictions. Unfortunately, people with disabilities and their advocates often encounter bureaucratic obstacles that prevent timely (or any) completion of necessary environmental modifications.

Use of Caregivers

Another strategy available to clients is to train family members and other caregivers to assist in the performance of various ADLs and IADLs. To help caregivers be effective, the occupational therapist needs to determine which activities require assistance and how much. For some activities, the client may need total assistance; with others, only standby assistance is indicated. The level of assistance might vary according to time of day, fatigue or pain level, or context of the performance. Changes in health status or activity priorities also might lead to the need for different levels of assistance. For instance, the time and energy available for occupational performance may be limited. The client may prefer to have a personal care assistant do most of his or her hygiene and dressing activities in order to conserve energy for more enjoyable activities, such as cooking or shopping. Because therapy timeframes probably limit the involvement of the therapist in determining all the assistance needs and how they might vary, it is important to help the client gain a realistic and thorough understanding of his or her strengths and limitations related to ADLs and IADLs.

Prevent (Disability Prevention)

Prevention as a primary category of intervention promotes safety and prevents health problems. The occupational therapist seeks to identify risk factors before an accident occurs to improve safety and reduce the risk of injury, hospitalization, chronic disability, or death. It should be noted that ADLs and IADLs can be considered preventive because they support social participation, promote nutrition and hygiene, and prevent specific health problems (e.g., by ensuring medication to control diabetes, HIV, or epilepsy is taken). By enabling the client to complete ADLs, prevention is taking place. The occupational therapist must always emphasize safety in the performance of activities and tasks. For people with visual difficulties, sensory deficits, balance disorders, or other conditions that place them at risk of personal injury, such as falls and slips, attention must be paid to object placement, environmental design (lighting and non-slip surfaces), location of safety apparatus (e.g., grab bars), and use of safe task methods.

Choosing Specific Types of Intervention

Once approaches are chosen, the occupational therapist, in collaboration with the client and caregivers, selects (from the approaches described previously) the types of intervention that are effective in leading to the desired changes in occupational performance. Intervention types include therapeutic use of self (i.e., planned use of personality, insights, perceptions, and judgments), therapeutic use of occupations and activ-

ities, consultation, education, and advocacy (AOTA, 2008). In terms of therapeutic occupations, the therapist most likely will use a combination of occupation-based activity (i.e., meaningful activities within the client's own context), purposeful activity (i.e., goal-directed activities within a therapeutic context), and preparatory methods (e.g., sensory input, physical agent modalities, splinting, and exercise).

Table 4.6 illustrates a sample intervention plan designed for a person with a CVA. Types of intervention can be delineated for clients with mental illness, as well as for those with physical and cognitive impairments. For instance, a remediation or restoration approach may be needed if the focus of intervention is on changing the client's addictive substance use pattern. The therapist may use an education process that helps the client identify his or her addictive habit patterns and create healthy replacements (Moyers & Stoffel, 2001). During this process, the therapist may adopt a therapeutic use of self that accepts the client's responsibility for leading the change process and that facilitates the client's belief in the likelihood of success (Miller & Rollnick, 2002). In addition, a prevention approach that focuses on engagement in both occupation-based and purposeful activity may be required so that the client does not relapse into addictive behavior. The education process facilitates the client's use of coping skills during occupational performance (Stoffel & Moyers, 2001). The therapist can also modify the client's social context so he or she spends less time with substance users and more time with people who model effective recovery habits, routines, and skills. This modification could be achieved by using the occupation-based activity of attending Alcoholics Anonymous (AA) social events and activities, which include AA support groups that teach the client about a recovery lifestyle. An advocacy type of intervention may involve the client learning how to refuse engagement in occupations and activities that involve the use of drugs and alcohol. The client may also have to advocate for himself or herself in terms of obtaining employment with a new or previous employer.

Formulating a Successful Plan of Care

Theory- and Evidence-Based Intervention

To achieve the desired outcomes of occupational therapy intervention, the therapist not only relies on client and caregiver collaboration but also is aware of the way in which current theories and evidence support the recommended approaches and interventions. With the focus of intervention on oc-

Table 4.6. Sample Occupational Therapy Intervention Plan

Problem Statement	Goals	Approaches	Types of Intervention
Medical • Right cerebrovascular accident • Depression *Performance* • Unable to initiate complete dressing or bathing tasks without verbal cues and physical assistance *Underlying factors* • Mental functions • Sensory functions • Neuromusculoskeletal	• Within 4 weeks, client will demonstrate the upper extremity strength and endurance to use assistive devices and a modified task procedure to dress independently within 30 minutes • Within 4 weeks, client will demonstrate the motor planning to shower independently using adaptive equipment	• Education of clients and caregivers • Restoration of motor skill and habit patterns and routines • Remediation of strength and endurance • Use of adaptive equipment, context modifications, and safe practices • Modification of activity demands • Remediation of motor planning physical context • Prevention of safety error	• Consultation with caregivers about physical context modifications for home and bathroom • Use of neuromotor techniques to facilitate normal tone, strength, and range of motion • Use of purposeful activity and occupation-based activity to restore skills and habits and to remediate motor planning

cupational areas, performance skills, and performance patterns, the occupational therapist must use practice models and theories that address successful changes, not only in underlying factors but also in current occupational performance (Baum & Baptiste, 2002). The use of multiple practice models may be necessary because some models address only underlying factors and some address only occupational performance. Some theories and practice models are specific to certain approaches or intervention types, such as learning theories that guide the use of education as a type of intervention.

The occupational therapist should use theory to guide intervention planning; in addition, he or she must critically appraise the latest research that demonstrates the efficacy and effectiveness of approaches and types of intervention. Effective interventions may be found in evidence-based practice products or clearinghouses, such as critically appraised topics, practice guidelines, and systematic evidence reviews.

The therapist also should analyze the outcomes he or she typically achieves when using a specific approach and type of intervention. In the absence of research, the therapist needs current knowledge of the latest expert opinions and theoretical developments supporting these approaches and types of interventions.

Mechanisms of Service Delivery

Once the intervention approach and intervention types are selected, the occupational therapist determines the mechanisms of service delivery. Several people may provide the intervention, including the therapist and the occupational therapy assistant. The practitioners may train the client to implement home programs or train the caregivers to assist. The location of intervention is an important consideration. It that may include clinical sites, such as a hospital room, clinic, or agency; key occupation contexts, such as the home, work sites, or schools; and community settings, such as where the client shops, eats in restaurants, or goes to church. The frequency of intervention and the duration of therapy required to achieve its goals are determined on the basis of the therapist's experience with other clients, outcomes data, research studies, expert opinion, and client preference.

Discharge Plans

Another important aspect of an effective intervention plan is that it be consistent with the context or the environment to which the client is discharged. After hospitalization, for instance, the client may prefer to return home and live independently and want an intervention plan based on that wish. After the occupational therapist conducts a realistic evaluation and develops an understanding of the client's prognosis, however, it may be apparent that discharge to the home is inappropriate—it might require a clinical environment providing more intensive therapy before discharge to home.

The context often dictates the intervention priorities and intervention approaches, particularly when the therapist decides to emphasize modification over remediation. If a client is home alone during a major part of the day, the more immediate need might be to ensure that he or she has access to prepared meals or light snacks, so the remediation of range of motion, strength, and coordination needed to use the oven can come later. Being alone may require learning kitchen habits that make meal preparation safer, such as using the microwave instead of the stove. This would allow the client to cook when alone, even though body functions have not improved adequately for oven operation.

Referral

A successful plan includes referrals to other occupational therapy practitioners with specific expertise (e.g., splinting, therapy for eating and swallowing, hand therapy, driving, or low vision rehabilitation). Referral to other professionals also may be needed— physical therapists, physicians, psychologists, social workers, dieticians, or speech and language pathologists. The occupational therapist can recommend involvement in specific support groups, fitness centers, or other activity groups that support engagement in enjoyable and healthy activities. To additionally support engagement in occupation, the therapist ensures the client is aware of community resources such as parks, museums, universities, volunteer opportunities, and funding sources.

Summary

The mainstay of occupational therapy practice consists of strategies that enable people to engage in daily occupations. Intervention planning is a process that bridges evaluation and intervention and requires a careful, analytical process of professional reasoning.

The evaluation phase includes an occupational profile and analysis of occupational performance, derived from interviews, the client's medical and occupational history, observations, and results from specific assessment instruments. The occupational therapist then generates a performance problem statement that indicates the client's occupational performance status and occupational performance problem priorities and lists the underlying factors contributing to the performance problem. The performance problem statement is the basis for intervention planning. It is part of a plan of care that delineates measurable goals that indicate the outcomes expected by the end of therapy.

Outcome measures are chosen early in intervention planning to guide selection of interventions that will most likely lead to the planned re-

sult. These measures should demonstrate to the client whether occupational performance and participation have improved or have been enhanced; whether disability has been prevented; whether changes have occurred in role competence, ability to adapt to occupational challenges, health and wellness, and quality of life; and whether the client receives occupational justice through self-advocacy and contextual or environmental modification.

Given the goals of the intervention, therapists work with the client to select the most appropriate mixture of intervention approaches and types. This process is based on a critical appraisal of the evidence; on the use of evidence-based practice products; and on the therapist's current knowledge of relevant theories and practice models. A successful intervention plan uses the appropriate mechanisms of service delivery and reflects understanding of the discharge context. The plan includes recommendations regarding the use of community resources and referrals to appropriate professionals.

Study Questions

1. What are the components of an occupational therapy performance problem statement?
2. What measurement parameters are useful in writing measurable goals?
3. Write some measurable intervention goals that include all the necessary aspects.
4. What is the difference between intervention approach and type of intervention? Give examples of each.
5. Compare and contrast remediation, restoration, and establishment.
6. Describe the aspects of a successful intervention plan.
7. How does the occupational therapist know which outcome measure to select?

References

American Occupational Therapy Association. (2008). Occupational therapy practice framework: Domain and process (2nd ed.). *American Journal of Occupational Therapy, 62,* 625–683.

American Occupational Therapy Association. (2009). Guidelines for supervision, roles, and responsibilities during the delivery of occupational therapy services. *American Journal of Occupational Therapy, 63,* 797–803.

Americans with Disabilities Act of 1990, Pub. Law 101–336, 104 Stat. 327.

Andresen, E. M. (2000). Criteria for assessing the tools of disability outcomes research. *Archives of Physical Medicine Rehabilitation, 81*(Suppl. 2), S15–S20.

Baum, C. M., & Baptiste, S. (2002). Reframing occupational therapy practice. In M. Law, C. M. Baum, &

S. Baptiste (Eds.), *Occupation-based practice: Fostering performance and participation* (pp. 3–16). Thorofare, NJ: Slack.

Cohen, M. E., & Marino, R. J. (2000). The tools of disability outcomes research functional status measures. *Archives of Physical Medicine and Rehabilitation, 81*(Suppl. 2), S21–S29.

Coster, W. J., Haley, S. M., & Jette, A. M. (2006). Measuring patient-reported outcomes after discharge from inpatient rehabilitation settings. *Journal of Rehabilitation Medicine, 38,* 237–242.

Coster, W., Haley, S. M., Jette, A., Tao, W., & Siebens, H. (2007). Predictors of basic and instrumental activities of daily living performance in persons receiving rehabilitation services. *Archives of Physical Medicine and Rehabilitation, 88,* 928–935.

Coster, W. J., Haley, S. M., Ludlow, L. H., Andres, P. L., & Ni, P. S. (2004). Development of an applied cognition scale to measure rehabilitation outcomes. *Archives of Physical Medicine and Rehabilitation, 85,* 2030–2035.

Falvey, J. E., Bray, T. E., & Hebert, D. J. (2005). Case conceptualization and treatment planning: Investigation of problem-solving and clinical judgment. *Journal of Mental Health Counseling, 27*(4), 348–372.

Finch, E., Brooks, D., Stratford, P. W., & Mayo, N. E. (2002). *Physical rehabilitation outcome measures: A guide to enhanced clinical decision making* (2nd ed.). Toronto, Ontario: Canadian Physiotherapy Association.

Haley, S. M., Coster, W. J., Andres, P. L., Ludlow, L. H., Ni, P., Bond, T. L. Y., et al. (2004). Activity outcome measurement for postacute care. *Medical Care, 42,* 149–161.

Haywood, K. L., Garratt, A. M., & Fitzpatrick, R. (2005). Quality of life in older people: A structured review of generic self-assessed health instruments. *Quality of Life Research, 14,* 1651–1668.

Jette, A. M., Keysor, J., Coster, W., Ni, P., & Haley, S. (2005). Beyond function: Predicting participation in a rehabilitation cohort. *Archives of Physical Medicine and Rehabilitation, 86,* 2087–2094.

Law, M., Baum, C. M., & Dunn, W. (2005). Occupational performance assessment. In C. H. Christiansen & C. M. Baum (Eds.), *Occupational therapy performance, participation, and well-being* (2nd ed., pp. 338–371). Thorofare, NJ: Slack.

Law, M., & Mills, J. (1998). Client-centered occupational therapy. In M. Law (Ed.), *Client-centered occupational therapy* (pp. 107–122). Thorofare, NJ: Slack.

Miller, W. R., & Rollnick, S. (2002). *Motivational interviewing: Preparing people to change addictive behavior* (2nd ed.) New York: Guilford.

Moyers, P. A., & Stoffel, V. C. (2001). Community-based approaches for substance use disorders. In M. Scaffa (Ed.), *Occupational therapy in community-based practice settings* (pp. 318–342). Philadelphia: F. A. Davis.

Pierce, D. (2001). Untangling occupation and activity. *American Journal of Occupational Therapy, 55,* 138–146.

Prvu Bettger, J. A., Coster, W. J., Latham, N. K., & Keysor, J. J. (2008). Analyzing change in recovery patterns in the year after acute hospitalization. *Archives of Physical Medicine Rehabilitation, 89,* 1267–1275.

Rogers, J. C., & Holm, M. B. (2009). The occupational therapy process. In E. B. Crepeau, E. S. Cohn, & B. A. Boyt Schell (Eds.), *Willard & Spackman's occupational therapy* (11th ed., pp. 478–518). Philadelphia: Lippincott Williams & Wilkins.

Salter, K., Jutai, J. W., Teasell, R., Foley, N. C., Bitensky, J., & Bayley M. (2005). Issues for selection of outcome measures in stroke rehabilitation: ICF activity. *Disability and Rehabilitation 27*(6), 315–340.

Sautter, K. M., Bokhour, B. C., White, B., Young, G. J., Burgess, J. F., Berlowitz, D., et al. (2007). The early experience of a hospital-based pay-for-performance program. *Journal of Healthcare Management, 52*(2), 95–107.

Stoffel, V. C., & Moyers, P. A. (2001). *AOTA Evidence-Based Practice Project: Treatment effectiveness as applied to substance use disorders in adolescents and adults.* Bethesda, MD: American Occupational Therapy Association.

Strzelecki, M. V. (2009). AOTA endorses outcomes measurement tool. *OT Practice, 14*(8), 5.

Tomlin, G. S. (2008). Scientific reasoning. In B. A. Boyt Schell & J. W. Schell (Eds.), *Clinical and professional reasoning in occupational therapy* (pp. 91–124). Philadelphia: Wolters Kluwer/ Lippincott, Williams & Wilkins.

Valderas, J. M., & Alonso, J. (2008). Patient reported outcome measures: A model-based classification system for research and clinical practice. *Quality of Life Research, 17,* 1125–1135.

Vess, J. (2001). Implementation of a computer-assisted treatment planning and outcome evaluation system in a forensic psychiatric hospital. *Psychiatric Rehabilitation Journal, 25*(2), 124–132.

Von Krogh, G., & Naden, D. (2008). Implementation of a documentation model comprising nursing terminologies—Theoretical and methodological issues. *Journal of Nursing Management, 16,* 275–283.

Wang, W. M., Cheung, C. F., Lee, W. B., & Kwok, S. K. (2007). Knowledge-based treatment planning for adolescent early intervention of mental healthcare: A hybrid case-based reasoning approach. *Expert Systems, 24*(4), 232–251.

Wilcock, A. A. (2006). *An occupational perspective of health* (2nd ed.). Thorofare, NJ: Slack.

World Health Organization. (2001). *International classification of functioning, disability and health.* Geneva: Author.

Wressle, E., Lindstrand, J., Neher, M., Marcusson, J., & Henriksson, C. (2003). The Canadian Occupational Performance Measure as an outcome measure and team tool in a day treatment programme. *Disability and Rehabilitation, 25*(10), 497–506.

Chapter 5

Methods for Teaching Basic and Instrumental Activities of Daily Living

LAURA K. VOGTLE, PHD, OTR/L, ATP, AND MARTHA E. SNELL, PHD

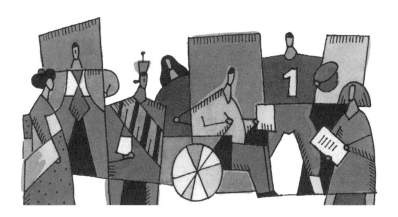

KEY WORDS

acquisition	participation
age appropriate	probe data
antecedent events	response prompts
baseline data	stages of learning
consequences	stimulus prompts
fluency	system of least prompts
generalization	time delay
graduated guidance	training data
maintenance	
partial participation	

HIGHLIGHTS

- A multidisciplinary team approach involving professionals and family members can often strengthen teaching and create practical opportunities for clients.

- Learning occurs in a sequence of stages beginning with skill acquisition through maintenance, proficiency, and generalization.

- Intervention approaches and learning criteria should match learning stages.

- Skills should be taught in settings or contexts that are as natural as possible.

- Prompts must be selected to fit the client, the situation, and the activity.

- During early learning or acquisition, reinforcement following correct and approximate responses (even when prompted) facilitates learning.

OBJECTIVES

After reading this material, readers will be able to

- Discuss the need for age-appropriate, client-centered occupations for clients in their care;

- Describe the stages of learning, and relate them to age-appropriate and occupationally relevant goals;

- Discuss how task and activity analysis are used in teaching activities of daily living skills;

- Describe the different components of teaching strategies, including the use of prompts and feedback, and different kinds of antecedents and consequences for these activities;

- Understand the need for systematic evaluation of teaching strategies used with clients; and

- Understand the importance of careful documentation and graphing of baseline and training data in measuring change and supporting reimbursement requests.

Regardless of what occupations are being taught to whom, there are general principles and methods of good instruction that should be used in interventions. When the client has cognitive limitations, additional guidelines and strategies should be reflected in teaching, and supplementary methods should be considered. This chapter describes some of the principles and methods occupational therapists can use when working with persons with cognitive limitations.

Initial Planning of Goals and Intervention

Guiding Principles for Selecting Appropriate Intervention

The occupational therapist should select interventions that

- Are suited to the client's chronological age,
- Create outcomes that the client needs now and later in life,
- Are valued by the client and/or by his or her family and peers,
- Are likely to be achieved with or without task or contextual modifications,
- Can be integrated into daily routines and become useful habits,

- Can be supported by the contexts within which the individual functions,
- Will meaningfully contribute to the individual's independence,
- May improve his or her positive self-image, and
- Are supported by evidence in peer-reviewed journals or policies advocated by law or professional organizations.

Perhaps the most important aspect of occupational therapy intervention is the choice of appropriate occupational outcomes, in collaboration with the client and his or her family or the client's organization. While it is possible to devise strategies to develop just about any occupational skill, if inappropriate long-term goals are the focus of therapy, the learner's time—whether client, student, family member, other caregiver, or organization—and the therapist's time are wasted. For example, when modifications such as hook-and-loop fasteners or elastic laces are available and preferred by the client, teaching shoe-tying can be an inappropriate goal. Therapists should consider the principles listed below when selecting therapy goals for occupational performance areas:

- Occupations chosen for intervention need to consider the temporal context of the client's chronological age.
- Selected goals should be useful to the person in both current and future life environments, roles, and contexts.
- Goals should be chosen by the individual, the family, or organization and deemed important.
- Goals should enable the person to achieve occupations carried out by the general population, such as basic and instrumental activities of daily living, sleep and rest, education, leisure, work, play, and social participation.
- Even if partial participation, rather than independent occupational performance, is the goal, objectives that are realistic for the learner and suited to his or her life setting should be selected.

When providing services for individuals with cognitive impairments, therapists often target narrow aspects of performance, such as motor or process skills, using activities appropriate for persons younger than the individual for whom intervention is being planned. This violates the first principle cited above. Sometimes the occupation or outcome targeted is valid (meaningful and age-appropriate), but the activities, materials, or methods used during the intervention are not. For example, teenagers with apraxia may be asked to toss bean bags into bean bag targets to improve eye–hand coordination so that they can participate in computer games with friends. This kind of intervention is not occupation-based and could be construed as culturally, socially, or temporally demeaning. Incorporating the computer game itself as the intervention rather than focusing on the motor skills needed to perform the occupation is more meaningful and more likely to build the performance needed to incorporate the occupation into routines later in life (Law, 2002).

The second through the fifth principles address other aspects of *occupations* and *participation:* Goals or activities selected for intervention should be meaningful to the person; be commonly performed in familiar contexts; and, if not learned, can be performed by someone else. These same principles are required in early intervention programs and mandated by law under Part C requirements of Individuals with Disabilities Education Improvement Act (IDEA, 2004).

Client-centered occupational goals are more likely to be integrated into daily routines and promote less dependence on others. Evidence suggests that goals written by families and clients promote "ownership" of the goal and are more likely to result in long-term success (American Occupational Therapy Association [AOTA], 2008; Doig, Fleming, Cornwell, & Kuipers, 2009; Trohanis, 2008). Such outcomes have purpose in daily contexts and therefore are valued by others. Learning to perform occupations that are valued by people in the client's social and cultural environments improves the way the client is viewed by others and by himself or herself (Lancioni et al., 2006; Wilson, Reid, & Green, 2006). Goals that have little value to the client mean the occupations taught will not be used once learned.

Some clients have significant limitations in performance skills, making it more practical to learn to perform part of the activity rather than the entire task. This practice, known as *partial participation,* was identified some years ago and reviewed more recently (Ferguson & Baumgart, 1991; Fisher & Frey, 2001) and includes the following:

- Help from others on difficult steps (the caregiver gets the clothes that Amanda selects from the closet and helps her put them on);
- Changing the order of the steps of the activity (John puts his bathing suit on before going to the pool area);
- Changing the rules of the activity (Elliott bats for Tim, then pushes him in his wheelchair to the bases); and

- Adding assistive technology (Don uses a device to speak and activates it with a head-tracker system).

Careful selection of activities that require partial participation is important so that the skills learned will fit into individual and caregiver's various contexts and thus become part of daily routines (Kottorp, Hällgren, Bernspå, & Fisher, 2003). Review of intervention progress and therapy outcomes at later dates is important; the client may learn more steps of the activity over time, requiring further modifications or adjustments in occupational performance, habits, and routines (AOTA, 2008).

Occupations important to the client and family often involve part of a daily schedule or routine and thus may include more instrumental activities of daily living (IADLs). Brown and her colleagues (Brown, Evans, Weed, & Owen, 1987) describe two types of related skills that can help occupational therapy practitioners build core activities of daily living (ADL) tasks to become part of a larger routine or role: (1) extension skills, and (2) enrichment skills. *Extension skills* include the ability to initiate a routine, prepare for the activity, monitor its speed and quality, problem-solve, and terminate the activity or clean up when done. *Enrichment skills* involve expressive communication (through non-symbolic or symbolic means), social behavior, and choice making. The first two columns in Table 5.1 illustrate how this component model is applied to the task of grooming one's nails. (The remaining columns show component analysis of skills and will be discussed later in this chapter.)

Depending on the intervention context, a number of people (staff, peers, family members) may contribute to teaching a daily living activity. Combining their professional expertise will strengthen teaching strategies and increase practice opportunities for the client. However, practitioners working in a team setting need to avoid "dividing up" the client into parts that reflect each member's professional territory. All who assist in teaching or supervising task or activity performance should be alert to the variety of extension skills (e.g., initiate, prepare, monitor tempo) and expansion skills (communication, choice-making, and social) that are embedded in basic and IADLs.

Ecological Inventories

How does one determine which occupations are important to the client? The most important sources of this information are the client and family. If at all able to give information through interview or direct

Table 5.1. Task Analysis Illustrating the Sensorimotor Task Component Model Used for Treatment Planning

Task Step	Task Component	Sensory Component	Motor Component	Grasp Component
Inspects nails to see if dirty or jagged	Initiation of task	Vision, light touch	Finger extension, wrist extension, forearm supination and pronation	N/A
Finds and select materials	Preparation for task	Vision, light touch, pressure discrimination	Finger flexion and extension, wrist extension, elbow flexion and extension, possible shoulder action	Radial digital grasp, lateral tip pinch, pad-to-pad pinch
Cleans and trims nails	Core steps of task	Vision, pain, light touch, pressure discrimination	MCP and IP flexion, extension, and abduction for all digits, including the thumb; wrist flexion and extension; ulnar and radial deviation; isolated finger control	Lateral tip pinch, pad-to-pad pinch, possible gross grasp
Checks nails for cleanliness and neatness	Quality monitoring	Vision	MCP and IP flexion and wrist extension, possible shoulder action	N/A
Grooms nails within an acceptable amount of time	Tempo monitoring	Rapid motor response to sensory input	Use of feedforward and feedback mechanisms to ensure motor efficiency, finger flexion and extension, possible shoulder action	Rapid change of grasp patterns as required by the task
Resolves problems that arise (such as locating materials)	Problem solving	Variable	Variable	Variable
Puts trimming supplies away	Termination of task	Vision, light touch, pressure discrimination	Finger flexion and extension, wrist extension, elbow flexion and extension, possible shoulder action	Radial digital grasp, lateral tip pinch, pad-to-pad pinch
Communications about any aspect of nail grooming (such as length of nails, hang-nail)	Communication	Variable	Variable	N/A
Makes choices within task (such as to polish or not)	Choice-making	Variable	Variable	Variable
Performs routine at appropriate time and location	Social aspect of task	Variable	Variable	Variable

Note. IP = interphalangeal; MCP = metacarpophalangeal; N/A = not applicable.

assessment, the client needs to contribute to the initial assessment. Skill checklists, such as ADL inventories, are often used to assess current abilities and to identify target goals. Standardized tools for ADL assessment include

- Klein–Bell Activities of Daily Living Scale (Law & Usher, 1988),
- Functional Independence Measure (Hamilton, Laughlin, Fiedler, & Granger, 1994),
- Functional Independence Measure for Children (McCabe & Granger, 1990), and
- Pediatric Evaluation of Disability Inventory (Haley, Ludlow, & Coster, 1993).

ADL checklists can be particularly valuable with clients who are unable to contribute to interviews. However, although checklists can help determine if a person has the obvious prerequisite skills, they also can lead practitioners to focus on skills that are not needed or less needed than others. Sometimes, as well, the sequential nature of a checklist causes therapists to regard tasks appearing earlier on the list as prerequisites to later skills, when they may not be. This is particularly true for early childhood assessments, such as the Denver II (Frankenburg, Dodds, Archer, Shapiro, & Bresnick, 1992). To avoid this problem and to develop a more comprehensive picture of the client in his or her routine environments, occupational therapists can use indirect methods of assessment, such as interviewing those directly involved with the client: those who know most about the individual's current performance needs (parents and family members, past teachers, peers, and practitioners) and those familiar with upcoming participation needs (the next teacher or practitioner, peers, job coaches, and so forth).

One example of these indirect methods of functional assessment is the Canadian Occupational Performance Measure (Law, Baptiste, Carswell, Polatajko, & Pollack, 1998). Comparable assessments exist in special education and are called *ecological inventories* and *environmental assessments* (Brown & Snell, 2000; Giangreco, Cloninger, & Iverson, 1993; Haney & Cavallaro, 1996). Using these tools, reference points for goals are assessed through direct interview or by observation. "Informants" who know the client or the settings the client will use in the future are asked questions such as

- What skills do you think are important for _____ [fill in name] _____ to learn?
- What skills are required of _____ that he or she does not know or that others must perform regularly?

- Are there some skills critical to _____'s safety and health that he or she might learn partially or totally?
- What skills are expected of _____'s peers in the same activities and places?
- Could _____ learn to assist with this skill [partial participation] or to perform the skill with adaptations? Without adaptations?

The client may be asked (or observed with input from those who know him or her to deduce the answers),

- What occupations do you want to learn?
- What part of this occupation is hard for you? Is easy for you?

Therapists may also review program requirements, visit settings where the client currently goes or could go in the future, such as desired places of employment or future residences, to understand what occupations the client needs to participate and to consider creative interventions or modifications. Once complete information is obtained, the therapist works with the client and his or her team to set priorities, considering assessment information from all team members. The skills that seem most needed and functional for the person typically become intervention objectives or goals for particular settings.

Stage of Learning

Learning is often seen as occurring in stages, from initial instruction to expanded instruction or generalized skills (Snell & Brown, 2000). During the initial phase of intervention, learners receive assistance and feedback (reinforcement and error correction) as they progress to the stage where occupations are self-regulated and successful. *Prompting* refers to the assistance provided to move a learner from initial learning to mastery of a skill. Others call this assistance *scaffolding* (Wang, Bernas, & Eberhard, 2001). Regardless of the term, most agree that some assistance should be provided initially to decrease a learner's frustration with new or difficult activities, to facilitate success and reduce errors. The type and amount of assistance depend on the learner's cognitive, sensory, and motor abilities, the contexts in which they function, and personal preferences. As the learner's competence increases, assistance is reduced. Figure 5.1 illustrates the relationship among the following four stages of learning (Snell & Brown, 2000):

1. *Acquisition learning* involves initial learning of an activity. In this stage, learners may not be able to perform the target activity at all or

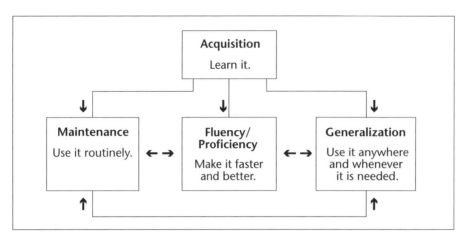

Figure 5.1. Four stages of learning.

may perform with limited competence (performance accuracy ranges from 0% to 60%).

2. *Maintenance learning* involves the routine use of an occupation and improving its accuracy under fairly stable and familiar conditions. At this stage, learners perform the target activity with limited competence but do not initiate the task during typical daily routines (roughly 60% accuracy or better during maintenance).

3. *Fluency or proficiency learning* involves improving the accuracy, quality, and speed of performance. At this stage, learners perform the activity with limited competence in that they may be too slow, careless, or inattentive to detail (roughly 60% accuracy or better).

4. *Generalization learning* involves performance under changing conditions (e.g., location, materials, time, task variation). At this stage, learners perform the activity with limited competence, that is, they fail to initiate or are unable to complete the task when the performance context changes in some way (roughly 60% or better accuracy).

Based on these brief descriptions, it becomes clear that intervention approaches and criteria should vary somewhat to match the different stages of learning. When therapy personnel view learning as progressing through these four stages, they are more likely to

• Adjust their intervention methods as they shift their focus from one stage to another;
• Avoid overemphasizing new activities; and
• Broaden their intervention focus so maintenance, fluency, and generalization into daily routines are considered as valuable as acquisition or performance of new activities.

While changes in performance skills are targeted across the stages of learning, strategies to promote engagement in targeted occupations can focus concur-rently on maintenance, fluency, and gener-alization—if practitioners are clear about their goals, if instruc-tion does not get too complex, and if performance data are available to see whether learning is occurring. The following case may help clarify this process.

Following a head injury, 13-year-old April wanted to learn to put on her shoes, socks, and AFOs (ankle foot orthoses) quickly enough so that she could do it every day before school rather than have her parents do it for her. This project was undertaken in June with hopes for proficiency by early September. The final goal of 10 to 15 minutes for putting the items on was decided on with input from the parents. In the acquisition learning phase, the therapist worked with April on accuracy: getting shoes and socks on over her heels and putting the AFOs on correctly. Once she could perform these difficult steps about two-thirds of the time, the focus shifted to maintenance (performance of the activity ino her daily routine). Her parents agreed she could perform the activity by herself on weekends; they would simply check whether items were on correctly when she was done and document her speed. April was working on independent maintenance of her skills. Her parents agreed to purchase touch-fastener shoes to eliminate lacing and tying, which could improve her speed from her initial 40 minutes. Throughout the summer, she worked hard and used a clock to time herself. Her efforts to use touch-fastener shoes and her daily monitoring of performance time represented a focus on fluency learning. By mid-July, she was able to get the AFOs on tight enough that her family no longer worried about blisters. Her time was reduced to 25 minutes—good, but still short of her goal. April and her parents made several additional task improvements aimed at further improving fluency and improving her timing while still getting her AFOs on tight enough. First, she would get up early enough to put her shoes on before her parents left for work. With this arrangement, she usually managed to get up 4 or 5 days a week to work on speed. Second, the therapist made improvements in the AFOs' touch fasteners, which made the task easier. By the start of school, April was able to get all items on in 15 minutes and was willing to get up early enough to put them on by herself each day. Once back in school, April requested that she work on generalizing the skill from home to the physical context of school. At the end of October, she was able to change her shoes for physical education in 10 minutes without help.

Maintenance and generalization are promoted even during initial learning (acquisition) when therapists select activities that are functional, needed, or valued by others, because they will be routinely used in multiple contexts. By targeting activities suited to the individual's age, he or she will be more inclined to develop habits using them. At the same time, peers, family members, or practitioners will tend to encourage appropriate activities more than they would occupations or behaviors that stigmatize the person in some way. When skill at performing selected activities is not fluent or proficient, others involved in the intervention are not likely to incorporate their use into routines. For example,

- A fifth-grade boy writes so slowly that the parents always do his assigned homework.
- Caregivers for a 30-year-old woman with cerebral palsy living in a group home often bathe her because it is faster than the client bathing herself.
- A young woman who knows how to make up beds but cannot be hired for motel housekeeping, because sheets and blankets are draped unevenly, and none of the wrinkles are smoothed.

These are fluency and generalization problems (performance skills, activity demands, and performance patterns). Unless the intervention addresses them, regular performance of occupations that others will value does not occur. Stated another way, activities will not be incorporated into daily routines if they cannot be performed at a reasonable speed, with the required accuracy and quality, or cannot be used when changes occur in activity demands and context.

During the acquisition stage, practitioners can also build some elements into the intervention plan that will promote generalization to multiple physical or social contexts from early on. Ways to do this include

- Providing intervention in natural or as close to natural contexts as possible;
- Using real (i.e., not simulated) materials (e.g., real shoes to teach dressing and shoe tying, real clothes to teach dressing and buttoning [not button boards or dolls], although larger clothes may be used during early instruction);
- Involving multiple teaching examples (e.g., staff members, peers, physical and social contexts, materials); and
- Selecting multiple examples carefully, starting with those that best sample the range of variation (e.g., for upper body dressing, a turtleneck, tank top, and T-shirt are used first because they best sample the range of variations in collar, sleeve length, fit, and fabric for shirts; Finnie, 1997).

This strategy of teaching the general case first teaches individuals how to perform occupations that are durable across commonly expected changes in contextual and activity demand requirements.

Target objectives or goals must specify the occupation or *behavior*, the desired outcome or *criterion* for performance, and the *conditions* or *context* under which the behavior or activity will be performed. The conditions for successful occupational performance include temporal and physical context, who is present, what activity demands are involved, and what assistance or adaptations are allowed or possible. A general rule to follow is to let the client's or family's realities dictate the context for learning. If the individual shows little or no learning under natural conditions, the conditions or activity demands may be simplified, for example, fewer variations in materials, location, times, and practitioners; less background noise, visual distraction; and so forth. Eventually, however, the individual must learn to perform the activity in typical contexts or the occupation will not become part of habits, routines, roles, or rituals.

The occupational therapist collaborates with other team members to rewrite selected intervention goals as *instructional objectives*. In April's case, this is the objective her team wrote for the skill of putting on shoes and socks:

- *Target objective*: April will be able to put on her touch-fastening shoes, socks, and AFOs on in 10 minutes each morning at home before school without assistance from her parents.

- *Behavior*: Putting on touch-fastening shoes, socks, and AFOs
- *Performance criterion*: In 10 minutes
- *Conditions or context*: Sitting on the floor in her bedroom
- *When*: Each morning before school
- *Where*: At home
- *Who is present*: No one
- *Materials*: Shoes, socks, and AFOs
- *Assistance*: None
- *Modifications*: Touch-fastening.

Direct Evaluation of Skills

We often have referred to assessment and data collection as an "evil necessity." We use the "evil" label for several reasons:

- Individuals seldom learn during evaluation, so it seems like wasted time.
- Many therapists find assessment or data collection tedious and time-consuming, especially when time with a client is restricted by reimbursement or caseload size.
- Many therapists are less experienced in specific details of data collection and in the use of the data gathered, thus cannot justify the effort it takes.

Performance data are necessary because only information relevant to the performance of the target goal can provide the objective information required to judge the success of intervention. For instruction during therapy to be efficient and effective, therapists need to gather and analyze performance on goals and outcomes. When data indicate minimal or slower progress than expected, the therapy approach or conditions (activity demands, modifications, etc.) need to be changed. Likewise, if the data indicate that the goal has been met, intervention can be directed toward a different stage of learning for the same occupation or toward other occupations. For example, Pete, an adolescent with spina bifida, has learned to perform his own intermittent self-catheterization with 60% consistency every 4 hours during the school day. Based on these data, his therapist might direct therapy toward improved consistency of performance while also shifting the focus of intervention toward several new goals. These goals might include promoting routine and spontaneous use of the skill in all the situations where training has occurred (maintenance) and extending the expectation for routine performance of self-catheterization to the home or other settings (generalization).

Observational Data

There are many kinds of data pertinent to therapy intervention. This discussion primarily addresses client performance data that measure some aspect of occupational performance relevant to the goals set by the therapist, client, and family. These data are mainly collected through direct observation of the client during performance of the activity. However, valuable data also can be collected after the skill has been performed. There are at least three different ways to do this:

1. Measure the *permanent products* resulting from the performance (checking to see if Lynn washes her hands and face after eating; estimating the spillage on the table and floor after she finishes eating).
2. *Socially validate* the client's performance by seeking the opinions of peers or caregivers on the success of instruction of a skill they regularly see (is Lynn's clean-up neat enough?)
3. Socially validate the client's performance outcomes by comparing them with her peers' performance of the same skill (how well groomed are Lynn's peers after eating?)

These comparisons can be made by

- Obtaining the subjective opinions of peers (in sensitive ways, ask peers to help by suggesting how Lynn could "fit in" better at lunch), or
- Comparing the client's performance to the peers' performance (note the food on Lynn's face compared to her peers or observe to see if peers clean themselves after lunch).

Evaluation: Test and Training Data

Observational data on occupational performance are collected under either training (intervention) or test (assessment) conditions. Both types of evaluation data can be useful. *Training* or *intervention data* reflect student performance during training or treatment sessions (for example, when assistance, cor–rective feedback, and reinforcement are provided according to the therapy plan). *Test* or *assessment data* reflect performance during non-training conditions such as daily routines (also referred to as "criterion conditions") when little or no assistance or feedback are available other than what naturally occurs in the environment. Test data often show lower performance than do training data.

Types of Activities

Discrete and Chained Behaviors

Target behaviors or specific occupations can be thought of as being either discrete behaviors (individually distinctive behaviors that stand alone) or chained behaviors (a routine or skill involving a sequence of discrete behaviors or steps).

Therapists target many types of discrete behaviors (performance skills), including lip closure, steps taken during walking, ability to grasp during household chores, and time it takes to get dressed. Discrete behavior or skill targets are typically defined in observable terms, then counted during a fixed period of time or over a set number of opportunities. For example, a therapist defines successful grasping behaviors as targeted performance skill goals for Muriel, a 5-year-old with cerebral palsy. Grasp is the "correct response," and failure to grasp during the occupation of play is an "incorrect response." Then the daily activities during which grasping occurs and can be measured are identified, along with the length of the observation period. Data gathered might be rate of performance, for instance, the number of successful and unsuccessful grasping behaviors Muriel makes in kindergarten during 10 minutes of toy and block play with peers. Because this example might be highly variable, due to changing activity demands during play, a better measurement procedure might be to count her successful and unsuccessful attempts at grasping during the first ten opportunities during playtime and determine the proportion of successful and unsuccessful grasps out of the total number of opportunities.

Chained behaviors are those involving a sequence of behaviors or skills that constitute a single activity or are needed to complete the activity. The sequence of behaviors often is identified as steps in a task or activity analysis of the skill. Examples include dressing tasks; standing and transfer tasks; some vocational skills; and most grooming, housekeeping, and cooking tasks. Frequently, activity analyses serve as the guide for intervention and evaluation because they list the behaviors and the sequence involved in performing activities targeted for intervention.

Activity Analyses

Preparing an Activity Analysis

Activity analysis can be broadly defined as breaking down routines or relationships into their components and their influences on an activity. Another commonly used term for this process is *task analysis*. Often

the occupations that therapists identify for intervention are analyzed into steps based on the occupational profile (Watson & Wilson, 2003). Commercially available activity analyses may seem to be time savers; we do not recommend them, because they fail to individualize the activity to the important contexts, individual client factors, performance skills, and activity demands. Developing good activity analyses involves several steps:

- Spend time observing the individual and others performing the activity.
- Develop the best approaches to completing the activity.
- Ask others' opinions about the activity performance (including the person who will learn it or family members who will support it).
- Field test the activity analyses, and revise them as needed.

To promote generalization across contexts, develop an activity analysis that is relatively generic or suits a number of situations where the learner will need to perform the activity (see Table 5.2).

There are many ways to analyze activities. For example, the approach illustrated in Table 5.1 focuses on component or performance skills analysis involved in the skill or activity—an analysis of the sensory, motor, and grasp components in addition to the behavior chain or core steps involved in the skill or activity. The activity analysis in Table 5.2 breaks eating, drinking, and wiping with a napkin into response steps and identifies the relevant stimuli (discriminative stimuli) that generate each response. What activity analysis methods have in common is the delineation of sequenced, observable behaviors that lead to the accomplishment of an activity. The kind of analysis used will depend on the needs of the client, the user (therapist, teacher, or parent), and the therapeutic goals identified.

We have found the following guidelines valuable in the development of activity analyses:

- Use steps of fairly even "size" (duration, accomplishment).
- Be sure each step is observable and results in visible progress toward activity completion.
- Order the steps in a logical sequence, but indicate when the sequence is optional.
- Distinguish any steps requiring another person's assistance and those parts of the activity performed by people other than the student or client.
- Write the specific steps in second-person singular (so they can be used as verbal prompts).

Table 5.2. Task Analysis for Teaching Spoon, Cup, and Napkin Use

Behavior	Discriminative Stimuli	Response
Spoon	"Eat" Spoon in hand Food in spoon Spoon touching lips Mouth open Food in mouth Spoon on table	Grasp spoon Scoop food Raise spoon to lips Open mouth Put spoon in mouth Remove spoon Release grasp
Cup	"Drink" Cup in hand Cup touching lips Liquid in mouth Liquid swallowed Cup on table	Grasp cup Raise cup to lips Tilt cup to mouth Close mouth and drink Lower cup to table Release grasp
Napkin	"Wipe" Napkin in hand Napkin touching face Face wiped Napkin on table	Grasp napkin Raise hand to face Wipe face Lower napkin Release grasp

Note. From "Using constant time delay to teach self-feeding to young students with severe/profound handicaps: Evidence of limited effectiveness," by B. C. Collins, D. L. Gast, M. Wolery, A. Holcombe, and J. Letherby, 1991. *Journal of Developmental and Physical Difficulties, 3,* p. 163. Copyright © 1991 by Plenum Publishing. Reprinted by permission.

- Use language meaningful to the person with whom it will be used, and place in parentheses any additional information that may be difficult to understand, but that is needed for the observer (e.g., "using a pincer grasp").
- Place the steps on an activity analytic data sheet, which allows recording of step-by-step data over a number of days (see Figure 5.2) (Snell & Brown, 2000).

Conducting Activity Analytic Assessments

Once a good activity analysis is prepared, the therapist uses it as a guide to to teaching the activity or task and measuring the client's performance. As the client performs the activity, each behavior or step in the activity analysis is then observed and scored as correct or incorrect. For example, Figure 5.2 contains the teaching objective and activity analysis for the routine tasks Chris needs to gain independence in sitting down on a chair in the example described below.

Chris is a 3½-year-old boy who attends a preschool 5 mornings a week. His therapy is integrated into daily activities in order to address performance skill needs and improve the likelihood that he will generalize his learning to his daily routine. Before being taught the activity indicated in Figure 5.2, Chris waited for help to sit down and stand up from a chair, as his balance was unsteady, and he sometimes fell when not assisted. His thera-

pists and teachers planned to use a total task approach to develop the ability to both sit in and stand up from a chair, so that whenever training and practice occurred, each step would be performed in order and with the needed assistance. His teachers used the task analysis to guide their observation of his performance on each step.

Two general methods of observation can be used:

1. *Single opportunity activity analytic assessment.* The learner is asked to perform the activity. Assessment stops after the first error, with all remaining steps scored as errors. Errors include performing the wrong step, making a mistake on a step, taking too long (if time is important), or not performing the step.
2. *Multiple opportunity activity analytic assessment.* The learner is asked to perform the activity. Each step is observed. Whenever an error occurs, it is recorded, and the evaluator positions the student for the next step. Positioning for testing a step is done without comment or instruction because this is a testing context, not a teaching one.

Chris's teacher and therapist decided to use a multiple opportunity activity analytic assessment approach so they could observe his performance on all steps during each test. His baseline performance over 5 days of assessment was collected and graphed

Name: Chris
Instructor: Maura
Instructional Cue: "Find your chair"
Program: Sitting
Method: Least to Most/4-sec latency

Objective: Given a natural opportunity or a request to sit in a preschool cube chair for an activity and a response latency of 4 seconds, Chris will perform correctly on at least 88% (7 of 8 steps) of the task analysis without assistance for three consecutive training opportunities and one probe.

	Date Baseline*					Date Training																	Probe
	2/27*	3/4*	3/5*	3/6*	3/7*	3/18	3/19	3/20	3/21	3/22	3/25	4/8	4/11	4/12	4/16	4/17	4/18	4/22	4/23	4/26	4/29	4/30	5/1	5/2*
1. Face cube chair	—	—	—	—	—	P	P	P	P	P	V	+	+	+	+	+	+	+	+	+	+	+	+	+
2. Bend forward	—	—	—	—	—	P	P	P	P	P	V	+	+	+	+	+	+	+	+	+	+	+	+	+
3. Grip arm handles	—	—	—	—	—	G	+	G	G	G	V	+	+	+	+	+	+	V	+	+	+	+	+	+
4. Shift right arm to left arm handle	—	—	—	—	—	P	P	P	P	P	P	+	+	+	+	+	G	+	+	+	+	+	+	+
5. Twist trunk and hips	—	—	—	—	—	P	P	P	+	+	V	+	+	V	V	+	+	+	+	+	+	+	+	+
6. Lower bottom to chair	—	—	—	—	+	+	+	+	+	+	+	+	+	+	+	+	+	+	+	+	+	+	+	+
7. Reposition hands and feet	+	—	+	+	+	+	+	+	+	+	+	+	+	+	+	+	+	+	+	P	+	+	+	+
8. Push bottom to back of chair using feet and hands	+	+	+	+	+	+	+	+	+	+	+	+	+	+	+	+	+	+	+	P	+	+	+	+
	25	13	25	25	38	58	50	38	50	50	38	100	100	88	88	100	88	88	100	75	100	100	100	100*

Key:

Baseline*
(+) independent
(—) error

Training
(+) independent
(V) verbal prompt
(G) gestural prompt
(P) physical prompt

Figure 5.2. Task analysis data sheet for Chris's objective of sitting down in a chair. Created by Maura Burke. Used by permission.

(Figures 5.2 and 5.3). He consistently missed the first 5 steps but was successful on the last 3, though inconsistently and with slightly improving performance over the 5 days. His baseline performance seems to indicate that Chris did not know how to perform the activity and that selecting the task as a goal was appropriate. His parents and teacher also indicated independent sitting and standing were much needed skills for many daily activities at home and at school.

When enrichment goals (communication, choice-making, social) are addressed at the same time as the original or core skills, they can simply be placed on the activity analysis sheet. For example, if the teacher and therapist want to include making a choice about which chair to sit in or verbalizing his success (Chris sometimes says "Sit!" when he is successful), these choice-making and communication goals could go directly into the activity sequence (if that can be predicted). Alternatively, they could simply be listed at the end of the activity analysis with frequency count entered for each observation. It may be helpful for therapists to keep a record of significant problem behaviors that occur (e.g., tantrums, falling down, or legs giving out); these behaviors can be defined and added to the end of the activity steps as well.

The graph of Chris's performance data (Figure 5.3) is summarized in percentage form; the percentage of 8 steps performed correctly during each observation. Because Chris is still in the acquisition stage of learning (less than 60% correct), his team decided to include only core behaviors in the activity analysis, and not extension skills (initiate, prepare, problem-solve, monitor tempo and quality, and terminate). These might be added later, along with enrichment skills (communication, choice making, social). However, if enrichment behaviors are added to an activity analysis, they are graphed separately from the core skill steps or from the core steps plus extension skills. Any problem behaviors added to the end of the activity analysis also need to be analyzed separately, because the intended goal is to decrease their frequency by replacing them with more appropriate behaviors. The use of data and graphing is discussed further in the last section of this chapter.

Intervention Strategies

Before discussing general teaching strategies, it might be helpful to review Table 5.3, which illustrates the events that may take place before and after the targeted self-care behavior. Antecedent events are those that occur before the target behavior or

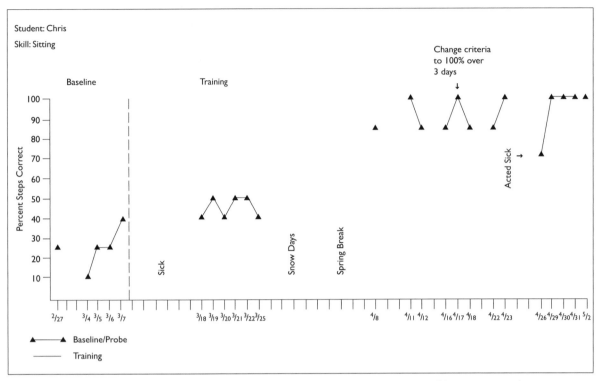

Figure 5.3. Chris's performance during baseline and training of sitting. Created by Maura Burke. Used with permission.

goal; some are intentionally arranged while others may not be under the practitioner's control. For example: just before learning spoon, cup, and napkin use at lunch (see the activity analysis in Table 5.2), Sam, who has autism, is hungry. Hunger serves as a powerful internal antecedent stimulus. The school bell ringing at lunchtime and classmates rushing to their lockers to get packed lunches are also stimuli that set the occasion for lunchtime. Once the children are seated in the lunchroom, more specific stimuli are present: the therapist's request to Sam "Let's eat," and task-discriminative stimuli (S^D) created by performing each response in the chain of taking a spoonful of food.

As shown in Table 5.3, performance of each response (right column) creates an antecedent discriminative stimulus (middle column) relevant to the next or upcoming response in the chain.

To teach Sam the three targeted mealtime skills (Table 5.2), his therapists decided to use physical prompts such as hand-over-hand assists, or planned antecedent events; they used only as much hand-over-hand assistance as was needed to get him to demonstrate each behavior in the three targeted task chains. The physical prompt worked for Sam; that is, the physical assistance prompts controlled his behavior, but the discriminative stimuli that

resulted from performing each step of the task did not yet control the responses that they preceded. When the therapist placed the spoon in Sam's hand, he seemed to know he needed to scoop some food, but he did not yet respond in a way that got food on the spoon. One major goal of instruction was to fade out the controlling antecedents that were provided by teachers or practitioners (for example, requests to "eat" and physical prompts). At the same time, Sam was taught to attend to the relevant antecedent stimuli (for example, food on his plate, with a spoon, napkin, and filled glass beside it; spoon in hand, food on spoon, spoon touching lips, etc.).

Also shown in Table 5.3 are consequences, or the events (planned or unplanned) that may be employed by the therapist following a target response. During intervention sessions, consequences include

- Comments or affirmation given about the accuracy or success of the response (confirmation of accuracy, e.g., "that's right");
- Feedback about an error ("You forgot to hold the bottom of the zipper" while pointing to the end of the zipper);
- Reinforcement (approval, praise, pat on the back, activity choice, tangibles);

- Correction (model missed step and give opportunity to perform with help);
- Extinction or ignoring errors, withholding comments when performance is not adequate; and
- Punishing consequences (withholding reinforcement, giving sharp criticism, requiring excessive practice following an error, time out).

We offer here a few comments on punishing consequences. Much of the early research on special education practices involved self-care instruction for individuals with developmental disabilities that employed punishing consequences or intensive teaching practices (for example, excessively lengthy training sessions; Farlow & Snell, 2000). Now, however, punishing consequences are regarded as unethical and socially invalid practices. We know that for most individuals, punishment does not contribute to creating good learning conditions.

- Punishment does not teach skills; nor does it always reduce problem behaviors.
- The therapist is put into a position of "me against you" control, emphasizing the negative aspects of a therapeutic relationship, which may hinder his or her effectiveness.
- Punitive methods are usually socially invalid or unacceptable to professionals, peers, or care providers and may violate the learner's basic rights.
- Problem behaviors that are not serious are best ignored, with redirection of the learner, focusing on teaching needed skills or replacement skills. If the problem behavior harms the learner, others, or task materials, a careful study of the situation (functional assessment) is called for with the possible development of a behavior support plan.

This chapter cannot deal adequately with this important topic. The reader is referred to a variety of useful references on problem behavior (Carr et al., 1994; Janney & Snell, 2000; O'Neill et al., 1997).

Artificial and Natural Prompts and Feedback

Antecedent events and consequences can be naturally occurring or intentionally arranged by a therapist. They also can either help or hinder learning. As clients advance into different stages of learning for specified occupations, artificial antecedent events and consequences should be faded out, leaving only those consequences that are natural, because these are the stimuli or activity demands that clients must attend to and incorporate into routine occupational

performance. The intervention task becomes one of directing clients to attend to things in the environment that assist them in performing activities. Whenever possible, natural cues should be emphasized as prompts from the onset of learning.

- **Sam**, who has autism, is learning to use a spoon and napkin and will benefit from having his teachers call attention to his peers, who sit nearby and can remind him to wipe his face clean.
- **Rose**, an older woman who has recently had a stroke, is relearning many of the daily living skills she once performed with ease. The therapist's verbal, gestural, and physical assists will be helpful, as will confirmations about her performance and help with her errors. However, Rose must learn to pay attention to the visual and tactile cues from the left side of her body and the cues of material placement. This will permit her to self-regulate and recognize whether or not her body is moving as it should be while she is dressing or helping her daughter with meal preparation. In place of the therapist's consequences (praise and approval), the comments and reactions of others that naturally occur will become the corrective and reinforcing consequences.

For many children, adolescents, and adult clients, the natural antecedents of peer modeling and the consequences of peer approval provide important means for learners to judge their own performance (Bass & Mulick, 2007; Betz, Higbee, & Reagon, 2008). Other studies have incorporated a process called *peer mediation* to successfully deliver interventions using peer modeling, natural cues and prompts, and feedback in natural environments (Odom et al., 2003; Robertson, Green, Alper, Schloss, & Kohler, 2003).

Antecedents: Instructional Cues

An instructional cue can be a request to perform a target skill or goal ("Get your lunch" or "Find your chair"), or it may be other stimuli that alert the learner to perform the activity without a request. When Sam follows his peers to the cafeteria line, for example, their actions of lining up, getting a tray, taking a spoon and fork, etc., cue him to begin the activity of moving through the line to get his lunch.

A common error of therapists and teachers is saying too much. When the instructional cue is a request, it should be stated once in a way that the client understands. Instructional cues should not be questions ("Do you want to tie your shoes?") unless

Table 5.3. Possible Antecedent and Consequence Events That May Precede and Follow the Target Response

Antecedent Events			
New Stimuli "To Be Learned"	Controlling Stimuli or Prompts	Response	Consequence

Teacher's request	Response prompts
	  Verbal instructions
		Correct response	Positive reinforcement
			  Self-reinforcement

Task materials	Pictorial prompts
	  Gestures/pointing
		Approximation	Confirmation
			  Give praise and approval

Time of day	Modeling Physical assistance	Incorrect response	Give a choice
Location	Partial	No response	Give preferred activity Give tangible reinforcer
Persons present	Full	Inappropriate behavior	

Internal stimuli	Stimulus prompts
	Stimulus fading
	Stimulus superimposition
	Stimulus shaping
			Error feedback
			  Pause for self-correction
			  Ignore, withhold positive
			   reinforcement
			  Provide gentle correction

the client is being given an option to do the task. To make cues understandable, the therapist must be familiar with the client's level of comprehension. Spoken instructional cues may be accompanied by gestures signs, pictures, or symbols if the learners use these to augment or replace verbal communication. When the individual does not give the desired response, assistance or prompts are given to encourage his or her performance rather than just repeating the cue.

The best conditions for teaching most people involve embedding instruction within the activity or routine, thus providing many natural cues for the learner, for example, location, activity materials, time of day, others performing a similar activity, and the need for the activity to be completed.

For Chris, who is learning to sit and stand by himself during preschool activities, the natural cues include his peers getting cube chairs, the teacher calling for circle time, and others taking a seat. His performance after several weeks of training was good enough for his therapist to replace the instructional cue "Find your chair" with directing his attention to natural cues. Whenever Chris failed to perform the first activity step, the teacher and therapist used one of three prompts, given in order of increasing assistance, and only as needed.

Antecedents: Prompts

As shown in Table 5.3, there are two general types of prompts—response prompts and stimulus prompts. We will limit our detailed discussion to response prompts, as they are more versatile in self-care activities and require less effort to use. *Stimulus prompts*, also called *stimulus modification procedures* (Wolery, Ault, & Doyle, 1992), are elements in the environment or context that are used to prompt the

individual. They require a gradual change from easy to hard over time, as performance improves, for example, fading out color-coding to teach a child to discriminate her grooming items from those of her classmates and family members or teaching a person to write his or her name by fading the stimulus prompts from tracing letters to thickly dotted letters, to thinly dotted letters, and finally to no dotted guidelines.

By comparison, *response prompts* encompass various types of therapist assistance that are directed toward the client responding. In order of increasing assistance, they include

- Specific verbal instructions ("open the shampoo");
- Pictorial or two-dimensional prompts, such as showing the learner photos of activity steps (see Lancioni & O'Reilly, 2001, for a review of the effectiveness of picture cues and others);
- Gestures such as pointing to needed materials or gesturing toward children's seats when it is time to begin class;
- Models or demonstrations of the target response; and
- Physical assistance, either partial (nudging a client's hand toward the toothpaste) or full assistance (using hand-over-hand assistance to get the client to pick up the toothpaste) (Garfinkle & Schwartz, 2002).

Prompts can be given individually (verbal request to pick up the soap in a hand-washing task or demonstrating the first step in a job task); in combinations (verbal request plus pointing to the soap, or therapist shows a photo that illustrates the step required); or as part of a planned hierarchy of prompts given one at a time, as needed.

Latency

With many prompts, a short period of time *(latency)* is given before and after prompting a client to initiate an activity step without help. This allows the client time to initiate the prompted performance. The latency may be as short as 2–3 or as long as 15 seconds; it will be determined depending on the client's natural response latency on known activities (how long it takes him or her to initiate a fairly familiar task step). Response latency will be slower when performance skills are impaired. When muscle tone is atypical, for example, volitional movement is delayed, or vision is limited. Zhang, Cote, Chen, and Liu (2005) describe an example of successful use of prompts followed by latency to teach a 39-year old adult with developmental delay to bowl.

Selection of Prompts

Prompts must be selected to fit the client, the situation, and the activity. For example, some students or clients with cerebral palsy or other neurological conditions may understand the activity and the order of its steps but need to learn to organize and grade movement. For these learners, sensory prompts such as deep pressure on an extremity may be far more effective than verbal or model prompts. For example, in a three-step task analysis for Chris of standing up from sitting, the therapist provides support at the knees after Chris scoots to the edge of the chair and then positions his hands on the arm rests. At this point, Chris can push up to stand.

Some prompts depend on the learner having certain kinds of performance skills before they can be used; if the learner does not have these skills, the prompt is not a "controlling stimulus" for a given response. For example, Rose's therapist made some activity step photos to prompt her completion of daily living tasks, but because Rose has very limited vision and does not readily associate pictured items with three-dimensional items, the photos will not prompt the required response. Her therapist will need to select another prompt that works for Rose or enlarge the photos and teach her to associate them with objects first.

Some kinds of assistance for steps clients cannot master independently may be more permanently added to the activity (permanent assistance or partial participation). This may involve prolonged personal assistance in that it may include various therapy techniques, such as cues to initiate motion or during a movement, support at a point of control (e.g., the hips, elbow), or even the performance of one or several entire steps. For example, the occupational therapist applies a tactile cue at the forearm and wrist whenever working with John on dressing skills. This personal assistance or permanent prompt is continued (rather than faded out) because it cues John to move his or her arm forward to initiate donning a shirt. In the same dressing activity, the therapist completes several very difficult nontarget steps (places the shirt over John's head and holds one sleeve out) but teaches the remaining activity steps.

Fading

There are many ways to prompt someone who does not know the steps of a particular activity. However, because all prompts will need to be faded out for the person to achieve complete independence, prompts must be added to instruction with care. Unnecessary or excessive assistance will only create more dependency on the therapist or caregiver. In the sections that follow, we describe four effective prompting procedures, roughly in order of increasing intrusiveness and difficulty: (1) observation learning or modeling, (2) time delay, (3) system of least prompts, and (4) graduated guidance. The last three approaches incorporate fading strategies. Therapists can also simply apply prompts singly or in combination without any organized approach for eliminating them, with the caveat that abrupt fading may result in performance setbacks for many learners with developmental disabilities.

Observation Learning or Modeling

Recent studies support the use of modeling or learning by watching another person perform a target activity in part or in full, either in real time or on video/DVD (Alonna & Wilder, 2009). This approach to teaching or intervention has been referred to as *observation learning* (Ledford, Gast, Luscre, & Ayres, 2008) and has been effective with a wide range of clients who have disabilities and a for wide range of functional tasks. Since modeling is a fairly nonintrusive, natural approach that has a good success record, it might be used as a prompting method before other more complex methods are chosen.

Learning through observation of models or demonstrations requires focused attention, memory, and the ability to imitate. Some have referred to this type of learning as a "see–then do" method. With observational learning, students may be praised (or prompted if necessary) for attending to the model, as they must see it before they can learn. If clients lack some of these skills, the approach can be simplified and coupled with reinforcement for improved attending or imitating. Model prompts also may be repeated, exaggerated, or given partially and may be paired with other prompts (gestures or partial physical prompts). Uncomplicated modeling of entire activities can also be effective. For example, modeling of the whole activity without verbal prompting was successful in teaching social skills and coffee making to three adults with severe developmental delay (Bidwell & Rehfeldt, 2004). Praise after successful completion of each step of the activity was used to reinforce skill acquisition.

Garfinkle and Schwartz (2002) demonstrated the use of observational learning in children with autism and other developmental delays. The intervention took place in the children's classroom and consisted of structured leadership to promote imitation, using prompts to facilitate imitation. Praise was given when successful imitations were performed.

Simultaneous Prompting

Simultaneous prompting involves the providing both teaching (intervention) trials and testing (probe) trials during daily ADL routines. Prompts are not gradually faded but simply present during teaching trials and absent during probe trials. This method has been applied more often to academic tasks and less often in teaching ADL occupations (Sewell, Collins, Hemmeter, & Schuster, 1998). Because it is simple to use and has support, we present it here.

To use simultaneous prompting, in teaching trials the therapist gives the controlling prompt (one that is known) at the same time as the target stimulus (one that is not known) is being taught. In this activity-based example with a preschooler, physical prompts are the controlling stimuli or prompt as the target stimulus is putting on a pullover, which involved 10 steps: Robbin, who is almost 3 and developmentally delayed, chooses dress-up play and selects a green pullover shirt from the clothing box. The therapist points to it, saying, "Put on your shirt." At the command, the therapist immediately places her hands over Robbin's and physically guides her through each step in the task until the shirt is on. The therapist explains in simple language what is happening as it is performed and delivers praise after each activity step as long as Robbin allows her guidance. When done, the therapist offers Robbin an activity-based choice while holding up materials: "Do you want to cook something or should we sweep?"

During intermittently given probe trials, therapists simply withhold prompts or physical assistance, give 5 seconds for the client to initiate the activity step, 25 seconds to complete a step, and praise when the step is completed. Errors and failures to respond are ignored, but the therapist performs the activity step and repeats the specific direction, giving the client an opportunity to perform each activity step in sequence. Criterion is reached when clients perform the activity completely during several consecutive probes: After Robbin could complete all dressing steps during three probe trials in a row, her team regarded her performance as meeting criterion, and the skill became one to maintain and to be generalized to her home environment.

Time Delay

Another approach for giving and fading assistance is to pause or add a delay period before giving a prompt. During delay periods, the client may either wait for assistance or try the response on his or her own. If the learner tries, the response may be correct or incorrect. For example, Sam is learning some basic self-feeding skills (Figure 5.2). His therapists decide that a physical prompt is best for him and plan to fade the prompt using time delay. They start teaching each skill using a no-delay period (0 seconds) between the discriminative stimulus (S^D) and the prompt, so Sam gets physical prompts continuously through each spoon, napkin, and cup cycle for several meals. Then his therapist inserts a 4-second pause between each S^D and the prompt, allowing Sam time to attempt the response without help. For some steps in the tasks, Sam waits for assistance (prompted correct responses); for others, he completes the steps (independent responses). On a few steps he tries on his own and makes errors, the therapist immediately repeats that step with help. Because Sam can eat faster when he tries on his own rather than waiting out the delay for help, time delay seems to motivate him to initiate without help, but because help is forthcoming at the end of a delay period, uncertain learners can simply wait.

Therapists using time delay more often adopt the simpler constant delay approach (for example, no delay followed by delays of 4 seconds). They also may use progressive delay trials, where a delay is gradually increased from 0 to 6 or 8 seconds or longer, depending on the client's natural response latency (e.g., 0, 2, 4, 6, or 8 seconds) (Graff & Green, 2004; Snell & Brown, 2000). Time delay has been found effective across many academic tasks as well as IADLs (preparing snacks, making beds, etc.) and social engagement activities like learning activities taught by peer tutors (Jameson, McDonnell, Polychronis, & Riesen, 2008) and leisure skills (Kurt & Tekin-Iftar, 2008; Zhang et al., 2005). Progressive time delay is more complicated than constant delay; applying either time delay to a chained activity like eating or dressing is more complicated than applying it to discrete or isolated responses, such as lip closure and grasping, or repeated responses, such as stepping. Balancing the effectiveness of a teaching approach with staff requirements is something teams need to consider in their choice of prompting methods. The principle of *parsimony*—to seek the simplest but still effective method—is the one to heed as teams make these choices (Etzel & LeBlanc, 1979).

When using either delay approach, the therapist needs to select a single or a combined prompt rather than a hierarchy of prompts and should plan how or when to increase the delay. The best guide is to increase the delay only after a period of several sessions or trials of successful waiting responses (the client does not make an error but allows himself or herself to be prompted) or correct responses (the client makes the response during the delay without help). If the client makes errors before the prompt, the delay might be shortened for several trials. If the client makes an error after the prompt, the prompt may not work for that person. If this happens repeatedly, another prompt should be considered. The delay should not be increased following errors; instead, the therapist should determine what type of error has occurred and address it accordingly. These decisions rely on the team's thinking about the task, the client, and the client's performance.

System of Least Prompts

Chris, the preschooler learning to sit in and stand up from a chair, did not readily perform the steps in these activities. His therapist planned to use a prompting procedure and discussed the options with his team. Because he could follow some verbal–gestural directions and often imitated models, they chose a prompting procedure with a "built-in" means for fading: a system of least intrusive prompts, also called *least prompts*. This involves selecting a hierarchy of prompts that work both for the client and the activity. These are used one at a time, starting with less assistance and moving to more. Therapists select a latency period and the student initiates the response with no help or with no additional help. For example, Chris has high tone and a movement disorder due to cerebral palsy, which slow his response time. With Chris's preschool teachers, his therapist decides to use a slightly longer latency of 5 seconds, that is, the therapist will pause for 5 seconds following her instructional cue to let Chris initiate the first step in the target task, before giving any assistance (unless

he begins making an error, at which point she will interrupt the error with the least intrusive level of assistance). She will pause for the 5-second latency after giving assistance, or prompt to allow Chris to initiate the step with a certain amount of assistance.

Typically, the following three levels of prompts are used (though only two may also be used):

1. Verbal instructions (simple statements for each activity step);
2. Verbal instructions plus a model or gesture (depending on the step, the therapist will point to the materials needed; for other activities a brief, partial model or demonstration of the movement required may be used);
3. Verbal instructions plus physical assistance (the therapist provides only as much guidance as is needed, placing a hand on the person's hand, wrist, forearm, or elbow or at control points such as the knees, shoulders, waist, or hips).

With Chris, the therapist decides to use only two levels of prompt (verbal plus gesture and verbal plus physical assist) but starts with the least intrusive prompt and proceeds to the more intrusive prompts if Chris cannot complete a particular step of the task or makes an error and needs more help. For each step, the therapist will wait for Chris's initiation during the latency before giving help, then, if he does not initiate or makes an error, offer a verbal prompt plus a pointing gesture, and wait. If he does not initiate the step within 4 seconds or does not complete the response (or makes an error), the therapist will move to the most intrusive prompt and physically help him to complete the step.

A least-prompts system is adaptable to many activities and individuals; it has been effective for people with mental retardation and other disabilities across many daily living tasks (Snell, 1997). On the negative side, this system is initially a bit complex for therapists to learn. It employs artificial instructor prompts rather than natural ones and can seem quite intrusive to clients. Examples include physically helping a person move through the step of opening the toothpaste or grasping a box of cereal in the grocery store.

A least-prompts system that uses modeling and physical prompts is better during the acquisition phase of learning, while more subtle prompts are better during later stages of learning. Examples of subtle prompts include an initial nod to encourage a hesitant student to keep going, followed by a nonspecific verbal prompt of "What's next?" followed finally, if needed, by gestures toward relevant stimuli (e.g., materials needed, location to move to, part of body to move).

Client factors need to be considered when choosing prompts. Some individuals are tactually defensive and do not like to be touched; others cannot use certain prompts due to skill limitations (not everyone can imitate a model prompt or follow verbal instructions). Therefore, the therapist needs to select prompts that work for the individual or select prompts, such as simple verbal instructions or pictures of activity steps, that could be learned after being associated with established prompts. Least-prompts systems require at least two levels of prompts, arranged in a hierarchy from least to most intrusive and preceded by a latency period. The later, more intrusive prompts in the hierarchy might be more consistently effective than the earlier, less intrusive prompts. This is acceptable as long as all the selected prompts are at least partially effective. Given these basic characteristics, the least-prompts system can be adapted to suit many different clients and activities (Richman, Wacker, Cooper-Brown, & Kayser, 2001).

Prompt systems, especially least prompts and time delay, offer several advantages; they have a built-in plan for fading out assistance, result in fewer errors than most teaching methods, and have a research basis of demonstrated effectiveness. When therapists rely only on consequences to teach new skills, students may become discouraged by their errors and fail to make progress. The combined use of antecedent-prompt strategies with planned consequences is the best teaching approach.

Graduated Guidance

Therapists using graduated guidance apply more intrusive physical prompts first, then fade them out. Several variations of graduated guidance have been used in teaching ADL skills to individuals with disabilities. In a hand-to-shoulder approach, therapists initially provide full hand-over-hand guidance throughout the activity but give only the amount of assistance that is needed for the learner to complete the activity. This requirement—"to give only as much help as is needed"—means that therapists must become highly sensitive to the pressure cues learners give back as they are being assisted. If the client's hands move in the desired direction during a dressing task, the therapist tries to back off and give less guidance. But if the client stops forward movement before he or she should, the therapist provides the movement. The general order of fading assistance is from the client's hands upward to the shoulder and then to omit physical assistance altogether. This approach has been used to teach eating behaviors (Saloviita, 2002).

One difficulty with graduated guidance is deciding when to reduce assistance. The best approach is to try reducing assistance periodically while encouraging the student or client to perform with less assistance. The client's own movements are the best guides to where less assistance is needed. Another approach is to use a brief waiting period before physically assisting each step (or some steps) in the activity, thus giving the client opportunities to initiate each step before being prompted. Watching the client perform without any help (such as testing performance) can also help determine what steps may need less assistance.

A second general graduated guidance approach involves using three different levels of physical assistance, varying again from more assistance to less assistance during training:

1. Full hand-over-hand assist,
2. Two-finger assist, and
3. "Shadowing" the person's hand from about 1–2 inches.

This approach has been used to teach self-care skills (Farlow & Snell, 2000). In both graduated guidance approaches, if the client resists the prompted movement, the therapist may maintain contact with the client but simply wait until there is no resistance before continuing to assist. When the therapist has successfully reduced assistance, praise for the client's increased effort should be increased. When the client seems to require more assistance, it can be given.

Graduated guidance allows the client to "get the feel" of the movement required by a skill and gradually to take more responsibility for making the movement without the therapist's guidance. This method does not work for individuals who are tactually defensive, do not like to be guided, or choose to move very quickly, nor will it work for those who become dependent on physical assistance. Often unnaturally intensive training and punitive correction methods have been coupled with graduated guidance; these are strategies that we do not recommend. Graduated guidance may be appropriate when it is suited to the learner and if less intrusive prompting methods have not been successful.

Consequences

Reinforcing Consequences Following Correct or Approximate Responses

Table 5.3 shows some of the consequences that adults and peers can offer to a learner after a target response. The following practices for using positive consequences are recommended for most learners.

Reinforcement Schedule

During early learning or acquisition, reinforcement following correct and approximate responses (even when prompted) facilitates learning. Reinforcement will occur more frequently during acquisition than during later stages of learning but should be "thinned" to an intermittent frequency so the student learns to perform without continuous reinforcement from others. If continuous schedules are not reduced over time, students may fail to use the skill under natural conditions when little reinforcement is forthcoming.

Appropriate to Learner

Reinforcing consequences should suit the client's chronological age, preferences, level of understanding, and learning situation. Some clients find simple confirmation reinforcing ("That's right"); others benefit more from task-specific praise ("Good job sweeping in the corner"). For some students, a choice of preferred activities can be provided at the end of a relatively long activity during the acquisition stage. Letting the client have a choice about the reinforcing consequence is always better than trying to anticipate what he or she might find enjoyable.

Natural Reinforcers

During later stages of learning, it is good to teach the client to self-monitor his or her performance by asking and answering "How well did I do this time?" It is also helpful to teach clients to look to more natural forms of self-reinforcement, such as having Sam eat a preferred finger food after a session of teaching spoon use, letting April choose the preferred activities whenever she reaches her time goals for putting on her shoes and AFOs, or letting Chris participate in the next activity once seated in circle at preschool.

Consequences are also part of prompt systems. For least prompts and graduated guidance, and when single prompts are used (with time delay or simply with a fixed latency), praise is the typical consequence given for completing a step. Only when more concrete reinforcers are needed should they be added, and then they should meet the "appropriateness" criteria. Early in learning, praise can be given following the completion of every step, whether or not the step was prompted. As learning progresses, the reinforcing consequences need to be decreased, so praise and other reinforcing consequences are reserved for progress made on more difficult steps, and is not given for steps completed with the most intrusive prompts.

Consequences Following Errors

When clients make errors, there are many different ways to respond. The stage of learning and the type of error made will influence the consequence, as will many of the client's characteristics (e.g., age, disabilities, skills). Consider Chris, the preschooler who is learning to sit and stand up from sitting. Before he has learned these tasks to about 60% accuracy, the therapist will need to correct any errors (e.g., "Grab the chair right here," while pointing to the chair arms) by showing Chris how to respond.

Corrections typically involve giving assistance following mistakes. Some prompt systems provide clear ways to respond to errors. For example, in a least-prompts approach, the therapist interrupts any mistakes with the next prompt in the hierarchy. However, if the incorrect response is simply a failure to respond, then the next prompt in the hierarchy is given, following the latency. In graduated guidance, the therapist also responds to errors by giving more assistance but typically more physical assistance. For example, if Linda, who is learning to brush her teeth, fails to remove the cap before squeezing the tube of toothpaste, the therapist may move her guiding hand away from Linda's elbow (a point of less assistance) to the wrist or hand (points of greater assistance) and ask Linda to repeat the missed step. Once Linda has learned more of the tooth brushing activity, the therapist might ask her "What's next?" (nonspecific verbal prompt) when Linda hesitates on a step she has done before without help. Alternately, the therapist may simply wait longer, giving Linda time to self-correct.

Both of these approaches encourage more self-correction and independence by the client, something that is especially desirable during the later stages of learning. People in these stages of learning a skill may simply check with the therapist when they've completed the activity; if it has not been done adequately, the therapist might withhold approval or ask them to try again. As we have noted earlier, the use of punitive consequences for errors is inappropriate.

Review of Progress and Intervention

This section discusses procedures for reviewing outcomes of therapeutic intervention. Therapists may not always have the opportunity to follow up on specific process recommendations. This happens, for instance, when return visits to occupational therapy are not approved by reimbursement agencies or in early intervention or school settings where therapists commonly treat children once a week for short periods of time.

Under these circumstances, opportunities for review of intervention outcomes may be restricted by time constraints or may not be possible at all. These are unfortunate realities in the current practice environment. It is our recommendation that therapists take time to read the following sections and consider ways to modify the review methods to suit individual settings and needs. For instance, when the therapist is not routinely present in a classroom setting, the teacher or aide may be able to collect information. Transdisciplinary settings, such as early intervention programs, present many opportunities for other professionals to collect outcome information. Some families are good at such details as well.

Client performance data (from testing and training) are used in a number of ways. Test data help teachers and therapists:

- Make decisions about what learning areas to target, depending on the client's *baseline data* (performance before instruction begins);
- Judge progress, once training has begun, by monitoring the client's progress using criterion or test conditions (referred to as *probing* or collecting *probe performance data*). Whenever possible, probes taken in the context where the goal behavior is used (e.g., desk work, lunchroom) are best, as they give a realistic picture of learning.
- Make decisions about environmental changes, such as hospital discharge or transition to another unit or service.

Baseline and Probe Data

Baseline data should be collected over at least two sessions or until they seem fairly stable, not varying by 40% or more in either direction (Farlow & Snell, 1994). If only one assessment is possible, therapists might ask family members, the client, or others familiar with the client's performance how well he or she currently performs the activity and estimate if performance is stable. When these data are relatively representative of the client's performance, instruction can begin, with baseline performance serving as a comparative guide for judging progress made during training. Chris's baseline performance, for example, (Figure 5.2), was measured over a week and indicated some improvement. Probe data involved repeating the test observation after teaching had begun.

Many therapists have found that probe observations need not be taken more than once every

5 training days (when training/therapy is daily) unless progress is poor. Even then, training data, rather than probe data, are more useful when analyzing the reasons for lack of progress (Farlow & Snell, 1994). Test data (both baseline and probe) typically are recorded using symbols for correct and incorrect responses (see Figure 5.2). They may be summarized as the percentage or number correct out of the total opportunities. It is useful to record these data on the same graph as training data but to use different symbols to distinguish between them (see Figure 5.3). Ungraphed or step-by-step task analytic data also should be saved and dated; they show which steps were correct and which were missed. Chris's trial-by-trial data are shown in Figure 5.2, and his percentage of correct performance is graphed in Figure 5.3.

Training Data

Training data are collected during the intervention session. Typically, clients perform a given activity better during training than during test conditions. This can be painfully obvious to therapists who treat in one-on-one intervention sessions, then find task performance plummets in contexts such as the classroom or home.

When recording training data, use of symbols is recommended for correct responses and for the types and amounts of assistance needed by the client to complete the behavior or step in the activity. Thus, steps in the three activities in Table 5.2 (spoon, cup, and napkin use) could be rated either "correct" or noted with a *P* to indicate that a physical prompt was given (see Figure 5.2). If several prompts are possible, different symbols may indicate which prompt obtained the response (e.g., *V* for verbal, *G* for gestural, *M* for model, *P* for physical assist).

If parents, caregivers, teachers, or spouses will be collecting data, they should be taught how to record correctly. Training data give the therapist objective information about how the learner responds to the therapy program and can be used to support requests from reimbursement sources for further sessions. Like test data, training data should be both preserved in an ungraphed form (so the information on individual steps is not lost) and graphed using the percentage correct or the number of steps correct. Note that in Figure 5.2, Chris's baseline and probe data are indicated with an asterisk.

Using Data

In addition to scanning graphs for the trend in progress and for variability, therapists can examine "raw" or ungraphed (step-by-step) data for specific error patterns or problem areas that provide clues to needed changes if progress is poor. Dated anecdotal records about student behavior, interfering circumstances, and illnesses may also help resolve why progress is inadequate. These data are particularly helpful for clients with complex problems, such as sensory disturbances. For example, Chris's data (Figure 5.2) indicate steady progress with less and less assistance on the first five steps of the task during March and April. On April 26, he required some physical assistance on steps he usually got correct, and the teacher noted on the graph that he did not appear to feel well that day. Since his performance was soon back to its higher level, the teachers made no changes in the program.

Farlow and Snell (1994) provide a detailed method for using data effectively; Brown and Snell (2000) also give some guidelines for this approach. Ottenbacher's (1986) book, *Evaluating Clinical Change: Strategies for Occupational and Physical Therapists*, gives similar information.

Several general steps are involved in analyzing data to improve treatment programming:

- *Collect data relevant to the treatment goals.* Collect training data whenever the client is seen. Several times a week is optimal but is not usual in most therapy settings. Collect probe data in other settings periodically, or have others involved in the client's life do so.
- *Preserve step-by-step data and graph data.* Indicate dates and types of data on the graph; baseline, intervention, test, and training data. In addition, on the back or front of the graph, note (and date) any relevant anecdotal comments pertinent to the performance data. Use graphs that show all attendance dates so absences, vacations, and other missed days are clear (see Figure 5.3). Connect data from continuous periods of time.
- *Determine trend if unclear.* If the data seem to be reliable and representative of the client's performance, determine the trend after graphing 6–8 data points. It will be ascending, flat, or descending. If the data are not representative (e.g., if the client has been sick) or not reliable (e.g., for three of the data points, the aide "recalled" the performance rather than recording the data during the performance), examine the trend after more data have been collected.

To illustrate, in the example of the preschooler given earlier, Chris's initial flat progress in March was followed after spring break by perfect performance during training. This higher-than-criterion performance caused the therapist and teacher to increase the criterion to 100% (Figure 5.3).

- *Ascending trends.* If the trend is ascending, continue the program unless the criterion (intervention) goal has been met, whereupon the goal needs to be changed.
- *Flat or descending trends.* If the trend is flat or descending, work with the client, the client's team, or both, depending upon the setting, to determine the possible reason(s) for the lack of progress.
  - o Is there a cyclical variability related to time—some days or sessions are worse due to a weekend, the therapist or the therapy assistant, a prescribed medication, or other changing factors?
  - o Are test data better than training data? If so, what are the differences between the two situations?
  - o Does the client have difficulty with the same step(s) across sessions?
  - o What are the reasons for errors? Is it a specific step? Are the errors setting-, time-, or staff-specific? Are they due to the learner not attempting the activity or performing incorrectly? Is the learner reinforced after making errors?
  - o Compare performance on other activities and behaviors with this performance. Are the errors similar? Does the target behavior interact with other behaviors (e.g., interfering behavior)? Are problem behaviors increasing? Does the program prevent access to other interactions and activities?
  - o Develop a possible explanation. Working with the client or client's team to develop a feasible explanation(s) for the lack of progress.
  - o Plan program improvements. As a team, decide on programmatic changes that will address the potential reasons for the behavior. If more than one explanation is developed, determine which one(s) should dictate program change, perhaps by making more observations.

Consider the example of Millie, an adolescent who is working on improving her use of a power wheelchair at school. Her lack of progress seems cyclical or related to sessions that isolate her from peers, but she is improving during training sessions held during physical education class with peers and at lunchtime in the cafeteria. Anecdotal records indicate that Millie often refuses to try driving during these sessions where no progress is being made and has cried several times.

Two potential explanations could be developed:

1. During the time periods when there is progress, Millie's trainers are doing something different (and more effective) than are her trainers at other times.
2. Millie enjoys instruction in the context of her peers—perhaps it's the cheering they sometimes give her when she tries harder to drive.

The first explanation was ruled out after team members realized that instructors during physical education and lunch were rotated and not specific to those times. Millie's team then decided to focus on the second explanation. They asked Millie if she might prefer to have a peer volunteer help during the times of the day when peers had not been present. When Millie indicated she would like this, they recruited volunteers and included them in all training sessions where little progress had been occurring. Data collected after this change indicated that her progress showed ascending trends in all sessions.

In current practice settings, ongoing evaluation is usually required by reimbursement sources. Therapists gather and examine client performance data to address program evaluation steps (Centers for Disease Control and Prevention, 1999). Relevant data include probes or intermittent test data (during baseline and probes of training progress) and training data supplemented by anecdotal notes about the client's performance and social validation of the progress attained. To validate client progress socially, one can

- Query learners themselves, their peers or family members, and teachers and therapists to obtain subjective opinions about progress and
- Compare clients' performance to their peers' performance. Though learning evaluation is never simple, it need not be overly complex to provide information pertinent to the effectiveness of a therapy program. The evaluation process should be ongoing, where and when possible, not applied at the conclusion of a program or a school year. Ongoing evaluation means that if the data indicate the client's progress is below expectations, the data are analyzed to clarify the reasons and to design the needed program changes. The data

are then used to monitor whether program changes actually lead to performance improvements.

Application of Strategies to Instrumental Activities

This chapter up to now has detailed strategies for providing ADL interventions. Most of the activities described incorporate basic ADL tasks, such as self-feeding, dressing, and drinking. The next part of this chapter will focus on use of the same strategies to teach IADLs.

Meal Preparation

To live independently with minimal support, adults with developmental disabilities need to be able to perform IADL tasks such as meal preparation. Rehfeldt, Dahman, Young, Cherry, and Davis (2003) provided an IADL intervention on a simple level, teaching three persons to make peanut butter and jelly sandwiches in their day treatment setting. They used observational learning through the use of video, accompanied by verbal praise for successful performance. After task analysis was carried out on sandwich making and videotaped following the task analysis steps, they used probes before and after the men watched the video to determine the impact of observation. Generalization of skills was studied by having the adults perform the tasks in probe phase at the kitchen of the sheltered workshop. Two of the three adults (two men and a woman) were unable to complete the task prior to training. The woman could perform some of the steps but not consistently. Verbal reminders were required by two participants during probe phases.

Health Behavior

One element of occupational therapy practice outcomes is health behavior, including prevention (AOTA, 2008). Providing interventions that will help clients who are vulnerable to risk protect themselves falls within the *Framework* and is an important aspect of community participation for adults with developmental disabilities.

One health concern is the vulerability of adults with developmental disabilities to sexual assault. This has led to emerging efforts to provide safety training to prevent such assaults. One effort was carried out by Egemo-Helm et al. (2007), with seven adult women with mild to moderate cognitive impairments, living in apartments with supports and in group homes, participating.

Interventions were held in both types of home, including scenarios, reports on behavioral responses to scenarios, role playing, and responses to verbal approaches from research assistants (in situ intervention). Training staff modeled appropriate responses to sexual suggestions and videotaped client responses to point out ineffective responses. Modeling was accompanied by praise when appropriate responses resulted. Additional role playing and instruction were the consequences used when clients responded inappropriately. Staff also tracked negative side effects by filling out surveys on a regular basis. Social validation studies were carried out with staff and caregivers. While three of the seven women dropped out of the study, the remaining four were able to demonstrate skills maintenance at 1 month. Two clients needed retraining at the 3-month follow-up.

Bosner and Belfiore (2001) demonstrated another example of health behavior training in their study of a 16-year-old girl with Down syndrome and diabetes who learned to give herself her own insulin injections. Two task analyses were developed, one for gathering materials needed and one for the actual injection process. A simulated injection procedure was used initially for safety reasons. A least-prompts system, combined with a time delay, was incorporated for training, allowing the researcher to intervene if safety concerns were observed. The young woman quickly mastered gathering materials for her injections. Learning to fill the syringe and inserting and removing the needle took some program modifications and required partial participation. While not completely independent when the study was completed, the girl needed assistance only in insertion and removal of the needle.

Leisure Activities

Leisure skills are another important occupation that contribute to life satisfaction. Wilson and colleagues (2006) assessed current levels of leisure activity of three women living in group homes, then carried out a process where family, staff members, and others in the community developed a list of age-appropriate leisure activities. The women were taught to make choices between pairs of activities, then were engaged in the activity of their choice using a least-to-most assistive prompt process. A timer was used to facilitate activity participation for short periods of time.

One focus of the process was to expand leisure opportunities for the clients; another was to train staff how to present possible leisure activities to people living in the group homes. Social validation procedures were carried out on the process. Two of the three participants continued to demonstrate high levels of leisure participation in the follow-up period.

This section of the chapter has been used to discuss different kinds of activities that can be taught using the strategies detailed earlier. The people cited have taught and maintained a broad range of occupations that are age-appropriate, socially valued, and important to the lives of persons with cognitive limitations. Occupational therapists need to think broadly and not limit the goals they choose for clients with cognitive impairments because they appear too complex. The intricacy of the occupations cited here prove that these clients are often capable of more than initially meets the eye.

Summary

Often the goal of occupational therapy intervention is to promote learning and thus enable occupational performance during daily routines, often involving basic and IADLs. Ideally, training occurs in the client's usual physical and social environments. To facilitate goal attainment, therapists need to target goals that will be meaningful to each individual learner, to use methods that are relatively uncomplicated but effective, to respect the client, and to review the client's progress on an ongoing basis. Training strategies for achieving goals with clients having intellectual disabilities may require the careful selection and use of cues and prompts as well as performance feedback. During the intervention process, training strategies and client behaviors should be carefully observed, documented, and analyzed. This process of data collection and analysis should be ongoing so that intervention can be modified if necessary.

Study Questions

1. Identify the principles that should be incorporated when identifying appropriate interventions, and discuss their relationship to the occupational therapy values of client-centered practice.
2. Explain how extension and enrichment skills can be embedded into routines in those intervention goals where partial participation is the outcome.
3. Consider the complex process of assessment of persons with intellectual disability, and discuss the importance and limitations of standardized assessments and how these factors can be enhanced through family/caregiver input.

4. Explain the use of single- and multiple-opportunity activity analytic assessments and their use as a basis for intervention with clients with intellectual disability.

5. Discuss the role of antecedent events and consequences on targeted behaviors and how they can be integrated into occupational therapy interventions.

6. Explain the difference between artificial and natural prompts, and discuss their use in building routines for clients with intellectual disability.

7. Identify the 4 kinds of prompts discussed in the chapter, and describe the benefits and challenges of using them in interventions.

8. Define the differences between baseline and training data collection processes and their uses in evaluating interventions.

References

Alonna, M., & Wilder, D. A. (2009). A comparison of peer video modeling and self video modeling to teach textual responses in children with autism. *Journal of Applied Behavior Analysis, 32,* 345–341.

American Occupational Therapy Association. (2008). Occupational therapy domain and process: Domain and process (2nd ed.). *American Journal of Occupational Therapy, 62,* 625–683.

Bass, J. D., & Mulick, R. A. (2007). Social play skill enhancement of children with autism using peers and siblings as therapists. *Psychology in the Schools, 44,* 727–735.

Betz, A., Higbee, T. S., & Reagon, K. A. (2008). Using joint activity schedules to promote peer engagement in preschoolers with autism. *Journal of Applied Behavior Analysis, 41,* 237–241.

Bidwell, M. A., & Rehfeldt, R. A. (2004). Using video modeling to teach a domestic skill with an embedded social skill to adults with severe mental retardation. *Behavioral Interventions, 19,* 263–274.

Bosner, S. M., & Belfiore, P. J. (2001). Strategies and considerations for teaching an adolescent with Down syndrome and Type I diabetes to self-administer insulin. *Education and Training in Mental Retardation and Developmental Disabilities, 36*(1), 94–102.

Brown, F., Evans, I., Weed, K., & Owen, V. (1987). Delineating functional competency: A component model. *Journal of the Association for Persons With Severe Handicaps, 12,* 117–124.

Brown, F., & Snell, M. E. (2000). Meaningful assessment. In M. E. Snell & F. Brown (Eds.), *Instruction of students with severe disabilities* (5th ed., pp. 67–110). Columbus, OH: Merrill.

Carr, E. G., Levin, L., McConnachie, G., Carlson, J. I., Kemp, D. C., & Smith, C. E. (1994). *Communication-based intervention for problem behavior. A user's guide for producing positive change.* Baltimore: Paul H. Brookes.

Centers for Disease Control and Prevention. (1999). *Framework for program evaluation in public health.* MMWR 48 (No. RR-11). Retrieved from http://www.cdc.gov/eval/framework.htm

Collins, B. C., Coast, D. L., Wolery, M., Holcombe, A., & Letherby, J. (1981). Using constant time delay to teach self-feeding to young students with severe/profound handicaps: Evidence of limited effectiveness. *Journal of Developmental and Physical Difficulties, 3,* 157–179.

Doig, E., Fleming, J., Cornwell, P., & Kuipers, P. (2009). Qualitative exploration of client-centered, goal-directed approach to community-based occupational therapy for adults with traumatic brain injury. *American Journal of Occupational Therapy, 63,* 559–569.

Egemo-Helm, K. R., Miltenberger, R. G., Knudson, P., Finstrom, N., Jostad, C., & Johnson, C. (2007). An evaluation of *in situ* training to teach sexual abuse prevention skills to women with mental retardation. *Behavioral Interventions, 22,* 99–119.

Etzel, B. C., & LeBlanc, J. M. (1979). The simplest treatment alternative: Appropriate instructional control and errorless learning procedures for the difficult-to-teach child. *Journal of Autism and Developmental Disorders, 9,* 361–382.

Farlow, L. J., & Snell, M. E. (1994). *Making the most of student performance data* (Research to Practice Series). Washington, DC: American Association on Mental Retardation.

Farlow, L., & Snell, M. E. (2000). Teaching self-care skills. In M. E. Snell & F. Brown (Eds.), *Instruction of students with severe disabilities* (5th ed., pp. 331–380). Columbus, OH: Merrill.

Ferguson, D. L., & Baumgart, D. (1991). Partial participation revisited. *Journal of the Association for Persons With Severe Handicaps, 16,* 218–227.

Finnie, N. (1997). Dressing. In N. Finnie (Ed.), *Handling the young child with cerebral palsy at Home* (3rd ed., pp. 190–208). Philadelphia: Butterworth-Heinemann.

Fisher, D., & Frey, N. (2001). Access to the core curriculum: Critical ingredients for student success. *Remedial and Special Education, 22,* 148–157.

Frankenburg, W. K., Dodds, J., Archer, P., Shapiro, H., & Bresnick, B. (1992). The Denver II: A major revision and re-standardization of the Denver Developmental Sceening Test. *Pediatrics, 89*(1), 91–96.

Garfinkle, A. N., & Schwartz, I. S. (2002). Peer imitation: Increasing social interactions in children with autism and other developmental disabilities in inclusive preschool classrooms. *Topics in Early Childhood Special Education, 22,* 26–38.

Giangreco, M. F., Cloninger, C. J., & Iverson, V. S. (1993). *C.O.A.C.H.: Choosing options and accommodations for children.* Baltimore: Paul H. Brookes.

Graff, R. B., & Green, G. (2004). Two methods for teaching simple visual discriminations to learners with severe disabilities. *Research in Developmental Disabilities, 25,* 295–307.

Haley, S. M., Ludlow, L. H., & Coster, W. J. (1993). Pediatric Evaluation of Disability Inventory: Clinical interpretation of summary scores using Rasch rating scale methodology. *Physical Medicine and Rehabilitation Clinics of North America, 4,* 529–540.

Haney, M., & Cavallaro, C. C. (1996). Using ecological assessment in daily program planning for children with disabilities in typical preschool settings. *Topics in Early Childhood Special Education, 16,* 66–82.

Hamilton, B. L., Laughlin, J. A., Fiedler, R. C., & Granger, C. V. (1994). Interrater reliability of the 7-level Functional Independence Measure (FIM). *Scandinavian Journal of Rehabilitation Medicine, 26,* 115–116.

Individuals with Disabilities Education Improvement Act of 2004, Pub. L. 108–446, 20 U.S.C. § 1400 *et seq.*

Jameson, M., McDonnell, J., Polychronis, S., & Riesen, T. (2008). Embedded constant time delay instruction by peers without disabilities in general education classrooms. *Intellectual and Developmental Disabilities, 46,* 346–363.

Janney, R. E., & Snell, M. E. (2000). *Teacher's guide to inclusive practices: Behavioral support.* Baltimore: Paul H. Brookes.

Kottorp, A. Hällgren, M., Bernspå, B., & Fisher, A. G. (2003). Client-centred occupational therapy for persons with mental retardation: Implementation of an intervention programme in activities of daily living tasks. *Scandinavian Journal of Occupational Therapy, 10,* 51–61.

Kurt, O., & Tekin-Iftar, E. (2008). A comparison of constant time delay and simultaneous prompting within embedded instruction on teaching leisure skills to children with autism. *Topics in Early Childhood Special Education, 28,* 53–64.

Lancioni, G. E., & O'Reilly, M. F. (2001). Self-management of instruction cues for occupation: Review of studies with people with severe and profound disabilities. *Research in Developmental Disabilities, 22,* 41–65.

Lancioni, G. E., O'Reilly, M. F., Singh, N. N., Groeneweg, J., Bosco, A., Tota, A., et al. (2006). A social validation assessment of microswitch-based programs for persons with multiple disabilities employing teacher trainees and parents as raters. *Journal of Developmental and Physical Disabilities, 18,* 383–391.

Law, M. (2002). Participation in the occupations of everyday life. *American Journal of Occupational Therapy, 56,* 640–649.

Law, M., Baptiste, S., Carswell, A., Polatajko, H., & Pollack, N. (1998). *Canadian Occupational Performance Measure* (3rd ed.). Ottawa, Ontario: Canadian Occupational Therapy Association Publications.

Law, M., & Usher, P. (1988). Validation of the Klein–Bell Activities of Daily Living Scale for Children. *Canadian Journal of Occupational Therapy, 55,* 63–68.

Ledford, J. R., Gast, D. L., Luscre, D., & Ayers, K. M. (2008). Observational and incidental learning by children with autism during small group instruction. *Journal of Autism and Developmental Disorders, 38,* 86–103.

McCabe, M. A., & Granger, C. V. (1990). Content validity of a pediatric functional independence measure. *Applied Nursing Research, 3*(3), 120–122.

Odom, S., Brown, W. H., Frey, T., Karasu, N., Smith-Canter, L., & Strain, P. (2003). Evidence-based practices for young children with autism: Contributions for single-subject design research. *Focus on Autism and Other Developmental Disabilities, 18*(3), 166–176.

O'Neill, R. E., Horner, R. H., Albin, R. W., Sprague, J. R., Storey, K., & Newton, J. S. (1997). *Functional assessment and program development for problem behavior.* Pacific Grove, CA: Brooks/Cole.

Ottenbacher, K. J. (1986). *Evaluating clinical change. Strategies for occupational and physical therapists.* Baltimore: Williams & Wilkins.

Rehfeldt, R. A., Dahman, D., Young, A., Cherry, H., & Davis, P. (2003). Teaching a simple meal preparation skill to adults with moderate and severe mental retardation using videomodeling. *Behavioral Interventions, 18,* 209–218.

Richman, D. M., Wacker, D. P., Cooper-Brown, L. J., & Kayser, K. (2001). Stimulus characteristics within directives: Effects on accuracy of task completion. *Journal of Applied Behavior Analysis, 34,* 289–312.

Robertson, J., Green, K., Alper, S., Schloss, P., & Kohler, F. (2003). Using a peer-mediated intervention to facilitate children's participation in inclusive child daycare activities. *Education and Treatment of Children, 26*(2), 182–197.

Saloviita, T. (2002). Behavioural treatment of improper eating by an institutionalised woman with profound intellectual disability—A description of a successful intervention. *Journal of Intellectual and Developmental Disability, 27,* 15–20.

Sewell, T. J., Collins, B. C., Hemmeter, M. L., & Schuster, J. W. (1998). Using simultaneous prompting within an activity-based format to teach dressing skills to preschoolers with developmental delays. *Journal of Early Intervention, 21,* 132–145.

Snell, M. E. (1997). Teaching children and young adults with mental retardation in school programs: Current research. *Behaviour Change, 14,* 73–105.

Snell, M. E., & Brown, F. (2000). Measurement, analysis, and evaluation. In M. E. Snell & F. Brown (Eds.), *Instruction of students with severe disabilities* (5th ed., pp. 173–206). Upper Saddle River, NJ: Merrill/Prentice-Hall.

Trohanis, P. (2008). Progress in providing services to young children with special needs and their families: An overview to and update of the Individuals with Disabilities Education Act (IDEA). *Journal of Early Intervention, 30,* 140–151.

Wang, X. HL., Bernas, R., & Eberhard, P. (2001, April). *Children's early literacy environment in Chinese and American Indian families.* Paper presented at the Biennial Meeting of the Society for Research in Child Development, Minneapolis, MN.

Watson, D. E., & Wilson, S. E. (2003). *Task analysis: An individual and population approach* (2nd ed.). Bethesda, MD: AOTA Press.

Wilson, P. G., Reid, D. H., & Green, C. W. (2006). Evaluating and increasing in-home leisure activity among adults with severe disabilities in supported independent living. *Research in Developmental Disabilities, 27,* 93–107.

Wolery, M., Ault, M. J., & Doyle, P. M. (1992). *Teaching students with moderate to severe disabilities.* White Plains, NY: Longman.

Zhang, J., Cote, B., Chen, S., & Liu, J. (2005). The effect of a constant time delay procedure on teaching an adult with severe mental retardation a recreation bowling skill. *Physical Educator, 61*(2), 63–74.

Chapter 6

Enabling Performance and Participation for Children With Developmental Disabilities

KARIN J. BARNES, PHD, OTR, AND ALISON J. BECK, PHD, OTR

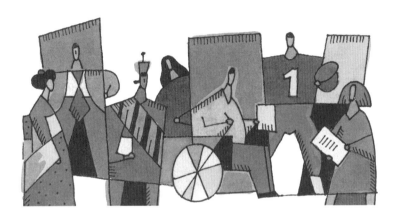

KEY TERMS

adaptive
  equipment

augmentative and
  alternative
  communication
  (AAC)

cerebral palsy

developmental
  disabilities

functional
  mobility

handling

intervention

positioning

HIGHLIGHTS

- Effective intervention requires consideration of the multiple factors influencing performance and participation, including the child, family, home, and school environments.

- Intervention for participation in the school setting involves collaboration with the family and educational staff.

- Attention to the elements of the sensory environment may improve a child's participation across areas of occupation.

- Modification of activity demands is an important approach in intervention.

Objectives

On completion of this chapter, readers will be able to

- Discuss children's school, home, and play contexts and environments and provide examples of occupational therapy processes designed to support participation by children with developmental disabilities within these contexts;
- Describe the developmental sequences of feeding, dressing, bathing, toileting, communication, and mobility skills;
- Explain the performance skills, client factors, and contextual concerns that influence children's achievement of feeding, dressing, bathing, toileting, communication, and mobility skills;
- Describe intervention strategies to improve mealtime skills of children with impairments in motor, sensory processing, and behavioral skills;
- Explain intervention strategies to improve dressing performance of children with motor, sensory processing, and cognitive impairments;
- Explain intervention strategies to improve bathing skills of children with motor, sensory processing, and cognitive impairments;
- Explain intervention strategies to improve toileting skills of children with motor and cognitive impairments;
- Describe the selection of and interventions to promote the use of augmentative and alternative communication systems; and
- Describe the types and selection of mobility devices and interventions to promote independent mobility for children with motor impairments.

Addressing the occupations (activities of daily living [ADLs], instrumental activities of daily living [IADLs], education, and play) of children with disabilities requires consideration of all aspects of the occupational therapy domain. The factors influencing the child's performance must be viewed in the personal and cultural context of the family and with full consideration of the physical and social environments of home, school, and play areas. Children learn and develop as a part of everyday family and community life. Thus, the occupational therapy process designed to improve children's meaningful participation in daily life requires considering the multiple factors that influence such performance (American Occupational Therapy Association [AOTA], 2008).

For example, the childhood activity of playing in the playground sandbox requires responding to the other children in the sandbox (social environment), playing with the sand (physical environment), and taking turns driving the toy truck through the sand (social and space demands and sequencing the activity). When an occupational therapist provides intervention for a boy with autism who wishes to play in a sandbox, he or she must consider the child's difficulty in coping with the tactile sensory environment and with comprehending the concepts involved in sharing, turn-taking and social space, and the unpredictable auditory stimuli of the playground.

In the United States, more than 7 million children with disabilities were served by the educational systems (public schools and early childhood intervention) in 2004 (U.S. Department of Education, 2006). Full participation in the ordinary activities of life cannot be taken for granted for this large group. At home, children learn appropriate ADLs, play, and leisure activities. In school, children develop academic skills; learn to socialize with peers; and interact with educators, including occupational therapists. The development of these important occupations may be impeded among children with disabilities.

Occupational therapists can provide interventions to support the child with disabilities, his or her family, other professionals, and community and school organizations so that the child can develop the skills necessary for participation in meaningful occupations. This chapter discusses the occupational therapy process for such children. The *Occupational Therapy Practice Framework* (AOTA, 2008)—hereinafter the *Framework*—provides the structure for discussion of therapy practices. It is used to help understand how specific daily occupations of children with disabilities are considered by the occupational therapy process, including home, school, and play environments, and the occupations of eating, dressing, bathing, toilet hygiene, communication management, and functional mobility. Also discussed are intervention principles, based on the occupational therapy process of analysis of the child; his or her occupations; and the context and environment. Case studies illustrate the therapy process.

Home Contexts and Environments

The cultural, personal, economic, physical, and social contexts and environments of the home and the family are vitally important and must be taken into account throughout the occupational therapy process. These profoundly affect the child's engagement in occupations and activities and shape the outcomes of any intervention.

Occupational therapists recognize the vast range of homes and the diverse family groupings that influence children's participation in meaningful occupations and activities. Homes can be small apartments, large houses, or mobile homes, in rural or urban settings. Families vary in size, familial relationships, family member age, ethnicity, sexual orientation, and socioeconomic status. The importance placed on the attainment of specific childhood occupations will vary according to these differences, as will the expectations placed on children. According to Hanson (2004), "Expectations for children concerning feeding, sleeping, and speaking, as well as the use of discipline, to mention only a few, vary widely across cultural groups" (p. 12). For example, mealtime routines differ among ethnic groups and according to the family's values. Some families have no established mealtimes; others see the family's evening meal as the most important time of the day. Table 6.1 provides examples of family conditions that highly influence a child's participation in occupations.

School Contexts and Environments

Schools typically have classrooms, halls, gyms, cafeterias, libraries, playgrounds, buses, and offices, involving a host of different people, including students, teachers, occupational therapists, bus drivers, and parents. These settings and people influence children's learning and shape their developing occupations and activities. School serves as the place where children learn academic, sport, vocational, social, and community skills. Participation in schools is considered an important right for children with disabilities in the United States under Individuals With Disabilities Education Improvement Act (P.L. 108–446) (Jackson, 2007; U.S. Department of Education, 2006).

The physical context of a school setting can play a major role in the success for a child with a disability. For example, a youth with cerebral palsy who uses a wheelchair may not be able to complete a vocational assembly task if he or she becomes too tired wheeling back and forth among different workstations spaced several feet apart. The occupational therapist can evaluate school environments as they influence the school occupations of specific students with disabilities. Hanft and Shepherd (2008) list physical contexts that should be observed in all relevant school settings, including "accessibility of building, objects, tools, devices, terrain, plants, animals," "space dimensions," and "sensory characteristics" (pp. 235–236).

The elements of the sensory environment may be evaluated informally or formally to determine their impact on student occupations. The Sensory Profile School Companion (Dunn, 2006) and the Sensory Processing Measure: Main Classroom and School Environments (Kuhaneck, Henry, & Glennon, 2007) are two occupational therapy assessment tools that evaluate the child's ability to process sensory information in the school environment. This type of information can be useful for the therapist as she or he develops an intervention plan for a child's classroom activities. This may be especially important for children with disabilities who have sensory processing impairments, such as autism or Fragile X syndrome (Roley, Blanche, & Schaaf, 2001).

Education, ADLs, IADLs, social participation, activity demands, and performance patterns all should be considered in the occupational therapy process for children with disabilities in schools. The School Functional Assessment is a comprehensive assessment of the child's skills within the school's physical context, including the activity demands (Coster, Deeney, Haltiwanger, & Haley, 1998). The tool is designed to help occupational therapists evaluate an elementary school student's participation in various school-related activity settings, his or her support needs, and his or her performance of school activities (Coster et al., 1998). The School Setting Interview (Hoffman, Hemmingsson, & Kielhofner, 1999) is another occupational therapy instrument designed to determine the student and environmental fit, focusing on accommodation needs of students with disabilities. For example, a student with spastic diplegia may have difficulty participating in art class. The use of the School Setting Interview could help determine that, for example, limited reach and poor balance are the reasons why. The occupational therapist could

Table 6.1. Family Aspects That Influence a Child's Participation

Aspects	Influence on Development
Culture	Does the family value independence? What mealtime customs are practices? What clothing is appropriate? Is assistive technology accepted? What family routines and rituals must be respected in designing intervention?
Time	Are family members able to extend the time required in care of the child? When in the family's daily routine can self-care skills be practiced?
Commitment	Are the parents committed to the effort needed to promote independence? Can family members apply the self-care interventions with consistency and regularity?
Communication	Do family members communicate daily problems and successes with each other?
Adaptability and flexibility	Can family roles adapt to changes in routines? Can family members share caregiving responsibilities?

then adjust the angle and width of the table to compensate for reaching limitations, and provide a chair with lateral support for balance. The student would then concentrate on his or her artistic endeavors instead of physical abilities.

In determining the needs of a student with a disability, the therapist considers social and cultural environment and context. Students usually want to perform occupations that align with the social expectations of other students—peer support is critical for social and academic inclusion of students with disabilities (Thousand, Villa, & Nevin, 1994). Evaluation and intervention strategies must include these contextual and environmental conditions. Townsend et al. (1999) developed an occupational therapy evaluation tool, the Occupational Therapy Psychosocial Assessment of Learning, that addresses psychosocial skills and the match between the student and the environment.

Play Contexts and Environments

Play, an important childhood occupation, is affected by the environment and context in which it occurs. This vital occupation can be compromised when the child does not have the physical, social, or cultural support needed to nurture it (Law, 2002). For example, when the parents of a child with spina bifida are busy taking care of their child's health maintenance, play development may be impeded because the parents lack sufficient time to play with him or her. The physical environment of the home impacts the child's play as well. Children who use

walking devices may have difficulty engaging in play activities when small or crowded home environments limit functional mobility.

Limited access to community or school playgrounds affects play opportunities for children with disabilities by decreasing social participation, development of motor skills, exploration of the environment, and opportunities for personal achievement (Frost, 1992). Occupational therapists may evaluate the contextual and environmental aspects of play for children with disabilities in order to provide interventions designed to encourage playground use. Holmstrand (2003) recommends several features necessary to increase the accessibility of playground equipment for children with disabilities, including

- Elevated sandboxes so children in wheelchairs can roll up to them;
- Overhead bars and rings that have been lowered so children in wheelchairs can reach them;
- Bridges wide enough for wheelchairs and children who use crutches;
- Swings with adequate trunk support; and
- Easy-to-reach manipulatives (objects and toys used with the hands) and activities, such as tic-tac-toe, on panels and tables that can be used by children with and without disabilities.

Accessibility guidelines for play areas, playgrounds, and play equipment have been developed by the U.S. Architectural and Transportation Barriers Compliance Board (2005) and are availalble at http://www.access-board.gov/play/guide/intro.htm.

The occupational therapist can identify intervention strategies that help the child meet his or her individual home, school, and play goals by considering the multiple factors that influence performance and participation in these settings. The therapist, child, parents, and teachers then develop intervention plans and strategies to support participation in the desired activities and occupations (Figure 6.1). Interventions that target contextual factors may involve approaches that create, establish, maintain, modify, and prevent activities and occupations as outlined in the *Framework* (see Table 6.2 for examples). Strategies to improve contextual and environmental factors may be used along with interventions focused on performance skill and patterns, activity demands, and client factors.

Eating and Self-Feeding

Development of Eating and Self-Feeding

Client Factors and Performance Skills

Full-term infants are born with the ability to consume nutrition, thereby sustaining life and growth. They first accomplish eating using *rooting* (to find the nipple) and *sucking* (to express liquid from the nipple). The gag reflex and automatic cough are also present (to prevent aspiration of liquids), ensuring that the ingested liquid moves through the correct passageway to the stomach. These early reflexes are integrated at 2 to 3 months of age, and in-

fants develop rhythmic sucking movements at this point. From sucking, the development of more advanced eating proceeds rapidly; by 2 years of age, children are proficient in drinking, chewing, and biting. Typical development of eating is presented in Table 6.3.

Not all children follow a typical sequence in developing self-feeding, but it is helpful to identify the usual sequence to provide general guidelines for the expected order in which skills develop. The ages listed next are approximate ages because all children are different. Infants practice self-feeding for many months before they accomplish independence at mealtimes. Bringing the hand to the mouth is one of the first motor behaviors that an infant demonstrates, and he or she may hold a bottle by 6 months. Finger-feeding a cracker or soft cookie is generally accomplished by 8 months.

By 7 to 8 months of age, an infant usually can sit in a high chair with the family at the dinner table. While observing the other family members, he or she engages in food play or finger feeding. An infant may play with a spoon by banging it on the high-chair tray. Dried cereal or small bits of soft foods provide entertainment and multiple opportunities to practice pincer grasp and finger skills. The selection of finger foods should match the child's oral–motor skills. Nuts, hard candy, popcorn, grapes, and hot dogs cut width-wise are not recommended, because they can totally occlude the airway if aspirated. Soft foods that dissolve in the mouth or

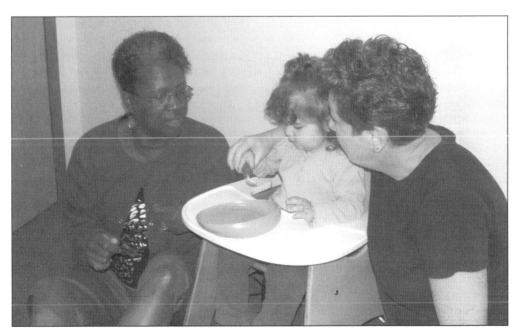

Figure 6.1. Occupational therapist advising teacher in mealtime strategies with a child.

Table 6.2. Examples of Occupational Therapy Contextual and Environmental Interventions for Children

Intervention Approaches	Examples
Create, Promote	**School:** Strategically place child with an attention deficit in classroom to optimize visual perception and learning.
	Home: Arrange bedroom to reduce sensory distractions and provide a calming environment for an adolescent with Fragile X Syndrome.
	Play Area: Create play area that allows child in a wheelchair easy access.
Maintain	**School:** Maintain handwriting skills by providing visual reminders of letter formation in the front of the classroom.
	Home: Maintain acquired social awareness and skills of a child with Conduct Disorder by placing behavioral reminder signs in the dining and TV rooms.
	Play Area: Maintain acquired play skills of child with cerebral palsy by removal of potentially hazardous equipment in the gymnasium.
Modify	**School:** Change circle time from a floor activity to a chair sitting activity for all students so that the student in a wheelchair will be at the same height as the other students.
	Home: Remove a bathroom wall so that the child in a wheelchair has easier access to the toilet and bathtub.
	Play Area: Provide additional space between pieces of backyard play equipment for easier access by children using walking devices.
Prevent	**School:** Prevent social ridicule of a student who sits on a ball seat to improve self-regulation by allowing all students the opportunity to use the special seat at other times.
	Home: Prevent parental back injuries by removal of architectural barriers at the house entrance for a youth in a wheelchair.
	Play Area: Prevent over-stimulation and possible socially unacceptable behavior of a child with autism by allowing only small groups of children in the play area.

require minimal chewing and cannot block the airway are appropriate for first finger feeding.

To develop independent spoon-feeding, an infant must understand the use of a tool and must have control of mid-range elbow, forearm, and wrist movements, including supination and pronation. Spoon-feeding often develops between 15 and 18 months of age. At this time, shoulder and wrist stability are adequate for holding the spoon to scoop the food and bring it to the mouth with minimal spillage. The child holds the spoon in a pronated gross grasp and brings the spoon to the mouth using exaggerated shoulder and elbow movements.

By 24 months of age, the child uses a supinated grasp of the spoon, holding it in the radial fingers. The subtle movements at the wrist and forearm needed to obtain the food and efficiently place the spoon in the mouth also emerge at this age. With this increased control, the child may begin to use a fork and to eat foods that are more difficult to handle (e.g., peas, corn, rice, cold cereal).

For cup drinking, the child begins initially between 6 and 12 months of age with a cup that has a lid and a spout. Some children can best manage a cup with handles; others prefer a small plastic cup without handles. A child tends to spill from a cup until 24 months of age, when jaw stability and hand control increase (Case-Smith & Humphry, 2005; Morris & Klein, 2000).

Performance Variables That Influence Eating and Self-Feeding

Problems With Motor Skills

Eating requires coordination, strength, and energy. The child must use a versatile sequence of oral movements in which tongue, cheek, jaw, and lip movements are coordinated. Children with significant motor problems (e.g., cerebral palsy or Down syndrome) often have difficulty coordinating the sequence of oral movements necessary for successful feeding. Children with cerebral palsy and Down

Table 6.3. Typical Development of Oral Eating

Age	Eating Skill	Type of Food and Utensil
Neonate	Oral reflexes of rooting and sucking; sucking is strong and rhythmic.	Breast or bottle
1 month	Sucking: rhythmic back-and-forth tongue movement with jaw opening and closing.	Breast or bottle
4 months	Strong sucking: tongue moves up and down, good lip seal.	Breast or bottle
6 months	Efficient sucking, good jaw stability and lip seal.	Breast or bottle, may introduce the cup, may begin pureed foods
9 months	Long sequence of continuous sucking; jaw stability improves on cup; uses a munching pattern with pureed foods; beginning of diagonal jaw movements; lateral tongue movements.	Pureed and soft foods, bottle or breast, cup
12 months	Rotary chewing movements; active upper lip in removing food; licking present.	Soft foods, some table foods, bottle or breast, cup
18 months	Well-coordinated rotary chewing; controlled and sustained biting; mobile tongue, including tongue elevation.	Table foods, soft meat
24 months	Well-graded and sustained bite; circular rotary jaw movements; tongue reaches lips and all gum surfaces; good lip closure; good jaw stabilization on cup.	Most meats and soft vegetables, cup without lid

syndrome frequently exhibit low muscle tone (i.e., hypotonia) in the face, neck, and trunk, which results in instability of the head and trunk. This postural instability may cause poor postural alignment; the child may fall into trunk and cervical flexion unless properly positioned. The child may also demonstrate hyperextension of the neck, thereby placing him or her at risk for aspiration due to improper alignment of the pharynx.

The jaw of a child with low muscle tone often moves in wide excursions, completely open or closed, without controlled mid-range movement; the graded jaw mobility and stability needed for chewing and cup drinking are lacking. The child's mouth is often open, which makes swallowing difficult and may result in drooling.

In a child with hypotonia, the tongue may be inactive, moving primarily with the movement of the lower jaw. The tongue may exhibit primitive extension and retraction (i.e., it extends beyond the lips and is held in the back of the mouth) rather than move up and down or side to side. Extreme movements of the jaw and tongue can disrupt coordination of the suck–swallow–breathe pattern. Extreme movement of the tongue may relate to poor neck and jaw stability, because the tongue does not

have a sufficient base of stability for controlled movement. Hypotonia also may involve the lips, rendering them relatively inactive. As a result, the child's ability to seal the lips on a bottle's nipple, a cup's rim, or a spoon is inadequate and results in food loss or air intake. Hypotonic cheeks create difficulty maintaining food on the chewing surfaces of the teeth or gathered together in the tongue's center for swallowing.

Alternatively, a child can demonstrate excess muscle tone (i.e., hypertonicity or spasticity) or fluctuating muscle tone in the face and oral area. A child with excess or fluctuating muscle tone may exhibit tonic oral reflexes or abnormal motor patterns that disrupt the rhythm and sequence of eating and put the child at risk for aspiration. Table 6.4 lists some of the functional problems associated with developmental disabilities.

Problems With Sensory Processing Skills

The sensory systems also contribute to the development of feeding skills. Introduction of new textures usually results in aversive responses in any young infant. For the child with hypersensitivity to touch, feeding is associated with genuine discomfort. A child with tactile defensiveness of the face and oral

Table 6.4. Problems in Eating and Self-Feeding Associated With Developmental Disabilities

Condition	Associated Eating Problems
Cerebral palsy	• Primitive sucking and chewing • Hyper- or hypotonia • Difficulty sequencing suck, swallow, and breathe • Difficulty coordinating lip, tongue, and jaw mobility • Postural instability
Sensory processing dysfunction	• Poor tolerance of tactile input • Limited chewing and biting skills • Oral–motor planning problems • Sensory defensiveness
Autism spectrum disorders	• Sensory defensiveness • Poor tolerance of specific tastes • Difficulty in communicating about feeding • Mealtime rituals
Respiratory or cardiac problems	• Poor endurance • Difficulty coordinating between swallowing and breathing • Purposely limits intake to limit workload of eating and digestion
Severe sensorimotor disabilities	• Poor stability and mobility of oral structures • Limited control of chewing and drinking • Swallowing problems and risk of aspiration • Nutritionally at risk due to oral–motor and communication problems
Failure to thrive	• Negative interactions between feeder/caregiver and child • Behavioral problems associated with feeding

areas demonstrates aversion to touch on or in the mouth and to textured foods inside the mouth. Such children may spit, choke, or gag when food is placed in the mouth, particularly if the food's texture is unfamiliar. When the child has hypersensitivity to oral touch, however, these responses continue well beyond the time usually required for children to develop tolerance. Hypersensitivity to oral touch can limit the child's nutritional intake and the variety of foods accepted. It also can result in negative or oppositional behaviors at mealtime. For, example, children with autism may experience this discomfort and have no method of communicating their dislike other than through negative or disruptive behaviors (Klein & Delaney, 1994).

Problems With Social, Emotional, and Communication Skills

Feeding difficulties are often accompanied by social, emotional, and communication problems. The child may not engage in feeding and may disengage by refusing to eat, throwing food, spitting food, or crying. These behaviors inevitably create stress for the family members, disrupt an important family routine, and can limit essential nutritional intake. Parents often misunderstand the child's negative responses and become anxious about the child's limited nutritional intake and negative behavior. This increased attention can be rewarding to the child, encouraging him or her to repeat the disruptive behaviors to again gain the parents' attention and emotional response. Mealtime scenarios of the child refusing to participate in eating can become routine if appropriate interventions are not implemented.

Contextual and Environmental Variables Influencing Eating and Self-Feeding

Social Environment

Eating and feeding almost always involve interaction with others. Initially, feeding is an intimate experience between caregiver and child (Humphry, 1991; Humphry & Thigpen-Beck, 1998). The give-and-take and communication between parent and child during eating contribute to building their relationship. Early in development, the parent establishes an eating rhythm, making sustained eye contact, holding and patting the child, and initiating first communications (e.g., when the infant signals hunger and satiation). Therefore, this is an initial time for responsive give-and-take between parent and child (Kelly & Barnard, 2000).

When the child makes an attempt to interact but receives no response, he or she may become passive, and no longer initiate communication. In infants with failure to thrive, the parent may not respond to the infant's signals or may not read the infant's cues.

A medical problem associated with interactional problems during feeding is congenital heart disease (CHD). Infants with CHD often refuse to eat, and parents report that feeding their infants is difficult and produces anxiety (Clemente, Baines, Shinebourne, & Stein, 2001), particularly when they become breathless and fatigued during the process. Parents of children with CHD and other significant health problems frequently worry about feeding safety and the adequacy of nutritional intake, often reporting that feeding their children with medical problems is a stressful rather than pleasurable task.

The family structure influences the child's development of eating skills (Case-Smith & Humphry, 2005). In single-parent families or when one parent is frequently away from home, feeding responsibilities may fall to one person. This responsibility can be overwhelming if a child must be fed four to five meals per day, each requiring an hour. One mother explained "I am the only one who can feed him. The staff at the child care center tries to feed him, but they worry when he chokes, and they do not know how to hold him and place the spoon so that he can swallow. He is starving when he comes home from child care, so I feed him a small meal then and dinner later. Since his birth 4 years ago, I have fed him almost every meal."

Although parents often bottle-feed infants on their laps and, later, face to face in the high chair, preschool children generally participate in family mealtime by sitting with other family members at the dinner table. Family mealtimes can help a child build skills, because he or she now has multiple role models and is usually highly motivated to become a full participant in the family meal. This social environment can reinforce the child's efforts to eat, but it can also compound his or her frustrations about eating, resulting in disruptive, acting-out behaviors.

Most families establish a routine that allows the child to participate in the family mealtime, thereby maintaining the social benefits of family gatherings and promoting the child's mealtime skills. If the child requires supportive seating, the wheelchair can be placed near to the table. When specific handling techniques are required, the child may be fed before the mealtime and be allowed to play with food on the tray while the other family members eat. Establishing eating as a social event is an important goal for every child, even when oral–motor skills are limited.

Cultural Context

Cultural background highly influences the eating routine, the amounts and types of food given to the child, how the child is served, and how much independence is valued. In certain cultures, large amounts of food are served, which can be overwhelming to a young child who struggles to eat. Although every culture has certain foods that are easier to masticate (e.g., rice, curry, cornmeal, yogurt), some cultures have standard food items that consist of fatty meats or foods that are difficult to chew.

Cultural context can affect feeding practices of families that have continued through generations. Schulze, Harwood, and Schoelmerich (2001) compared the feeding practices of Anglo-American and Puerto Rican–American mothers whose infants were 12 months of age. Anglo mothers encouraged their infants to self-feed; Puerto Rican mothers spoon- or bottle-fed their infants. Only one in 28 Puerto Rican infants self-fed, but 26 of 32 Anglos infant self-fed. Anglo mothers reported that they expected their infants to self-feed earlier and expressed the importance of autonomy. Puerto Rican mothers placed more emphasis on maintaining close interpersonal relationships with their children.

Physical Environment

Home and child care environments may either promote or inhibit the development of eating and feeding skills. Sensory aspects of the environment, such as noise level, amount of visual stimuli, and lighting can interfere with child's ability to eat. Quiet, nonstimulating, and calming environments can allow the child to concentrate and perform at optimal levels. Music can promote a level of arousal that is optimal for eating. For example, calming music that has one beat per second can promote sucking (Morris & Klein, 2000).

The physical arrangement of the home can also either promote or discourage development of feeding skills. Tables and chairs should be modified to meet the needs of children with disabilities. A comfortable and adaptable arrangement for feeding is required, particularly when a child requires physical support and adapted equipment for success in feeding.

Interventions for Eating Problems

The following sections describe interventions for eating disorders of children with motor performance problems, sensory processing problems, and interaction and communication problems.

Motor Performance Problems

Intervention for motor performance problems falls into two categories: positioning and oral–motor strategies.

Positioning

During eating, postural alignment and stability must be adequate to support oral–motor control. Full external support is required when postural stability is low. For example, a high-back chair with lateral supports and straps may be recommended for a child with severe cerebral palsy. The goal of any positioning device is to provide the level of head and

trunk support that will allow the child to demonstrate the highest level of oral motor control (Logemann, 1998).

For the child who has not developed head control, slightly reclining the chair while maintaining 90° of hip flexion can help the child with head control and facilitate oral movements for feeding. A slightly reclined position (30°) also lets the child use gravity to assist in the suck–swallow sequence (Morris & Klein, 2000). Whether the chair is tilted backward or is upright, neck alignment in neutral (with head directly over shoulders) or in slight flexion is critical so that the throat structures are in optimal alignment for efficient swallowing. A slightly forward position of the head appears to facilitate swallowing by bringing the throat structures closer together, and making closure of the trachea easier. Figure 6.2 shows an occupational therapist's use of positioning a child's head while drinking from a cup. This position of slight flexion should be considered for children with swallowing problems (Logemann, 1998). If the child is at risk for aspiration, a video

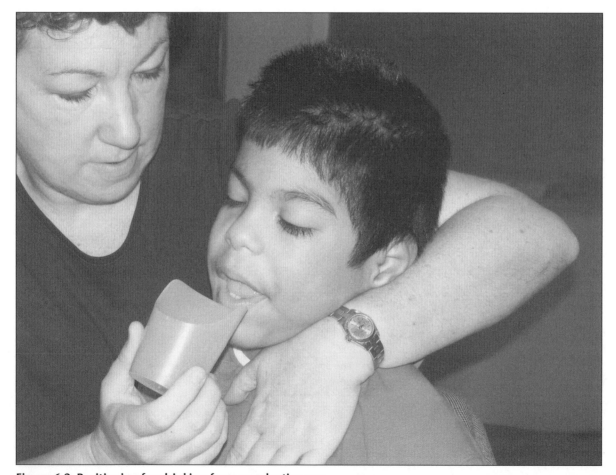

Figure 6.2. Positioning for drinking from an adaptive cup.

fluoroscopic swallow study should be conducted and can reveal the head and neck position that results in optimal swallowing and alert the health care provider to further swallowing problems or dangers.

Oral–Motor Strategies

With the head well supported, the therapist's or parent's fingers, or cupped hand, can be placed under or around the child's chin to enhance jaw stability. One finger exerts pressure through the front of the chin to promote chin tuck; another provides support under the jaw. The goal of this support is to assist in jaw stability and to provide support for the tongue's movement. This technique appears to be effective with premature infants (Einarisson-Backes, Deitz, Price, Glass, & Hays, 1994) and with children who have cerebral palsy (Gisel, Applegate-Ferrante, Benson, & Bosma, 1995).

When spoon feeding, downward pressure on the tongue with the bowl of the spoon or the nipple can inhibit tongue retraction or protraction and facilitate sucking. This gentle pressure, rhythmically applied with a spoon, promotes a cupped tongue and an organized suck–swallow pattern.

When the occupational therapist determines a technique effective, he or she recommends that it be implemented on a regular basis. Instruction to parents and other care providers is essential and should be reinforced with modeling, pictures, and feedback as the caregiver learns the techniques. Given the stress often involved in feeding a child who requires specific handling techniques, feeding techniques should be taught to multiple family members and child care providers so that responsibility can be shared. Continual monitoring of the child's response to the eating intervention is critical to assist in problem solving and to help the caregivers adapt the techniques when needed (see Case Study 6.1).

Sensory Processing Problems

Modifying Sensory Aspects of Food

Altering the sensory qualities of food is another way to improve eating performance (Case-Smith & Humphry, 2005). A child's tongue movement is guided by the texture of food or drink and responds to the sensory stimulus in the mouth. Foods that are smooth and stick together can facilitate organized tongue responses. Thick, heavy, and cohesive foods (e.g., oatmeal, puddings) tend to facilitate an efficient suck–swallow pattern. Highly textured foods result in increased tongue movements. Foods that break apart and fill the mouth with sensory input can cause disorganized responses, coughing, or choking.

To promote more mature oral movements, the occupational therapist carefully selects appropriate food textures to use in therapy sessions and to recommend to the family, based on the child's level of oral–motor skill and sensory tolerance. Some guidelines for texture selection are provided in Table 6.5. A combination of strategies can be more successful than selecting a single one. Foods that are contraindicated for a child with severe oral–motor problems are those that break apart into small pieces that are difficult to manage (e.g., raw carrots, crisp cookies) and those that are tough and require a grinding motion to masticate (e.g., some meats, chewy candies).

Strategies for Sensitivity to Touch

When a child has hypersensitivity to touch (or tactile defensiveness), the face and oral areas often are particularly sensitive. Hypersensitivity of the oral area may be a result of an extended period of non-oral feeding or of lack of appropriate oral experiences. The occupational therapist evaluates the child's sensory function through a combination of observation and parent and other caregiver interviews. The therapist asks about the food textures the child tolerates and then observes as he or she is offered a variety of textures. Aversive responses, choking, gagging, or expressions of discomfort all can indicate sensory processing problems.

When the child has oral tactile hypersensitivity, multisensory experiences at times other than mealtime can decrease the child's response to touch. Oral play with rubber toys and a warm, wet washcloth can be helpful; children generally enjoy these textures. In particular, rubber toys promote tongue and jaw movements and are an acceptable method of desensitizing the oral area. Brushing with a regular or NUK toothbrush helps to desensitize the child's mouth (Schubert, Amirault, & Case-Smith, 2010) (Figure 6.3). Asking the parent to brush the child's teeth and gums twice a day may easily fit into the family's daily routine. Routines vary, however, and parents may select more playful methods of oral stimulation.

Just before mealtime is an optimal time to desensitize the oral area to improve acceptance and tolerance of the meal. The amount and type of sensory input must depend on the child's responses to touch. In children with severe tactile hypersensitivity, the therapist should begin with application of deep pressure around and in the mouth, stroking with the finger inside a nipple or a washcloth. Taste

Table 6.5. Guidelines for Selection of Food Texture

Developmental Level	Recommendation
Child demonstrates a munching pattern and does not have lateral tongue movements.	Use pureed, smooth foods.
Child has poor tongue control and an inefficient suck–swallow pattern.	Avoid thin liquids and thicken liquids when possible.
Child is demonstrating beginning chewing skills.	Use soft foods that have cohesion (e.g., cheeses, chicken, well-cooked vegetables with no skins). Graham crackers, butter cookies, and some cereals are good foods for chewing because they dissolve quickly once inside the mouth, presenting less risk of choking.
Child maintains a munching or sucking pattern for an extended period of time.	A food grinder is an excellent method for varying the texture of food and allowing the child to eat a variety of foods despite low level oral–motor skills.
Child demonstrates beginning chewing skills but tends to mash foods between the tongue and upper pallet.	Grainy breads and crackers are better than soft white breads or white crackers, which tend to stick to the upper pallet.
Child demonstrates some lateral movement of the tongue.	Add foods with texture (e.g., peas, beans) to smooth and cohesive foods (e.g., mashed potatoes). Thicker foods tend to stay in the mouth longer and increase the work of the tongue, and they are easier to control. Peanut butter is an example of a food that is generally too thick when consumed by itself.
Child needs additional muscle tone and strength for effective biting and chewing.	Some foods can increase muscle tone for improved chewing. Viscous foods promote rotary chewing and graded jaw movements. Some dried fruits (e.g., apricots, apples) can be used to increase chewing. Tough or fibrous meats are contraindicated in children without basic chewing skills.
Child with beginning chewing skills has not yet developed controlled bite.	The therapist holds a long piece of vegetable or meat between the side teeth to promote graded biting. Strips of cheese or lunch meat can be used. Soft cookies and crackers placed to the side can also promote controlled biting. Pretzels and apple slices require more jaw strength and may be tried as a next step in biting skill.

experiences can be added by dipping the washcloth or nipple in juice or strained fruits. Tooth brushing, with extra input to the gums and sides of the tongue, also can help prepare the child for feeding. Prior to each meal, the parent or therapist should provide the same sensory preparation routine for the child to increase the success of the eating experience (Morris & Klein, 2000). Guidelines for introducing food textures to the child with sensory processing problems are presented in Table 6.6. Among the most difficult textures to tolerate are small, discrete bits of food, such as small pieces of meat, corn, or raisins. With some children, incorporating textured food into smooth food substances like pudding or applesauce may make the texture tolerable. Other children, however, expel any discrete bit of food from the mouth.

Understanding the basis of the child's oral hypersensitivity is important when planning an intervention program. Oral hypersensitivity related to neurological impairment is often among the most difficult to overcome. When sensory intolerance appears related to lack of oral sensory experience, such as with a child who is fed with a gastrostomy tube, the hypersensitivity may be easier to overcome. This child generally improves rapidly when given graded sensory experiences. Although the guidelines in Table 6.6 apply to many children, every child is unique and has individual preferences for oral sensory experience, food textures, and tastes.

Interaction and Communication Problems

Interaction problems during feeding are not easily solved. Often these problems reflect long-standing

Case Study 6.1. Trevor: A Child With Oral–Motor Dysfunction

Occupational Profile

Trevor had a history of neonatal asphyxia. Initially, he was extremely hypotonic and moved little. He was given liquids through an oral–gastric tube, but his oral sucking was adequate for oral feeding by 3 weeks of age. During bottle-feeding, he was positioned upright with head well supported, jaw support was applied, and a soft preemie nipple was used. This method was slow, but his growth was adequate with nutritional supplements. Trevor was held in his mother's arms for feeding, and she was the primary person responsible for feeding him.

Analysis of Occupational Performance

Trevor was bottle-fed until 10 months, when his mother expressed interest in attempting pureed foods. At this point several problems had to be overcome:

- He exhibited a pattern of spastic quadriparesis;
- He demonstrated extreme hypersensitivity because he had not experienced texture in his mouth;
- When textures were attempted, he spit them out and turned his head;
- His head and trunk control remained poor;
- He required full support to sit.

When a spoon was introduced, Trevor demonstrated wide jaw excursions: His mouth opened to its full range and then clamped shut on the spoon in a tonic bite. His tongue moved in extension–retraction and was not effective in taking the food from the spoon. Lateral tongue movement was poorly controlled. He gagged easily if the spoon was placed in the center of his tongue. His suck–swallow was disorganized, and he often coughed when given small amounts of food.

Intervention

Positioning. Trevor required full head and trunk support for feeding. A feeder chair was used because it provided complete support, had a strapping system, and helped maintain a position of 90° hip flexion. He tended to arch in all positions; therefore, additional support was provided at the anterior upper trunk to maintain his alignment. Backward pressure on the front of his chest helped maintain a position of chin tuck, which is important for efficient suck–swallow. Although the strapping helped with his postural alignment, he attempted to arch and hyperextend his head. A small pad was placed behind his head to prevent hyperextension and to promote chin tuck. The feeding chair was placed at a 60° angle so that gravity assisted his oral movements and swallow. This angle also prevented food loss from his mouth.

Handling. To decrease his sensory defensiveness before to feeding, his mother gently stroked the area around his mouth and his lips with a warm washcloth. She also stroked his gums and rubbed his tongue. Trevor liked this input and would frequently bite the washcloth and smile.

During feeding the mother was instructed to use jaw control. She placed her hand around his jaw with her third finger under his mandible, her index finger along his cheek, and her thumb on his front mandible to reinforce his chin tuck. Her hand prevented his wide jaw movement and gave support to his tongue to move the food back in his mouth for swallowing. She placed the spoon in the center of his tongue and pressed down gently to facilitate a suck–swallow response. Smooth pureed foods were used; textured food was avoided until his suck–swallow became more reliable.

Family Variables. Trevor's mother frequently asked the therapist if she was applying the techniques correctly. The therapist reassured her often that her gentle touches and careful attention to his responses were important to the success of the feeding efforts. She was always responsive to his cues and waited patiently for his responses. Although her hesitancy established a comfortable pace for Trevor, the time required for a meal was not realistic in the family's busy daily schedule. The therapist encouraged her to place slightly more food on the spoon and to establish a somewhat quicker pace. This was possible after Trevor's initial hypersensitivity was reduced. The therapist reassured the mother that Trevor would indicate if the amount or pace exceeded his capability. With practice, she became more comfortable and feeding became more efficient.

The therapist discussed with the mother who else could be trained to feed Trevor and who might give her respite from this responsibility. She identified her mother as someone else who could help and the best candidate for learning the techniques.

Outcomes

These methods worked fairly well; however, Trevor could only take in small amounts of food on the spoon, and his suck–swallow response was slow and inefficient, thereby requiring several attempts. He required 15 minutes to eat a bowl of pureed food. This level of oral feeding was acceptable, since his primary nutritional source was formula from the bottle. The mother's goal in the following 6 months was to increase the amount of food he could take by mouth and to increase the textures that were acceptable to him. The grandmother attended the following therapy sessions and learned how to position and handle Trevor for feeding. One day each week, she helped care for Trevor, giving his mother a day of respite.

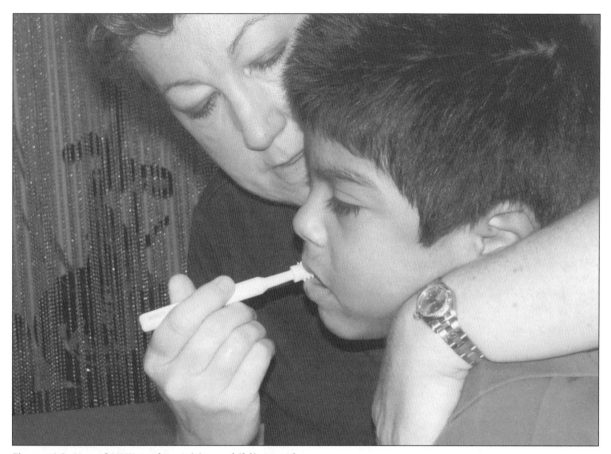

Figure 6.3. Use of NUK to desensitize a child's mouth.

concerns. Negative feeding interactions can indicate the child's frustration and distress related to hunger or discomfort when eating. However, negative feeding interactions may also reflect habits and routines that the child has adopted because he or she has been rewarded with attention when practicing negative behaviors. The following guidelines for occupational therapists can help improve children's behaviors during mealtime and snacks:

- Perform a functional analysis of the problem. What initiates the negative behaviors? Often the behavior is a form of communication— What is the child attempting to communicate by his or her behaviors?
- When the source of disruptive behaviors is identified, discuss with the parent or caregiver how that situation can be avoided or modified so the disruptive behavior is not needed.
- Help the parent or caregiver read the child's cues. Problems often occur when a child's gestures and speech are difficult to understand and cues are subtle. Help the parent or caregiver become more sensitive to the gestures or facial expressions that indicate the child's discomfort, satiation, or dislike of a food.

- Recommend that the feeders give the child choices during feeding so that he or she participates in the meal and gains a sense of being in control. The child can select which food to eat or indicate when a bite is desired. He or she should direct the pace and sequence of the meal (e.g., choosing a drink over solid food, meat instead of a vegetable).
- Explain to the family that a child who struggles to eat or has oral hypersensitivity needs consistent praise and positive feedback. Positive interaction between the child and parent or other family members can be as important as the amount of nutritional intake. Each influences the other.
- Teach the family to use behavioral management techniques when behaviors become disruptive. A regimen can be established that defines limits to the child's behavior and specific consequences when the limits are exceeded. When the discipline technique is consistently applied, the child learns which behaviors are allowed and which are not. "Time out" or elimination of something desired can be effective consequences of disruptive behaviors (Lee & Axelrod, 2005).

Table 6.6. Food Texture Progression

Recommendations	Examples	Nutritional Value	Precautions
1. To facilitate sucking and swallowing, use pureed or soft foods.	Gelatin	High sugar Limited protein value	Avoid gelatin with fruit pieces.
	Pureed meats and vegetables	Good variety of vitamins and protein	Avoid using baby foods for extended periods.
	Pudding or custard	High carbohydrates; milk provides calcium and protein	Tapioca pudding can be very offensive to hyper-sensitive children and may provide extra stimulus to hyposensitive children.
	Applesauce	Low calorie; high fluid content	
2. To facilitate sucking and swallowing, use a heavy food that easily forms a bolus and gives proprioceptive input.	Mashed potatoes (excellent consistency for providing proprioceptive input)	High carbohydrate; adding margarine provides calories; adding powdered milk adds protein and calcium	Mixing firm bits of food with mashed potatoes may not be tolerated by sensitive children; incon-sistency in texture may cause choking.
	Oatmeal	High carbohydrate; milk adds calcium and protein	
3. Liquids may need to be thickened to improve and facilitate swallowing.	Liquids may be thickened with yogurt, wheat germ, gelatin, cereal, carrageen	*Yogurt:* protein and calcium *Wheat germ:* carbohydrates and fiber *Gelatin:* see above *Cereal:* carbohydrates, vitamins (depends on the type of cereal)	Avoid high carbohydrates to thicken liquids; when food pools in the back of mouth, alternate with thinner liquids; avoid cornstarch.
4. To promote chewing initially, use chewy or gummy foods that hold together to make a bolus.	Bananas; cheese; progress to chicken, lunch meat, marshmallows, soft vegetables, crackers, dried fruit, apples, zwieback toast, graham crackers	*Fruits:* carbohydrates and vitamins *Cheese:* protein and calcium *Meat:* protein *Vegetables:* vitamins and complex carbohydrates	Avoid foods and meats that break apart; avoid vegetables with skins unless well cooked.
5. To promote chewing when jaw is more stable but movement is primitive, use crispy or harder solids.	Crackers, graham crackers, dried fruit	*Crackers:* complex carbohydrates *Graham crackers:* complex carbohydrates and fiber *Dried fruit:* high-calorie carbohydrates	If you use carrots or beef jerky, avoid allowing child to bite off pieces. Use of tough meat may increase abnormal postures.
6. To desensitize the mouth, grade the texture of the food; use a blender, if possible, to make small variations in texture.	Begin with pureed, then progress to soft foods, then lumpy or solid	Different nutrients can be provided in a variety of textures	Do not begin with lumpy foods—A hypersensitive child will be intolerant of these. When blending foods, avoid mixing all foods together.
Use a variety of tastes, textures, and temperatures.	Be creative, given the above guidelines	Variety should improve the nutritional balance	Consult nutritionist and occupational or speech therapist for advice.

Interventions for Self-Feeding Problems Related to Motor Performance

When children have motor skill limitations that interfere with self-feeding, a variety of therapeutic interventions may be needed to increase their skills. The following sections describe positioning, handling, and adaptive equipment.

Positioning

Correct alignment and adequate support for stable trunk and head are essential for demonstration of eye–hand coordination in self-feeding and eventual independence in this occupation. The mid-range movement of the hand and arm through space require either well-developed trunk stability or sufficient external support to keep the trunk aligned and stable. The child must feel secure and relaxed during self-feeding to use the strength, control, and endurance needed to eat an entire meal. Correct positioning (i.e., the chin tucked, shoulders depressed and slightly forward, and the pelvis in neutral alignment) allows the child to use both hands at midline and in midspace for spoon-to-mouth feeding and cup drinking. This position can be maintained in a wheelchair or feeder chair with adequate pelvic, hip, and lateral trunk supports. If the child retracts his or her shoulders, supports may be added to the back of the chair to maintain the child's arms in a forward shoulder-protracted position.

When the shoulder is unstable, an external support for the upper arm or elbow can help the child control a hand-to-mouth pattern. The child can stabilize his or her arm on a small bolster placed under the arm. The bolster separates the child's elbow from the trunk, thereby maintaining a position of some shoulder abduction. Then, stabilizing the elbow on a tray or table, the child scoops food and reaches his or her mouth with minimal movement of the shoulder and elbow. The bolster, in combination with the tray surface, serves as a lever that helps the child effectively engage in hand-to-mouth motion.

Simply raising the tray or table surface can also assist the child whose hand-to-mouth pattern is unstable. With the child bearing weight on his or her elbows, raising the height of the wheelchair tray promotes upright sitting and humeral abduction (Morris & Klein, 2000). This postural help can improve hand-to-mouth control, as the child stabilizes the elbows on the tray and then uses simple elbow flexion and extension to feed. An elevated, well-fitting tray can enable the child with motor performance problems to gain the postural control needed to self-feed independently when given easily managed foods.

Handling

For the child with cerebral palsy and limited control of arms in space, handling during feeding should emphasize postural stability and proximal support of the arms (Boehme, 1988). An aide, parent, therapist, or assistant can provide shoulder depression and protraction and scapular stability during self-feeding. Support and guidance of the upper arm may be needed to establish a smooth hand-to-mouth pattern. This support should help the child stabilize his or her arm in space rather than move it through the range, allowing her or him to be an active participant in the feeding process. Therefore, the therapist should provide the least amount of support needed to allow the child to self-feed successfully. This support should be able to be reduced with practice.

To provide subtle guidance of the spoon to mouth, the therapist can hold the spoon handle between his or her own extended index and third fingers. The therapist slips these fingers holding the handle into the child's palm and places his or her thumb on the dorsum of the child's hand. Using a gross grasp, the child holds onto the therapist's fingers that align the spoon handle, and the therapist then facilitates a self-feeding pattern by subtly guiding the hand-to-mouth pattern. This strategy is particularly successful with a child who has developed a basic hand-to-mouth pattern but spills frequently. The therapist's or parent's fingers inside the child's hand support the small movements of hand and wrist needed to enter the spoon in the mouth and to reduce spillage.

The physical and social environments for implementing these handling strategies should be considered. Feeding strategies can limit face-to-face communication. The positions required to use these strategies makes implementation during family mealtime difficult (e.g., the feeder may have to sit beside rather than in front of the child). The techniques can be most appropriately implemented during snack time at school or at home. When using these techniques, the caregiver should work to decrease the amount of physical assistance, so that the child continually makes small gains in independence during the meal.

Adaptive Equipment

Adaptive equipment for feeding is readily available and is often helpful in enabling independent self-feeding. Adapted utensils, plates, and cups help increase the child's ability to self-feed and decrease spillage and frustration. Helpful equipment includes built-up handles; plates with high, curved rims and nonskid pads; and cups with handles and lids. Morris and Klein (2000) provide numerous examples of equipment that enable the child to self-feed successfully.

Spoons that assist the child in self-feeding generally have enlarged handles, flat bowls, and angled handles. Cups with lids reduce spillage. Lids without spouts may be helpful when the child exhibits suckling (in and out) tongue movement. Straws can promote the child's ability to suck and allow the child to drink without lifting the cup from the table surface. More sophisticated adaptive equipment, such as an electric feeder, may enable a child to self-feed without using his or her arms. However, the cost and difficulty of setup should be a consideration in the purchase of such devices. Criteria for selecting adaptive equipment include safety, durability, ease of cleaning and use, and developmental appropriateness.

Dressing

Development of Dressing Activities

Dressing proficiencies in typical children develop over a 4- to 5-year period, within the first 6 years of life. Their timing and pace depend on the child's interest and initiative and the value the family places on dressing independence.

The child first begins to participate in dressing at about 12 months, when she holds out her arm or leg to allow the parent to put the garment over the body part or when he decides that he will remove his shoes or pants on his own. It is not until 5 or 6 years of age that the child can accomplish the most difficult fasteners. The child will use the rest of the childhood years to refine dressing and develop clothing preferences in accordance with his or her cultural context and social environment. Table 6.7 provides some guidelines to the sequence and typical ages when specific dressing activities are accomplished.

Problems in Performance Skills

Dressing requires basic and complex motor and praxis skills. Balance, postural stability, and flexibility are needed to reach one's feet, head, and other body parts in order to put on pants, shoes, or belts. Strength is needed to fit tight clothing over body parts and pull on shoes. Pincer grasp, in-hand manipulation, and bilateral hand use are required to close fastenings, lace shoes, button shirts, and tie hair ribbons. Sensory–perceptual skills allow a child to direct buttoning with touch, vision, and proprioceptive skills.

For the child with a motor disability, such as cerebral palsy, independent participation in dressing may be difficult. Poor postural control, abnormal movement patterns, and slowness of movement may interfere with the development of dressing activities and performance patterns needed to get ready for school in the morning. Problems with dexterity and two-hand coordination may interfere with ability to zip pants and properly arrange clothing.

Problems in Client Factors

A child must be able to tolerate and accept the feel of clothing next to his or her skin. Most children tolerate touch, but some children do not tolerate certain textures. Infant's clothing is typically soft, but clothing for older children can be stiff or rough. Children usually learn to accept the increasing texture and variety in clothing materials.

Infants and children with problems in sensory function, such as sensitivity to touch, may not tolerate certain types of materials or clothing. They may become irritable when dressed or may resist dressing. For example, a child may insist on only wearing certain clothes based on his or her preferred texture (e.g., the girl who insists on wearing the same dress day after day).

Body awareness and body scheme are inherent in dressing activities. A child learns to match body parts to clothing pieces and in the process learns the important perceptual concepts of front, back, right, and left. Visual discrimination and sensory functions are important to recognize clothing characteristics and how they fit the body (Meriano & Latella, 2008).

Children with sensory processing disorders may have difficulties such as inadequate body scheme, difficulty using both hands together, visual discrimination problems, dyspraxia, and directionality problems (Miller, 2006). These problems can impede participation in dressing even when the neuromusculoskeletal and movement-related functions are relatively adequate. Children with difficulty with specific mental functions may also have difficulty in dressing. Tying or buckling shoes, putting the correct leg in the pant leg, and lining up buttons can be difficult tasks if a child has difficulty with concept formation, sustained attention, or motivation. Appropriate dressing, with clothing neatly arranged, also requires that the child can judge his or her appearance.

Contextual and Environmental Conditions That Influence Dressing

The degree to which a child participates in dressing is highly influenced by the family's social environment. Family economic status and available re-

Table 6.7. Sequence of Typical Development of Dressing

Age (in years)	Self-Dressing Skills	Age (in years)	Self-Dressing Skills
1	Cooperates with dressing (holds out arms and feet) Pulls off shoes, removes socks Pushes arms through sleeves and legs through pants	$3\frac{1}{2}$	Finds front of clothing Snaps or hooks front fastener Unzips front zipper on jacket, separating zipper Puts on mittens Buttons series of three or four buttons Unbuckles shoe or belt Dresses with supervision (help with front and back)
2	Removes unfastened coat Removes shoes if laces are untied Helps pull down pants Finds armholes in over-the-head shirt	4	Removes pullover garment independently Buckles shoes or belt Zips jacket zipper Puts on socks correctly Puts on shoes with assistance in tying laces Laces shoes Consistently identifies the front and back of garments
$2\frac{1}{2}$	Removes pull-down pants with elastic waist Assists in pulling on socks Puts on front-button coat, shirt Unbuttons large buttons		
3	Puts on over-the-head shirt with minimal assistance Puts on shoes without fasteners (may be on wrong foot) Puts on socks (may be with heel on top) Independent in pulling down pants Zips and unzips jacket once on track Needs assistance to remove over-the-head shirt Buttons large front buttons	$4\frac{1}{2}$	Puts belt in loops
		5	Ties and unties knots Dresses unsupervised
		6	Closes back zipper Ties bow knot Buttons back buttons Snaps back snaps

Note. From *Pre-Dressing Skills*, by M. D. Klein, 1988, Tucson, AZ: Therapy Skill Builders. Copyright © 1988 by Therapy Skill Builders. Adapted with permission.

sources for clothing also affect dressing performance. Parents' time resources (e.g., whether both parents work outside the home) also determine the morning and evening performance patterns and how much time can be devoted to dressing.

Cultural customs and beliefs often influence how much independence in dressing is valued. In some cultures, independence at early ages is highly valued, whereas in others, interdependence may be more valued, so a parent dressing a preschool child is not only accepted, it is seen as a demonstration of affection and care (Lynch & Hanson, 2004). Cultural customs and beliefs also influence dressing activities and the type of clothes worn. Individuals from Middle Eastern cultures may prefer to cover much of the body, including the head. Children may be required to wear multiple layers of clothing or can wear simple, one-piece clothing.

As in any ADL, parents of different cultures may show a continuum of preference for independence in their children (Lynch & Hanson, 2004), for example, parents may choose to dress their children until school age. It is important that the occupa-

tional therapist be sensitive to the family's values and beliefs about the child's independence in dressing. Families that value interdependence among its members may view dressing as an opportunity for engagement with the child and not necessarily expect independence. Parents of a child with disabilities may highly value their child's physical appearance as expressed in clothing. They may want their child to appear as typical or attractive as possible, to reduce stigma and increase others' acceptance. The therapist should understand these values and beliefs, and dressing intervention should accommodate them (see Case Study 6.2).

Interventions for Dressing

Dressing interventions should actively involve the parents and the child with a disability. Generally, the development of dressing skills involves gradually increasing the child's participation and gradually decreasing the parents' assistance. Interventions for children with developmental disabilities can utilize preparatory methods (improvement of motor skills), purposeful activities (dressing games and dressing dolls), and occupation-based engagement in donning clothing and making environmental modifications (use of pictorial directions and closet modifications). The therapist also may consult with the parents and the classroom teacher on the best methods for dressing at home and school.

Improving Motor Performance Skills

When a child has difficulty dressing because of movement problems, occupational therapy intervention may include the establishment of motor skills that support the occupation of dressing. For example, the young child with poor trunk control can be dressed while sitting between the parent's legs to support the pelvis and lower trunk. Seated behind the child, the parent guides the infant's movements as he or she pushes the arms and legs

---

Case Study 6.2. Megan: Family Values and Dressing

Megan was a beautiful 7-year-old girl who had cerebral palsy, and her mother always dressed her in the most fashionable styles. Megan's wardrobe included items such as blue denim overalls, which had multiple fasteners at the shoulder and waist, and short pants and dresses with tiny buttons in awkward positions. The outfits made it impossible for Megan to manage her clothing for independent toileting. The teaching staff members at school were frustrated because she remained dependent in dressing tasks when she could have been independent if she wore simpler, easy-to-manage clothes.

The occupational therapist suggested that Megan wear sweatshirts and sweatpants with an elastic waist to school so that she could be independent in toileting. This suggestion angered the parents because they highly valued Megan's appearance and beautifully tailored clothes. They valued how others at school perceived her appearance much more than how independently she was able to function at school. The occupational therapist provided suggestions for clothing that was both fashionable and easy to manage; however, the parents continued to primarily use clothing that created the image they held of their daughter as a beautiful, meticulously dressed child. The school-based team decided that respect for the parents' priorities was most important; therefore, throughout the school year, the teachers continued to help Megan with toileting and dressing.

---

through sleeves and pant legs. This occupation-based intervention allows the child to practice bilateral movements and develop trunk control, both motor skills needed to don shirts and pants. Table 6.8 presents a motor analysis for donning a t-shirt.

To improve dressing motor performance, occupational therapy interventions can include child-directed purposeful dressing activities (Figure 6.4). The therapist can make dressing a natural and fun part of the therapy session. For example, children may put on exercise clothing to "work out," dress up in silly clothes, or dress up to pretend to be someone else (e.g., a teacher, fire fighter, farmer, chef). Dressing interventions using therapeutic positioning allow focusing on the motor performance skills identified as missing or delayed. Practice on a low bench, with the therapist sitting behind the child, provides a dynamic interplay between the therapist and child during a dressing activity and helps the child develop needed motor performance skills. When practicing at home, dressing activities in a small chair with armrests or dressing on the floor with the child's back supported against a wall may provide adequate surfaces for trunk support and postural stabilization.

Upper body dressing interventions for children with movement disorders include enhancing postural stability and symmetry, bilateral coordination, controlled reach (including reach overhead and across midline), grasp and release, and use of hands in space. Interventions for lower body dressing require the above as well as well-developed trunk control, sitting balance, and controlled leg movements. For example, to place the feet through pants legs, a child must reach forward and across the midline with the arms extended while shifting weight and maintaining the upright position. This sequential activity is difficult for the child with abnormal muscle tone and movement patterns, such as in cerebral palsy, because it involves a combination of shoulder flexion and elbow extension with shoulder mobility, elbow stability, trunk control, and active leg movements.

Adaptive Techniques for Dressing

Occupational therapists have long studied the performance aspects of dressing to determine the best ways to modify the sequences and actions needed for children with disabilities ("Dressing Techniques of the Cerebral Palsied Child," 1954; Klein, 1988). Interventions may focus on ways to modify the performance patterns or activity demands of dressing; the therapist may modify the actions, steps, sequences, and timing required for dressing. For example, children may be taught a modified way to

Table 6.8. Motor Analysis for Donning a T-Shirt

Donning a T-Shirt	Observe
Reach for shirt	Shoulder stability in directed reach Trunk control in forward weight shift Quality of reach—smooth and directed Symmetry of bilateral reach
Grasp of shirt	Hand opening Grasping pattern and control Use of two hands together Isolated distal finger prehension
Bring t-shirt over head	Use of two hands together Ability to maintain grasp during active movement of shoulder and elbow Adequate shoulder range for bringing shirt over top of head Smooth bilateral shoulder flexion with elbow flexion Maintenance of head and trunk stability Resistive grasp and arm flexion during forceful movement of shirt opening over head
Right arm through sleeve	Ability to locate arm opening (using visual or tactile perception or both) Ability to stabilize shirt with left hand Shoulder extension with elbow flexion to position arm Shoulder abduction with elbow extension to push arm through sleeve
Left arm through sleeve	Same, location of the sleeve is usually easier May require slightly greater arm strength to push through sleeve if the t-shirt fits tightly

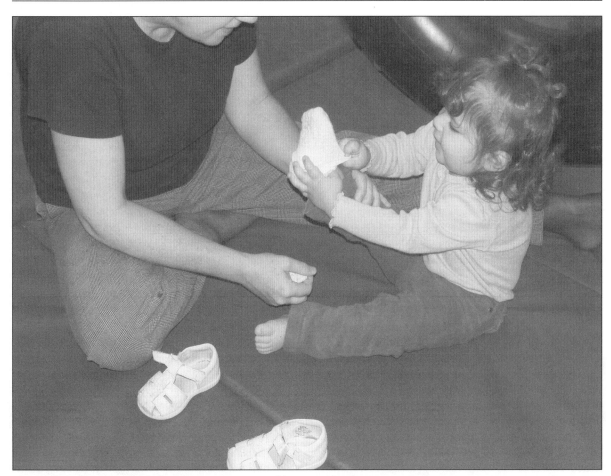

Figure 6.4. Child-directed dressing component of intervention.

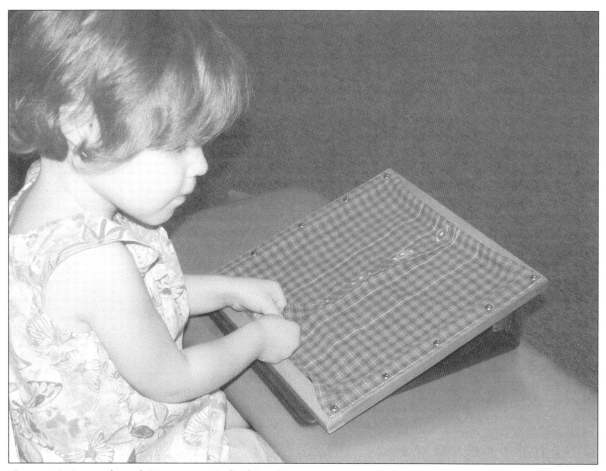

Figure 6.5. Button board (Patterson Medical Products, Inc., 2008) on slanted surface.

don their coats by laying the coat on the floor up-side down, pushing both hands through their sleeves while lifting the coat overhead. This tech-nique requires over-the-head arm movement but eliminates crossing the midline and reaching be-hind the trunk. One-hand tying techniques can be used for children with limited bilateral hand skills. Children with limited motor sequencing skills may learn to tie their shoes using the "bunny ear" method that requires simple, symmetrical, hand movements rather than the more complex and asymmetrical movements of the "over and around" method. Regardless of technique(s) utilized, parents should be advised to give their child sufficient time to work on dressing without rushing.

Adaptive Equipment for Dressing

Supportive positioning and/or sitting are methods to adapt dressing so that a child has the trunk sta-bility to become independent in this occupation. When a child with a movement disability is unsta-ble in sitting and lacks the balance needed to reach forward and to the sides, seating should be provided

that is safely supportive of the trunk, including the pelvis and shoulders. Some children may be taught to dress in their wheelchair so that they can shift their weight from side to side using the armrests for support. Dressing while sitting in the corner of a room, supported by the wall, will give the child trunk support for the side-to-side movements of dressing (Shepherd, 2001). Stools, bolsters, and rail-ings provide external support for the balancing, weight-shifting, and stabilizing needed during dressing. Additionally, equipment such as button boards and slanted table surfaces may help a child develop the body functions (visual perception and control of voluntary movement) to develop dressing independence (Figure 6.5)

Buttonhooks, long shoehorns, long-reach zipper aids, and adapted shoe ties can increase the child's dressing independence (Klein, 1988). Metal rings can be placed on the zipper. A dressing stick can aid in donning socks when range of motion is limited in the shoulder or the lower extremity. These devices are inexpensive and can be helpful in gaining dress-ing independence for the child and adolescent.

151

Modify Activity Demands Through Alternate Clothing

Clothing for children with movement impairments should be easy to don and doff. Pullover garments should have easy, wide openings with necklines that can stretch. Flexible, elasticized waistbands and large sleeve openings are helpful. Garments that enable the child to dress independently are loose-fitting, with stretchy (knit) fabrics, elastic waistbands, and few (or no) fastenings. Touch fastenings can replace buttons, zippers, and shoelaces.

Examples of clothing easy to don and doff are sweatshirts and pants, oversized t-shirts, and elastic-waist shorts and skirts. However, occupational therapists should be sensitive to the parents and child's preferences. Clothing selection is the family's choice, based on their likes and dislikes, their cultural background, how much they value style and the resources available to invest in clothing.

When children have hand skill difficulties fasteners should be avoided or replaced with Velcro® fasteners. For children who have difficulty identifying the front, back, right, and left sides of garments, tags can be sewn inside the garment to help in correct orientation for donning. Garments can be marked inside with permanent colors for right and left. Clothing is recommended in which the front and back and right and left can be easily distinguished. A selection of t-shirts and sweatshirts with designs on the front is recommended for this purpose. For the child with tactile hypersensitivity, clothes should "feel good." Soft, knit fabrics are generally easier to tolerate than stiff fabrics. However, children vary in their response to the texture of clothing; given the variety of fabrics available, children can be allowed to feel and select their clothes prior to purchase.

Therapeutic Use of Preparatory Methods in Dressing

Children with hypersensitivity to touch may benefit from preparatory methods prior to dressing. Joint compression, deep tactile pressure techniques or both may help calm or organize the child before dressing. If the parent is helping the child dress, firm touch and secure holding can help the child tolerate the tactile input of the material to his or her skin, as the sensation can be overwhelming. Establishing a set routine in dressing (e.g., always the pants first and the shirt last) can help to prepare and organize the child. Verbal cueing prior to dressing can also help the child know what touch inputs to expect. Children with visual perception problems, such as figure-ground problems, will benefit when the environment is well organized and uncluttered. The parents can place clothing so that it is sequenced in the order of donning and is oriented correctly (top to bottom, right to left).

Teaching Strategies

The child with developmental disabilities, such as motor planning or cognitive problems, can benefit from practicing dressing with feedback from the occupational therapist and parents. The steps of dressing activities can be verbally reinforced and verbal or gestural prompts can guide the child toward the next step (Van Houton, 1998). The backward chaining method can be effective in teaching a child to dress. In backward chaining, the parent performs most of the dressing task, allowing the child to complete the final steps. The parent systematically performs fewer of the beginning steps, allowing the child greater participation in completing the task (Klein, 1988). This results in successful task completion and a sense of accomplishment in dressing.

Bathing

Development of Bathing Skills

Bathing is a relaxing and pleasurable activity for most children and parents. Bath time generally includes playful interaction and learning about one's body, in addition to hygiene. It is important that children with disabilities experience bathing as a relaxing, enjoyable experience during which which they are comfortable and safe (Table 6.9).

A child is interested in participating in bathing by age 2 ½ years (Parks, 2004). At this age, the child has mastered postural control coupled with prehension skills, allowing water play and movement about the tub or shower. The child's participation indicates a tolerance and enjoyment of the sensory experience of bathing or showering. By 4 years of age, a child may wash and dry with supervision. The 5 to 6 year old is able to able to bathe with supervision and move in and out of the tub. Complete independence in bathing cannot be expected until 8 years of age (D'Eugenio & Moersch, 1981); however, the age of bathing independence depends on the parents' preference.

Problems in Performance Skills

Motor skills such as postural stability and sitting balance are required for the child to sit in the bathtub because the tub is slippery and hard, and the risk of injurious falls is great. In addition, reaching and adequately cleaning all body parts can be a formidable task. These motor skills are quite difficult for children with movement problems, such as cerebral palsy, ataxia, or Down syndrome. In order to take a washcloth or soap over the body, the child must maintain grasp during active range of the shoulder and arm, while maintaining an upright posture and shifting weight.

Problems in Client Factors

Bathing and showering are activities that have intense sensory components. These activities have temperature, tactile, auditory, visual, and proprioceptive components that are different from the other daily occupations of children. Children with difficulty in registration, modulation, and discrimination of the sensory environment may have low tolerance for bathing activities and respond negatively with temper tantrums and other behavioral disruptions. Difficulty in neuromuscular and movement-related functions, such as poor range of motion and abnormal muscle tone, may contribute to difficulty.

Problems in Mental Functions

Bathing is a complex activity that requires the cognitive ability to understand safety issues and actions, to plan and execute a series of motor tasks, to use the equipment and materials of the bathtub, and appreciate the concept of hygiene. Independence in bathing, as in other ADLs, requires adequate attention span, reasoning skills, social skills,

and understanding of personal welfare; adaptive and responsible behaviors are also required (Furuno et al., 1994). Children with mental retardation, attention deficit disorders, autism, or other difficulties in mental functions may struggle in the execution of bathing activities. For example, a child with mental retardation may not be able to carry out the series of tasks in using a washcloth to clean body parts. A child with attention deficit disorder may have difficulty completing bathing tasks because of distractibility. Children with body scheme difficulties may not understand the parents' verbal cues about washing specific body parts and may ignore some body parts.

Contexts and Environments Influencing Bathing

Cultural values influence how the family defines bathing, how often it is performed, and the importance of hygiene. In some cultures, bathing once a week is the norm; in others, a daily bath is expected. Some parents may choose sponge bathing outside a bathtub for the first 3 to 4 years of their child's life. Often families have routines for bathing (e.g., the same time of day or the regularity of hair washing) that are highly ingrained. Sensitive questioning about their bathing traditions or habits allows the occupational therapist to understand preferred routines and offer the most helpful intervention plan.

Table 6.9. Problems in Bathing

Diagnosis	Potential Problems
Cerebral palsy	Sitting balance in tub
	Easy startle
	Range-of-motion limitation affecting reach to all body parts
	Reaching and washing hair
	Transferring in and out of tub
	Poor control of the soap and washcloth in hands
Spina bifida	Sitting balance
	Sensation in legs
	Motor planning
	Tactile defensiveness
Hypersensitivities	Aversion to bathing; may have a tantrum at bath time
	Does not bathe thoroughly because uncomfortable
Cognitive delays	Has difficulty sequencing the bathing task
	Does not thoroughly complete task
	Limited dexterity and delayed fine motor skills

Interventions for Bathing

Improving Motor Performance Skills

Bath time may be a time when parents encourage the child with a movement disability to practice and develop desirable motor and praxis skills, such as the stability and mobility needed in washing. The occupational therapist's analysis of bathing activities can target specific motor skills as a focus of bathing activities. Often, the movements that limit bathing independence are reaching to the feet, back, and head. Intervention activities to improve reach to various body parts may be directed toward improving range of motion, bending, and postural stability. Obviously, close parental supervision is necessary to prevent falls or other injuries.

A child with cerebral palsy may have difficulty with the motor skills needed for bathing because of tight muscle groups and postural instability, for example, reaching his or her feet, top of head, and back. Preparatory intervention methods outside of bathing times may be used to target these motor skills to improve bathing activities. Methods can be used to increase range of motion at the hips, legs, and arms. Postural stability, with scapular stability and mobility, may be emphasized in purposeful and preparatory activities. For example, the child can be given opportunities to practice activities similar to the activities of bathing, such as grasping an object while rotating and moving the upper arm from side to side. These movements may help the child develop the active arm and hand control needed to manage a washcloth. Other occupation-based intervention activities may be used that use similar performance skills, such as removing items from varied heights in cabinets or rubbing body lotion on legs and face while sitting on the floor.

In addition to the development of the child's motor skills, the occupational therapist will address the issue of safe movement in and out of the tub or shower. These methods must keep in mind the physical safety of the parents as well as the child. The therapist can consult with the parents on safe methods of lifting the child into the tub and how to achieve sitting stability once in the tub. For example, the small child with cerebral palsy should be held symmetrically in slight trunk and neck flexion while being moved in and out of the tub. This method of securely holding reduces the possibility of the child exhibiting a startle response and falling backward or to the side.

Adaptive Equipment for Bathing

The average bathroom is filled with physical barriers for both small and large children with disabilities and their parents. The occupational therapist can help the family modify the environment or modify performance patterns by using adaptive equipment or devices.

When the family has the financial means, structural changes may be made to the bathtub or shower for easier and safer access. These include changes in the showerheads or faucets, replacement of traditional tubs or showers with wheelchair roll-in showers, tubs with nonskid surfaces, and the addition of permanent grab bars and rails. These costly modifications should be made in consultation with plumbers, architects, or contractors.

Various adaptations to assist in bathing can be made without structural modifications. Nonskid bath mats or rubber appliqués may be placed on the tub bottom and sides to prevent slips and aid in transfers. Numerous bath chairs are available that support the child during bathing and during transfers at the tub. Hammock chairs made of plastic netting stretched over PVC piping support the child's head and trunk in a semi-reclined position. These offer the child stability and safety and raise his or her position in the tub to ease the bathing task for the parent. Bathtub rings give children with head control, but poor sitting balance, an increased sense of security in the tub by securely holding the lower trunk upright (Shepherd, 2005). Tub benches that extend outside of the tub allow sliding into the tub to eliminate lifts and positioning by the parents. Wheeled shower chairs can be used to move an older child into an accessible shower stall. All bathtub equipment should be evaluated for safety and should be used with constant parental supervision (Juvenile Products Manufacturers Association, 2009).

Handheld showerhead extensions can be attached to bathtub facets, helping to direct water to different body parts without body movement or posture shifts. This helps the child who has limitations in balance and motor control and his or her parents reach all body parts and rinse without submersion (e.g., for the child in a tub chair). Parents may find that use of simple household equipment, such as sponges with handles, bath mitts, liquid soaps, and pitchers for rinsing may help decrease movement and reaching during bathing. Safety suggestions, such as antiscald devices, are described by the U.S. Consumer Product Safety Commission (2008).

Modifying Bathing Routines

Bathing is an ADL that is frequently routinized— Parents and children may use repetitive and regular patterns. However, the occupational therapist may recommend changing the bathing routines if ease and efficiency can be improved. For example, when sensory function problems such as tactile defensiveness or auditory hypersensitivity are present, bathing may have an unsatisfactory impact on routines. The therapist first helps the parent understand that the child's aversive response to bathing is a sensory processing problem. When the negative behaviors are understood as as such, parents can more readily add a positive, confident approach using verbal cueing, reassurance, and changes in the sensory environment in the bathing routine.

A child with tactile defensiveness can be given deep pressure prior to the bath to improve tolerance of tactile input. The washcloth and towel may be used with deep pressure to increase acceptance of the bathing activities. The extremities and back are less sensitive and should be washed prior to the stomach and face. After bathing, the child can be wrapped tightly in a towel and held snugly in the parent's lap. Children with auditory processing problems, as frequently seen in children with autism, may best respond to bathing if they enter the bathroom after the noise of water filling the tub is over and bathroom fans are turned off.

Toilet Hygiene

Development of Toilet Hygiene

The developmental process toward independence in toilet activities is initiated at age 12 to 15 months as the baby demonstrates recognition that he or she has had bladder or bowel elimination (Rogers & D'Eugenio, 1991). This recognition may be expressed, through verbalization or gesture, as displeasure about wet or soiled diapers. Gradually, the baby becomes increasingly more aware of the processes of elimination. He or she begins to show interest in the toileting of other family members and begins to associate the toilet with elimination. Toilet training begins by teaching the child to recognize that he or she needs to eliminate and goes to the toilet to do so. Success comes gradually by rewarding approximations and with the use of much prompting by the parents. The length of time to train a baby from diapers to the use of a toilet varies greatly among children, families, and cultures (Hanson, 2004). Most children have developed bladder and bowel control during day and night, with occasional accidents, by the age of 4 to 5 years (Brown et al., 1991). The manner in which parents and care providers train this ADL varies

considerably, depending on the methods chosen and the age when the process starts.

Problems in Motor Skills

Independent toileting requires numerous motor skills that vary by gender, type of clothing worn, and type of toilet used. The child has to be able to accomplish a series of varied motor activities: balancing skills to safely sit on the toilet, shifting weight to wipe, and moving on and off the toilet. The child must have the active range of motion needed for reaching for toilet tissue, wiping the perineal area, and flushing the toilet. Prehensile skills are needed to grasp toilet tissue, wipe, and flush. Additionally, the child requires motor skills to unfasten, remove, and refasten clothing and underwear.

Children with movement problems may struggle with toileting because of difficulty with the above motor skills. For example, a child with Down syndrome may have difficulty with clothing fasteners, with grasping the toilet and, and with wiping because of low muscle tone, poor bilateral coordination, and immature grasping patterns. A child with hypertonicity cerebral palsy may have difficulty balancing on the toilet, wiping, and handling clothing because of spasticity in the hips, lack of trunk stability, and poor hand skills. Boys who have motor difficulties and who wish to stand in front of the toilet to urinate may not be able to stand, balance, unfasten pants, and direct urine into the toilet.

Problems in Mental Functions

The numerous steps involved in toileting must be completed in a specific order to ensure elimination success. Children with mental retardation or other cognitive disabilities may have difficulty remembering these steps and their order or may have limited focus and concentration, preventing performance of all steps in a timely manner. They may lack the motivation to eliminate in a timely manner or fail to recognize the need to eliminate until it is urgent and convenient opportunities have passed. Whatever the cause or manifestations, difficulty in bowel and bladder control can affect the child's self-esteem and body image (Ganter, Erickson, Butters, Takata, & Noll, 2002).

Contexts and Environments Influencing Toilet Hygiene

Toileting is a personal and private activity; families have different opinions of how it is best or properly accomplished. Occupational therapists working

155

with the families of children with disabilities should consider cultural norms and social expectations surrounding toileting and sexuality so toileting interventions will be appropriate. The physical environment of the home, the location of the bathroom, and the type and size of toilet all affect the occupational therapy process.

Interventions for Toilet Hygiene

Improving Motor Performance Skills

Activities to improve the underlying movement problems associated with toileting problems may be an important focus in occupational therapy interventions. Through a carefully developed occupational profile and intervention plan, the occupational therapist can help develop activities to improve motor skills. For example, if a child with Fragile X syndrome has difficulty with the fasteners of clothing during toileting, this can be practiced at times other than toileting. Later, as the child improves this skill, it may be used in actual toileting. For a child with trunk balance instability, intervention may include balancing on a tilt table or ball to target this performance skill. Then, as trunk stability develops, it may enhance toileting success. Additionally, giving the child frequent opportunities to practice the correct activities of elimination at the actual toilet will help him or her develop the needed motor performance skills.

Modifying Performance Patterns

The motor steps of toileting may be modified to help the child successfully accomplish them. Children with trunk weakness can sit backward on the toilet seat, using the toilet tank as a support for the arms and trunk during elimination. Toilet tissue may be grasped and held prior to sitting on the toilet by children with balancing problems, thus reducing reaching while sitting on the toilet seat. Parents can completely remove pants and underwear before toileting to prevent soiling and reduce toileting time. For children with sequencing difficulties, pictures of the toileting sequence may be displayed by the toilet for them to follow. Pictures and/or Social Stories (Wrobel, 2003) may assist children with autism who may have fears associated with toileting or who may refuse to use bathrooms outside of their routine environments. Additionally, for children with cognitive or motivational difficulties, learning regular toilet hygiene may be reinforced through the use of appropriate reinforcements such as play privileges after successful elimination (Lee & Axelrod, 2005).

Educating Parents and Caregivers

An important component of toileting intervention is communicating helpful handling and transferring steps to parents and other caregivers. The occupational therapist can advise the best techniques for clothes handling, transferring at the toilet, and cleaning the perineal area. The therapist can also show the parents ways to accommodate poor balance and stability and compensate for limited range of motion and prehension skills. For example, a child with spastic diplegia may require parental assistance to pull down underwear and transfer safely onto the toilet seat. An occupational therapist can show the parents the best way to hold the child's arms so that she can assist in pulling down her underwear and can show them how to hold on to the child's hips during transfer to ensure safety and comfort. As the parents practice with the child, the occupational therapist will prompt and reinforce the parent's correct handling.

Adaptive Equipment for Toileting

Toileting is an occupation that should be accomplished with ease and with as little frustration as possible. The use of adapted equipment can help many children with disabilities reach this goal in their home and school environments.

Equipment for Sitting and Standing Stability

When a child has inadequate sitting balance to safely use a toilet, the use of external assistance can be considered. After the child is on the toilet, a table may be placed in front of the toilet on which the child can rest his or her arms, providing stability while while eliminating. Balancing during elimination, transferring on to and off of the toilet, and handling of clothing can be helped by rails or bars installed on the sides and back of the toilet. These allow the child to hold on as he or she uses the toilet and encourages independence and relaxation in the process (and should be installed by a carpenter to ensure durability and safety). Adaptive toilet seating, with back, sides, and armrests, can be placed over the toilet; making the seat smaller can help to provide sitting stability. If the child has poor head control, the seat back can include head wings for lateral stability. All toilet seat adaptations should be securely installed so that the moving on to and off of the toilet will not cause slippage.

Small children sitting on toilets should have adequate foot support. Foot rests or raised flooring surfaces around the toilet will help the child feel more secure and can help relax tight muscles in the legs and hips, which will aid in elimination and cleaning. These must be safely secured to prevent tripping. The use of smaller and lower toilets, particularly in school settings, can provide foot support and aid in transferring at the toilet.

Equipment for Reaching Difficulties

The occupational therapist and caregivers may consider using equipment to compensate for reaching problems in obtaining toilet tissue and wiping. Reachers may be used to obtain tissue and or wipe the perineum. The tissue dispenser can be moved to a location within the child's reach. Additionally, the use of disposable wipes that clean better than toilet tissue can be considered.

The therapist, parents, and other caregivers must weigh several considerations in the use of toileting adaptive equipment, including safety, speed of use, durability, ease of cleaning, flexibility, and cost. Occupational therapists have access to numerous rehabilitation catalogs containing adaptive toileting equipment. Comparing and evaluating options will help determine the best equipment for the needs of the child. If the equipment is for the child's school environment, use by other children must be taken into account.

Communication Management

Communication skill is essential to living in social groups. It begins with eye contact between parent and neonate and develops throughout childhood. General milestones in oral and gestural communication are presented in Table 6.10.

The variables that contribute to written and oral communication skills are complex and multifaceted. Augmentative and alternative communication (AAC) systems are available to increase or improve both conversational and graphic communication skills. When an AAC system is considered for a child, the occupational therapist will help determine which is most appropriate and help train the child to use it.

Client Factors and Performance Skills That Influence Use of AAC Systems

AAC systems are most often considered for children with moderate to severe cerebral palsy, when oral–motor delays interfere with speech production. When a child has a relatively high cognitive level and severe motor problems, simple communication by gesture is inadequate, and a communication method that simulates speech becomes a priority. When evaluating to determine whether or not AAC is appropriate, it is important to assess client factors (neuromusculoskeletal and mental functions), motor and praxis skills (mobility and manipulation), and sensory–perceptual skills (positioning, vision, hearing, location, and timing of movements). Assessment of motor and praxis and sensory–perceptual performance skills will help in selecting which device will work, how the child will access it, and what level of complexity is appropriate. In addition, assessment of cultural, social, virtual, and physical contexts is essential as contextual supports and accommodations are critical to effective use of AAC systems.

Neuromusculoskeletal Functions and Motor and Praxis Skills

To access AAC systems, the child needs to be in a position that optimizes his or her ability to control the device for the length of a communication interaction. If the trunk and/or head are unstable, external support is critical. In evaluating the child's posture and motor skills, the following questions should be asked:

- Is the child's head stable and in a position that allows complete viewing of the keyboard?
- Is the head sufficiently stable that he or she can control eye movements to scan the keys or track the cursor?
- Are the trunk and shoulders sufficiently stable for controlled arm movement and adequate active range of arms?
- Is trunk control adequate to maintain a midline position during arm and hand movements?
- Is trunk stability sufficient so the child can maintain upright posture through a communication exchange?
- What will be the means to control the device (hands, head, or eyes)?

Mental Functions and Cognitive Skills

Cognition is highly related to the individual's communication interests and needs. Operation of an AAC device can require only basic skills or highly sophisticated skills. The basic skills needed to operate AAC devices successfully include alertness, attention span, vigilance, understanding of cause and effect, ability to express preferences and make choices, understanding of object or pictorial permanence, and symbolic representation skills.

Cognitive skills that directly relate to AAC choice include understanding symbols, categorization, sequencing, matching, and sorting (Cook &

Table 6.10. Milestones in the Development of Communication

Age	Communication Skills	Age	Communication Skills
3 months	Quiets to voice Looks at person who is talking Reacts to tone of voice Smiles to person who is talking	18 months	Imitates environment sounds during play Retrieves objects on verbal request Uses inflection Greets familiar people with an appropriate vocalization
6 months	Repeats sounds that are imitated by a caregiver Imitates inflection Turns head when name is called Stops activity when name is called Begins to listen Requests a toy with a gesture	21 months	Identifies at least four animals Identifies 15 or more pictures of common objects Uses inflection patterns Experiments with two-word utterances
9 months	Imitates familiar two-syllable words (baba, dada) Makes gestures for "up" and "bye-bye" Responds to "no" Uses eye gaze during communication	24 months	Imitates three-syllable words Follows three-part commands Uses greetings and farewells appropriately Says "no" Uses words in play Uses words to describe remote events Uses words to request action Answers simple questions with a verbal response
12 months	Imitates two-syllable words (different sounds) Identifies three objects Responds to "give me" Takes turns		
15 months	Imitates new two-syllable words Follows simple commands Identifies most common objects when they are named Appropriately indicates "yes" or "no" in response to questions Identifies two body parts Uses words to express wants		

Note. From *The Carolina Curriculum for Infants and Toddlers With Special Needs, Third Edition,* by N. M. Johnson-Martin, S. M. Attermeier, and B. J. Hacker, 2004, Baltimore, Paul H. Brookes Publishing Company. Adapted with permission.

Hussey, 2008). Memory is important: The child must remember the meaning of the symbols on the keyboard, and many new devices require several steps to access the system and select a correct page for the topic of conversation. When an encoded or symbol system is used (most AAC systems involve encoding), the child must remember what each symbol represents and how combinations of symbols means different words.

Evaluation of cognition and language should include receptive- and expressive-language skills, level of problem-solving skills, and memory, with emphasis on the child's ability to understand and remember symbols. Children with severe cognitive disabilities who have extreme limitation in the abilities listed above may still be able to benefit from a simple ACC device; some have as few as 14 word choices. Appropriate systems for these children are those that enable the child to communi-cate basic needs and make simple decisions (Mirenda, 2003).

Sensory–Perceptual Skills

AAC devices require adequate visual acuity and perceptual skills. In addition, the child must be able to scan and track to follow the sequence of letters or symbols on the device. If the child has difficulty with visual scanning, the number and placement of keys must be considered. Increasing the size of the keys, increasing the contrast between the key and the background, and increasing the space between keys can accommodate problems in visual acuity. Various foreground–background combinations can be tried to improve the contrast. The issues of greatest concern in visual perception are spatial relationships, form recognition and constancy, and figure-ground discrimination (Cook & Hussey, 2008). Each area of visual perception has specific implications for the layout of keys and the system's configuration.

Contextual and Environmental Variables That Influence Use of AAC Systems

Family and Cultural Considerations

The family's interest in and enthusiasm for technology determine whether an AAC device will work for their child. If the family is comfortable with technology, a sophisticated device can be considered. Others should use a simple AAC device or method. All devices require training, problem solving when they do not work, and tolerance for learning new applications and systems. All require patience to operate, and most involve some programming to update the device and to meet the child's needs as they change.

Disorganized families may have difficulty maintaining the device in accessible places and keeping up with required maintenance and changes needed in vocabulary. Most often, the barriers to using augmentative communication are lack of knowledge; most families are unfamiliar with the equipment and need to learn how to operate it and to problem-solve when the device malfunctions.

Physical Environment

Aspects of the physical environment that are important to consider when evaluating for AAC include how the device will be transported and how the child will be assured of consistent access to it. If the child is mobile, a method for transporting the device is needed. Often it is placed on the wheelchair tray. Even if the child is ambulatory, however, he or she should not be the carrier. A system for carrying the device may include placement in a book bag or hanging it on a wheeled walker. The environments in which the child will use it may include the playground and the cafeteria; provisions must be made for use across environments.

Social Environment and Virtual Context

Use of an AAC device can greatly enhance a child's participation in his or her social environments. The explosion of technology has allowed AAC users to become full participants within a virtual context. Speech-generating devices allow literate children and adolescents to seamlessly access email, chat rooms, and a variety of social network applications (Cook & Hussey, 2008). This allows them to relate to other users as people first and positions their disability as secondary or completely hidden, if preferred.

In informal communication situations, such as birthday parties, the use of visual scene displays has been shown to be effective in encouraging communication among young children (Drager, 2003). In the more formal environment of the inclusive classroom, AAC devices can have both positive and negative results. When there is a long message generation time, the distraction to other students, and policy restrictions on the use of the AAC device may limit the child's social participation (Cook & Hussey, 2008). The acceptance or non-acceptance of the AAC device by the adults in the classroom is important in the social success of the user (Kent-Walsh & Light, 2003).

Users of AAC often use adaptive strategies as they communicate with the device. These may include hand signals, verbalizations, or eye movements. In conversations with the AAC user, the communication partner must be aware of and respond to these strategies in addition to the device's synthesized speech (Bruno & Dribbon, 1998).

Interventions for Communication Management

Occupational therapy's intervention approaches to assisting communication are in the areas of *modification* and *prevention*. To promote participation, the design, selection, and implementation of an AAC system involves modification of the child's performance patterns, contexts, and activity demands. Positioning the device and the child includes preventive strategies addressing client factors and activity demands.

Designing and Selecting an AAC System

Occupational therapists are part of the team that helps a family select an augmentative communication system. When the plan includes helping the family decide on and obtain an AAC device, the team must make the following decisions:

- What type of system will adequately meet the child's current communication needs?
- What system will be capable of growing with the child to meet future communication goals?
- How will the child access the system? What selection method is most appropriate, and what control interface is needed?
- What skills need to be supported and/or developed for the child to use the system successfully?
- What are the training needs of the family, caregivers, and teachers?

Among the range of devices available, the most sophisticated choice is not neccessarily the best choice. Nonelectronic devices, such as picture boards and books, may be most appropriate for some children (Cook & Hussey, 2008). In general, the advantages of nonelectronic devices are that they are inexpensive, easily transported, easily changed and adapted, nonthreatening, and comfortable for the communication partners to use. The child may use a head pointer, mouth stick, or hand to select pictures. Some disadvantages of these systems are that they do not provide audible or visible (onscreen) messages and have limited ability to adapt to the child's expanding vocabulary.

A variety of electronic devices are currently available. The current technology is versatile, flexible, and designed to grow with the child. Typically, newer devices are easier to program and reprogram, allowing the parent or teacher to regularly update the vocabulary and messages available to the child. In deciding which device to use and how to introduce it to the child, several features need to be considered:

- How will the child access the device (i.e., direct selection or scanning)?
- What vocabulary is needed? What prestored messages should be used? How much versatility in vocabulary is needed?
- What type of output does the device provide? Is the speech synthesized or digitized? Is written output provided?
- How portable is the device? Can it be easily transported? Can it be used on a wheelchair or on other surfaces?
- Does the device include environmental controls? Can it be used to operate the television or radio (Beukelman & Mirenda, 2005)?

Children can access electronic communication devices using direct selection or scanning. In direct selection, the child targets his choice by pointing directly to a key or symbol, then selects it by pointing or pressing. The hands are used most often, but the head also can be used with a head pointer. If the child has skills nearly or just adequate to use a direct selection device, adaptations may be made to improve accuracy and endurance. Increasing the child's postural support, adjusting the height or angle of the device, or using a variety of tools for access (a head stick or hand stick) may enable the child to use this method successfully.

In scanning, the child is presented with a display that is sequentially scanned by a cursor or light. The child selects a symbol or key by hitting a switch or clicking the mouse when the cursor or light reaches it. Various scanning methods are available, depending on the number of symbols the child requires for everyday communication. In item-by-item scanning, the cursor moves to all possible symbol choices one at a time. Item-by-item methods are simple but slow; therefore, this method is less than ideal when many choices are available. To increase the rate of selection, row–column scanning methods can be used. In row–column scanning, the rows are lighted sequentially, and the child selects the row with the desired item in it. Then the cursor scans the columns sequentially, and the child selects the item when the cursor reaches it. Most new devices offer both direct selection and scanning. Innovations in scanning allow the child to make selections using wireless infrared pointing systems that can be attached to the head or through eye-controlled systems.

Although scanning can be performed with minimal motor skill, it requires controlled visual tracking skills, attention skills, and an understanding of sequencing (Cook & Hussey, 2008). It also requires more time than direct selection but gives the user more access options. The system design can include a range of switches (control interfaces) to make selections; the goal is to provide optimal accuracy and speed. The following features should be considered in selecting a switch for a child:

- Type and size of activating surface,
- Force and pressure required to activate the switch,
- Range of motion required,
- Alternatives in positioning the device, and
- Sensory feedback provided by the switch.

Switch types that can be used with AAC systems are sip and puff, joystick, and proximity switches (for more information, see www.ablenetinc.com). Figure 6.6 shows the use of a dual selection switch. Switch selection should be based on what the child can use reliably with minimal effort for long periods of time.

Positioning the Device and the Child

Once a device has been selected, the occupational therapist offers recommendations on how it can be accessed throughout the day. If the child spends most of the day in a wheelchair that has a tray, it may be appropriate to mount the device and switch, if needed, on the tray or wheelchair. The mounting of the device can determine whether or not the child is able to use it efficiently or independently. Mounting the device at an angle is usually ideal for viewing and for hand control.

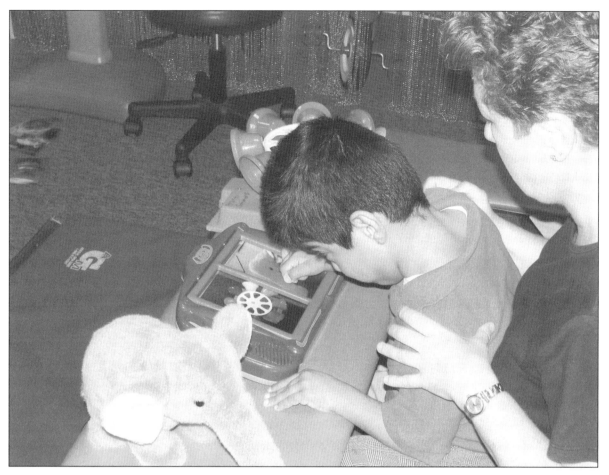

Figure 6.6. Dual selection switch.

Mountings can include hardware such as clamps or flexible mounting systems (e.g., gooseneck arms with clamps). The mounting should ensure the child has adequate range of motion, strength, visual field, and motor control to operate the device.

Most powered wheelchairs will accept a mount that can easily be adjusted and positioned for optimal viewing and access. The child's wheelchair must be considered when ordering an AAC device so an integrated system can be developed that considers interfaces with environmental control units, the wheelchair, and computers.

Positioning should consider the child's optimal posture for head, arm, and hand control, as well as issues related to endurance and effort. An optimal seating position offers maximum postural stability and alignment. In most cases, the feet should be flat, with the hips flexed at 90° and the trunk in good alignment. Correct posture can be maintained with straps, trays, and footrests.

Enhancing the Child's Performance With the Device

To help the child generalize his communication skills, it is important that he or she consistently use the AAC device in home, school, and community environments. A primary concern in choosing a system is the accuracy of arm movement for selecting the keys. Accuracy requires both eye–hand coordination (hitting the correct key) and timing (particularly when a scanning method is used and the child must hit a switch when the cursor signals the correct letter). It is also important to evaluate speed of movement to determine the most efficient method of communication. If the child's movements are delayed, then methods that select individual letters to spell words become impractical for producing conversational speech.

Generally, the child's arm and hand control the device and determine the type and size of keyboard that can be used. When hand movements are poorly controlled, the keys can be enlarged or a key guard can be used. When hand strength is weak, a membrane keyboard can enable the child to select items using minimal pressure. Various keyboard designs can accommodate a limited range of arm movement or excessive arm movement.

If the access point is the head or eyes, the range, speed, and accuracy of head and eye movements must be evaluated. Generally, methods of access using the head and eyes require visual scanning. Therefore, timing and accuracy are critical in establishing the most practical method of communication. Sometimes a hand or head pointer device can improve accuracy. For a hand pointer, sometimes a keyguard is helpful to improve the accuracy of hitting the correct key when hand stability is a problem.

Integrating the AAC System Into the Home and Classroom

An AAC device becomes fully integrated into the child's daily life when it is accepted in all environments and understood by all communication partners. Because communication needs are constant, the device should always be close to the child. Because extended downtime and repair time are unacceptable to the child and his or her communication partners, good-quality devices should be obtained.

An important focus of the occupational therapist's intervention is to help integrate use of the device into the child's daily life. The therapist helps parents, teachers, and aides learn to operate and program it because all communication partners should be able to solve problems to prevent device failure and downtime. The therapist can provide initial instruction and ongoing consultation so that all caregivers and teachers understand the child's skill level and working vocabulary, how the device operates, and the optimal setup for use. By assessing use of the device in a variety of environments, the professional team can solve problems related to setup and environmental barriers and determine how the people present in each environment can promote efficient use of the device. Daily caregivers play a critical role in ensuring that the child has immediate access to the device and that assistance is provided as needed. All caregivers should engage in ongoing efforts to create a vocabulary and system that enable the child to communicate at the level of his or her cognitive skills.

Because even the most proficient user produces communication that is slower than normal speech, the partners must adapt the pace and rhythm of a natural turn-taking interaction. Patience and attentiveness beyond that required in normal conversation are necessary. It may be tempting to speak for the child rather than allow him or her to use the device. Knowing the child's vocabulary and communication skills allows the therapist and teacher to provide appropriate assistance and support—without communicating for the child.

As much as possible, the child's skills should be developed in natural communication experiences with peers or family members. These experiences are meaningful and tremendously important in motivating the child to carry on the difficult work of learning and using the AAC system.

Functional Mobility

Development of Functional Mobility

Children become mobile at an early age. Purposeful rolling often begins at 6 to 7 months of age and crawling or pivoting on the abdomen by 6 months. Mobility milestones of the first 5 years are listed in Table 6.11. With these first forms of mobility, the child learns about the environment and begins to understand its sensory qualities, as well as sensing perceptual concepts such as depth, direction, space, and body scheme (Deitz, Swinth, & White, 2002). As children become mobile, they also develop an understanding of the activity demands within the environment. Butler (1997) indicated that the development of mobility is related to the development of cognitive and social skills. Specific client factors and performance skills that can be achieved through mobility include spatial awareness, increased speed and distance, perception of directionality, and greater participation in activities (Chiulli, Corradi-Scalise, & Donatelli-Schultheiss, 1988). The development of independent mobility seems to provide the child with a sense of mastery within the environment that is critical to self-esteem, self-image, and satisfactory participation in desired occupations and activities.

Aspects That Influence Mobility

Problems in Motor Skills

Children who have motor disabilities often require devices to achieve independent mobility. Wheelchair mobility should be considered for children with limitations in strength (muscular dystrophy, myotonia), paralysis (myelomeningocele), or poor motor control (cerebral palsy). The child with limited lower extremity strength or control, but adequate upper extremity strength and control may be a candidate for a self-propelled chair. When a child lacks postural and arm

Table 6.11. Typical Development of Mobility

Age	Mobility Milestone
3–4 months	Rolls accidentally
6–7 months	Rolls in both directions
	Roles sequentially and segmentally
7 months	Crawls forward on belly
8–9 months	Creeps on hands and knees
	Cruises sideways
11–15 months	Walks with one hand held
	Cruises in either direction
	Walks independently, stopping and starting
	Creeps up stairs
18 months	Walks independently, seldom falls
	Runs stiffly
	Walks up stairs while holding on
	Walks down stairs while holding on
24 months	Runs well
	Walks up stairs without support
	Jumps down from step

control, a transport chair, stroller, or power mobility need to be considered.

In all types of wheelchair, seating for optimal postural alignment and control is critical. Seating components (e.g., adapted cushions, lateral and head supports, strapping) assure that the child is comfortable, is in good alignment, has weight distributed evenly, and can participate in the environment. Children with severe or multiple disabilities or limited strength almost always need seating components that assist in postural stabilization and alignment. Appropriate seating generally allows for optimal control of arms and eyes, as well as good respiration and skin integrity (Colangelo & Shea, 2010).

Cognitive Functions

Purposeful and safe movement with mobility devices through environments requires cognition, or thinking and reasoning. In particular, power mobility requires that a child can follow instructions, understand indirect cause and effect, comprehend directions involving location (directionality), and show judgment (Currie, Hardwick, & Marburger, 1998). In general, a cognition level between 18 months and 2 years is needed before use of a mobility device should be considered. Diamond and Armento (2002) states the children as young as 3 years of age can be considered for power mobility. When children are provided with power mobility and become independent in mobility, they show increased self-initiated movement (Deitz et al., 2002), may make gains in cognition, and demonstrate increased motivation to explore and interact with the environment. Similarly, children needing self-propelled or power mobility devices must have sufficient visual acuity and perceptual abilities to control and direct the wheelchair. Visual and perceptual disorders may therefore mitigate against a child using power mobility.

Contexts and Environments That Influence Mobility

A family's cultural values influence their acceptance of a mobility device. In families who greatly value independence, the idea of a self-propelled or power wheelchair is enthusiastically accepted. Families that value interdependence of family members may consider a wheelchair unnecessary and a disruption of their family's interactions. These families may choose to carry or assist their child in walking. Some families also may be concerned about the appearance of the child when in a wheelchair. The wheelchair may signal to them that their child has a disability, thus carrying with it a stigma. This may lead some parents to use a stroller for several years to deemphasize the child's motor disability and nonambulatory status.

Important to the child's success in using a wheelchair is the accessibility of all of his or her environments. Parents are initially unprepared for the child's use of a wheelchair; therefore, the home may lack accessibility. All of the child's environments need to be assessed for accessibility. Transporting the wheelchair—a large and often heavy piece of equipment—also must be considered.

Choosing a Mobility Device

While the wheelchair is the most common solution to mobility limitation, a range of devices should be considered for the child. Play toys on wheels (e.g., carts or scooter boards) and strollers may be the first transportation devices for the child (Swinth, 1997). Powered mobility is considered when a child is unable to self propel a wheelchair manually or as an appropriate additional chair when a child must independently propel long distances, as in changing classrooms in middle or high school.

Identifying the mobility device that best matches the child's skills and needs requires collaboration among the family, occupational therapists, and other team members. Critical variables to discuss are the child's motor skills, visual perception, cognition, the family's values, resources and concerns, and the child's environments (Currie et al., 1998). These variables are discussed below as they relate to the following mobility devices: transport chairs, self-propelled wheelchairs, powered chairs, and scooters. The team also determines the child's positioning needs and helps the child perform desired occupations in the chair.

Strollers and Transport Chairs

Child Considerations

The first mobility device of the young child is usually a stroller, as it is lightweight and practical for community travel. Strollers with firm seats and backs that can be adjusted to different angles provide greater postural support and are appropriate for young children with trunk instability. Large, sturdy strollers offer a convenient means of transportation. If the child has poor trunk and head control, a seat insert can fit into the stroller to provide additional external support. Commercial seat inserts have secure strapping systems, footrests, and lateral supports if needed.

When the child reaches the age and size when a stroller is no longer appropriate or no longer offers adequate support, another mobility device is considered. If the child is unable to self-propel, a transport chair is recommended. Transport chairs can be customized to fit the needs of the child by selecting optional features that assist in maintaining postural stability and alignment. The options available include head and trunk supports, wedged or contoured seats, various strapping systems, and lap trays. Complete modular systems with replaceable and adjustable components can be modified to assist the child. These features allow for correct trunk and pelvic alignment and for postural stability (Bergen, 1990; Cook & Hussey, 2008). The entire seat may tilt from upright to various reclining angles ("tilt-in-space"), offering the child a variety of position options (Boninger, Cooper, Schmeler, & Cooper, 2005). The upright position is selected for most occupations and activities requiring hand motor and praxis skills, such as using scissors, crayons, and turning book pages. The semireclined position may be appropriate for some ADLs, such as buttoning, interaction with friends, and watching television, and can be used intermittently throughout the day to provide the child with rest in a relaxed position. Adjustable chair components allow improved fit and increased child participation.

Family and Environmental Considerations

Parents may prefer a stroller because a child in a stroller appears "normal" and does not carry the stigma of a child in a wheelchair. A stroller is also less expensive, lighter, folds up easily, and can be transported in a car, making it ideal for shopping, public events, or appointments away from home. If it provides security and good positioning, it can be a temporary option prior to considering purchase of a wheelchair.

A stroller is most appropriate for use outdoors on smooth surfaces; the rigid structure of the base prevents smooth travel over rough terrain—which can also damage a stroller's frame. Moreover, most strollers do not support trays and are usually fixed in a semi-reclined position, thus limiting their functional use at school or home.

While transport chairs are much more expensive than strollers, they are more durable, more versatile, and can grow with the child. They and their various special features allow for good fit and positioning. They also provide security and stability during mealtime and classroom activities, freeing parents and teachers from the need to provide postural support.

A possible problem for a parent who has physical limitations is that a transport chair is usually heavier than a stroller. Because it usually provides a better fit and optimal postural support, however, the child can stay in it for longer periods of time. This may be helpful during social and meal times, especially if the tilting feature is used to help the child shift his or her weight on the buttocks.

Some transport or travel chairs can be placed in car seats by collapsing the wheelbase; however, they do not always fit into small compact cars. They are also difficult to lift into vans and other high-based cars or trucks. The family and occupational therapist should evaluate the fit of the chair in their family automobile prior to purchase.

Transport chairs are versatile: They can serve as functional chairs within the home and classroom. They are usually sturdy and provide smooth riding over uneven terrain. They may require more space in the classroom, however, and be more difficult to maneuver than a small wheelchair. A tilting base feature offers the child an optimal view of the room based on his or her visual field. Transport chairs may be ordered with a tray. Large trays with bordering rims make ideal surfaces for play but are sometimes awkward in small spaces.

Self-Propelled Wheelchairs

Child Considerations

There is a wide variety of manual wheelchairs available. A manual wheelchair is considered for children who have the arm strength, control, and endurance for self-propulsion and who have the cognitive, perceptual, and visual skills to direct a chair within their environments. Most manual wheelchairs are lightweight and easily handled and transported. Small chairs that are low to the ground match the needs of the young child to be at the height of his or her peers. These small wheelchairs may not have the maneuverability of larger chairs, but they are appropriate for the classroom environments of young children.

Regular-sized wheelchairs offer a choice of seat and back sizes and shapes and may be ordered to fit the child with projected growth considered. Manual sport or ultralight wheelchairs are about half the weight of a standard chair (Cook & Hussey, 2008). The amount of support the chair provides can be adjusted by adding or eliminating lateral supports, trays, and strapping. Footrests, a firm back and seat, and armrests are standard items and are available with different features and functions. Armrests can be adjusted to change the height of a lap tray for various activities. For example, the tray may be raised during self-feeding to support the hand-to-mouth movement and then lowered when the child is engaged in arts and crafts. Most manufacturers also offer a variety of back and seat designs and dimensions. Companies specializing in designing and fabricating contour seating and wheelchair equipment may also customize seating. The ultralight chairs do not have as many seating options.

Family and Environment Considerations

Self-propelled wheelchairs, as with transport chairs and strollers, come in various weights, but are typically lightweight and are easily collapsed and lifted into a car. Cost is a consideration, particularly when evaluating optional features. The appearance of the chair is important, and the current chairs (e.g., the sports wheelchairs) are available in a range of colors and styles. The space and floor maneuverability available in the home, community locations, the child care center, and the school may be factors in wheelchair choice.

Powered Chairs

In general, children who do not have the upper extremity strength or control necessary to propel a chair but have the cognitive, problem-solving, and perceptual skills to plan and direct chair movement from one location to another are candidates for powered mobility. Advancements in technology allow children with severe physical disabilities to use this option (Wright-Ott, 2005).

Powered mobility can also be appropriate for children who can walk or propel a chair short distances but who have limited strength and endurance and cannot independently manage long distances. Powered mobility may be a choice for the older child who, on entrance to high school or college, has long distances to cover daily, sometimes over rough terrain. Below are several options for the child who would benefit from powered mobility.

Scooters

Motorized scooters are typically used as additional systems for long distances by children who have adequate upper body control to sit with minimal trunk support. While the scooter is usually considered a vehicle for community travel, it is available in a front-wheel drive, lightweight, model that has enhanced maneuverability for indoor use (Wright-Ott, 2005).

Standard Powered Chairs

The child can control or drive a power chair using a variety of input devices. Stoller (1998) lists a variety of methods to activate switches, including physical contact, muscle contraction, air pressure, light reception (infrared light switch), sound, gravitational changes (mercury switches), and magnetic fields (magnetic switches).

A common control for a power chair is the proportional joystick. The child moves the joystick in the direction he or she wants the chair to go. The chair's speed is proportional to the amount of joystick deflection. Digital control, using a microswitch, gives the child less control over direction, starting, and stopping the chair than the proportional joystick, but speed is usually programmed into the switch system. While switch systems offer less control, they also require less control. These systems include a press pad, arm slot, and individual switches (Cook & Hussey, 2008).

Switches enable the child to control the chair through sip and puff, or by the head, knee, arm, foot, or other body part, using different mounting of switches. The child with fair motor control, but poor strength and endurance, can easily operate and direct a chair using microswitch control. When the child has poor control but forceful movement, the switch can also correct for the degree of force by responding with a programmed speed and a limited choice of directions. Accurate knowledge of vision and cognition abilities can guide the occupational therapist in the selection of an appropriate control interface for the chair and in training the child to use the power mobility.

Family and Environmental Considerations

Although powered chairs may offer the child the first and only opportunity for independent mobility, a number of variables must be considered by the family prior to investing in this type of device. If the powered chair is an additional mobility device for the child who already has a manual chair, the cost of an additional chair may not be covered by insurance. Because powered chairs are heavy, transporting them may require a van and a lift even when the battery pack can be detached and lifted separately. Moreover, the home environment must be made accessible, with wide spaces to accommodate the chair's limited maneuverability. Overall, the expenses of powered mobility may be unmanageable for families and must be considered.

Literature has advocated use of powered mobility for the young child (aged 18 to 24 months) who is immobile and without cognitive impairment (Boninger et al., 2005; Butler, 1997; Deitz et al., 2002; Trefler & Taylor, 1988). While it may be developmentally appropriate to obtain power mobility for a young child, the family may not be ready to accept the need for mobility assistance—they may be reluctant to accept this physical symbol of their child's disability. In addition, given the expense of the chair, the growth and development of the child should be considered when ordering the size and features. The powered chair needs ongoing mainte-nance and may require relatively frequent repair. The family must be willing to undertake this ongoing responsibility.

Positioning and Fitting the Child to the Chair

Use of self-propelled or powered-mobility travel chairs requires correct positioning and seating in order to meet the activity demands of the child's environments and contexts. Occupational therapists and other team members evaluate the child's neuromotor, sensory, and orthopedic status in order to make recommendations regarding seating (Boninger et al., 2005; Wright-Ott, 2005). Outcomes for use of mobility chairs include promotion of normal muscle tone while inhibiting abnormal or primitive reflexes, preventing orthopedic deformities, accommodating impaired sensation, assuring comfort and safety, and increasing participation in meaningful occupations. An extensive range of commercial seating systems is available (Cook & Hussey, 2008). Taylor (1987) describes these components of evaluation for seating and positioning: "neuromotor and orthopedic summaries determine sensation status and gross/fine motor abilities, assess strength and activities of daily living status, and compile work/education and psychosocial histories" (p. 711).

Trunk support and pelvic alignment are critical to positioning in the chair. A child's pelvic tilt, lateral symmetry, and rotational position all must be evaluated in determining seating equipment (Currie et al., 1998). In general, the pelvis is placed in neutral alignment, with the back of the buttocks next to the chair back and the knees bent at least at 90° angles (Stoller, 1998). Straps for the trunk can provide support and stability when the child lacks postural control. Straps that cross the chest in a V, H, or X design can assist with alignment, upright posture, and maintenance of posture when fatigue becomes a factor. Straps that originate on the chair back below the level of the shoulders and fit over the top of the shoulders help maintain postural alignment.

The lower extremities should be well supported, with neutral rotation at the hips and usually 90° of flexion at the hips, knees, and ankles. This promotes neutral pelvic alignment and discourages posterior pelvic tilt and lower extremity extension. A contoured seat prevents the child from sliding forward in the chair (e.g., children with strong extensor tone).

Additional features may be added to the chair when shoulder retraction and head control are issues. Shoulder protraction wings encourage midline positioning of the upper extremities and encourage engagement in occupation. Head supports can assist the child in maintaining his or her head at midline. When head control is poor and frequently pulls into flexion, head straps or a cervical collar can be considered; however, these devices must be selected and used with extreme care as the head may slip into an undesirable and unsafe position, increasing, rather than helping, poor neck alignment. A better choice may be to tilt the seating unit backward, thus allowing gravity to assist in maintaining head alignment against the chair's back.

Use of Mobility Devices to Increase Participation in Occupation

Occupational therapists focus on improving participation and engagement in occupation while the child is seated in the chair (Deitz, Jaffe, Wolf, Massagli, & Anson, 1991). One primary method is to supply the child with a tray surface to support hand use in activities and occupations. Wheelchair trays are standard features with transport chairs and some powered chairs. Self-propelled chairs may come with desk arms to accommodate sitting at a table.

Wheelchair trays can provide a surface for eating, school or vocational activities, and play and leisure activities. The tray may also provide a surface for a communication device or a computer. Augmentative and alternative communication devices need to remain with the child; mounting them on the wheelchair tray may be a convenient solution. The tray has the additional benefit of helping the child maintain an upright posture by supporting the midtrunk and maintaining the upper extremities in a functional position (Colangelo & Shea, 2010). Other performance issues to be addressed with a child in a chair are

- Can the child reach with adequate range to manage the environment (e.g., turn faucets on and off; write on the blackboard; reach shelves, the floor, and a light switch)?
- Can the child turn the chair and maneuver it through rooms and hallways?
- Can the child propel or drive up to a table or desk and position himself or herself comfortably for tabletop activities?
- Can the child propel or drive the chair over grass, rough terrain, and other outdoor surfaces in his or her environment (Wolf, Massagli, Jaffe, & Deitz, 1991)?
- Can the child transfer in and out of the chair independently for toilet hygiene, rest, and car use?

- Can the child move his or her chair into close proximity with classmates and peers to participate in school and play activities?
- Can the child transport backpacks and other school supplies while in the wheelchair?

The child, family, occupational therapist, and other team members can identify the limitations in the environment that require accommodation. Together, the team helps the child overcome any performance limitations. In some cases, the physical environment can be adapted. For example, table heights can be adjusted and home or school modifications can be made. The child may become independent in transferring into the chair with adapted environmental supports and modified techniques. Additionally, social environments, personal contexts, and performance patterns may be modified. For example, the teacher can modify the sequencing of group games at recess to allow the child in the wheelchair to participate. The child can be supported for play in a small group by placing a table game on the wheelchair tray with friends seated around. These interventions allow the child using a mobility device to meet outcome goals for participation in desired occupations.

Summary

Children with developmental disabilities often require assistance with their daily occupations, such as eating, dressing, bathing, toilet hygiene, functional mobility, and communication management. The child's ability to achieve independence and mastery of these occupations is important for his or her well-being within his or her environments and contexts. Achieving individualized outcome goals can enhance the child's social participation with family members, school educators, and peers.

Occupational therapists are particularly skilled and resourceful in enhancing the child's engagement in occupations through the development of an occupational profile and analysis of occupational performance. The therapist analyzes the involved performance skills, patterns, and client factors; determines the performance patterns and activity demands of desired occupations; and maintains a perspective on the child's occupations as related to his or her culture, family, home, and school contexts and environments. Occupational therapists work closely with the child, family, and others to ensure that a consistent, comprehensive, and client-centered approach is implemented (Figure 6.7).

Intervention targets the priorities of the child and family and involves appropriate school and

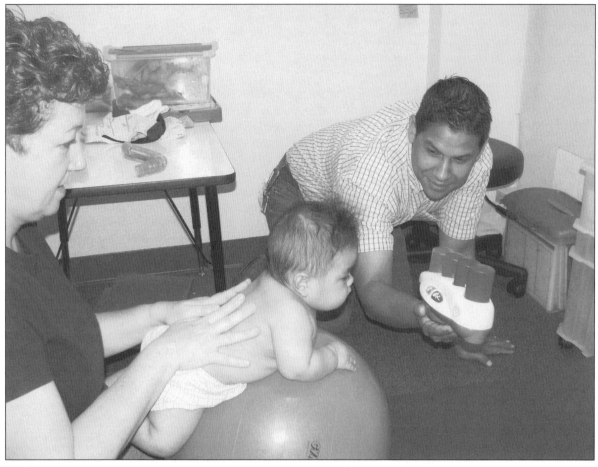

Figure 6.7. Parent collaboration in occupational therapy intervention.

community resources. Occupational therapists recognize that interventions targeting participation and engagement in occupations can be long-term, and sometimes even lifelong, for the child with developmental disabilities. The occupational therapist's comprehensive understanding of many aspects of the child creates the opportunity for increased mastery of desired occupations.

Study Questions

1. Describe those environmental and contextual factors that should be evaluated by an occupational therapist to determine their relationship to the child's success in school occupations.
2. What are the performance skills, client factors, and environmental/contextual conditions that affect the eating skills of children with disabilities?
3. How can sensory–perceptual problems cause difficulty in dressing and bathing?
4. What interventions improve toileting for children with problems in motor skills?

5. What recommendations should the occupational therapist make in selecting an AAC system for the child with poor motor skills?
6. What is the role of the occupational therapist in promoting a child's use of an AAC system across environments?
7. What variables need to be considered when recommending mobility devices to the family of a young child?

References

American Occupational Therapy Association. (2008). Occupational therapy practice framework: Domain and process (2nd ed.). *American Journal of Occupational Therapy, 62,* 625–683.

Bergen, A. F. (1990). *Positioning for function: Wheelchairs and other assistive devices.* Valhalla, NY: Valhalla Rehabilitation Publications.

Beukelman, D. R., & Mirenda, P. (2005). *Augmentative and alternative communication: Management of severe communication disorders in children and adults* (3rd ed.). Baltimore: Paul H. Brookes.

Boehme, R. (1988). *Improving upper body control.* Tucson, AZ: Therapy Skill Builders.

Boninger, M., Cooper, R., Schmeler, M., & Cooper, R. (2005). Wheelchairs. In J. DeLisa, B. Gans, & N. Walsh (Eds.), *Physical medicine and rehabilitation: Principles and practices* (4th ed., pp. 1289–1306). Philadelphia: Lippincott Williams & Wilkins.

Brown, S., D'Eugenio, D., Drews, J., Haskin, B., Lynch, E., Moersch, M., et al., (1991). *Developmental programming for infants and young children: Preschool developmental profile* (Vol. 8). Ann Arbor: University of Michigan Press.

Bruno, J., & Dribbon, M. (1998). Outcomes in AAC: Evaluating the effectiveness of a parent training program. *Augmentative and Alternative Communication, 14*(2), 59–70.

Butler, C. (1997). Wheelchair toddlers. In J. Furumasu (Ed.), *Pediatric powered mobility: Developmental perspective, technical issue, clinical approaches* (pp. 1–6). Arlington, VA: RESNA.

Case-Smith, J., & Humphry, R. (2005). Feeding interventions. In J. Case-Smith (Ed.), *Occupational therapy for children* (5th ed., pp. 481–520). St. Louis, MO: Mosby.

Chiulli, C., Corradi-Scalise, D., & Donatelli-Schultheiss, L. (1988). Powered mobility vehicles as aids in independent locomotion for young children. *Physical Therapy, 68*, 997–999.

Clemente, C., Baines, J., Shinebourne, E., & Stein, A. (2001). Are infant behavioural feeding difficulties associated with congenital heart disease? *Child: Case, Health, and Development, 27*(1), 47–59.

Colangelo, C., & Shea, M. (2010). A biomechanical frame of reference for positioning children for functioning. In P. Kramer & J. Hinojosa (Eds.), *Frames of reference for pediatric occupational therapy* (3rd ed., pp. 489–567). Philadelphia: Lippincott Williams & Wilkins.

Cook, A., & Hussey, S. (2008). *Assistive technologies: Principles and practice* (3rd ed.). St. Louis, MO: Mosby.

Coster, W., Deeney, T., Haltiwanger, J., & Haley, S. (1998). *School Function Assessment: User's manual.* San Antonio, TX: Psychological Corporation.

Currie, D., Hardwick, K., & Marburger, R. (1998). Wheelchair prescription and adaptive seating. In J. DeLisa et al. (Eds.), *Rehabilitation medicine: Principles and practices* (3rd ed., pp. 763–789). Philadelphia: Lippincott Williams & Wilkins.

Deitz, J., Jaffe, K. M., Wolf, L. S., Massagli, T. L., & Anson, D. (1991). Pediatric power wheelchairs: Evaluation of function in the home and school environments. *Assistive Technology, 3*, 24–31.

Deitz, J., Swinth, T., & White, O. (2002). Powered mobility and preschoolers with complex developmental delays. *American Journal of Occupational Therapy, 56*, 86–96.

D'Eugenio, D., & Moersch, M. (Eds.). (1981). *Developmental programming for infants and young children, Volume 4: Preschool assessment and application.* Ann Arbor: University of Michigan Press.

Diamond, M., & Armento, M. (2002). Children with disabilities. In J. DeLisa, B. Gans, & N. Walsh. (Eds.), *Physical medicine and rehabilitation: Principles and practices* (4th ed., pp. 1493–1517). Philadelphia: Lippincott Williams & Wilkins.

Drager, K. D. R. (2003). Light technologies with different system layouts and language organizations. *Journal of Speech Hearing Research, 46*, 289–312.

Dressing techniques for the cerebral palsied child. (1954). *American Journal of Occupational Therapy, 8*(1), 8–10, 37–38.

Dunn, W. (2006). *Sensory profile school companion: User's manual.* San Antonio, TX: Psychological Corporation.

Einarsson-Backes, L. M., Deitz, J., Price, R., Glass, R., & Hayes, T. (1994). Effect of oral support on feeding efficiency in preterm infants. *American Journal of Occupational Therapy, 46*, 490–498.

Furuno, S., O'Reilly, K., Hosaka, C., Inatsuka, T., Allman, T., & Zeisloft-Falbey, B. (1994). *Hawaii Early Learning Profile, revised.* Palo Alto, CA: VORT Corporation.

Frost, J. (1992). *Play and playscapes.* Albany, NY: Delmar.

Ganter, B., Erickson, R., Butters, M., Takata, J., & Noll, S. (2002). Clinical evaluation. In J. Delisa, B. Gans, & N. Walsh (Eds.), *Rehabilitation medicine: Principles and practice* (4th ed., pp. 1–48). Philadelphia: Lippincott Williams & Wilkins.

Gisel, E. G., Applegate-Ferrante, T., Benson, J., & Bosma, J. F. (1995). Effect of oral sensorimotor treatment on measures of growth, eating efficiency, and aspiration in the dysphagic child with cerebral palsy. *Developmental Medicine and Child Neurology, 37*, 528–543.

Hanft, B. & Shepherd, J. (2008). *Collaborating for student success: A guide for school-based occupational therapy.* Bethesda, MD: AOTA Press.

Hanson, M. J. (2004). Ethnic, cultural, and language diversity in service settings. In E. W. Lynch & M. J. Hanson (Eds.), *Developing cross-cultural competence: A guide for working with children and their families* (3rd ed., pp. 3–18). Baltimore: Paul H. Brookes.

Hoffman, O., Hemmingsson, H., & Kielhofner, G. (1999). *A user's manual for the school setting interview (SSI).* Chicago: University of Illinois at Chicago.

Holmstrand, K. (2003). *Guidelines for safe, accessible playgrounds.* Retrieved November 30, 2003, from http://life.familyeducation.com/safety/toy-safety/36204.html

Humphry, R. (1991). Impact of feeding problems on the parent–infant relationship. *Infants and Young Children, 3*(3), 30–38.

Humphry, R., & Thigpen-Beck, B. (1998). Parenting values and attitudes: Views of therapists and parents. *American Journal of Occupational Therapy, 52*, 835–843.

Jackson, L. (Ed.). (2007). *Occupational therapy services for children and youth under IDEA* (3rd ed.). Bethesda, MD: AOTA Press.

Johnson-Martin, N. M., Altermeier, S. M., & Hacker, B. J. (2004). *The Carolina Curriculum for infants and toddlers with special needs* (3rd ed.). Baltimore: Paul H. Brookes.

Juvenile Products Manufacturers Association. (2009). Retrieved May 22, 2009, from http://www.jpma.org/

Kelly, J. E., & Barnard, K. E. (2000). Assessment of parent–child interaction: Implications for early intervention. In J. P. Shonkoff & S. J. Meisels (Eds.), *Handbook of early childhood intervention* (pp. 258–289). Cambridge: Cambridge University Press.

Kent-Walsh, J. E., & Light, J. C. (2003). General education teachers' experiences with inclusion of students who use augmentative and alternative communication. *Augmentative Alternative Communication, 19,* 102–124.

Klein, M. D. (1988). *Pre-dressing skills.* Tucson, AZ: Therapy Skill Builders.

Klein, M. D., & Delaney, T. A. (1994). *Feeding and nutrition for the child with special needs.* Tucson, AZ: Therapy Skill Builders, Psychological Corporation.

Kuhaneck, H., Henry, D., & Glennon, T. (2007). *Sensory Processing Measure: Main classroom and school environments forms.* Los Angeles, CA: Western Psychological Services.

Law, M. (2002). Participation in the occupations of everyday life [Distinguished Scholar Lecture]. *American Journal of Occupational Therapy, 56,* 640–649.

Lee, D. L., & Axelrod, S. (2005). *Behavior modification: Basic principles* (3rd ed.). Austin, TX: Pro-Ed.

Logemann, J. A. (1998). *Evaluation and treatment of swallowing disorders* (2nd ed.). Austin, TX: Pro-Ed.

Lynch, E., & Hanson, M. (2004). *Developing cross-cultural competence* (3rd ed.). Baltimore: Paul H. Brookes.

Meriano, C., & Latella, D. (2008). Activities of daily living. In C. Meriano & D. Latella (Eds.), *Occupational therapy interventions: Function and occupations* (pp. 131–236). Thorofare, NJ: Slack.

Miller, L. J. (2006). *Sensational kids: Hope and help for children with sensory processing disorder (SPD).* New York: G.P. Putnam's Sons.

Mirenda, P. (2003). Toward functional augmentative and alternative communication for students with autism: Manual signs, graphic symbols, and voice output communication aids. *Language, Speech, and Hearing Services in Schools, 34,* pp. 203–216.

Morris, S. E., & Klein, M. D. (2000). *Pre-feeding skills* (2nd ed.). San Antonio, TX: Therapy Skill Builders.

Parks, S. (2004). *Inside HELP: Hawaii Early Learning Profile: Administration and reference manual.* Palo Alto, CA: VORT Corporation.

Rogers, S. & D'Eugenio, D. (1991). *Developmental programming for infants and young children: Assessment and application* (Vol. 1). Ann Arbor: University of Michigan Press.

Roley, S. S., Blanche, E. E., & Schaaf, R. C. (2001). *Understanding the nature of sensory integration with diverse populations.* San Antonio, TX: Therapy Skills Builders.

Schubert, L. M., Amirault, L. M., & Case-Smith, J. (2010). Feeding Intervention. In J. Case-Smith (Ed.), *Occupational therapy for children* (6th ed., pp. 446–473). St. Louis, MO: Elsevier/Mosby.

Schulze, P. A., Harwood, R. L., & Schoelmerich, A. (2001). Feeding practices and expectations among middle-class Anglo and Puerto Rican mothers of 12-month-old infants. *Journal of Cross-Cultural Psychology, 32*(4), 397–406.

Shepherd, J. (2001). Self-care and adaptations for independent living. In J. Case-Smith (Ed.), *Occupational therapy for children* (4th ed., pp. 489-527). St. Louis, MO: Mosby.

Shepherd, J. (2005). Activities of daily living and adaptations for independent living. In J. Case-Smith (Ed.), *Occupational therapy for children* (5th ed., pp. 521–579). St. Louis, MO: Elsevier/Mosby.

Stoller, L. (1998). *Low-tech assistive devices: A handbook for the school setting.* Farmingham, MA: Therapro.

Swinth, Y. (1997). Technology for young children with disabilities. In J. Case-Smith (Ed.), *Pediatric occupational therapy and early intervention* (pp. 277–300). Andover, MA: Andover Medical Publishers.

Taylor, S. J. (1987). Evaluating the client with physical disabilities for wheelchair seating. *American Journal of Occupational Therapy, 41,* 711–716.

Thousand, J., Villa, R., & Nevin, A. (Eds.). (1994). *Creativity and collaborative learning: A practical guide to empowering students and teachers.* Baltimore: Paul H. Brookes.

Townsend, S., Crey, P., Hollins, N., Helfrich, C., Blondis, M., Hoffman, A., et al. (1999). *A user's manual for Occupational Therapy Psychosocial Assessment of Learning (OT PAL).* Chicago: University of Illinois at Chicago.

Trefler, E., & Taylor, S. J. (1988). Power mobility for severely physically disabled children: Evaluation and provision practices. In K. M. Jaffe (Ed.), *Childhood power mobility: Developmental, technical, and clinical perspectives* (pp. 117–126). Washington, DC: RESNA.

U.S. Architectural and Transportation Barriers Compliance Board. (2005). *A guide to the ADA accessibility guidelines for play areas.* Retrieved June 7, 2009, from www.access-board.gov/play/guide/intro.htm

U.S. Consumer Product Safety Commission. (2008). *Childproofing your home: 12 safety devices to protect your children* (Publication 252). Bethesda, MD: Author.

U.S. Department of Education. (2006). *Twenty-sixth annual report to Congress on the implementation of the Individuals with Disabilities Education Act.* Washington, DC: Author.

Van Houton, R. (1998). *How to use prompts to initiate behavior.* Austin, TX: Pro-Ed.

Wolf, L. S., Massagli, T. L., Jaffe, K. M., & Deitz, J. (1991). Functional assessment of the Joncare Hi-Lo Master power wheelchair for children. *Physical and Occupational Therapy in Pediatrics, 11*(3), 57–72.

Wright-Ott, C. (2005). Mobility. In J. Case-Smith (Ed.), *Occupational therapy for children* (5th ed., pp. 657–687). St. Louis, MO: Mosby.

Wrobel, M. (2003). *Taking care of myself: A healthy hygiene, puberty, and personal curriculum for young people with autism.* Arlington, TX: Future Horizons.

Chapter 7

Strategies for Adults With Developmental Disabilities

KRISTINE HAERTL, PHD, OTR/L

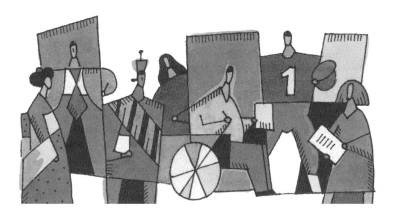

KEY TERMS

adaptive

client-centered
   occupation-
   based
   approaches

compensatory

developmental
   disabilities

extended care network

remedial

HIGHLIGHTS

- People with developmental disabilities often have physical and cognitive challenges that affect daily function.

- Theoretical models and frames of references often used with adults with developmental disabilities include behavioral, biomechanical, cognitive, sensory, and holistic approaches.

- Evaluation of adults with developmental disabilities includes an analysis of strengths and barriers to occupational performance in physical, mental, psychological, social–emotional, sensory–perceptual, and cognitive performance.

- Holistic evaluation should consider the client's quality of life and the dynamic interactions among the client, family, and extended care network.

- Occupational therapy intervention strategies include remedial and adaptive approaches.

- This chapter presents various approaches related to ADLs and IADLs.

OBJECTIVES

After reading this material, readers will be able to

- Describe some of the major challenges to occupational performance experienced by adults with developmental disabilities;

- Describe major considerations when selecting theoretical approaches to use for evaluation and intervention in adults with developmental disabilities;

- List commonly used evaluation methods and assessment tools when working with populations with developmental disabilities;

- Distinguish between remedial and adaptive intervention strategies when addressing occupational performance for adults with developmental disabilities;

- Describe specific remedial and adaptive intervention strategies that may be used by occupational therapists to enhance the occupational performance of adults with developmental disabilities; and

- Describe the integration of the client, family, therapist, extended care network, and context in providing holistic, client-centered occupational therapy for adults with developmental disabilities.

According to the Institute on Community Integration (2008), over 6 million people in the United States are affected by developmental disabilities. The term *developmental disabilities* often causes confusion. It is a term that may summon thoughts of mental retardation or cerebral palsy, but by definition and scope, the term also includes autism, autism spectrum disorders (ASD), spina bifida, learning disabilities, pervasive developmental disorders, fetal alcohol syndrome, developmental sensory losses, and a host of other developmental conditions that cause physical and mental impairments.

The term was originally used in the 1970s to denote chronic neurodevelopmental conditions affecting an individual's ability to function in daily life (Malone, McKinsey, Thyer, & Straka, 2000). As the terminology has expanded, however, a generally accepted definition arose in Western countries centering on a developmental cognitive deficit requiring an IQ less than or equal to 70 and some type of functional deficit (Sonander, 2000). In the United States, the current legal definition of

developmental disabilities has broadened and includes "a severe disability of an individual...that (a) is chronic; (b) is attributable to a mental and/or physical impairment manifested prior to age 22; (c) results in substantial functional limitations in three or more of the following: self-care, receptive and expressive language, self-direction, learning, capacity for independent living, economic self-sufficiency; and (d) requires interdisciplinary services" (Developmental Disabilities Assistance and Bill of Rights Act of 2000).

Within this legal definition, children from birth to age 9 may qualify as developmentally disabled without the above-stated functional deficits if they have a specific congenital or acquired condition along with a substantial developmental delay. Although the Developmental Disabilities Act is a federal law, within the guidelines of the act individual states and school districts may vary on qualifications for services and may expand services to include people with other related developmental conditions.

Canadians often use the definitions set forth by the American Association of Mental Retardation (2002), which refer to *developmental disabilities* as lifelong limitations identified before age 18 affecting both intellectual and adaptive function (Sullivan et al., 2006). Additional international definitions are categorized in the *Diagnostic and Statistical Manual of Mental Disorders (DSM-IV-TR;* American Psychiatric Association, 2000) and the *International Classification of Functioning, Disability and Health (ICF;* World Health Organization, 2002). Within these publications, classifications are given for specific developmental disabilities such as *pervasive developmental disorder, autism,* and *intellectual disorders.* The newest version of the *ICF* includes contextual variables that influence health in all conditions, including developmental disabilities. Given the broad scope of the conditions included in this definition, clients with developmental disabilities may have substantially different characteristics from one condition to another.

Therapists in nearly all areas of occupational therapy practice will provide services to people with developmental disabilities. Clients with developmental conditions may manifest physical, psychological, intellectual, sensory, perceptual, and emotional–behavioral difficulties. Evaluation and intervention for an ambulatory client who is nonverbal, mentally retarded, and has autism will require intervention techniques that vastly differ from those involved in evaluation and intervention with a nonambulatory, highly intelligent client who has spina bifida.

Given the broad spectrum of developmental disabilities, detailed information on evaluation and intervention techniques for every condition is well beyond the scope of this chapter. Rather, it presents a decision-making framework related to evaluation and intervention. It also provides general suggestions to maximize occupational performance in living skills. Information from this chapter should be considered along with techniques presented in Chapter 6 on self-care strategies for children with developmental disabilities.

Intervention Approaches

The occupational therapy literature provides a wide range of intervention approaches and frames of references for working with clients who have developmental disabilities. Therapists must use effective clinical reasoning skills to choose frames of reference appropriate to the client in order to maximize occupational performance. Integral to holistic practice is consideration of factors related to the client, family, context, activity, occupational therapist, team, and those in the extended care network (e.g., conservator, guardian, group home staff, employer).

Providing client-centered services to adults with developmental disabilities may prove challenging, particularly if the client has impairments that affect insight and judgment (Balboa, 2000). When working with such clients, emphasis should be placed on enhancing participation throughout the therapy process; efforts to maximize personal meaning and occupational engagement have been shown to have a positive influence on quality of life (Christiansen, Backman, Little, & Nguyen, 1999; Christiansen & Townsend, 2010).

The following section describes various frameworks used when working with adults with developmental disabilities and special considerations within each approach. The word *approach* is used to denote theoretical frameworks, models, and frames of reference that may be used with this population.

Client-Centered Occupation-Based Approaches

In the current health care environment of shorter stays and increased external regulatory requirements, occupational therapists may focus too heavily on problem areas and overlook client strengths, interests, and resources. According to Hale (2000),

little evidence exists that occupational therapists routinely incorporate client strengths and resources into the therapy process. A comprehensive, client-centered approach to working with adults with developmental disabilities should include an interface between the client's expressed desires (along with the family's priorities) and the views of the client's extended care network (e.g., conservators, guardians, group home staff, employers). Given the complexity of many developmental conditions, along with the number of services received, coordinating care may prove challenging.

Client-centered approaches in occupational therapy consider the client's views and attributes, along with the environmental context and occupational needs. Examples of such client–centered, occupation-based approaches include the Person–Environment Occupation–Performance Model (Baum & Christiansen, 2005; Christiansen & Baum, 1997), the Ecology of Human Performance Model (Dunn, Brown, & McGuigan, 1994), the Occupational Performance Process Model (Fearing, Law, & Clark, 1997), the Contemporary Task-Oriented Approach (Bass Haugen & Mathiowetz, 1995; Mathiowetz & Bass Haugen, 1994), the Canadian Model of Occupational Performance (Canadian Association of Occupational Therapists, 1997; Townsend, 2002), and the Model of Human Occupation (Kielhofner, 1995, 2008). These approaches share a client-centered focus that acknowledges the roles of the client, context, and desired outcomes in occupational therapy. Such a holistic approach to therapy requires comprehensive evaluation of the client's strengths and resources. (Box 7.1 summarizes useful questions about working with adults with developmental disabilities according to these general principles.)

Quality of Life

In recent years, renewed emphasis has been placed on maximizing quality of life for persons with disabilities (Brewin, Renwick, & Shormans, 2008; Brown, Raphael, & Renwick, 1999; Holburn, Cea, Coull, & Goode, 2008; Renwick, 2004). According to Schalock (2005), *quality of life* is (a) multidimensional and influenced by personal and environmental factors; (b) has similar objective and subjective components for all people; (c) is enhanced by self-determination, purpose, resources, and a sense of belonging; (d) reflects a full, interconnected life; (e) involves measurements that consider physical, social, and cultural environments; and (f) should be evidenced-based and drive intervention. The Centre for Health Promotion has developed a quality-of-life framework (Brown et

Box 7.1. Intervention Considerations in Adults With Developmental Disabilities

When working with adults with developmental disabilities within a holistic, client-centered approach, intervention should be guided by the following questions:

Client:

1. Who is the client, and what is his or her occupational performance profile? Occupational performance profiles summarize the client's occupational patterns, history, interests, values, and needs (AOTA, 2008).
2. What is the client's status in cognitive, physical, psychological, sensory–perceptual, social, and emotional performance? What is the prognosis for improvement and change within each of these areas?
3. What are the resources available for the client?
4. What are barriers to performance and means to address such barriers?
5. What are the client's strengths and needs? How can the strengths best be utilized, and what is the best way to meet the needs?

Family:

1. What is the family's role in the client's life?
2. How does the client view the role of the family? Do conflicts exist between the client and family members?
3. To what extent should the family be involved in the therapy process?
4. If the client currently lives with the family, are there expectations the client will transition to another place of residence?
5. If the client lives with the family, are there enough supports in place to maximize occupational performance?
6. Are the family's views consistent with those of the client, the interdisciplinary team, and other concerned individuals?
7. What are the family's resources, strengths, and needs? How can the strengths best be utilized, and what is the best way to meet the needs?

Therapist:

1. How can a therapeutic relationship best be developed with this client?
2. Which theoretical approaches and frames of references should be used?
3. What are the appropriate evaluation and intervention techniques?
4. What is the therapist's occupational therapy diagnosis (Rogers & Holm, 1989)? What is the client's current status in occupational performance, and what are the expectations for improvement?
5. Should remedial, adaptive, or compensatory strategies be utilized?
6. How best can the therapist collaborate with the client on evaluation, realistic goal development, intervention, and discharge? For example, if a client with mild mental retardation (IQ = 65) feels strongly that he or she wants to live in an apartment and the family and team believe it would be unwise to pursue independent living, what strategies may be used to come to agreement on the therapy process?
7. What are the therapist's strengths and needs? How can the strengths best be utilized, and what is the best way to meet the needs?

Extended Care Network:

1. Who are the other important individuals in the client's life, and how will their relationships with the client affect the therapy process (e.g., group home staff, conservator, guardian, friends, employers)?
2. If the client will be cared for by others (e.g., personal care attendant or group home staff), are they adequately trained, prepared, and willing to implement the therapy plan?
3. What are the extended care network resources, and how can they best be utilized in the therapy process?
4. What are the strengths and needs of the extended care network? How can the strengths best be utilized, and what is the best way to meet the needs?

Environment:

1. What are the client's cultural, physical, social, personal, spiritual, temporal, and virtual contexts (AOTA, 2008), and how will they affect the client's occupational performance?
2. What are the environmental demands for occupational performance? Are those performance outcomes reasonable? For example, will the client be required to independently make his or her own meals? If so, can the client reasonably be expected to perform the required tasks? If not, what supports are available?
3. Will the client's environment change? If so, what resources, adaptations, and outcomes are needed before the move? For example, will the client move to a different residence?
4. What are the environmental resources, strengths, and constraints? How can the strengths best be utilized, and what is the best way to overcome the constraints?
5. What are the short-term and long-term contextual needs of the client, and how can they best be met?

al., 1999) that emphasizes three domains: (a) being, (b) belonging, and (c) becoming. Within the domains, nine subdomains provide a framework for consideration in providing services to people with disabilities (Renwick, 2004):

- Physical being, psychological being, spiritual being;
- Physical belonging, social belonging, community belonging; and
- Practical becoming, leisure becoming, growth becoming.

This framework may be used to guide intervention within a variety of theoretical approaches. Intervention principles follow the quality-of-life guidelines in *Occupational Therapy Practice Framework*, American Occupational Therapy Association ([AOTA], 2008) (hereinafter the *Framework*) in order to reach goals in conjunction with the subdomains (Renwick, 2004). For example, a client may be given a choice of how or when to complete activities of daily living (ADL) tasks related to self-care. The therapist explores with the client which goals related to self-care would enhance personal choice, meaning, and quality of life. Focus on client-centered approaches with consideration of the client's health, well-being, and quality of life is crucial to holistic care.

Commonly Used Theoretical Approaches

In conjunction with a holistic client-centered approach, occupational therapists use theoretical frameworks to guide their evaluation and intervention. The following section provides a summary of commonly used approaches in working with adults with developmental disabilities, along with a discussion of general considerations for therapists within each approach. The examples are not meant to be inclusive of all approaches but represent examples of approaches to practice.

Remedial vs. Adaptive Approaches

For people with developmental disabilities, therapy often focuses on remedial and adaptive approaches (Neistadt, 1990). *Remedial approaches* are aimed at changing underlying structural or functional problems. Such approaches may be used when there is expectation for neuroplasticity and structural change, and the client has a demonstrated ability to learn. Remedial interventions are planned based on the expectation of recovery through retraining of specific underlying deficits (Unsworth, 1999, 2007). It is assumed that improvement in underlying cognitive perceptual function will have a

greater influence on skill development because of the potential for generalization, that is, applying a skill learned in one area to others (Toglia, Golisz, & Goverover, 2009). Although much of the literature focuses on remediation with head injury, use of such approaches is also common in developmental disabilities, particularly in relation to sensory integration and sensory processing intervention.

Whereas remedial approaches emphasize fixing the underlying problem, *adaptive approaches* incorporate alterations to the environment or an activity in order to optimize occupational performance. Rather than direct intervention, adaptation often includes use of compensation, support, education, and training of family and caregivers (Latham, 2008; Toglia et al., 2009). Adaptations may also include use of compensatory techniques in order to compensate for underlying deficits that impair occupational performance. Occupational therapists selecting an intervention approach for an adult with developmental disabilities should

- Review the client's therapeutic history and goals,
- Assess the client's likely response to various approaches,
- Consider the suitability and timing of combined approaches, and
- Match client factors to prospects for change (as in remedial approaches) or need for compensation (as in adaptive approaches).

Clients with chronic developmental conditions will likely respond to remedial techniques differently from clients with acute conditions who require an intensive rehabilitative approach. The occupational therapist should carefully consider how and when to apply remedial approaches in conjunction with adaptive and compensatory strategies. If a client has a longstanding underlying deficit that is intrinsic to the developmental disability, prospects for remediation may be slim, and use of adaptive and compensatory strategies may be more appropriate. For example, if a client with a long history of mild mental retardation has chronic difficulties with monthly budgeting skills, it may make more sense to use adaptive strategies and external supports, such as using a financial payee with client spending privileges, rather than try to remediate the underlying cognitive and skill deficit. Such decisions are based on the desired task and activity demands and on the client's needs, context, the capabilities, and potential for remediation.

The term *age-appropriate* is often used in discussions of activities with clients who have developmental disabilities. Occupational therapists must take care not to imply value judgments on the age appropriateness of an activity. Sociocultural and personal value systems drive concepts of age appropriateness. When using activities as interventions within therapy, the meaning of the activity and the functional status of the client should be considered in conjunction with the developmentally appropriate selection of activities. For example, some individuals may equate coloring with crayons to a developmental level of an elementary school child. While coloring is certainly an activity used in the elementary years, it does not warrant discounting coloring as an activity that may be meaningful to older adult clients as well. For example, John, age 42, had moderate mental retardation and obsessive qualities. The therapy team reported that he frequently engaged in self-injurious behaviors and property destruction. Attempts were made to engage John in age-appropriate activities such as involvement in sporting activities, household maintenance, and woodworking. John rejected all of these activities, yet when his 6-year-old niece came to visit him with a coloring book and crayons, he participated in parallel process and colored for 20 consecutive minutes. John's occupational therapist determined that this was an area of interest and therefore encouraged him to explore coloring of other media such as posters and designs. Although the activity of coloring was not initially identified as an appropriate activity for someone John's age, it provided meaning and satisfaction to him.

Behavioral Approaches

Occupational therapists often use behavioral approaches with people who have developmental disabilities, particularly with clients who have forms of mental retardation or conditions that result in problematic behaviors. Such approaches may be used in training a particular skill or addressing a target behavior.

As early as the 1960s, professions began using behavioral analysis in the treatment of developmental disabilities (Auburn University, 2008). Behavioral approaches draw on the works of theorists such as Ivan Pavlov and B. F. Skinner, focusing on behavior as a process of stimulus and response (Berger, 2008). Behavioral methods in therapy have emerged from applied behavioral analysis and use conditioning methods to influence client behaviors (Watling, 2004). Occupational therapists function as facilitators of desired behaviors by defining target behaviors, setting goals, and developing a plan to meet the goals through use of skill instruction,

modeling, coaching, and behavioral reinforcement. A successful outcome of the behavioral approach results in generalized learning to various environments in daily life and improved occupational performance. Examples of behavioral approaches include use of token environments, providing a positive reinforcement such as extra time with staff for good behavior, and use of extinction techniques such as ignoring negative behaviors.

When using behavioral approaches with clients with developmental disabilities, the occupational therapist must consider possible causes for any unwanted behaviors, the potential for shaping the client's behaviors, and the client's ability to generalize learning from setting to setting. To develop desired behaviors such as learning of a new skill, the therapist works with the interdisciplinary team to determine the client's physical and cognitive potential and his or her personal motivation to learn the skill. When a client has compromised cognition and difficulty with learning and generalization, the therapist must consider whether a behavioral approach will be useful. Toglia (1991, 2005) emphasized the fact that transfer of learning occurs in degrees and that generalization occurs along a continuum. When training clients in a specific living skill, consideration must be given not only to the task itself but also to the client's ability to transfer the skill across various contexts. People with profound cognitive deficits may not have the capacity to generalize learning of the task. Therefore, more realistic skill development should be the focus.

An influence on the success of behavioral approaches is client motivation; therapists should work with the client and caregivers to determine goal priorities and areas of personal meaning in order to enhance motivation. Bruce and Borg (2002) identified the following strategies to enhance client motivation in intervention:

- Give explanations to the client about his or her condition and expectations.
- Provide assurance and explain the purpose of therapeutic activities.
- Engage the client (and caregivers) in the goal-setting process.
- Ensure that the goals are appropriate to the client's functioning level.
- Offer support and affirmation during the therapy process.

An occupational therapist must also discern whether underlying reasons contribute to behaviors that interfere with a client's ability to learn a particular skill. For example, when teaching oral hygiene, if a client becomes self-abusive during the process of brushing his or her teeth, the therapist, before implementing a behavioral modification plan, should consider possible reasons for the behavior other than direct opposition. Reasons may include a physical problem, or sensory processing deficit. If the client has an underlying sensory defensiveness, perhaps other interventions such as sensorimotor or sensory processing techniques may be effective to decrease the self-injurious behavior and maximize function (Hanschu, 1998, 2004; Hirama, 1989; Stancliff, 1998).

Sensory Processing/ Sensory Integrative Approaches

Sensory-based approaches build on the work of A. Jean Ayres (e.g., 1972, 1979) and assume the ability to positively affect the central nervous system through use of organized sensory input. Since Ayres's pioneering work, additional, similar approaches have been developed both in the United States (Hanschu, 2004; Oetter, Laurel, & Cool, 1991; Oetter, Richter, & Frick, 1993; Wilbarger & Wilbarger, 1991; Williams & Shellenberger, 1994) and abroad (Portwood, 1996).

Occupational therapists have a long history of using sensory-based approaches with people with developmental disabilities (Spitzer & Roley, 2001). Application of these approaches is used for a wide variety of purposes, including

- Decreasing sensory defensiveness;
- Reducing negative behaviors, such as self-injurious behaviors;
- Improving underlying sensory processing and sensory integration; and
- Facilitating improved adaptive response to increase daily function.

Research has demonstrated the importance of sensory integrative functioning to perform a variety of daily occupations (Fanchiang, 1996; Kinnealey, Oliver, & Wilbarger, 1995; Pfeiffer, Kinnealey, Reed, & Herzberg, 2005; Spitzer & Roley, 2001). Therapists often use sensory-related approaches to improve nervous system functioning, which enhances adaptive responses and improves client performance in areas such as dressing, toileting, and eating. For example, a therapist may initiate a brushing program before working on dressing techniques with a client who exhibits sensory defensiveness. The rationale is that the brushing program may decrease the sensory defensiveness, thereby increasing the client's ability to tolerate various textures and fabrics. Other applications may include

use of a weighted vest to facilitate attention to task (Fertel-Daly, Bedell, & Hinojosa, 2001; VandenBerg, 2001) or use of tactile stimulation to the gums prior to brushing teeth.

Classic forms of sensory integration intervention, as developed by Ayres, emphasize client-centered therapy. Clients are encouraged, through use of an active therapeutic environment, to naturally seek out sensory experiences. Those who have serious developmental disabilities are at greater risk for self-harm; therefore, therapists need to provide maximal structure for the sensory stimulation yet seek to offer clients some choice in the context of treatment. Assumptions of this theoretical framework include an understanding that the brain is plastic throughout life (Bundy, Lane, & Murray, 2002), with plasticity decreasing with age. One must be cautious in predicting neurological change, as clients with major neurological damage will likely always have some form of damage. Bundy and colleagues emphasized that Ayres's theories were not intended to explain neurological deficits in developmental disabilities such as Down syndrome and cerebral palsy. Therefore, therapists should have a clear rationale for use of sensory processing techniques based on the client's diagnosis, goal areas, and evidenced-based practice. The authors did, however, emphasize the fact that sensory integration and sensory processing issues may occur along with developmental disabilities. Principles identified by Parham et al. (2007) as integral to sensory integration therapy include the following:

- The intervention plan is client- and family-centered and based on detailed evaluation.
- Therapy is delivered in a safe therapeutic environment that provides opportunities for motor planning and stimulation of the proximal senses (tactile, vestibular, proprioceptive).
- Therapy provides the "just-right challenge" for the client.
- Therapeutic environments are designed to support optimal arousal and increase motivation.
- Therapy encompasses a collaborative relationship between the therapist and client and encourages client-directed activities.
- The occupational therapist develops rapport and a trusting therapeutic alliance with the client and caregivers.

While there have been reports of success in applying sensory experiences with adolescents and adults (Hanschu, 1998, 2004; Reisman & Hanschu, 1992; Smith, Press, Koenig, & Kinnealey, 2005), much of the research on these approaches is focused on pediatric populations. Continued research is needed to improve validation of sensory-based intervention for adults with developmental disabilities. Given the chronic nature of developmental disabilities, clients will likely need ongoing intervention or home programs to promote organized sensory experiences throughout life. Wilbarger (1995) emphasized the importance of an ongoing "sensory diet" in order to promote adaptation and optimal occupational performance. Occupational therapists may need to train clients and caregivers to implement long-term sensory programs at home and in the community and periodically reevaluate to to monitor client progress and ensure the programs are implemented consistently and accurately. Adaptation of existing approaches such as the ALERT program (Williams & Shellenberger, 1994) and other psychoeducational methods may be used to teach clients and caregivers techniques to facilitate neurological readiness to participate in skill training and therapy.

Physical and Biomechanical Approaches

People with developmental disabilities often have accompanying physical dysfunction, particularly in disorders such as cerebral palsy and spina bifida. Occupational therapists often use rehabilitative biomechanical approaches to reduce physical deficits and maximize occupational performance. The biomechanical approach focuses on the remediation of underlying physical deficits and the prevention of additional problems that may affect occupational performance (Flinn, Jackson, Gray, & Zemke, 2008). Use of this model is largely remedial in nature and is more in line with a medical model approach (Pierce, 2003) than some of the other occupation-based models. Key areas of intervention include preventing deformity, maintaining capacity for motion, restoring motion, and compensating for limited mobility (Kielhofner, 2004). Therapeutic modalities include strength activities, stretching techniques, and exercises designed to increase range of motion and functional mobility. Biomechanical approaches should emphasize use of these techniques in order to enhance occupational performance. They should therefore incorporate meaningful occupations.

The biomechanical model is often used in response to loss of previous function. Rehabilitation efforts are therefore remedial in nature. When applying such models to populations with developmental disabilities, it is important to remember that many of the underlying physical problems are chronic; therefore, the potential for remediation should influence the intervention plan. If weakness or lack of read-

only memory affect independence in daily living or quality of life, the client may benefit from approaches that improve these components, such as strengthening and stretching. Since people with developmental disabilities often have multiple problems affecting their psychological, social–emotional, cognitive, and sensory systems, it is suggested that this approach be combined with other approaches. When possible, use of meaningful occupations should be included with biomechanical techniques. For example, rather than working on increasing shoulder flexion endurance through repetitive lifts of a weight, similar motions may be worked on while completing a meaningful activity such as painting a large wall mural. When planning the activity within the biomechanical approach, the level of understanding of the adult with a developmental disability and the perceived meaning of the activity should be considered.

Cognitive Disability Approaches

The cognitive disabilities model was originally designed by Claudia Allen (1985). It comprises six levels of cognitive function with specific skills identified in each level. The approach is based on matching activities to the adult client's cognitive function and uses detailed activity analysis to provide a framework for evaluation and intervention. Kielhofner (2004) identified three core aspects of intervention within the cognitive disabilities model:

1. Measuring and monitoring cognitive change in the client,
2. Adapting interventions and the environment to fit the cognitive level of the client, and
3. Considering that clients have fairly stable cognitive baseline abilities even after acute episodes or exacerbation of illness-related conditions.

Allen's original model focused on psychiatric populations but more recently has been applied to other populations, for example, those with various dementias (Burns, 1992). Allen and Blue's (1998) publication on how to make clinical judgments within the cognitive disabilities model further extended the model to two distinct sets of populations: (1) clients who are expected to have rapid improvement in function (e.g., clients with head injuries and stroke) and (2) clients with long-term cognitive disabilities who are expected to remain static or decline in cognitive function (e.g., regressed psychiatric populations, dementias). Because advances in neuroscience have demonstrated the plasticity of the brain throughout the life span, Levy and Burns (2005) have proposed a reconfigured cognitive disabilities model in order to align it more closely with information processing theory as currently understood.

Despite the broader application in Allen and Blue's (1998) publication of the cognitive disability model, research in this model has generally been focused on populations with psychiatric and dementing conditions and dementia. Harjamaki (2000) found that although limited research exists on the practical benefit of the Allen's assessments with populations with developmental disabilities, therapists working with this population reported using the Allen Assessments, particularly the Allen Cognitive Level Test, more frequently than other commonly used evaluation tools. Given the level of use of this model with these populations, therapist training and caregiver education are critical to enhancing understanding of levels of function and corresponding prognosis and precautions. Earhart (1992) created a detailed analysis of activities that describes a wide variety of daily living skills and client abilities at each cognitive level in relation to the skill. Such analysis may facilitate evaluation, intervention, and client and caregiver education.

Bruce and Borg (2002) identified limitations of the cognitive disabilities model as trying to treat too broad a range of problems, contradicting other models that assume an ability to remediate underlying problems, and that interventions using crafts as a medium will generalize to home and community environments. Given these limitations, occupational therapists should be careful to maintain a client-centered focus when determining the utility of the cognitive disabilities model for their clients. Although the cognitive disabilities model is helpful in providing a framework for understanding clients' general functioning level, one must be cautious in making a long-term prognosis on future capabilities in daily living skills.

Occupational therapists also use other cognitive approaches, including

- Quadraphonic approach (Abreu, 1992, 1998; Abreu & Peloquin, 2005);
- Multi-contextual approach (Toglia, 1991);
- Dynamic Interactional Model of Cognition (Toglia, 1998, 2005);
- Dynamic cognitive intervention approach (Hadas-Lidor & Weiss, 2005); and
- Cognitive–behavioral approaches built on the work of theorists such as Albert Ellis, Albert Bandura, and Donald Meichenbaum (Bruce & Borg, 2002).

Toglia and Abreu's works are often described in terms of rehabilitation after an acquired brain injury but may prove helpful in providing a framework for understanding cognition and its role in occupational therapy evaluation and intervention. Hadas-Lidor and Weiss's (2005) dynamic cognitive intervention approach draws upon classic theorists such as Lev Vygotsky and Reuven Feurestein and views the person as an open system. The dynamic cognitive intervention approach emphasizes the importance of mediated learning experiences through concepts of reciprocity, transcendence, and mediation of meaning. Efforts are made to increase the client's intentionality and raise awareness of personal behaviors and actions. Finally, cognitive–behavioral applications seek to change behaviors through education and skill building. Using the cognitive–behavioralist model, therapy may include work with the client and education of the client's family and caregivers regarding the client's disability, suggested techniques, specific home programs, and available resources.

When selecting theoretical approaches to address cognition in adults with developmental disabilities, it is important to consider the client's cognitive level, as well as his or her ability to learn and develop some level of insight. Kellogg (1998) described evaluation and intervention techniques for clients with severe disabilities or profound retardation and identified barriers to them, including significant difficulties in communication, mobility, interaction, and daily living skills. Clients were unlikely to respond well to traditional evaluation techniques or efforts aimed at client education. Because many clients with developmental disabilities have mental retardation in conjunction with other disabilities, selection of approaches to address cognition should consider the learning potential of the client as well as priorities for therapy.

Evaluation and Assessment

The *Framework* (AOTA, 2008) describes *evaluation* as a process that includes identification of occupational needs, problems, and concerns. Clients are identified within the *Framework* as people, organizations, and populations, and the aim of the occupational therapy process is to promote health and participation through engagement in occupation. When working with adults with developmental disabilities, formal standardized methods of evaluation may not always be appropriate, particularly with populations with profound disabilities. Therefore, identification of occupational needs will often include observation, historical records, and caregiver reports. Evaluation involves an analysis of strengths and barriers to occupational performance in physical, mental, psychological, social–emotional, sensory–perceptual, and cognitive performance.

Before selecting tools and methods, therapists must consider the purpose of the evaluation and the ability of the client to engage in the evaluation process. Common reasons for evaluation include

- Initial identification of occupational needs and strengths;
- Identification of intervention goals;
- Monitoring change over time;
- Monitoring response to therapy;
- Recommendation for discharge placement;
- Recommendation for special programming, home programming, or specific interventions; and
- Evaluation for court purposes (i.e., to determine the client's functioning level in order to qualify to receive funds through developmental disabilities services).

While the evaluation for court purposes is not as common—because the definition of developmental disabilities includes criteria for a functional deficit—therapists may be invited to testify as expert witnesses for the court to determine the extent of a functional deficit. Therapists may also perform evaluations in legal situations involving petitions for guardians or conservators; consideration of the need for a court-appointed payee; or, less commonly, determination of parental rights. Since evaluation for court purposes occurs less frequently than other types of therapy evaluation, discussion of evaluation with the developmentally disabled adult will focus on evaluation for therapy purposes.

The *Framework* (AOTA, 2008) identifies two substeps of evaluation: (a) to produce a client occupational profile identifying needs and priorities and (b) to conduct an analysis identifying issues and factors that support or hinder occupational performance. Evaluations often include use of formal and informal assessments. Standardized tools may not work well with clients who have extensive developmental disabilities, in part because standardized tests often require rigid testing circumstances and procedures. Many adults with developmental disabilities require adaptations to perform the test, which makes accurate testing using standardized procedures difficult (Bachner, 1998, 2004). As a result, when standardized instruments are used, they are often structured inter-

views of caregivers or observations of clients in natural contexts.

When working with adults with developmental disabilities, occupational therapists commonly use one or more assessment instruments (Table 7.1) to develop an occupational profile and determine strengths and needs in occupational performance. Examples of such instruments commonly used with this population are

- AAMR Adaptive Behavior Scales (Nihara, Leland, & Lambert, 1993),
- Adult/Adolescent Sensory Profile (Brown & Dunn, 2002),
- Assessment of Motor and Process Skills (Fisher, 2006),
- Functional Independence Measure (now the FIM™; *Guide for the Uniform Data Set for Medical Rehabilitation,* 1999),
- Scales of Independent Behavior–Revised (Bruininks, Woodcock, Weatherman, & Hill, 1996),
- Sensory Integration Inventory–Revised for Individuals With Developmental Disabilities (Reisman & Hanschu, 1992), and
- Vineland Adaptive Behavior Scales–Revised (Sparrow, Bella, & Cicchetti, 1984).

An occupational therapist, caregiver, or someone very familiar with the individual completes these instruments. The therapist then scores the responses, producing a standardized score along a continuum of performance. This type of instrument is often beneficial in the intervention process but should be used in conjunction with additional evaluation techniques (see Table 7.1).

Selection of assessment tools for individuals with developmental disabilities should take into account the client's diagnosis, areas identified for assessment, and appropriate selection of tools based on their utility, psychometric properties, and ability to accurately test the client. In selecting appropriate assessments, therapists must consider whether top-down, holistic, occupation-based tools should be used or bottom-up, component-based assessments that seek to identify underlying problems. In both instances, consideration should be given to specific barriers to occupational performance and to whether remedial or adaptive approaches will be selected for intervention purposes. Various standardized developmental assessments may also be used with adults who have developmental disabilities (Table 7.1). However, since many such tools are normed for pediatric populations, therapists should take care in selecting appropriate assessment methods.

Observation; history-taking; checklists; and client, family, and caregivers interviews are crucial in the evaluation process. Balboa (2000) identified performance inventories recommended by Spencer and Sample (1993) as possible interview/observation tools that may be helpful with developmentally disabled populations (see Appendix 7.A). This tool identifies current levels of functioning and priorities of intervention in five domains: (a) domestic/home, (b) general community, (c) vocation, (d) recreation and leisure, and (e) school. Another tool identified as useful is the nonstandardized Let's Do Lunch assessment that provides a framework for assessing strengths and difficulties in eating (Bachner, 1998, 2004). This assessment is administered during mealtime; client performance is coded through task analysis in sensory, perceptual, neuromuscular, motor, cognitive, and psychosocial functions. This information may prove useful in considering the implications of occupational performance in other areas of daily living skills. Appendix 7.B provides an example of the tool.

Client-centered, occupation-based assessments such as the Occupational Performance History Interview II (Kielhofner et al., 2004), the Occupational Circumstances Assessment Interview and Rating Scale (Forsyth et al., 2005), and the Canadian Occupational Performance Measure (Law et al., 2005) are also useful with clients with developmental disabilities. Because they yield information about the client's perspective on perceived skill, function, and importance in areas of occupational performance, these tools facilitate client engagement throughout the therapy process. Therapists should consider the cognitive ability of the client to engage in this type of assessment and should use the information in conjunction with other assessment methods.

A final consideration for assessment and evaluation is analysis of the environmental context. Clients with developmental disabilities may have limited abilities to participate in standardized assessment methods, making additional evaluation techniques important, for example, review of the client's context and environment. Traditionally, therapists have considered physical, social, cultural, and temporal elements when assessing contexts. More recently the *Framework* (AOTA, 2008) has added personal, spiritual, and virtual dimensions as aspects of context. Use of ecological environmental assessment tools is often useful to identify needs, assess resources, and develop intervention priorities. Dunn (1998) identified the most important aspects of context-based evaluations as determination of the meaning of occupational performance to the client in a given context and development of provisions to maximize quality of life within that context. Making an accurate analysis of a client's performance context requires the therapist to collaborate with the client, the client's family, and the care network.

Intervention

The *Framework* defines an *intervention plan* as "a plan that will guide actions taken and that is developed in collaboration with the client . . . based on selected theories, frames of reference, and evidence outcomes to be targeted " (AOTA, 2008, p. 646). Development of the intervention plan is based on information from the evaluation and identification of priorities. The therapist collaborates with the client, family, interdisciplinary team, and care network to optimize the client's occupational performance and maximize quality of life. Collaboration during the intervention phase of therapy may be challenging, particularly when working with people with severe disabilities. Such clients may have compromised intellectual and communication skills, and, therefore, identifying their interests, likes, and dislikes might require information provided by caregivers and direct observation.

The Centre for Health Promotion's (CHP) framework for quality of life, presented earlier in the chapter (Renwick, 2004), may be applied to occupation-based intervention by identifying areas that decrease quality of life, then developing goals to maximize occupational performance and enhance quality of life. The occupational therapist considers priorities established in the intervention plan in conjunction with the client profile and develops a holistic plan based on the three areas of the CHP framework: being (physical being, psychological being and spiritual being), belonging (physical belonging, social belonging, and community belonging), and becoming (practical becoming, leisure becoming, and growth becoming). For example, consider an adult client with severe physical dysfunction who requires 2 hours to dress each morning, which often makes him late for work. His quality of life could be enhanced by adaptations or physical assistance to help him dress more quickly, leaving more time to enjoy breakfast and get to work. In this example, rather than identifying dressing independently as the end goal of therapy, the intervention focuses on quality of life and occupational balance as priorities. Occupational therapists should consider quality-of-life issues throughout the therapy process.

Table 7.1. Examples of Assessments Used in Adult Populations With Developmental Disabilities

Assessment Tool	Type	Description
AAMR Adaptive Behavior Scale–Residential and Community (Nihara et al., 1993)	Observational rating scale	Observational rating scale filled out by caregiver in domains of living skills and social behavior
Adolescent/Adult Sensory Profile (Brown & Dunn, 2002)	Self-report	Interview tool designed to detect possible sensory processing difficulties
Assessment of Motor and Process Skills (Fisher, 2006)	Objective observation based	A structured occupation based tool that evaluates clients during IADL performance
Canadian Occupational Performance Measure (Law et al., 2005)	Interview	Individualized client-centered interview evaluating self-perception of occupational performance
Dysphagia Evaluation Protocol (Avery-Smith et al., 1997)	Interview history-taking	Protocol designed to summarize functional status
Functional Evaluation for Assistive Technology	Observation and interview	A checklist designed to determine the use and utility of technology as related to functional tasks
The FIM™ (Guide,1999)	Observation/ history-taking	Widely used tool designed to assess areas of self-care and social cognition
Independent Living Scales (Loeb, 1996)	Observation task assessment	General assessment of IADLs to facilitate appropriate intervention
Jacobs Pre-Vocational Assessment (Jacobs, 1991)	Structured observation	Assesses work-related tasks in preparation for employment
Katz Index of ADL (Katz et al., 1963, 1970)	Observation and interview	An index rating of level of independence in areas of bathing, dressing, toileting, transferring, and eating
Klein–Bell ADL Scale (Klein & Bell, 1982)	Observational rating scale	Provides a comprehensive 170-item scale to rate the level of assistance needed in ADLs
Occupational Circumstances Assessment Interview Rating Scale (Forsyth et al., 2005)	Interview	Interview of personal perception of occupational adaptation
Occupational Performance History Interview–II (Kielhofner et al., 2004)	History-taking interview	Assesses roles, routines, and goals based on the Model of Human Occupation
Oral Function in Feeding (Stratton, 1981)	Structured observation	Provides a structured format to evaluate oral function during eating
Performance Assessment in Self-Care Skills (Rogers & Holm, 1994)	Task assessment/ observation	Evaluation of self-care ADLs and IADLs in 26 tasks
Scales of Independent Behavior–Revised (Bruininks et al., 1996)	Observational rating scale	Provides standardized scores on function and behavior (short-form and long-form versions)
Sensory Integration Inventory–Revised (Reisman & Hanschu, 1992)	Observational checklist	General inventory of 4 areas of sensory integration function that may affect occupational performance
Supports Intensity Scale (Thomson et al., 2004)	Interview	Interview designed to detect supports needed for persons with intellectual disability
Swallowing Ability and Function Evaluation (Kipping et al., 2003)	Observational task assessment	Measure of swallowing function as related to feeding and eating

Table 7.1. Examples of Assessments Used in Adult Populations With Developmental Disabilities *(cont.)*

Assessment Tool	Type	Description
Vineland Adaptive Behavior Scales–Revised (Sparrow et al., 1984)	Structured interview/ rating scale	Interdisciplinary tool that rates clients in ADLs, socialization, communication, and motor skills
Vocational Adaptation Rating Scales (Malgady & Barcher, 1982)	Observational rating scale	Emphasizes work-related behaviors in order to assess work readiness
Volitional Questionnaire 4.0 (de Las Heras et al., 2003)	Observational checklist	Questionnaire designed for those who are not able to partake in self-assessment. Composed of 14 items that identify behaviors related to values, interests, and personal causation
Work Adjustment Inventory	Self-report scale	Assesses work-related temperament to assist in job placement for persons with disabilities

Note: ADLs = activities of daily living; IADLs = instrumental activites of daily living.

General Intervention Strategies

Several intervention strategies outlined earlier may be useful with adults who have various developmental disabilities. Intervention with this population should include

- Determination of barriers and supports to occupational performance;
- Interpretation of evaluation data, development of an occupational profile, and application to intervention planning;
- Identification of priorities for intervention;
- Identification of the client's strengths and needs in the targeted areas;
- Development of a plan to address occupational needs;
- Consideration of the need for remedial intervention, adaptation, and compensation;
- Development of goals related to health promotion, establishment and restoration of function, maintenance of occupational performance, modification, and prevention (AOTA, 2008);
- Implementation of learning strategies such as backward and forward chaining, step-by-step directions, use of direct training and practice (if the client has the learning capacity), initially in a familiar environment and gradually in various environments, and use of hand-over-hand techniques when appropriate;
- Establishment of routines and habits;
- Identification of resource needs such as assistive technology, adaptive equipment, and environmental modification; and
- Implementation of training and education for caregivers and the care network.

The following sections provide an overview of ADLs, instrumental activities of daily living (IADLs), rest and sleep, education, work, play and leisure, and social participation. Each section identifies general barriers that may be encountered in the adult population with developmental disabilities and examples of intervention strategies that may be used. Strategies presented are aimed at the individual with the disability but will often include training and education of caregivers and the care network.

Bathing

As a person with a developmental disability advances through teenage years, there may be an increased desire for independence during bathing, particularly if the individual has been dependent on others for bathing in the past. If maximizing independence in bathing is determined a priority, consideration should be given to current performance, safety issues, and supports needed to achieve the desired outcome (see Box 7.2).

Difficulties with bathing may include transfer in and out of the tub; lack of balance and coordination (James, 2008); bathing skill and knowledge deficits; and sensory processing concerns and sensory defensiveness. Also, difficulties with cognition that may affect safety, such as adjusting the temperature and use of bath mats. When developing intervention strategies, the occupational therapist considers the client's knowledge of the bathing task itself along with whether the client has the physical and mental capacity to perform the skill safely and effectively.

Remedial Strategies

- If the client is able learn and retain information, skill training may be used through use of

183

videos and pictures, discussions, role-plays with the clothes or bathing suit on, and direct observation to ensure the client fully understands all areas to be washed, how to apply soap, the procedure for shampooing, how to thoroughly rinse one's body, and how to get in and out of the bath and shower safely.

- Underlying gross and fine motor, postural, and balance issues may need to be addressed for the client to bathe safely and effectively.

Adaptive/Compensatory Strategies

The therapist should consider the level of supervision and assistance needed to ensure safety. For example, the temperature of the water heater may need to be lower to prevent accidental burns.

- Tear-free shampoo may be advisable if the client has difficulty shampooing hair.
- Use of nonallergenic and mild soaps is advisable for those with allergies or sensory sensitivities.
- A bath mitt, soap on a rope, and bath organizers can be helpful to minimize the chance of dropping soap, shampoo, and other bathing items.
- The environmental assessment should determine whether grab bars, a bath mat, a tub seat, a handheld showerhead, or any other specialized equipment are needed for positioning.
- Those with obsessive traits, fear of bathing, or sensory sensitivity may need rituals and transitions built around scheduled bathing times. It may be helpful to follow the bath time with a desired activity with meaning for the client.

Dressing

Dressing is a complex activity requiring postural control, motor planning, strength, flexibility, dexterity, cognition, and sensory–perceptual awareness. Value judgments and cultural norms affect clothing style; climate and activity influence the type of clothing worn.

People with developmental disabilities may have difficulties dressing in any number of areas. Individuals with fragile X syndrome may have hypotonicity, which causes barriers to dressing and other self-care tasks (Moor, 2000), and those with cerebral palsy often have hypertonicity (increased muscle tone), which presents a different set of problems in successfully extending the limbs as needed for dressing.

Many people with developmental disabilities become completely independent in dressing; however, those with profound retardation and severe disabili-

---

Box 7.2. Case Example—Mark

Mark, a 34-year-old male with mild mental retardation and depression was admitted to a group home. Despite daily showers the group home staff reported that Mark consistently had strong offensive body odor. He was referred to the occupational therapist for skill training in grooming and hygiene. During the evaluation phase of therapy, the therapist asked Mark to demonstrate with his bathing suit on his showering procedure. Mark proceeded to stand in the shower, run the water, and turn it off after a couple of minutes. After further exploration the therapist realized that Mark's concept of a shower was to stand under the water for a few minutes without applying shampoo or soap. Skill and knowledge deficits were determined to be primary barriers to successful occupational performance in this activity.

The therapist chose a combination of behavioral and cognitive behavioral approaches to take on the roles of educator, facilitator, and reinforcer. The therapist trained Mark in his bathing suit how to properly take a shower. After a few sessions Mark demonstrated the ability to use soap and shampoo independently. He was put on a token program and received weekly points for completion of his grooming and hygiene routine. Points were redeemed for items such as magazines, 1:1 time with staff, and food items. Staff were trained to follow through with Mark's behavior program. Following 3 weeks on the program, staff reported a significant decrease in body odor and problems with grooming and hygiene.

---

ties may be dependent in this area throughout life. Those with cognitive difficulties may have difficulty with adaptive equipment and selection of appropriate attire. As the client enters adulthood, size and positioning must be considered in order to protect the caregiver from injury. If the client can be trained to help (e.g., by independently moving body parts), the caregiver burden may be eased, and the level of dependence on others decreased.

An additional dressing challenge for adults with developmental disabilities is that they may be prone to sensory processing difficulties (Baranek et al., 2002; Dunn, Miles, & Orr, 2002). These clients may not want to wear certain types of clothing or may be prone to taking off clothing that feels uncomfortable. For the individual with sensory processing difficulties, techniques to decrease sensitivities are often helpful prior to dressing, as is selecting of clothing in comfortable fabrics and materials, such as cotton and flannel.

Remedial Strategies

- Provide skill training in clothing selection and dressing techniques using the strategies suggested earlier in this chapter and the text.
- Use hand-over-hand, interactive guiding (e.g., the Affolter Approach; Affolter, 1987).
- Address underlying flexibility, strength, dexterity, praxis, sensory, and postural concerns that may pose barriers to dressing.
- Use relaxation, calming, and desensitization techniques prior to dressing with clients prone to high tonicity , sensory sensitivity, or anxiety during dressing.

Adaptive/Compensatory Strategies

- Choose adaptable, loose-fitting, comfortable clothing. Remember that as individuals become adults, style and type of clothing may become more important. Some adaptive clothing is unappealing, making consideration of style as well as utility important.
- Choose attractive, wrinkle-free clothing that is durable, washable, allows ease of movement, and has fasteners that are easy to manipulate.
- Use adaptive dressing aids when appropriate. Remember that clients with cognitive difficulties may have limited capacity to independently use adaptive devices.
- If the client has difficulty with buttons but the buttoned look is desired, hook-and-loop fasteners may be used on the interior of the fabric and buttons attached externally.
- Use tube socks without heels to decrease problems with the heel ending up on the foot and causing discomfort.

Toileting and Bladder/Bowel Management

Several toileting and bowel or bladder concerns may arise in adults with developmental disabilities. Physical problems, dietary concerns, and cognitive problems all interfere with independence in this area. Prescribed medications may have unwanted side effects of constipation or diarrhea and may affect bladder control. Collaborating with the client's physician and a nutritionist is wise in order to assure proper dietary intake and consider whether medical intervention is needed.

Incontinence often causes embarrassing situations and social dilemmas for people with developmental disabilities. The National Institute on Clinical Education in London (2007) has set forth guidelines suggesting that underlying reasons for incontinence should be addressed prior to more invasive strategies. Major areas of consideration in developing systems of training, including bowel and bladder management, include

- Maintaining client dignity,
- Protecting skin integrity,
- Preventing the spread of disease-causing organisms,
- Reducing caregiver exposure, and
- Reducing cleaning and management costs (Rees & Sharpe, 2009).

Before developing intervention techniques, the occupational therapist must determine whether or not the client can be trained in toileting and bowel/bladder management. Foxx and Azrin (1973) established a detailed toilet-training procedure for working with people with mental retardation. The authors identified key client requirements for training, including

- Some level of vision (or visual aids) to navigate to the bathroom;
- The ability to get to the toilet;
- Some level of motor control, including control over hand movements; and
- Some receptive language and ability to understand the training procedures.

The therapist should evaluate client motivation and self-awareness before intervention. People with developmental disabilities may have impaired cognition and self-awareness that significantly delay or even preclude toilet training. To achieve bladder control, clients must have the following abilities (Miller & Bachrach, 1995):

- An awareness that the bladder contracts,
- The ability to recognize when the bladder is full,
- The ability to inhibit contractions and wait for urination,
- An awareness of when the bladder is empty,
- The ability to hold urine during stress and high fluid intake, and
- The ability to inhibit urination during sleep.

People with developmental disabilities may have impaired cognition and self-perception, resulting in significantly delayed toilet training, or they may never develop the ability at all. Similar to bladder control, bowel management requires an internal awareness of the ability to hold and to move the bowels. When considering bowel management programs, identified key intervention techniques include habit training, dietary modifications, biofeedback training, and medical interventions (Mason, Santoro, & Kaull, 1999).

Establishing a routine for toileting is often helpful in order to maximize independence. Additional adaptive equipment may be needed for toileting in people with physical disabilities, strength, and postural concerns. Intervention plans involving toilet training and bowel/bladder management require collaboration of the client with all caregivers. It is important that caregivers be trained in specific programs in order to be consistent and to maximize the learning process.

Remedial Strategies

- Obtain medical and dietary consultations to address underlying physical and nutritional concerns.
- Begin skill and habit training during daytime hours, and use a routine.
- Use techniques to develop self-awareness of physical sensations related to bowel and bladder control.
- Administer behavioral reinforcement and shaping techniques.
- Implement the use of charts such as an "accident" chart to monitor times that incontinence is most likely to occur, followed by a plan for intervention in response to the incontinence.
- Use techniques to address underlying postural and strength considerations for toileting.

Adaptive/Compensatory Techniques

- Use disposable training pants and similar products to address bowel and bladder concerns.
- Use clothing that is easily removed for toileting purposes.
- Use flushable wet wipes or other cleaning pads to assist in the cleaning process.
- Offset physical impairments with adaptive aids such as raised toilet seats; grab bars; low mirrors to check for hygiene; and accessible, nonslippery surfaces.

Grooming and Hygiene

Personal hygiene and grooming are affected by cultural norms and personal and family values. Physical, cognitive, and sensory–perceptual difficulties may all impair an individual's ability to successfully participate in daily grooming; adults with developmental disabilities may need cues and prompts to fully participate. For example, a client with moderate mental retardation may daily brush the front of her hair but forget to brush the back. Less obvious tasks such as caring for fingernails may be left undone without cues and assistance. Clients with sensory sensitivities may refuse to brush teeth, resulting in compromised oral hygiene. Occupational therapists should identify underlying barriers to grooming and hygiene before developing specific intervention strategies.

Remedial Strategies

- Address underlying sensory sensitivities, physical barriers, and knowledge deficits that interfere with grooming.
- Provide skill training through role-plays, videotapes, direct practice, hand-over-hand approaches, and other techniques described in this text.
- If needed, use a mounted wall mirror to facilitate training and self-awareness.
- Use weighted wrist cuffs, and add proprioceptive cues to minimize dyscoordination and enhance motor planning.

Adaptive/Compensatory Strategies

- For individuals with sensory sensitivities, textured toothbrushes or electric toothbrushes may be helpful.
- Use a toothpaste pump rather than a tube.
- Consider which type of deodorant and personal care items are easiest for the client to handle and use.
- Use liquid soap.
- Guide the caregiver in controlling the amounts used of personal care items such as toothpaste and shampoo.
- Use adaptive equipment such as long-handled brushes, suction cups to secure small items such as fingernail brushes and other grooming aids.
- Use checklists, pictures, and cues for completion of tasks.

Feeding/Eating

Although sometimes used interchangeably, the terms *feeding* and *eating* are different from one another. Eating involves the ability to keep and manipulate food in the mouth and swallow it; feeding refers to the process of bringing food from the plate or cup to the mouth (AOTA, 2007). People with developmental conditions often have eating, feeding, and swallowing issues related to anatomical, medical, physiological, and behavioral factors (Cooper-Brown et al., 2008). A dysfunction of eating, *dysphagia*, is one of the most common associated conditions for people with intellectual and communication disorders (Petersen & Rogers, 2008). Physical, cognitive, and sensory–perceptual problems may impair an individual ability to self-feed independently and may impair the oral–motor function, causing problems with dysphagia. Food allergies, restrictions, sensitivities, and preferences further confound feeding and eating for people with developmental disabilities. Avery-Smith (2002) identified indirect strategies that may be used with people with dysphagia prior to evaluation including

- Using a quiet environment,
- Paying careful attention to positioning,
- Completing oral stimulation before eating,
- Presenting appetizing food in an appealing manner, and
- Using adaptive equipment and feeding utensils as necessary to maximize performance.

Therapists may also apply these techniques during the intervention phase when working with adults with developmental disabilities. Stratton (1989) stressed the importance of positioning, food presentation, use of adaptive utensils, and careful attention to diet as key areas of concern. The work further emphasized that because of difficulty with generalization, skill training should occur during mealtimes in the client's natural context.

Additional considerations include the type of foods served and how often they are served. People with oral sensitivities may only eat specific textures of food. Avery (2008) suggested consideration of food progressions based on levels of thickness ranging from thick purees to thin flavored foods and water. Foods may be thickened by adding, for example, pudding, milk, or commercial thickeners.

Use of oral–motor stimulation programs and gradually introducing foods are additional techniques used to enhance variety in the diet. For individuals with attention and task completion difficulties, sitting at mealtimes may be a challenge. Scheduling shorter but more frequent meals or augmenting small meals with nutritious snacks can alleviate behavior difficulties at mealtime.

An additional area of difficulty often encountered in populations with developmental disabilities is self-monitoring of intake. Clients may lack internal controls to address the amount of intake. In addition to teaching clients about food portions (provided they have the cognitive ability), external controls on portions and types of foods may be needed.

A final consideration is training in the social behavior required in public settings. Therapists may plan additional interventions to address issues such as maintaining attention, appropriate behavior in public settings, the ability to patiently wait for meals in restaurants, and awareness of culturally and contextually specific mealtime manners. Discussing specific intervention techniques for these areas is beyond the scope of this chapter. The following general strategies may be useful in working with adults who have developmental disabilities.

Remedial Strategies

- Address underlying oral–motor or swallowing difficulties and weaknesses through techniques such as vibration, tapping, oral–motor exercises, and stretching (Avery-Smith, 2002).
- Address postural and range of motion concerns that inhibit proper feeding and eating.
- Use desensitization, calming, and sensory stimulation techniques to address oral–motor hypo- and hypersensitivities.
- Provide a sensory diet with heightened tactile and proprioceptive input to stimulate sensation and movement prior to eating (Avery, 2008).
- Provide mealtime training regarding proper food portions, social behaviors, and nutrition, possibly using modeling, practice, and role-playing techniques.
- Provide individual and small-group training on mealtime manners and public etiquette.

Adaptive/Compensatory Strategies

- Adjust length of mealtimes according to the client's needs. If appropriate, supplement small meals with nutritious snacks.
- Use adaptive equipment such as built-up and weighted utensils, Dycem,™ plate guards, and adapted cups.
- Select food textures and types based on the client's preferences and needs (e.g., soft foods, liquid-based foods, small pieces).
- Schedule visits to public eating places during quieter times.
- Provide meaningful activities during wait periods in public restaurants.

Functional Mobility

As people with developmental disabilities enter adolescence and adulthood, functional mobility extends beyond the home and into the community. Adults with developmental disabilities will have established a pattern of mobility throughout the childhood years (see Chapter 6). As they reach adulthood, the occupational therapist should reassess their occupational needs regarding functional mobility. Expanded occupations and activities outside the home require careful planning to ensure that the necessary resources and supports are available. In conjunction with remedial approaches, occupational therapy evaluation and intervention for mobility concerns often include orthotic prescription, positioning, adaptation of movement patterns, and use of assistive technology (Gillen, 2002).

The *Framework* (AOTA, 2008) identifies functional mobility as relating to mobility from one position to another, functional ambulation, and transport of objects. Pierce (2008) proposed a hierarchy that suggests that foundational mobility needs for basic ADLs, such as personal hygiene and grooming, must be met prior to mobility needs for higher level IADLs. As the mobility requirements become more complex (e.g., community mobility and driving), the client is required to use increased cognitive and motor functions to accomplish the tasks involved. Therefore, skills for the lower level of mobility (e.g., transfer out of a bed) must be in place before higher level skills (e.g., transfer into a car). Mobility may be impaired for the adult with developmental disabilities by issues of strength, range of motion, coordination, motor control, and sensory–perceptual problems. Additional concerns about cognitive awareness, safety, and judgment may further affect the client's ability to make wise choices on how and where to ambulate. For people with epilepsy, seizures are a safety concern, particularly grand mal seizures in which the client loses conscious control of motor functions. Other developmental disabilities, such as spina bifida and severe cerebral palsy, often require special mobility equipment such as wheelchairs and walkers. Intervention planning for functional mobility combines remedial skill training with adaptive strategies and equipment in order to match the client's strengths and needs to the environmental context and daily occupational requirements.

Interventions for adults with developmental disabilities include training for the client, caregivers, and care network. For example, establishing health maintenance and exercise routines may facilitate adequate strength and fitness to manage and maintain functional mobility. Clients should also be taught proper body mechanics, particularly if muscle imbalances, coordination, and balance issues are of concern. Caregivers may also need education regarding safe transfers, particularly as an adolescent or young adult client gains height and weight.

Comprehensive evaluation of and intervention for functional mobility take into consideration individual client factors, along with the environmental context and daily occupational patterns. Equipment may include wheelchairs, scooters, walkers, canes, crutches, and other ambulatory devices. Consideration should be given to the environment, equipment demands (e.g., type of wheelchair), occupational needs, and ability of the client to use the equipment or learn the techniques and skills for desired outcomes. If clients have expectations of increasing independence and motility, a motorized wheelchair may be advantageous, particularly in the community. Use of a power wheelchair has been found to enhance occupational performance, adaptability, competence, and self-esteem in clients with severe mobility impairments (Buning, Angelo, & Schmeler, 2001).

Remedial Strategies

- Promote balance, flexibility, and strength training to enhance personal mobility.
- Provide skill training in the use of mobility equipment, the proper way to make transfers, and basic body mechanics.
- Provide skill training using simulated situations, videos, pictures, and in vivo training related to safe ambulation in a variety of environments.

Adaptive/Compensatory Strategies

- Use wheelchair bags, walker bags, duffels on wheels, and other means to carry items safely and effectively.
- Provide safety training for caregivers.
- Evaluate and recommend equipment that matches the needs of the client and environmental demands.

Sexuality

Occupational therapists may address the topic of sexuality with adolescents and adults who have developmental disabilities. Issues of sexuality include sexual expression, love, intimacy, boundaries, and personal protection. Sexual relationships are often tied to self-worth, and it is important to educate the client on healthy relationships. Individuals with developmental and physical disabilities have a basic right to sexual expression and intimate relationships (Sullivan & Caterino, 2008), yet many of the settings in which they are treated pose barriers to formation of healthy intimate relationships.

Few programs for people with developmental disabilities directly address sexuality, and therefore, teens and young adults may not have adequate knowledge in this area. A Danish survey of people with an ASD revealed higher levels of socially inappropriate expressions of sexuality, social deficits, and deviant sexual behavior (Waltz, 2002). The authors attributed the differences to unnatural environmental exposure to sexuality (e.g., atypical means of learning about sexuality) as well as to sensory differences. Research by Stokes and Kaur (2005) indicated people with high-functioning ASD often wish for intimate relationships, yet their social disabilities often prevented formation of healthy relationships due to poor prosocial behaviors and lack of knowledge related to privacy and sexual issues. Such difficulties may be minimized through carefully planned interventions and education.

Issues of sexuality in adults with developmental disabilities are complex. For example, people with an ASD may be prone to sensory processing difficulties (Dunn et al., 2002), and therefore, therapists must determine whether behaviors such as public masturbation are due to sexual expression, or sensory self-stimulation. Often the question of sexual vulnerability arises and interdisciplinary teams have to work with the client, family, and extended care network to determine means of healthy sexual expression while at the same time protecting individuals against exploitation. In addition to vulnerabilities and sensory processing disturbances, individuals with physical disabilities, such as those with spina bifida, may have problems with lubrication or other sexual difficulties (Brei, 1999). Additional difficulties may be encountered through the side effects of medications (Waltz, 2002). In conjunction with general education on sexuality and healthy relationships, clients may benefit from education on sexual options for people with disabilities. Further information on this topic can be found in Chapter 17.

Remedial Strategies

- Provide education to the client, caregivers, and extended care network, using techniques such as role-plays, videotapes, group discussions, and contextual training about healthy relationships, sexuality, and boundaries.
- Use health promotion and prevention techniques to inform the client about safe sexual and relationship practices.
- Provide education and intervention specially designed to address sexual expression for people with physical disabilities.

- Use intervention strategies to address underlying sensory processing problems that may cause inappropriate public sexual stimulation and exposure.

Adaptive/Compensatory Strategies

- Use adaptive sexual aids and techniques (see Chapter 17).
- Provide for alternative sources of stimulation.
- Facilitate environmental accommodations and private spaces for clients with specific sexual needs.
- Implement behavioral plans and vulnerable adult plans for clients deemed at risk for sexual exploitation.

Assistive Technology and Personal Device Use

Assistive technology is often used to facilitate the occupational performance of and increase the level of independence of people with developmental disabilities. Although often referred to as *assistive devices,* Cook and Hussey (2002) defined *assistive technology* as "a broad range of devices, services, strategies, and practices that are conceived and applied to ameliorate the problems faced by individuals who have disabilities" (p. 5). This definition broadens the scope of assistive technology to include not only physical devices but also the application of knowledge and development of strategies to enhance client function. A comprehensive discussion of this topic is beyond the scope of this chapter, but the following provides some basic considerations in use of assistive technology with populations with developmental disabilities.

The interactions among the person, environment, tasks, and devices is important to evaluate when determinig the appropriateness of assistive technology for adults with developmental disabilites (Mann & Beaver, 1995). In this approach, occupational therapists consider the client's current function and desired outcome, the tasks and environmental context, and the selection of technology. An important consideration is whether the client has the ability to learn to use the device. Additional selection criteria include

- The appearance of the device,
- The cost–benefit ratio of the device,
- The ability of the device to complete the desired task, and
- The availability of a selection of custom-made versus off-the-shelf items (Mann & Beaver, 1995).

Given the diverse environmental contexts of many adults with developmental disabilities, the occupational therapy process focuses on technology needs in the home, school, work, and community (Buning, 2009). Assistive technologies often used with adults with developmental disabilities include keyboard and computer technologies (see Figure 7.1), communication systems, mobility devices for functional and transportation mobility, robotic aids, and sensory aids. It is recommended that clients be given a chance to try a particular technology in order to assess whether it is an appropriate fit. Some clients may resist using some types of technology; before investing in a costly item, the client's motivation and ability to use the technology should be assessed. Finally, the training needs of a client must be determined. Trefler and Hobson (1997) recommended that the training occur in the context in which the technology will be used. This is especially important for an adult client with a developmental disability, as concerns may arise regarding his or her ability to transfer learning and use of the assistive technology from one environment to another. Training of the family, caregivers, and care network is often necessary to ensure consistent skill training, reinforcement, and training among individuals who are interacting with the client.

Instrumental Activities of Daily Living (IADLs)

While adults with physical disabilities along with their developmental disability are more readily recognized as disabled by others, those with more subtle, hidden disabilities such as fetal alcohol effects, borderline retardation, or learning disabilities may initially appear unaffected. Often these individuals are fairly independent with basic ADLs but have difficulty in other tasks such as writing a paper, managing a checkbook, or filling out a job application. These individuals may struggle to meet the demands of the external world. Occupational therapists identify the barriers to client performance and develop intervention strategies to maximize performance and quality of life in IADLs, work, play/leisure, social settings, and educational performance.

Home Management and Care of Self, Others, Including Children), and Pets

According to Mulcahey (1999), a healthy, well-adjusted adult has the ability to interact comfortably with others, respect authority, respect himself or herself, solve problems with confidence, and ask for help when needed. Adults with developmental disabilities need to employ strategies to perform daily chores and meet responsibilities, such as skill train-

ing, use of adaptive equipment, and development of daily routines. Some clients hire personal care attendants or other helpers to assist with chores, cleaning, and cooking. One area of concern, particularly with clients with cognitive impairments, is the ability to use good judgment and adhere to safety procedures when completing such daily routines. Formal and informal living skills evaluations in the client's residence are often helpful to evaluate needs and develop intervention strategies.

Perhaps one of the most neglected areas of skill training in occupational therapy is parenting skills. A review of the occupational therapy literature (Cohn, 2001; Cohn, Miller, & Tickle-Degnen, 2000; Humphry & Thigpen-Beck, 1998) revealed that therapists often focus on parenting from the perspective of the parent of a child with a disability but infrequently from the perspective of the parent with a disability. Parents with physical disabilities may require compensatory techniques and household adaptations; those with cognitive deficits often require basic training in child development and parenting skills. In cases of more severe developmental disabilities, issues of competence and safety may be of concern, in which case care must be taken to involve the family and extended care network in determining supports needed to ensure the well-being of the client, the spouse (if the client is married), and the children.

Despite an increase in the number of people with major cognitive issues in parenting roles, services to these populations have not corresponded with the increased need (Kirkpatrick, 2008). The Social Care Institute for Excellence (2007) suggested a systems perspective, involving clarity of responsibility among the caregiver with the disability, the family system, and the service providers. The occupational therapist is a vital part of the interdisciplinary team in providing services to the client with disabilities and the family system.

Remedial Strategies

- Provide skills training in household maintenance and caring for the self, for others, and for pets (see Figure 7.2).
- Provide education for the entire family on safety, adaptation, and home management techniques.
- Pursue remediation of underlying strength, endurance, and range-of-motion difficulties to ease the client's physical burden.
- Conduct interactive parenting sessions along with training in child development and parenting skills.

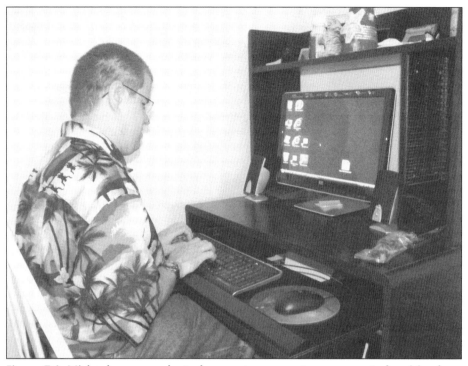

Figure 7.1. Michael uses an adapted computer screen to compensate for vision loss.

Adaptive/Compensatory Strategies

- Use adaptive equipment for daily chores, such as long-handled brooms, reachers, and mops.
- Select lightweight small appliances.
- Use daily reminders, schedules, and white-boards for self-organization.
- Add necessary support systems, such as a nanny or housekeeper.
- Use sensory aids such as talking clocks, visual aids, and teletype systems.
- Provide training in energy conservation and efficiency techniques (e.g., use of schedules, ergonomics, establishment of routines).

Shopping, Meal Preparation, Safety, and Emergency Management

Shopping and meal preparation require a high level of cognitive ability. These activities involve community mobility, budgeting, planning, organization, and adherence to safety procedures.

Accurate evaluation of the client's safety and judgment during meal preparation is important to ensure that the client understands the safe, proper use of appliances and to identify the supports needed to minimize risks. Clients with physical and sensory impairments may benefit from using adapted appliances and utensils, such as enlarged stove knobs, high-contrast items (for people with low vision), and

ergonomic aids. Clients with subtle cognitive disabilities who present safety risks may learn to prepare meals primarily in a microwave to reduce the risk of fire and other hazards. Emergency response and crisis management preparations should include clear displays of emergency telephone numbers and training in first-aid and safety principles. Some adult clients with developmental disabilities may have limited ability to generalize emergency procedures to other environments; occupational therapists should evaluate supports and provide experiential training using role-plays and scenarios.

Remedial Strategies

- Use skill training in shopping, meal preparation, and emergency response in the client's community and place of residence.
- Provide practice opportunities in preparation of a few nutritious meals.
- Use skill training, including role-plays, video-tapes, training aids, and simulated situations to educate the client in emergency response practices in the client's community and place of residence.
- Use therapeutic interventions to remediate underlying physical and sensory deficits that impair client occupational performance in this area.

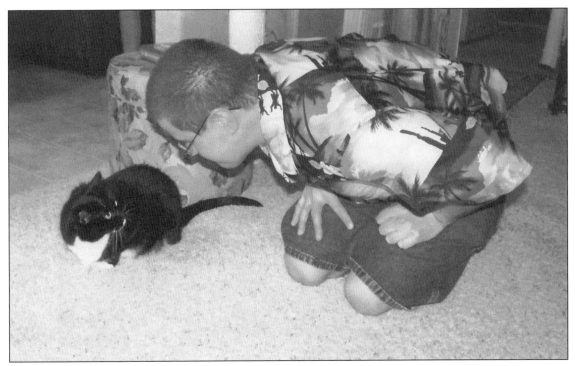

Figure 7.2. Increasingly, animals and pets are used as part of therapy.

Adaptive/Compensatory Strategies

- Use adapted appliances and ergonomic aids.
- If safety is a concern, use safer cooking methods (e.g., a microwave oven).
- Recommend shopping at smaller stores and stores near the client's place of residence.
- Use grocery or meal delivery services if transportation is problematic.
- Provide for external supports such as a housekeeper or aide to prepare meals.
- Use charts and visible aids to cue the client on safety and emergency procedures and on important emergency telephone numbers.

Financial Management

The area of financial management is considered one of the most important outcome areas for people with disabilities (Dowrick, 2004). Decisions regarding finances should involve the client, to the extent possible, based on his or her cognitive ability.

There are various levels of independence in financial management. As the adolescent with developmental disabilities enters adulthood, decisions must be made about his or her level of competence and ability to manage his or her own finances. Parents may continue to manage the client's finances, a conservator may be appointed, or the client may get assistance from external sources or may manage his or her finances independently.

Basic money management skills include counting change, making change from a transaction, budgeting, and banking. People with developmental disabilities may be at risk of financial exploitation and must have protection as prescribed by laws regarding vulnerable adults. People with cognitive and attention disorders may also be prone to impulse control issues that may affect spending habits. In those with attention deficit disorders, impulsivity and inattention may cause impaired occupational functioning (Weiss, 1997) that affects higher level living skills such as money management. Other developmental disabilities such as ASDs affect executive functions, resulting in problems with organization, problem solving, impulse control issues, and poor memory (Bolick, 2001). All of these symptoms affect a client's ability to effectively manage finances and make responsible spending decisions. In addition to external assistance, the following strategies may prove effective in promoting money management skills and financial responsibility.

Remedial Strategies

- Scaffold the teaching of monetary systems through the use of token-based behavioral programs and rewards systems.
- Allow for mastery of money management skills on a developmental level, from simple

tasks to more complex banking skills, starting with basic tasks such as counting and making change. Use role-plays and experiential sessions to practice assertive behaviors and social responsibility to prevent financial exploitation.

- When possible, work with parents of adolescents with developmental disabilities on estate and financial planning before the client enters adulthood.
- Provide opportunities for practice of basic money management through use of vocational programs; hospital-, clinic-, day treatment–, and program-based stores; and trips into the community.
- Teach the client the value of items in order to promote wise spending decisions.

Adaptive/Compensatory Strategies

- Provide for a financial conservator and external supports when needed.
- Use simplified weekly budgets (e.g., the client may have a conservator but is given responsibility to budget for a nominal amount on a daily or weekly basis).
- Have the client manage only one account (e.g., a savings account) and another individual manage the checking account.
- Use accounts that require cosignatures.
- Develop external supports, and when feasible, arrange with the employer that the client receive a weekly, as opposed to a biweekly or monthly, check, as such payment schedules are often easier to manage.

Health Management and Maintenance

Health management and maintenance involve health promotion, health-enhancing behaviors, and health prevention. People with intellectual disabilities have greater unmet health needs than those of the general population (Cooper et al., 2006). In addition to cognitive issues, people with developmental conditions often have physical and sensory disabilities that require ongoing health management. Problems occur when clients do not follow through with health maintenance and management and engage in health-compromising behaviors such as smoking, drug use, and other negative behaviors (Taylor, 1999). Further difficulties may result when clients have additional disability-related concerns such as special nutritional requirements, daily medications, and exercise regimens designed to preserve and enhance physical and emotional functioning. For therapeutic interven-

tions to be of benefit, the client must be willing and motivated to adhere to the therapy program and recommendations. The therapy must fit the needs of the client and must be presented at a level where the client can fully understand and follow through with the recommendations. Key need areas in developmental disabilities include proper use of assistive technology, maintenance of exercise programs, adherence to nutritional recommendations, and medication compliance.

Many adult clients with developmental disabilities are prescribed multiple medications. According to Haynes, McKibbon, and Kanani (1996), follow-through on prescriptions and health advice is low (about 50%) in the general population. Clients with compromised cognition often struggle even more with compliance, not only because of motivational issues but also because of a lack of understanding and ability to follow the medication regimen. More complex treatments have been found to lower treatment compliance rates (Brannon & Feist, 2000). The use of external supports and assistance, along with with pill boxes and other aids, helps ease the burden of medication compliance; additional strategies that may encourage health-promoting behaviors include establishing norms in group facilities (e.g., group exercises), developing routines and habits, and using educational and behavioral strategies.

Remedial Strategies

- Implement health prevention and screening programs designed to identify and meet client needs (Cooper et al., 2006).
- Educate the client, family, and extended care network in medication management, nutritional requirements, and therapy regimens.
- Provide group and individual therapy sessions to enable the client to practice health management skills and develop habits and routines (e.g., cooking nutritious meals compliant with specialized or diabetic diets).
- Use peer support to promote healthy behaviors.

Adaptive/Compensatory Strategies

- Use external supports such as a visiting nurse or attendant to assist with follow-through.
- Use adaptive strategies and equipment (e.g., pill boxes, premeasured food, talking clocks).
- Use posted reminders regarding daily health routines.
- Adjust schedules to give the client cues (e.g., taking medications before each meal, receiving a phone call from an individual to remind the client about an appointment).

Sleep and Rest

Client-centered approaches should focus on the client's lifestyle balance and how it is affected by sleep–wake–rest cycles. People with developmental disabilities may have unusual sleep and wake patterns or disturbances that affect the daily routine (Waltz, 2002). Sleep difficulties may affect their level of alertness, productivity, efficiency, and occupational performance. Transitions from an arousing alerting activity to a restful activity or bedtime may be difficult, particularly for individuals who have difficulty regulating their arousal systems.

Additional difficulties in sleep–wake cycles, arousal, and energy level may be caused by medications, energy expenditure, stress, and medical conditions. As the occupational therapist considers the client's daily activity profile, identification of problems should include sleep or arousal difficulties. As problems are reported to the interdisciplinary teams, efforts should be made to determine the underlying problem(s) and develop intervention strategies. In addition to medical interventions, calming techniques and relaxation exercises may prove helpful based on the client's cognitive level. To promote a balance of activity and a transition to bedtime, use of daily routines, schedules, and transition techniques may be helpful (Moor, 2000). Additional considerations should include the sleeping environment, the type of bedding, sleep habits and practices, and physiological factors that affect sleep (Jan et al., 2008).

Remedial Strategies

- Educate the client in use of relaxation and calming techniques prior to bedtime.
- Address underlying physiological and sensory processing difficulties that affect arousal and inhibit sleep.

Box 7.3. Case Example—Joy

Joy has developmental disabilities and mental health concerns. Throughout her childhood and adolescence, she received multiple services and lived in structured, institutionalized settings. In addition to developmental concerns, barriers to Joy's occupational performance included

1. Poor sensory integration, including dyspraxia and sensory defensiveness;
2. Cognitive difficulties, such as poor planning, organization, and abstraction; and
3. Deficits in living skills and socialization skills.

Joy was totally dependent in all IADLs and required prompts and minimal assistance with basic ADLs. Joy had hypo- and hypersensitivity to incoming stimulation and required cues, prompts, and assistance in meeting daily grooming needs. She sought out social relationships, but she frequently was unaware of boundary issues and proper assertiveness. Her difficulties with planning and organization complicated her efforts to meet daily needs, as did her over- and underarousal, which resulted in either hyper- or hypoactivity.

Beginning at age 18, in conjunction with a multidisciplinary approach, Joy received intensive occupational therapy services that included sensory integration therapy, living skills training, social skills training, and modification of her environment. Within a year of intensive intervention, she showed significant gains in occupational performance. With environmental adaptations and built-in supports, Joy has lived in her own apartment for more than 10 years without rehospitalization. Initially, Joy received fairly intensive case management and therapy services. With a daily routine, development of calming and alerting strategies, and establishment of living and social skills, she progressed to the point that she has now lived over 10 years independently without case management assistance.

Joy works part-time, maintains active involvement in her church, and engages in socialization through local community events. Examples of the daily adaptations and strategies Joy uses include working part-time on an adapted work schedule; using whiteboards in her apartment to help her stay organized; and scheduling her days to stay busy, manage anxiety, and allow time for relaxation. Joy works part-time during the late morning, her hours of personal peak performance. She uses strategies such as brushing for calming and sour candies for alerting to regulate her arousal state for maximal function (see Figure 7.3). Keeping whiteboards in her apartment helps her maintain a daily routine, schedule her day, and note reminders of important appointments and strategies to meet personal needs (see Figure 7.4). She uses the public transit system, takes weekly trips into the city, and frequently walks to the library and local shopping center. She also manages her routine to allow periods of calming and adjusts her physical environment to help her meet personal goals.

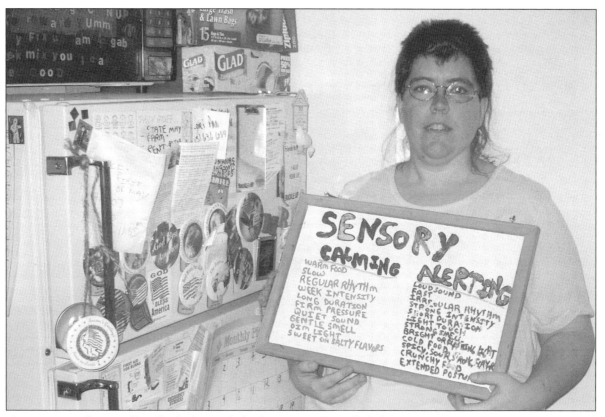

Figure 7.3. Joy keeps a list of calming and alerting strategies to help her through the day.

- Plan schedules carefully, considering the levels of energy expenditure required by daily activities and adjusting activities to balance energy expenditures throughout the day (see Box 7.3).
- Implement stress reduction techniques and self-awareness strategies to address underlying stress and anxiety.
- Plan interventions using a holistic approach that includes health promotion, good nutrition, and exercise.

Adaptive/Compensatory Strategies

- Establish a routine with careful transition plans prior to bedtime.
- Adjust the client's schedule and daily activity requirements on the basis of his or her natural sleep–wake–rest cycles. For example, if the client naturally goes to bed late and gets up late in the morning, then do not schedule early morning appointments.
- Adapt the environment in order to promote rest and sleep (e.g., use of lights with dimmer switches, creation of calming rather than stimulating environments).

Community Mobility

As the client with developmental disabilities enters adulthood, community mobility becomes increasingly important for educational, vocational, and social reasons. In addition to mobility provided by wheelchairs and ambulatory equipment, issues of transportation, driving, and travel aids should be addressed. Depending on state requirements, driving evaluations may be recommended in order to ensure that the client is able to drive safely. Occupational therapists may use driving evaluations in the clinic prior to formal evaluations in the community. Increasingly, simulators and virtual reality applications are used to train and educate the client in driving, safety, and traffic laws.

Driving evaluation includes both client evaluation and an assessment of the vehicle and the appropriate client–vehicle fit (Pierce, 2008). Cook and Hussey (2002) identified a set of predriving evaluation items, including evaluation of visual and perceptual skills, hearing reaction time, cognitive skills, and physical skills. The evaluation should determine needs related to competence, special vehicle modifications, vehicle selection, and vehicle access. For clients who are unable to drive, medical trans-

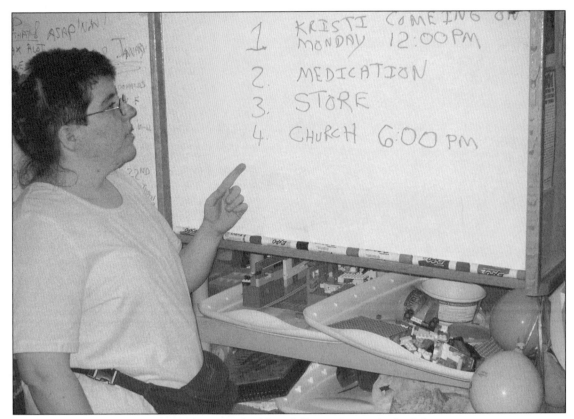

Figure 7.4. Joy uses a whiteboard to keep track of her daily routine and schedule.

portation systems may be useful as well as training in the use of public transit systems.

Remedial Strategies

- Reassess and prescribe any changes in ambulatory aids. Some clients may need electric wheelchairs or scooters to enhance community mobility; others may require a lighter weight, more easily propelled wheelchair.
- Use driver simulation and training prior to the actual state driving test.
- Implement bus training, including the use of public transit systems and medical transportation systems. For clients with cognitive issues, it is recommended that training begin with only one route and involve repeated practice under therapist supervision before generalizing to other routes.

Adaptive/Compensatory Strategies

- Use adaptive aids such as secondary vehicle controls, lifts, wheelchair restraint systems, and adapted driving controls (e.g., adapted handles, blinkers, brakes).
- Use restricted licenses as available (e.g., the client can drive only during the day, or only within a certain distance from home).

- Use volunteer drivers and other assistive transportation systems.

Communication

Clients with cognitive impairments or ASDs often have compromised language capabilities. Other people with central nervous system involvement of the speech centers, such as those with cerebral palsy, may have disjointed or difficult-to-understand speech. As these clients age, traditional low-technology communication aids may no longer suit their needs, at which point the team must determine the best communication system to maximize performance. The first decision should be to determine the primary mode of communication (Harden, 2001) so that the team, family, and extended care network can work with it consistently. Additional decisions include where communication needs to occur, how effective the technology will be within the environment, the client's ability and motivation to use the system, and the opportunities for others to use it system with the client.

In addition to communication aids, clients with developmental disabilities often need to learn communication skills related to social interaction, assertiveness skills, and the difference between private and public conversation. Due to difficulty with generalization, the client may need repeated practice both at home and in the community. Additional strategies that may be helpful include the use of role-plays, videos, and feedback following social interaction.

Remedial Strategies

- Use social skills training groups and therapy techniques designed to enhance the client's ability to communicate in a variety of public situations.
- Use role-plays, modeling, practice, Social Stories, and feedback to enhance oral and written communication skills.
- Provide skills training for the client, family, and extended care network in the use of communication devices in multiple contexts.

Adaptive/Compensatory Strategies

- Use communication devices, picture boards, and sign language.
- Use simplified language, yes-or-no questions, and brief sentences.
- Use adapted household equipment such as teletype systems, phones with enhanced volume, hearing aids, and voice recognition software.

Play, Leisure, and Social Participation

The emergence of the community participation movement emphasizes the importance for people with disabilities of promoting skill training and community development to foster community participation (Wituk, Pearson, Bomhoft, Hinde, & Meissn, 2007). Bhattacharyya (2004) proposed three principles of community development—(a) self-help, (b) felt needs, and (c) participation—in order to promote shared identity and community participation. The occupational therapist works with individuals and communities to promote healthy environments to maximize occupational participation (see Figures 7.5 and 7.6).

Development of social skills affects every area of an individual's life, including the ability to secure employment, participate in community events, and engage in play or leisure activities with others. Several developmental disorders have accompanying symptoms causing difficulties with social interactions and participation. The *Diagnostic and Statistical Manual of Mental Disorders* (American Psychiatric Association, 2000) includes the following diagnostic criteria for autistic and Asperger's disorders:

- Marked impairment in the use of nonverbal behaviors such as eye-to-eye gaze, facial expression, body postures, and gestures to regulate social interaction;
- Failure to develop peer relationships appropriate to developmental level;
- Lack of spontaneous seeking to share enjoyment, interests, or achievements with other people; and
- Lack of social or emotional reciprocity.

Other disorders such as childhood disintegrative disorder, Rett's disorder, and attentional disorders all have criteria that indicate potential difficulties in social interactions, difficulty with engagement in leisure and social activities, or both. Additional occupational barriers are encountered for clients with cognitive deficits, as the ability to explore and identify meaningful activities may be impaired.

Intervention techniques designed to enhance social skills and social participation may include the use of social skills curricula, Social Stories, and activity groups. Greene (2001) presented social modeling as an effective tool in teaching social skills. The author identified modeling as a cognitive–behavioral approach that includes verbal modeling, skill performance, practice, and feedback.

Programs that incorporate social modeling often include use of role-plays, stories, and discussions. Social skills may also be practiced while working on goals related to play and leisure. The use of games, community outings, and exploration of interests are suitable for intervention and serve a dual purpose in giving the client opportunities to work on social skills. Clients may need cues and reminders regarding social behaviors in a variety of situations (e.g., personal vs. public social interaction, maintenance of boundaries, and use of personal space). Occupational therapists should emphasize developing leisure interests that are appropriate to the client's skill level, interests, and context.

Remedial Strategies

- Provide social skills training using psychoeducation, behavioral modification, and cognitive–behavioral programs.
- Use interest checklists and opportunities to explore and develop play and leisure interests.
- Use activity groups, task groups, community outings, and structured play opportunities.

Adaptive/Compensatory Strategies

- Educate caregivers and the extended care network in modification of communication and social interaction to facilitate social exchange.
- Focus on mastery of one or two social skills at a time.

- Use adapted play/leisure equipment (e.g., adapted sports, bicycles, games).
- Modify rules to the cognitive level of the client.
- Use schedules to promote daily leisure time.

Education and Work

Young adults with developmental disabilities who are involved in meaningful activity such as work or volunteer opportunities report a higher level of life satisfaction (Salkever, 2000). Transition planning for the client with developmental disabilities occurs as the adolescent enters adulthood. After high school, decisions must be made whether he or she will pursue vocational training, an education toward a degree, or employment. Many students with developmental disabilities do well in vocational training programs; these often result in increased attendance, provide practical experience toward a vocation, and facilitate exploration of a particular type of career or job (American Academy of Pediatrics, 2000). Others, especially those with milder forms of disabilities and higher cognitive abilities, choose college. For those who are unlikely to pursue educa-

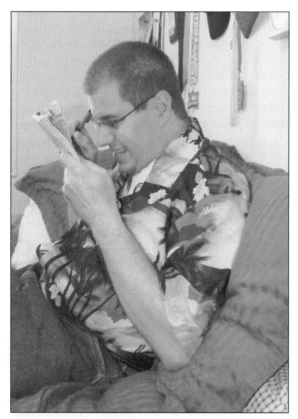

Figure 7.5. Michael uses a large-print word finder to adapt for vision loss; the wall behind him displays his medals from active involvement in adapted sports and Special Olympics.

tion beyond high school, the client and team must work together to determine a plan to pursue vocational goals.

Selection of the appropriate work and educational environment for a client with developmental disabilities should consider his or her interests, skills, performance level, and occupational needs. The American Academy of Pediatrics (2000) recommends the following for adolescents and young adults with developmental disabilities:

- Teach adolescents about public laws (e.g., American with Disabilities Act [ADA], Individuals with Disabilities Education Improvement Act [IDEA]) and their implications for education and career opportunities.
- Provide opportunities for volunteer work and internships.
- Provide opportunities for career exploration.
- Emphasize independence at their place of residence.
- Provide opportunities for meaningful employment.

Giving the client personal choice in vocational participation has been shown to promote increased satisfaction (Siporin & Lysack, 2004). Intervention for work and education goals should focus not only on vocational skill training but also on the ability to search and apply for employment, engage in the interview process, and determine applicability to the client's skills and interests. Dolyniuk et al. (2002) emphasize the importance of training the individual in social along with vocational and educational skills in order to promote self-efficacy and increased awareness of social context within vocational and educational settings. The authors stressed the value of role-playing, perspective taking, and direct experience in social settings in developing the skills necessary for success in vocational settings.

Remedial Strategies

- Direct training in educational and vocational skill areas, including (a) getting to and from school or work, (b) social behaviors, (c) study and work habits, (d) work routines, (e) understanding rules and regulations, (f) ability to take feedback and make changes as necessary, (g) follow-through with safety procedures, and (h) ability to obtain necessary resources and external supports for success in the work and school environments.
- Use of Social Stories, role-playing, videos, and direct practice to teach problem-solving

and adaptive behaviors in work and school settings.

- Use internships and volunteer experiences to develop work skills.
- Develop prevocational skills.

Adaptive/Compensatory Strategies

- Match the work or education setting to the client's skills (e.g., sheltered workshop, enclaves, supported employment, transitional employment, competitive employment).
- Educate the academic and vocational staff working with the client (in compliance with ADA and IDEA and other regulatory practices).
- Use adaptive equipment as needed (e.g., adaptive keyboards, voice recognition software, ergonomic aids).
- Adapt the routine of the day to accommodate the disability through use of extended or more frequent breaks, extended test-taking time, extended deadlines, or shorter hours.
- Adapt the work environment and job tasks to the skill and needs of the client.

Summary

This chapter presented a framework for approaching clients with developmental disabilities, along with strategies for evaluation and intervention. Occupational therapists apply diverse approaches to evaluation of and interventions for adults with developmental disabilities. Evaluation of the client's needs for intervention requires determining the level of cognition, current performance capacity, situational context, and other factors that pertain to the peformance of tasks required for everyday living. Intervention then typically involves a wide range of remedial or adaptive/compensatory strategies. For clients with the capacity to learn, careful selection of learning strategies involving chaining or other techniques, opportunities for direct practice in natural settings, and establishing routines are essential for success. The selection of a particular approach requires clinical reasoning that is based on the needs and therapeutic goals of the client. Therapists should use client-centered, holistic practices to focus on quality of life to maximize the client's occupational performance.

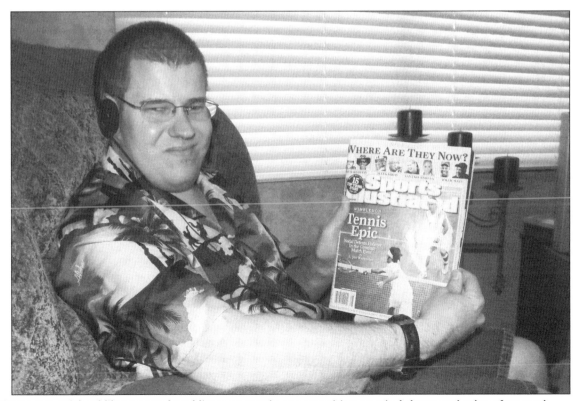

Figure 7.6. Michael likes to read and listen to music as a transition to wind down and relax after work.

Study Questions

1. Describe some of the major approaches used in evaluation of and intervention for people with developmental disabilities.

2. What is a client-centered, occupation-based approach? How is it used with people with developmental disabilities?

3. What are some common areas for evaluation of people with developmental disabilities?

4. What measurement tools are available for evaluating ADLs in adults with developmental disabilities?

5. What is the difference between a remedial and an adaptive approach to evaluation and intervention? When would you use these approaches in treating a client with disabilities?

6. List examples of intervention techniques using remedial and adaptive strategies for adults with developmental disabilities.

7. How would you involve the family and extended care network in caring for a person with developmental disabilities?

References

Abreu, B. C. (1992). The quadraphonic approach: Management of cognitive–perceptual and postural control dysfunction. *Occupational Therapy Practice, 3,* 12–29.

Abreu, B. C. (1998). The quadraphonic approach: Holistic rehabilitation for brain injury. In N. Katz (Ed.), *Cognition and occupation in rehabilitation: Cognitive models for intervention in occupational therapy* (pp. 51–123). Rockville, MD: American Occupational Therapy Association.

Abreu, B. C., & Peloquin, S. M. (2005). The Quadraphonic Approach: A holistic rehabilitation model for brain injury. In N. Katz (Ed.), *Cognition and occupation across the lifespan* (2nd ed., pp. 73–112). Bethesda, MD: AOTA Press.

Affolter, F. D. (1987). *Perception, interaction, and language: Interaction of daily living: The root of development.* Berlin: Springer-Verlag.

Allen, C. K. (1985). *Occupational therapy for psychiatric diseases: Measurement and management of cognitive disabilities.* Boston: Little, Brown.

Allen, C. K., & Blue, T. (1998). Cognitive disabilities model: How to make clinical judgments. In N. Katz, (Ed.), *Cognition and occupation in rehabilitation* (pp. 225–279). Rockville, MD: American Occupational Therapy Association.

American Academy of Pediatrics. (2000). The role of the pediatrician in transitioning children and adolescents with developmental disabilities and chronic illnesses from school to work or college. *Pediatrics, 106,* 854–856.

American Association of Mental Retardation. (2002). *Mental retardation definition, classification, and systems of support* (10th ed.). Washington, DC: Author.

American Occupational Therapy Association. (2007). Specialized knowledge and skills in feeding, eating, and swallowing for occupational therapy practice. *American Journal of Occupational Therapy, 61,* 686–700.

American Occupational Therapy Association. (2008). Occupational therapy practice framework: Domain and process (2nd ed.). *American Journal of Occupational Therapy, 62,* 625–683.

American Psychiatric Association. (2000). *Desk reference to the diagnostic criteria from DSM-IV-TR.* Washington, DC: Author.

Auburn University, Department of Psychology. (2008). *Behavioral analysis in developmental disabilities.* Retrieved May 8, 2009, from http://media.cla.auburn.edu/psychology/gs/masters/b_analysis_bb.cfm

Avery, W. (2008). Dysphagia. In M. V. Radomski & C. A. Latham (Eds.), *Occupational therapy for physical dysfunction* (6th ed., pp. 1321–1344). Philadelphia: Lippincott Williams & Wilkins.

Avery-Smith, W. (2002). Dysphagia. In C. A. Trombly & M. V. Radomski (Eds.), *Occupational therapy for physical dysfunction* (5th ed., pp. 1091–1109). Philadelphia: Lippincott Williams & Wilkins.

Avery-Smith, W., Rosen, A. B., Dellarosa, D. M. (1997). *Dysphagia evaluation protocol.* San Antonio, TX: Harcourt Assessment.

Ayres, A. J. (1972). *Sensory integration and learning disorders.* Los Angeles: Western Psychological Services.

Ayres, A. J. (1979). *Sensory integration and the child.* Los Angeles: Western Psychological Services.

Bachner, S. (1998). Let's do lunch: A comprehensive nonstandardized assessment tool. In M. Ross & S. Bachner (Eds.), *Adults with developmental disabilities: Current approaches in occupational therapy* (pp. 263–306). Bethesda, MD: American Occupational Therapy Association.

Bachner, S. (2004). Lets do lunch: A comprehensive nonstandardized assessment tool. In M. Ross & S. Bachner (Eds.), *Adults with developmental disabilities: Current approaches in occupational therapy* (rev. ed., pp. 166–205). Bethesda, MD: AOTA Press.

Balboa, K. T. (2000). Independent living strategies for adults with developmental disabilities. In C. Christiansen (Ed.), *Ways of living* (2nd ed., pp. 123–140). Rockville, MD: American Occupational Therapy Association.

Baranek, G. T., Chin, Y. H., Hess, L. M., Yankee, J. G., Hatton, D. D., & Hooper, S. R. (2002). Sensory processing correlates of occupational performance in children with Fragile X syndrome: Preliminary findings. *American Journal of Occupational Therapy, 56,* 538–546.

Bass Haugen, J. B., & Mathiowetz, V. (1995). Contemporary task-oriented approach. In C. A. Trombly (Ed.), *Occupational therapy for physical dysfunction* (4th ed., pp. 510–527). Baltimore: Williams & Wilkins.

Baum, C. M., & Christiansen, C. H. (2005). Person–environment–occupation–performance: An occupation-based framework for practice. In C. H. Christiansen, C. M. Baum, & J. Bass-Haugen (Eds.), *Occupational therapy: Performance participation and well-being* (3rd ed., pp. 242–266). Thorofare, NJ: Slack.

Berger, K. (2008). *The developing person through the life span* (7th ed.). New York: Worth.

Bhattacharyya, J. (2004). Theorizing community development. *Journal of Community Development Society, 34,* 5–35.

Bolick, T. (2001). *Asperger syndrome and adolescence: Helping preteens and teens get ready for the real world.* Gloucester, MA: Fair Winds Press.

Brannon, L., & Feist, J. (2000). *Health psychology: An introduction to behavior and health.* Stamford, CT: Wadsworth.

Brei, T. (1999). The adult with spina bifida. In M. Lutkenhoff (Ed.), *Children with spina bifida: A parent's guide* (pp. 313–328). Bethesda, MD: Woodbine House.

Brewin, B. J., Renwick, R., & Shormans, A. F. (2008). Parental perspectives of the quality of life in school environments for children with Asperger syndrome. *Focus on Autism and Other Developmental Disabilities, 23,* 242–252.

Brown, C., & Dunn, W. (2002). *Adolescent/Adult Sensory Profile user's manual.* San Antonio, TX: Psychological Corporation.

Brown, I., Raphael, D., & Renwick, R. (1999). *Quality of life and life changes for adults with developmental disabilities in Ontario.* Toronto, Ontario: Centre for Health Promotion.

Bruce, M. A., & Borg, B. (2002). *Psychosocial frames of reference: Core for occupation-based practice.* Thorofare, NJ: Slack.

Bruininks, R. H., Woodcock, R. W., Weatherman, R. F., & Hill, B. K. (1996). *SIB–R: Scales of Independent Behavior–Revised.* Itasca, IL: Riverside.

Bundy, A. C. Lane, S. J., & Murray, E. A. (2002), *Sensory integration: Theory and practice.* Philadelphia: F. A. Davis.

Buning, M. E. (2009). Assistive technology and wheeled mobility. In E. B. Crepeau, E. S. Cohn, & B. A. Schell (Eds.), *Willard and Spackman's occupational therapy* (11th ed., pp. 850–867). Philadelphia: Wolters Kluwer Health/Lippincott Williams & Wilkins.

Buning, M. E., Angelo, J. A., & Schmeler, M. R. (2001). Occupational performance and the transition to powered mobility: A pilot study. *American Journal of Occupational Therapy, 55,* 339–344.

Burns, T. (1992). Cognitive Performance Test. In C. K. Allen, C. A. Earhart, & T. Blue (Eds.), *Occupational therapy treatment goals for the physically and cognitively disabled* (pp. 46–50). Bethesda, MD: American Occupational Therapy Association.

Canadian Association of Occupational Therapists. (1997). *Enabling occupation: An occupational therapy perspective.* Ottawa, Ontario: CAOT Publications.

Christiansen, C., Backman, C., Little, B. R., & Nguyen, A. (1999). Occupations and subjective well-being: A study of personal projects. *American Journal of Occupational Therapy, 53,* 91–100.

Christiansen, C., & Baum, C. (1997). Person–environment–occupational performance: A conceptual model for practice. In C. Christiansen & C. Baum (Eds.), *Occupational therapy: Enabling function and*

well-being (2nd ed., pp. 47–70). Thorofare, NJ: Slack.

Christiansen, C. H., & Townsend, E. A. (2010). An introduction to occupation. In C. H. Christiansen & E. A. Townsend (Eds.), *Intoroduction to occupation: The art and science of living* (2nd ed., pp. 1–34). Boston: Pearson.

Cohn, E. S. (2001). From waiting to relating: Parents' experiences in the waiting room of an occupational therapy clinic. *American Journal of Occupational Therapy, 55,* 167–174.

Cohn, E. S., Miller, L. J., & Tickle-Degnen, L. (2000). Parental hopes for therapy outcomes: Children with sensory modulation disorders. *American Journal of Occupational Therapy, 54,* 36–43.

Cook, A. M., & Hussey, S. M. (2002). *Assistive technologies: Principles and practice* (2nd ed.). St. Louis, MO: Mosby.

Cooper, S. A., Morrison, J., Melville, C., Finlayson, J., Allan, L., Martin, G., et al. (2006). Improving the health of people with intellectual disabilities: Outcomes of a health screening programme after one year. *Journal of Intellectual Disability Research, 50,* 667–677.

Cooper-Brown, L., Copeland, S., Dailey, S., Downey, D., Petersen, M. C., Stimson, C., et al. (2008). Feeding and swallowing dysfunction in genetic syndromes. *Developmental Disabilities Research Reviews, 14,* 147–157.

de las Heras, C. G., Geist, R., Kielhofner, G., & Li, Y. (2003). *The Volitional Questionnairie (VQ)* (Version 4.0). Chicago: Model of Human Occupational Clearinghouse, Department of Occupational Therapy, College of Applied Health Sciences, University of Illinois.

Developmental Disabilities Assistance and Bill of Rights Act of 2000, P. L. 106–402, Stat. 1677.

Dolyniuk, A., Kamens, M. W., Corman, H., Dinardo, P. O., Totaro, R. M., & Rockoff, J. C. (2002). Students with developmental disabilities go to college: Description of a collaborative transition project on a regular college campus. *Focus on Autism and Other Developmental Disabilities, 17,* 236–239.

Dowrick, M. K. (2004). Learning outcomes for students of school learning age in special schools: A preliminary study of stakeholder's perceptions. *Journal of Intellectual and Developmental Disability, 29,* 293–305.

Dunn, W. (1998). Person-centered and contextually relevant evaluation. In J. Hinojosa & P. Kramer (Eds.), *Evaluation: Obtaining and interpreting data* (pp. 47–76). Rockville, MD: American Occupational Therapy Association.

Dunn, W., Brown, C., & McGuigan, A. (1994). The ecology of human performance: A framework for considering the effect of context. *American Journal of Occupational Therapy, 48,* 595–607.

Dunn, W., Miles, S. M., & Orr, S. (2002). Sensory processing issues associated with Asperger's syndrome: A preliminary investigation. *American Journal of Occupational Therapy, 56,* 97–102.

Earhart, C. A. (1992). Analysis of Activities. In C. K. Allen, C. A. Earhart, & T. Blue (Eds.), *Occupational therapy treatment goals for the physically and cognitively disabled* (pp. 125–305). Bethesda, MD: American Occupational Therapy Association.

Fanchiang, S. C. (1996). The other side of the coin: Growing up with a learning disability. *American Journal of Occupational Therapy, 50,* 277–285.

Fearing, V. G., Law, M., & Clark, J. (1997). An occupational performance process model: Fostering client and therapist alliances. *Canadian Journal of Occupational Therapy, 64,* 7–15.

Fertel-Daly, D., Bedell, G., & Hinojosa, J. (2001). Effects of a weighted vest on attention to task and self-stimulatory behaviors in preschoolers with pervasive developmental disorders. *American Journal of Occupational Therapy, 55,* 629–640.

Fisher, A. G. (2006). *Assessment of Motor and Process Skills: Volume 1: Development standardization and administration manual* (6th ed.). Fort Collins, CO: Three Star Press.

Flinn, N. A., Jackson, J., Gray, J. M., & Zemke, R. (2008). Optimizing abilities and capacities: Range of motion, strength, and endurance. In M. V. Radomski & C. A. Latham (Eds.), *Occupational therapy for physical dysfunction* (6th ed., pp. 573–597). Philadelphia: Lippincott Williams & Wilkins.

Forsyth, K., Deshpande, S., Kielhofner, G., Henriksson, C., Haglund, L., Olson, L., et al. (2005). The *Occupational Circumstances Assessment Interview and Rating Scale (OCAIRS)* (Version 4.0). Chicago: Model of Human Occupation Clearing House.

Foxx, R. M., & Azrin, N. H. (1973). *Toilet training the retarded: A rapid program for day and nighttime independent toileting.* Champaign, IL: Research Press.

Gillam, J. E. (1994). *Work Adjustment Inventory: Measures of job-related temperament (WAI).* Austin, TX: Pro-Ed.

Gillen, G. (2002). Improving mobility and community access in an adult with ataxia. *American Journal of Occupational Therapy, 56,* 462–466.

Greene, S. (2001). Social skills intervention for children with autism and Asperger's disorder. In H. Miller-Kuhaneck (Ed.), *Autism: A comprehensive occupational therapy approach* (pp. 153–171). Rockville, MD: American Occupational Therapy Association.

Guide for the Uniform Data Set for Medical Rehabilitation. (1999). *FIM™, Version 5: Australia.* Buffalo, NY: University at Buffalo.

Hadas-Lidor, N., & Weiss, P. (2005). Dynamic cognitive intervention. In N. Katz (Ed.), *Cognition and occupation across the lifespan: Models for intervention in occupational therapy* (2nd ed., pp. 391–412). Rockville, MD: AOTA Press.

Hale, S. (2000). Naming strengths and resources of the client and therapist. In V. G. Fearing & J. Clark (Eds.), *Individuals in context* (pp. 69–78). Thorofare, NJ: Slack.

Hanschu, B. (1998). Using a sensory approach to serve adults who have developmental disabilities. In M. Ross & S. Bachner (Eds.), *Adults with developmental disabilities: Current approaches in occupational therapy* (pp. 165–211). Rockville, MD: American Occupational Therapy Association.

Hanschu, B. (2004). Using a sensory approach for adults with developmental disabilities. In M. Ross & S.

Bachner (Eds.), *Adults with developmental disabilities: Current approaches in occupational therapy* (rev. ed., pp. 71–113). Bethesda, MD: AOTA Press.

Harden, B. (2001). Assistive technology for students with autism. In H. Miller-Kuhaneck (Ed.), *Autism: A comprehensive occupational therapy approach* (pp. 201–223). Rockville, MD: American Occupational Therapy Association.

Harjamaki, K. (2000). *Assessing cognitive abilities of adults with developmental disabilities: A survey of current practice.* Unpublished master's thesis, College of St. Catherine, St. Paul, MN.

Haynes, R. B., McKibbon, K. A., & Kanani, R. (1996). Systematic review of randomized trials of interventions to assist patients to follow prescriptions for medications. *Lancet, 348,* 383–386.

Hirama, H. (1989). *Self-injurious behavior: A somatosensory treatment approach.* Baltimore: Chess.

Holburn, S., Cea, C. D., Coull, L., & Goode, D. (2008). What is working and not working: Using focus groups to address quality of life for people living in group homes. *Journal of Developmental and Physical Disabilities, 20,* 1–9.

Humphry, R., & Thigpen-Beck, B. (1998). Parenting values and attitudes: View of therapists and parents. *American Journal of Occupational Therapy, 52,* 835–842.

Institute on Community Integration. (2008). *About developmental disabilities.* Retrieved May 2, 2008, from http://ici.umn.edu/relatedresources/definition.html

Jacobs, K. (1991). *Occupational therapy: Work-related programs and assessment* (2nd ed.) Boston: Little, Brown.

James, A. B. (2008). Restoring the role of independent person. In. M. V. Radomski & C. A. Latham (Eds.), *Occupational therapy for physical dysfunction* (6th ed., pp. 774–816). Philadelphia: Lippincott Williams & Wilkins.

Jan, J. E., Owens, J. A., Weiss, M. D., Johnson, K. P., Wasdall, M. B., Freeman, R. D., et al. (2008). Sleep hygiene for children with neurodevelopmental disabilities. *Pediatrics, 122,* 1343–1350.

Katz, S., Downs, T. D., Cash, H. R., & Grotz, R. C. (1970). Progress in development of index of ADL. *Gerontologist, 10,* 20–30.

Katz, S., Ford, A. B., Moskowitz, M., Jackson, B. A., & Jaffe, M. W. (1963). Studies of illness in the aged. The index of ADL: A standardized measure of biological and psychosocial function. *Journal of the American Medical Association, 185,* 914–919.

Kellogg, H. A. (1998). An OTR's description of the legacy, current environment, and clinical issues characterizing adults with profound disabilities. In M. Ross & S. Bachner (Eds.), *Adults with developmental disabilities: Current approaches in occupational therapy* (pp. 90–122). Rockville, MD: American Occupational Therapy Association.

Kielhofner, G. (1995). *A Model of Human Occupation: Theory and application* (2nd ed.). Baltimore: Lippincott Williams & Wilkins.

Kielhofner, G. (2004). *Conceptual foundations of occupational therapy* (3rd ed.). Philadelphia: F. A. Davis.

Kielhofner, G. (2008). *A Model of Human Occupation: Theory and application* (4th ed.). Baltimore: Lippincott Williams & Wilkins.

Kielhofner, G., Mallinson, T., Crawford, C., Nowak, M., Rigby, M., Henry, A., et al. (2004). *Occupational Performance History Interview–II (OPHI–II)* (version 2.1). Chicago: Model of Human Occupation Clearinghouse, University of Illinois at Chicago.

Kinnealey, M., Oliver, B., & Wilbarger, P. (1995). A phenomenological study of sensory defensiveness in adults. *American Journal of Occupational Therapy, 49,* 444–451.

Kipping, P., Ross-Swain, D., & Yee, P. (2003). *Swallowing Ability and Function Evaluation (SAFE).* Austin, TX: Pro-Ed.

Kirkpatrick, K. (2008). Working with parents with a learning disability. *Learning Disability Today, 8,* 8–11.

Klein, R. M., & Bell, B. (1982). Self-care skills: Behavioral measurement with Klein–Bell ADL Scale. *Archives of Physicial Medicine and Rehabilitation, 63,* 335–338.

Latham, C. A. (2008). Occupation as therapy: Selection, gradation, analysis, and adaptation. In M. V. Radomski & C. A. Latham (Eds.), *Occupational therapy for physical dysfunction* (6th ed., pp. 358–381). Philadelphia: Lippincott Williams & Wilkins.

Law, M., Baptiste, S., Carswell, A., McColl, M. A., Polatajko, H., & Pollock, N. (2005). *Canadian occupational performance measure* (4th ed.). Ottawa, Ontario: Canadian Association of Occupational Therapists.

Levy, L. L., & Burns, T. (2005). Cognitive disabilities reconsidered: Rehabilitation of older adults with dementia. In N. Katz (Ed.), *Cognition and occupation across the life span* (2nd ed., pp. 347–388). Bethesda, MD: AOTA Press.

Loeb, P. A. (1996). *Independent Living Scales (ILS).* San Antonio, TX: Psychological Corporation.

Malgady, R. G., & Barcher, P. R. (1982). The vocational adaptation rating scales. *Applied Research in Mental Retardation, 3*(4), 335–344.

Malone, D. M., McKinsey, P. D., Thyer, B. A., & Straka, E. (2000). Social work early intervention for young children with developmental disabilities. *Health and Social Work, 25,* 169–180.

Mann, W. C., & Beaver, K. A. (1995). Assessment services: Person, device, family, and environment. In W. C. Mann & J. P. Lane (Eds.), *Assistive technology for people with disabilities* (2nd ed., pp. 219–317). Rockville, MD: American Occupational Therapy Association.

Mason, D. B., Santoro, K., & Kaull, A. (1999). Bowel management. In M. Lutkenhoff (Ed.), *Children with spina bifida: A parent's guide* (pp. 87–105). Bethesda, MD: Woodbine House.

Mathiowetz, V., & Bass Haugen, J. (1994). Motor behavior research: Implications for therapeutic approaches to central nervous system dysfunction. *American Journal of Occupational Therapy, 48,* 733–745.

Miller, F., & Bachrach, S. J. (1995). *Cerebral palsy: A complete guide for caregiving.* Baltimore: Johns Hopkins University Press.

Moor, D. Y. (2000). Daily care. In J. D. Weber (Ed.), *Children with Fragile X syndrome: A parent's guide.* (pp. 121–154). Bethesda, MD: Woodbine House.

Mulcahey, M. A. (1999). Nurturing an emotionally healthy child. In M. Lutkenhoff (Ed.), *Children with spina bifida: A parent's guide* (pp. 257–271). Bethesda, MD: Woodbine House.

National Institute on Clinical Education. (2007). *Faecal incontinence: The management of faecal incontinence in adults.* London: Author.

Neistadt, M. E. (1990). A critical analysis of occupational therapy approaches for perceptual deficits for adults with brain injury. *American Journal of Occupational Therapy, 44,* 299–304.

Nihira, K., Leland, H., & Lambert, N. (1993). *AAMR Adaptive Behavior Scale–Residential and Community* (2nd ed.). Austin, TX: Pro-Ed.

Oetter, P., Laurel, M., & Cool, S. (1991). Sensory motor foundations of communication. In C. B. Royeen (Ed.), *Neuroscience foundations of human performance.* Rockville, MD: American Occupational Therapy Association.

Oetter, P., Richter, E., & Frick, S. (1993). *M.O.R.E. integrating the mouth with sensory and postural functions* (2nd ed.). Hugo, MN: PDP Publications.

Parham, D., Cohn, E. S., Spitzer, S., Koomar, J. A., Miller, L. J., & Burke, J. P. (2007). Fidelity in sensory integration intervention research. *American Journal of Occupational Therapy, 61,* 216–227.

Petersen, M. C., & Rogers, B. T. (2008). Introduction: Feeding and swallowing and developmental disabilities. *Developmental Disabilities Research Reviews, 14,* 75–76.

Pfeiffer, B., Kinnealey, M., Reed, C., & Herzberg, G. (2005). Sensory modulation and affective disorders in children and adolescents with Asperger's disorder. *American Journal of Occupational Therapy, 59,* 335–345.

Pierce, D. E. (2003). *Occupation by design: Building therapeutic power.* Philadelphia: F. A. Davis.

Pierce, S. L. (2008). *Restoring mobility.* In M. V. Radomski & C. A. Latham (Eds.), *Occupational therapy for physical dysfunction* (6th ed., pp. 817–853). Philadelphia: Lippincott Williams & Wilkins.

Portwood, M. (1996). *Developmental dyspraxia: A practice manual for parents and professionals* (2nd ed.). Durham, England: Educational Psychology Service.

Rees, J., & Sharpe, A. (2009). The use of bowel management systems in the high-dependency setting. *British Journal of Nursing* (Continence Suppl.), *18,* S19–S24.

Reisman, J. E., & Hanschu, B. (1992). *Sensory Integration Inventory–Revised for individuals with developmental disabilities.* Hugo, MN: PDP Press.

Renwick, R. (2004). Quality of life: A guiding framework for practice with adults with developmental disabilities. In M. R. Ross & S. Bachner (Eds.), *Adults with developmental disabilities: Current approaches in occupational therapy* (rev. ed., pp. 20–38). Bethesda, MD: AOTA Press.

Rogers, J. C., & Holm, M. B. (1989). The therapist's thinking behind functional assessment I. In *AOTA Self-Study Series: Assessing function.* Rockville, MD: American Occupational Therapy Association.

Rogers, J. C., & Holm, M. B. (1994). *Performance Assessment of Self-Care Skills (PASS)* (Version 3.1). Unpublished manuscript, University of Pittsburgh at Pittsburgh.

Salkever, D. S. (2000). Activity status, life satisfaction, and perceived productivity for young adults with developmental disabilities. *The Free Library*, Retrieved September 9, 2003, from http://www.the freelibrary.com

Schalock, R. L. (2005). Guest Editorial—Introduction and overview. *Journal of Intellectual Disability Research, 49,* 695–698.

Siporin, S., & Lysack, C. (2004). Quality of life and supported employment: A case study of three women with developmental disabilities. *American Journal of Occupational Therapy, 58,* 455–465.

Smith, S. A., Press, B., Koenig, K. P., & Kinnealey, M. (2005). Effects of sensory integration intervention on self-stimulating and self-injurious behaviors. *American Journal of Occupational Thearapy, 59,* 418–425.

Social Care Institute for Excellence. (2007). *The adult services resource guide 9: Working together to support disabled parents.* London: Social Care Institute for Excellence.

Sonander, K. (2000). Early identification of children with developmental disabilities. *Acta Paediatrica, 89,* 17–23.

Sparrow, S. S., Bella, D., & Cicchetti, D. V. (1984), *Vineland Adaptive Behavior Scales.* Circle Pines, MN: American Guidance Service.

Spencer, K. C., & Sample, P. L. (1993). Transition planning services. In C. B. Royeen (Ed.), *AOTA self-study series: Classroom applications for school based practice* (Lesson 10). Rockville, MD: American Occupational Therapy Association.

Spitzer, S., & Roley, S. S. (2001). Sensory integration revisited: A philosophy of practice. In S. S. Roley, E. I. Blache, & R. C. Schaaf (Eds.), *Sensory integration with diverse populations* (pp. 3–27). San Antonio, TX: Therapy Skill Builders.

Stancliff, B. L. (1998). Play with a purpose: Sensory integration treatment and developmental disabilities. *OT Practice, 3,* 34–40.

Stokes, M. A., & Kaur, A. (2005). High-functioning autism and sexuality: A parental perspective. *Autism, 9,* 266–289.

Stratton, M. (1981). Reliability of the behavioral assessment scale of oral functions in feeding. *American Journal of Occupational Therapy, 39,* 436–440.

Stratton, M. (1989). Clinical management of dysphagia in the developmentally disabled adult. In J. A. Johnson & D. A. Ethridge (Eds.), *Developmental disabilities: A handbook for occupational therapists.* New York: Haworth Press.

Sullivan, A., & Caterino, L. C. (2008). Addressing the sexuality and sex education of people individuals with autism spectrum disorders. *Education and Treatment of Children, 31,* 381–394.

Sullivan, W. F., Heng, J., Cameron, D., Lunsky, Y., Cheetham, T., Hennen, B., et al. (2006). Consensus guidelines for primary health care of adults with developmental disabilities. *Canadian Family Physician, 52,* 1410–1418.

Taylor, S. (1999). *Health psychology* (4th ed.). Boston: McGraw Hill.

Thomson, J., Bryant, B., Campbell, E., Craig, E., & Hughes, C. (2004). *Supports Intensity Scale manual.* Washington, DC: American Association on Intellectual and Developmental Disabilities.

Toglia, J. P. (1991). Generalization of treatment: A multi-context approach to cognitive perceptual impairments in adults with brain injury. *American Journal of Occupational Therapy, 45,* 505–516.

Toglia, J. P. (1998). A dyanamic interactional model to cognitive rehabilitation. In N. Katz (Ed.), *Cognition and occupation in rehabilitation: Cognitive models for intervention in occupational therapy* (pp. 51–123). Rockville, MD: American Occupational Therapy Association.

Toglia, J. P. (2005). A dynamic interactional model to cognitive rehabilitation. In N. Katz (Ed.), *Cognition and occupation across the life span* (2nd ed., pp. 29–72). Bethesda, MD: AOTA Press.

Toglia, J. P., Golisz, K. M., & Goverover, Y. (2009). Evaluation and intervention for cognitive perceptual impairments. In E. B. Crepeau, E. S. Cohn, & B. A. Schell (Eds.), *Willard and Spackman's occupational therapy* (11th ed., pp. 739–776). Philadelphia: Wolters Kluwer Health/Lippincott Williams & Wilkins.

Townsend, E. (Ed.). (2002). *Enabling occupation: An occupational therapy perspective.* Ottawa, Ontario: Canadian Association of Occupational Therapists.

Trefler, E., & Hobson, D. (1997). Assistive technology. In C. Christiansen & C. Baum (Eds.), *Occupational therapy: Enabling function and well-being* (2nd ed., pp. 483–506). Thorofare, NJ: Slack.

Unsworth, C. (1999). *Cognitive and perceptual dysfunction.* Philadelphia: F. A. Davis.

Unsworth, C. (2007). Cognitive and perceptual dysfunction. In S. B. O'Sullivan & T. J. Schmitz (Eds.), *Physical rehabilitation* (5th ed., pp. 1151–1188). Philadelphia: F. A. Davis.

VandenBerg, N. L. (2001). The use of a weighted vest to increase on-task behavior in children with attention difficulties. *American Journal of Occupational Therapy, 55,* 621–628.

Waltz, M. (2002). *Autistic spectrum disorders: Understanding the diagnosis and getting help* (2nd ed.). Sebastopol, CA: O'Reilly.

Watling, R. (2004). Behavioral and educational intervention approaches for the child with an autism spectrum disorder. In H. Miller-Kuhaneck (Ed.), *Autism: A comprehensive occupational therapy approach* (2nd ed., pp. 245–271). Bethesda, MD: AOTA Press.

Weiss, L. (1997). *Attention deficit disorder in adults: Practical help and understanding.* Dallas, TX: Taylor.

Wilbarger, P. (1995). The sensory diet: Activity programs based on sensory processing theory. *Sensory Integration Special Interest Section Newsletter.*

Wilbarger, P., & Willbarger, J. (1991). *Sensory defensiveness in children aged 2–12.* Santa Barbara, CA: Avanti Educational Publications.

Williams, M. S., & Shellenberger, S. (1994). *How does your engine run? Leader's guide to the ALERT program for self-regulations.* Albuquerque, NM: Therapy Works.

Wituk, S., Pearson, R., Bomhoff, K., Hinde, M., & Meissn, G. (2007). A participatory process involving people with developmental disabilities in com-

munity involvement. *Journal of Developmental and Physical Disabilities, 19,* 323–335.

World Health Organization. (2001). *International classification of functioning, disability and health.* Geneva: Author.

Appendix 7.A. Performance Inventories

Performance Inventory
Performance Domain: Domestic/Home

School: _____   Student: _____

Age: _____   Date: _____

Directions: Address the following areas through interviews with the student, family members, or others as appropriate, or through student observation.

Goal Area	Activity	Current Level of Functioning
Eating and food preparation	1. Meal planning	
Interview with parents and school cafeteria staff	2. Preparing meals and snacks • gathers ingredients and equipment • opens containers (e.g., soda cans, milk cartons, cereal box) • follows recipes • uses microwave • uses stove top • uses oven • users other appliances	
Observation of student's home kitchen layout	3. Eating a meal/snack • oral–motor skills (e.g., swallowing, chewing) • uses utensils • uses manners	
	4. Preparing eating area • sets table • gets condiments	

	5. Cleaning up after meal
	• puts away leftovers
	• wipes off work surface
	• washes dishes
	  – handwashing
	  – using dishwasher	

	6. Accessibility to kitchen • uses adaptive equipment	
Priorities		
Grooming and dressing	1. Grooming • brushes teeth • uses mouthwash • brushes/combs hair • styles hair • skin care • maintains appearance	
Interview with parents/ caregivers and student	2. Dressing/undressing • undresses self • chooses appropriate clothes • dresses self • dresses appropriate for season/weather conditions	
Priorities		
Hygiene and toileting Interview with parents, caregivers, and student	1. Using private and public toilets • wipes self • flushes toilet • washes hands 2. Washing hands and face 3. Bathing/showering 4. Shampooing/rinsing hair 5. Shaving (for men) 6. Using deodorant	
Priorities		

Domestic/Home Domain (cont.)

Goal Area	Activity	Current Level of Functioning
Houshold maintenance	1. Keeping room neat • makes bed • changes bed linens • straightens room	
Interview with parents/ caregivers	2. Handling household chores • does laundry • vacuums/dusts • cleans bathroom • sweeps	
	3. Maintaining outdoors • rakes leaves • mows lawn • weeds • waters lawn • cleans up after animals	
Priorities		
Social skills	1. Telephone use • telephone etiquette • takes message • dials telephone • can use telephone for emergency • can use assistive devices if necessary • can use telephone directory	
Interview with parents/ caregivers	2. Caring for others • pet care • sibling care • babysitting • care of elderly	
	3. Reciprocal relationships • gift giving • remembers birthdays • sends thank you cards	
Priorities		
Sexuality/health/safety Hygiene and toileting	1. Awareness of public versus private sexual activities • closes door for bathing, toileting, dressing, etc. • chooses appropriate place to masturbate	
Interview with parents/ caregivers	2. Appropriate show of affection	
	3. Awareness of bodily and sexual functions	
	4. Knowledge and use of birth control methods	
	5. Knowledge of sexually transmitted diseases	
	6. Knowledge of general health concerns • disease transmission (e.g., covers mouth when sneezing, coughing; controls drooling; blows nose) • health concerns specific to disability (e.g., skin care, range of motion, positioning of weight) • takes medication (e.g., knows medication schedule, ability to swallow, related behavioral concerns) • cares for minor injury	
	7. Awareness of home hazards and emergency procedures • poisons • fire • accidents	
Priorities		

Performance Inventory
Performance Domain: General Community

School: _____   Student: _____

Age: _____   Date: _____

Directions: Address the following areas through interviews with the student, family members, or others as appropriate, or through student observation.

Goal Area	Activity	Current Level of Functioning
Travel	1. "Walking" (wheeling) to and from destination • safety when crossing streets • arrives at destination	
	2. Riding bicycle • knows safety rules • able to find way • locks bicycle	
	3. Riding school bus/city bus • demonstrates appropriate behavior when on bus • communicates with bus driver • can find appropriate bus • can read bus map • can make a transfer • knows how to pay an appropriate amount • shows bus pass	
	4. Driving own vehicle • knows laws • demonstrates safe and defensive technique • can physically handle task • uses appropriate adaptive equipment • uses seat belts	
	5. Orienting skills • identifies signs • carries identification • asks for help • responsible for possessions • uses caution with strangers • reads maps	
Priorities		
General shopping	1. Handling money/budgeting • makes shopping lists • recognizes budget constraints • handles money exchanges	
	2. Locating/getting items • pushes cart • uses store directory • asks for help • follows list • makes choices • does cost comparisons	
	3. Clothes/personal items • plans for trip • selects appropriate store • selects items within budget • makes wise choices • handles money exchanges	
Priorities		
Restaurant	1. Reading menu (or alternative) 2. Communicating to wait person 3. Using manners 4. Locating restrooms 5. Totaling bill (including tip) 6. Handling money exchanges	
Priorities		

General Community Domain (cont.)

Goal Area	Activity	Current Level of Functioning
Using services	1. Using pay telephone 2. Using relay system (if hearing impaired) 3. Using beauty parlor 4. Making appointments 5. Using banking services 6. Using/communicates with dentist, doctor, etc. 7. Using laundromat/drycleaner	
Priorities:		

Note. From "Transition Planning Services," by K. C. Spencer and P. L. Sample, 1993, in C. B. Royeen (Ed.), *AOTA Self-Study Series: Classroom Applications for School-Based Practice* (Lesson 10), Rockville, MD: American Occupational Therapy Association. Copyright © 1993 by the American Occupational Therapy Association. Reprinted with permission.

Appendix 7.B. "Let's Do Lunch" Assessment Tool
Task Analysis: Eating in the Lodge

Resident: _____*Helen*_____ Therapist: ___*S. Bachner, OTR/L*___ Date: _____*11/13/96*_____

Scoring Codes:
S = Sensory = tactile, proprioceptive, vestibular, visual, auditory, gustatory, olfactory
P = Perceptual = stereognosis, pain response, body scheme, visual perceptual, visual acuity
N = Neuromuscular = reflex, ROM, muscle tone, endurance, postural control
M = Motor = gross coordination, crosses midline, laterality, praxis, oral motor control
C = Cognitive Integration = level of arousal, attention span, initiation, problem solving
P = Psychosocial = social conduct, self-expression, self-management

TASK 0 = independent, 1 = verbal cue, 2 = physical assist, 3 = total assist		S	P	N	M	C	P
1. Enters Dining Room	0 1 ②3	✔	✔				
2. Locates End of Line	0 1 2 ③	✔	✔				
3. Stands on Line	⓪1 2 3						
4. Collects a Tray	0 1 2 ③		✔			✔	
5. Puts Tray on Counter	0 1 2 ③		✔			✔	
6. Faces Correct Direction	0 1 2 ③						
7. Moves "Forward"	0 ①2 3						
8. Balances on Two Feet	⓪1 2 3						
9. Sees Food Items	0 1 2 ③		✔				
10. Reaches for Food Items	0 1 2 ③		✔			✔	
11. Inhibits Impulse to Take All Food	⓪1 2 3						
12. Makes Food Choice Decisions *N.A.*	0 1 2 ③					✔	
13. Holds Loaded Tray With Two Hands	0 1 2 ③					✔	
14. Navigates Turn Off of Line to Seating Area	0 1 2 ③		✔			✔	
15. Ambulates Efficiently With Tray and Contents	0 1 2 ③	✔	✔				
16. Visually Scans Room *Only responds to stimuli in central visual field*	0 1 2 ③		✔				
17. Visually Targets an Available Seat *Guided to table c̄ available seat*	0 1 ②3						
18. Visually Targets an Available Seat With Friends *Stands beside chair per escort #17*	0 1 ②3						
19. Gets to a Targeted Seat	0 1 ②3						
20. Puts Tray on Table	0 1 2 ③						
21. Pulls Chair Out *Refuses*	0 1 2 3						
22. Sits Down and Positions Legs Under the Table *Refuses to sit*	0 1 2 3						
23. Achieves Good Upper Body Posture in Seat *N.A.*	0 1 2 3						
24. Achieves Good Lower Body Posture in Seat *Wants to eat while standing*	0 1 2 3						
25. Aligns Self With Tray at Midline *Continues to resist sitting in chair*	0 1 2 3						
26. Acknowledges Peers at Table (or Nearby) *Smiles at peers if in her central vision (20"–30" central)*	0 1 2 3		✔				

Appendix 7.B. "Let's Do Lunch" Assessment Tool
Task Analysis: Eating in the Lodge *(cont.)*

	Score	S	P	N	M	C	P
27. Visually Attends to Tray/Contents *Moves visual target to 4" from eyes*	0 1 2 ③						
28. Reaches for Utensils (Wrapped in Napkin)	0 1 2 ③						
29. Uses Two Hands to Unwrap Utensils *If given to her*	⓪ 1 2 3						
30. Places Napkins in Lap *Still standing—N.A.*	0 1 2 3						
31. Uses Bilateral Hand Movements to Open Packets *Fine-motor O.K.—Doesn't coordinate c̄ eyes*	0 1 ② 3						
32. Seasons Food With Salt and Pepper *N.A.*	0 1 2 3						
33. Holds Knife by the Handle *Only uses spoon*	⓪ 1 2 3						
34. Spreads Butter With Knife *N.A.*	0 1 2 3						
35. Cuts Food With Knife *N.A.*	0 1 2 3						
36. Grasps Eating Utensils With Functional Grip (R or L) *Only briefly—prefers to use fingers*	⓪ 1 2 3						
37. Visually Targets Desired Food Items *Seems to need high contrast, central 20"–30", 4" from eyes*	0 1 2 3						
38. Initiates Movement of Utensils Toward Food Item *Prefers fingers for food exploration*	⓪ 1 2 3						
39. Loads Spoon/Pieces With Fork *Can use spoon but likes fingers*	⓪ 1 2 3						
40. Contains Food Items on Plate/Bowl *Given hi-sided plate to assist c̄ containment— did better*	0 1 ② 3		✔				
41. Brings Food to Mouth With Utensil *Holds bowl at 4" from face c̄ Ⓛ hand*	⓪ 1 2 3		✔				
42. Closes Lips to Contain Food in Mouth	⓪ 1 2 3						
43. Chews Bolus With Teeth *Needs mechanical-soft/ground meat for safety*	0 1 2 3						
44. Swallows Bolus	⓪ 1 2 3						
45. Safe Chewing and Swallowing—*Not when eating regular diet (consistency)*	0 1 2 3						
46. Wipes Mouth as Needed	⓪ 1 2 3					✔	
47. Targets Drinking Glass *Having Trouble Locating it*	0 1 2 ③		✔				
48. Crosses Midline (R/L) With Hands as Needed	⓪ 1 2 3						
49. Reaches/Grasps/Lifts Glass to Mouth *Needs to be placed in her hand*	0 1 2 ③		✔				
50. Drinks Liquid With a Safe Pace and Adequate Swallow *Doesn't tip head back. Why?*	⓪ 1 2 3						
51. Finishes All Food Items on Plate *Required verbal and physical prompts to locate food*	0 1 2 ③		✔				
52. Pushes Chair Back *N.A.*	0 1 2 3						

(Continued)

Appendix 7.B. "Let's Do Lunch" Assessment Tool
Task Analysis: Eating in the Lodge *(cont.)*

		S	P	N	M	C	P
53. Sitting to Standing With Adequate Balance	⓪ 1 2 3						
54. Reaches to Table and Picks up Tray	0 1 2 ③						
55. Re-Aligns Body for Ambulation	⓪ 1 2 3						
56. Carries Tray Without Spilling	0 1 2 ③						
57. Determines Where to Return Tray	0 1 2 ③		✔			✔	
58. Reaches Location for Tray Deposit	0 1 2 ③						
59. Deposits Tray in Return Window	0 1 2 ③						
60. Locates Exit Door From Dining Room	0 1 2 ③						
Summary of Components: Lack of Familiarity			✔				
Needs (Least Functional)						✔	
Strengths (Most Functional)		✔		✔	✔		✔

Item Numbers Identified for TX: _____

COMMENTS: *If bowl remains on tray, client stretches head forward—obvious muscle strain, tension.*
Tension disappeared when bowl lifted 4" from eyes/mouth. Needs eye exam. ••previous socialization to
people ••

Chapter 8

Enabling Performance and Participation for Persons With Rheumatic Diseases

CATHERINE L. BACKMAN, PHD, OT(C), FCAOT

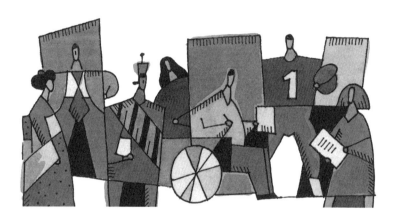

KEY TERMS

ankylosing
  spondylitis (AS)

fibromyalgia (FM)

hand function

joint protection
  and energy
  conservation
  principles

juvenile idiopathic
  arthritis (JIA)

osteoarthritis
  (OA)

osteoporosis (OP)

rheumatoid arthritis (RA)

self-management
  principles

systemic lupus
  erythematosus (SLE)

systemic sclerosis
  (scleroderma, SSc)

HIGHLIGHTS

- Evidence is accumulating to support specific occupational therapy interventions to improve health and functional outcomes for people with arthritis.

- Work disability occurs early and affects one-third of people with inflammatory arthritis (e.g., rheumatoid arthritis, ankylosing spondylitis). Ergonomic modifications and targeted application of joint protection and energy conservation principles may help clients sustain employment.

- Self-management is a cornerstone to living well with chronic illness. Occupational therapists should tailor recommendations to support individuals in engaging in their chosen occupations while concurrently managing their arthritis.

- Rheumatic conditions may lead to participation restrictions that are associated with increased depression and decreased well-being. Strategies to preserve engagement in valued occupations may mediate well-being.

OBJECTIVES

After reading this material, readers will be able to

- Describe the impact of several rheumatic diseases on occupational performance;

- Explain factors to consider when recommending adaptive strategies, equipment, and environmental modifications for individuals with rheumatic diseases;

- Describe adaptive strategies, equipment, and environmental modifications for maintaining, restoring, or improving engagement in occupational areas (ADLs, IADLs, work, school, play, leisure, and social participation);

- Given a case example, apply joint protection and energy conservation principles to specific adaptive strategies to enhance the individual's occupational performance; and

- Summarize principles incorporated in arthritis self-management programs.

The term *rheumatic diseases* refers to over 100 different acute and chronic illnesses affecting the musculoskeletal system of bones, joints, muscles, tendons, and ligaments. Similarly, *arthritis* is a general term (*arthro* = joint, *itis* = inflammation) referring to the predominant characteristic of many rheumatic diseases: joint inflammation.

Rheumatic diseases affect people of all ages, from infancy to old age. While some rheumatic conditions are self-limiting and result in short-term, isolated problems, many are chronic, systemic illnesses resulting in life-long functional limitations of varying degrees. Arthritis disability reduces participation in employment, leisure, and social activities at all ages (Badley & DesMeules, 2003). Because it is common, even practitioners who do not work in arthritis clinics or programs will encounter clients with these conditions.

Occupational therapy is appropriate at any stage of disease activity, whenever clients experience difficulties in occupational performance or present with changes in body function that suggest they are at risk for limitations in occupational performance.

Epidemiology

Rheumatic and musculoskeletal conditions are among the most common chronic conditions and a leading cause of disability in both the United States

(Hannan, 2001) and Canada (Badley & DesMeules, 2003). Population-based studies indicate the prevalence of doctor-diagnosed arthritis is in the range of 15% to 24% (Helmick et al., 2008; Lagace, Perruccio, DesMeules, & Badley, 2003). Overall, about two-thirds of those affected by rheumatic diseases are girls and women. Aboriginal people are disproportionately affected (Lagace et al., 2003). Because many rheumatic diseases are chronic in nature, prevalence increases with age, and arthritis is the most common reason men and women over 65 visit a physician (Hannan, 2001). Put another way, more than 37 million Americans and more than 4 million Canadians have rheumatic disorders. These numbers are expected to increase to close to 60 million and 6 million, respectively, by 2020. Moreover, if arthritis were eradicated, the average life expectancy of the population would increase by almost 1 full year (Manuel, Lagace, DesMeules, Cho, & Power, 2003).

Rheumatic diseases create a tremendous economic burden on individuals and society. In the United States in 2003, direct costs from arthritis health care services amounted to over $80 billion, and indirect costs attributed to lost earnings added a further $47 billion (Yelin et al., 2007). Given that substantial costs are attributed to lost income, interventions that enable people with rheumatic diseases to maintain, improve, or restore their ability to participate in productive activities will decrease this burden. Table 8.1 summarizes pertinent features for some of the more common types of arthritis encountered in occupational therapy practice.

Osteoarthritis

Osteoarthritis (OA) is the most common type of arthritis. Pain from hip or knee OA may prevent individuals from engaging in physical activity, lead to deconditioning, and restrict participation in everyday activities—yet regular physical activity should be encouraged to maintain cartilage health, reduce pain, and maintain function. Over time, degenerative changes to cartilage and bone may progress to severe or "end-stage" joint disease, treated with reconstructive surgery. For example, hip and knee joint *arthroplasties* (total joint replacements) are a common and successful intervention to alleviate pain and restore function. Other surgical procedures include joint resurfacing, osteotomies, and joint fusions. Occupational therapy is indicated in pre- and postoperative management of OA when joint pain and limited mobility hamper ADLs or threaten participation in IADLs, work, and leisure. Typical preoperative therapy includes instruction in self-care

(Text continues on p. 218)

Table 8.1. Types of Rheumatic Conditions Commonly Encountered in Occupational Therapy Practice

Diagnosis	Approximate Prevalence[1]	Key Features	Risk Factors or Vulnerable Populations
Osteoarthritis (OA)	10%–12% overall In population studies of adults: Hand 27% Hip 27% Knee 13%–37%	• Mainly a disease of the cartilage, precise mechanism unknown • Tends to affect weight-bearing joints (hip, knee, feet, spine) and small joints of the hand (carpometacarpal joint of the thumb, proximal and distal interphalangeal joints of all fingers) • Characterized by joint pain, aching, stiffness, and decreased range of motion • Onset usually after age 45 • Fatigue may also be a concern, especially when pain is persistent	• Female • Older age • Obesity • History of joint trauma (injury, sports, occupations with repetitive joint stress) • African-Americans have higher rates of knee OA
Rheumatoid arthritis (RA)	0.6%–1.0%	• Chronic, systemic, inflammatory disease of unknown cause, characterized by exacerbations and remissions • Disorder of the immune system, with no known cure • Onset in adulthood, from late teens to over 60, with peak age of onset in 30s to 40s • Symmetrical involvement of the synovial joints, especially metacarpophalangeal, wrists, elbows, knees and feet, although any synovial joint may be affected • During exacerbations, joints are swollen and painful due to inflammation of the synovial lining of the joint capsule • Prolonged periods of inflammation lead to pannus formation, thinning cartilage, lax ligaments and capsule, muscle weakness, and instability of the joint • Systemic nature of RA means that other organs such as the heart, eyes, and lungs may be involved	• Female (affects women 3 times more than men) • Family history (people with a first-degree relative with RA are 3–4 times more likely) • Aboriginal peoples (American Indian, Canadian First Nations) have higher rates of RA
Ankylosing spondylitis (AS)	0.5%–1.0%	• Chronic inflammatory condition affecting spine and sacroiliac joints, at the insertion of ligaments to bones; heel spurs are common • May also affect peripheral joints such as the ankle or wrist • Characterized by exacerbations and remissions, and the severity of the disease varies widely • Histocompatibility antigen HLA-B27 is usually positive • Insidious, typically beginning as hip pain (from inflammation of the sacroiliac joint), between 16 and 35 years of age • Bony ankylosis may occur in later disease, severely limiting spinal mobility	• Male (affects men 3 times more than women • Family history • Higher rates among North American Aboriginal peoples, especially Haida and Pima nations

(Continued)

Table 8.1. Types of Rheumatic Conditions Commonly Encountered in Occupational Therapy Practice *(cont.)*

Diagnosis	Approximate Prevalence[1]	Key Features	Risk Factors or Vulnerable Populations
Fibromyalgia (FM)	~3%	• A syndrome of widespread, chronic pain near but not in the joints, usually worse in the neck and shoulder region • Accompanied by reports of sleep disturbance, persistent fatigue • A contested diagnosis of unknown etiology • Diagnostic criteria established by the American College of Rheumatology include a history of widespread pain for more than 3 months' duration and pain on direct pressure applied to at least 11 of 18 specified tender points in the body • Possible biological explanations include disordered central processing of pain stimuli, changes in the neurotransmitter systems of substance P and serotonin, low growth hormone levels, and decreased blood flow in the thalamus and caudate nuclei, which are involved in processing of pain stimuli (Burckhardt, Clark, & Bennett, 1991) • Unlike most rheumatic conditions, there is no joint or tissue damage resulting from FM, and it does not appear to progress over time	• Female (women affected 4–8 times more than men)
Juvenile idiopathic arthritis (JIA)	.04%–.06%	• Like RA, JIA is characterized by exacerbations and remissions of joint pain and inflammation • To be classified as juvenile disease, onset must occur before 16 years of age • 3 types of JIA: polyarticular (30%), pauciarticular (50%), systemic onset (20%) • Polyarticular JIA, at onset, involves 5 or more joints, usually in a symmetrical pattern, similar to adult RA. Fever and anemia may occur; disease course may be severe, resulting in joint damage requiring reconstructive surgery in young adulthood • Pauciarticular JIA presents as arthritis in 1–4 joints, usually asymmetrical, and without systemic features. Knee, ankle, and elbow are commonly affected. An associated risk of uveitis and iritis require regular ophthalmology examinations. • Systemic onset JIA is characterized by daily fever spikes, a classic pink rash, and inflammation in one or more joints. The fever and fatigue associated with systemic onset JIA may prevent children from feeling well enough to participate in school and play. Other organ systems may be involved, including the liver, spleen, heart, and lungs	• Polyarticular affects girls more than boys • Polyarticular—girls more likely to have an early onset (<5 yrs) and boys more likely to experience later onset (ages 10–12) • Systemic onset affects girls and boys equally

Disease	Prevalence	Description	
Lupus (SLE)	0.05%	• Chronic systemic condition, ranging from mild disease characterized by a rash, arthritis, and fatigue to a severe, life-threatening illness involving the kidneys, lungs, heart, and central nervous system • Affects both adults and children • Disease course marked by exacerbations and remissions, with skin rashes, photosensitivity, joint and muscle swelling, and pain • Joint involvement is symmetrical and similar in distribution to RA, but rarely do people with SLE develop severe joint limitations	• Affects women up to 10 times more often than men
Scleroderma (SSc)	0.02%	• Characterized by inflammatory, fibrotic, and degenerative changes of the skin, blood vessels, tendons, skeletal muscle, gastrointestinal tract, heart, and lungs • Skin appears edematous, shiny, feels rigid (it is hard to pinch the skin and subcutaneous tissue) • 2 subtypes: diffuse cutaneous SSc has higher likelihood of pulmonary fibrosis, myopathy, tendon friction rubs, renal crises, and lower survival rates than limited cutaneous SSc • Both types present with Raynaud's phenomenon, joint contractures, and gastrointestinal problems.	• Affects women 5 times more often than men
Osteoporosis (OP)	6% at 50 yrs 50% at >80 yrs	• Low bone mineral density and increased bone fragility leading to increased risk of fractures • Peak bone mass is attained in the third decade of life, is typically higher in men than women, slowly declines with age in both sexes, but there is a rapid decline in women during the first few years after menopause • Because corticosteroids are used to treat other rheumatic conditions (and at higher doses in the past than are used today), OP may be secondary to a primary rheumatic disease diagnosis that initiated the referral to occupational therapy.	• Affects women 4 times more than men • Prevalence highest in Caucasian and Asian women (20%) • Genetic predisposition for low bone mass • Long-term use of nicotine, alcohol, corticosteroids

[1]Estimates summarized from Badley & DesMeules, 2003; Ramsey-Goldman, 2001; Zhang & Jordan, 2008.

activities using alternate methods or assistive devices for the immediate postoperative period, such as walking aids, bathtub transfers, and long-handled sock aids. Occupational therapists may play a role in preventing the development of OA when they help clients minimize repetitive stress to joints at work or in sports, play, and recreational activities.

Rheumatoid Arthritis

Rheumatoid arthritis (RA) is less common than OA but can be much more disabling. Early diagnosis and treatment with disease-modifying antirheumatic drugs (DMARDs) within 3 months of onset helps prevent irreversible joint damage and improves health outcomes (Nell et al., 2004), yet those with limited access to health care or limited understanding of the risks and benefits often do not receive DMARDs this early (Lacaille, Anis, Guh, & Esdaile, 2005). DMARDs include methotrexate and gold (alone or in combination) and biologic response modifiers. Other medications that may be used in RA are nonsteroidal anti-inflammatory drugs (NSAIDs) and corticosteroids, but these act only on symptoms, whereas DMARDs delay disease progression. Some medications are taken orally and others are administered by injection. Being able to manage medications and staying informed and alert to potentially harmful side effects are part of the lifelong self-management of this illness. Hormonal factors are suspected to play a role because RA is more common in women, tends to remit during pregnancy and flare after delivery, and men with RA tend to have low levels of circulating testosterone (Hannan, 2001). There also appears to be a genetic marker predictive of disease severity (Khani-Hanjani et al., 2000).

When the disease is active (known as a *flare* or *exacerbation*), the person with RA may feel unwell, possibly with a fever, and will have acutely inflamed joints, more fatigue, and longer periods of morning stiffness. However, when the disease is well controlled with medications, or during remissions, they may resume many of the activities that were set aside during an exacerbation. These "ups and downs" in ability to perform daily activities can be very frustrating and may influence overall mood and sense of well-being. RA may run a mild course that is easily controlled, or be more severe, with progressive joint destruction, persistent fatigue, and subsequent disability.

For many people, RA leads to a number of functional limitations. Approximately one-third of people with RA will leave employment prematurely (Allaire, Wolfe, Niu, & LaValley, 2008; Lacaille, Sheps, Spinelli, Chalmers, & Esdaile, 2004). RA also limits performance of household work, home maintenance, caregiving, and volunteer work (Backman, Del Fabro Smith, Smith, Montie, & Suto, 2007; Backman, Kennedy, Chalmers, & Singer, 2004) and leisure and social activities (Katz & Yelin, 2001). The loss of valued life activities is strongly associated with psychosocial distress, such as depression (Katz & Yelin, 2001).

Occupational therapy interventions have the potential to minimize the pain and inflammation that restrict participation, as well as enhance function in all aspects of daily living. Most people with RA will have reduced strength and dexterity in the hands and wrists. This may be the cause of their difficulties with occupational performance, so particular attention is given to assessment and treatment of hand function.

Ankylosing Spondylitis

Ankylosing spondylitis (AS) is another type of inflammatory arthritis with exacerbations and remissions. It affects predominantly adults, with only about 5% of cases beginning in adolescence (Hannan, 2001). AS is the most common disease in a group of rheumatic conditions classified as *spondyloarthritides* (Helmick et al., 2008). Psoriatic arthritis and Reiter's syndrome are other spondyloarthritides.

The pain and stiffness associated with AS tend to be worse after a period of rest and improve with gentle physical activity. The limitations often associated with this type of arthritis include difficulty reaching the feet or floor: maintaining an effective posture at work and rest; and doing physically demanding work, home, or leisure activities. Therefore, occupational therapy includes the provision of long-handled assistive devices, advice on postural habits such as daily prone lying to minimize kyphosis, positioning devices such as ergonomic chairs, and problem-solving strategies specific to the client's daily occupations. Therapeutic exercise to maintain strength and mobility, and an erect posture if ankylosis occurs, are a mainstay of treatment.

Fibromyalgia

Fibromyalgia (FM) is a chronic pain syndrome typically affecting women in midlife. They report aches, pains, and tenderness throughout the body but not in the joints. Because of the difficulty diagnosing FM, many people spend considerable time and experience great frustration trying to identify the source of their pain. For some, the diagnosis may be a relief after being given any number of other diagnoses in the past, or worse, told that it was "all in their heads."

Pain and fatigue may limit physical activity, leading to decreased muscle strength and endurance. Clients with FM who are referred for rehabilitation interventions are often deconditioned and may be reluctant to engage in even modest physical activity. However, a cornerstone of managing fibromyalgia is physical activity, carefully graded to match the interests and physical capacity or fitness of the individual. In general, it is best to begin at a level below that which the person feels achievable and build on success. This concept of the "just-right challenge" is common in grading activities in occupational therapy and contributes to maintaining motivation and developing new habits.

Juvenile Idiopathic Arthritis

Juvenile idiopathic arthritis (JIA) is the term used to describe arthritis—inflammation (cellular damage) of the *synovium* (the lining of joints)—with onset before 16 years of age. Previously called *juvenile rheumatoid arthritis*, the name has been changed to reflect the difference between the juvenile (childhood) forms of arthritis and adult forms of arthritis. Although JIA is idiopathic (the cause is not known), it is likely the result of a combination of genetic, infectious, and environmental factors.

The three types of JIA (Cassidy & Petty, 2001; Taylor & Erlandson, 2001) are outlined in Table 8.1. All affect normal growth and development. The inflammation of joints and tendons may affect bone growth, and coping with pain, stiffness, decreased mobility, and fatigue limit participation in some age-appropriate activities. Joint contractures or subluxation are not uncommon and may require splinting, a visible sign of illness. Hospitalizations, outpatient treatments, and medications all have an impact on children's schedules. Where possible, therapy should be playful and integrated into the child's routine with the help of parents and other family members. At school, the occupational therapist may consult with teachers regarding ways to facilitate the child's participation in classroom and extracurricular activities.

Systemic Lupus Erythematosus and Systemic Sclerosis

Two of the main connective tissue diseases that occupational therapists may see are *systemic lupus erythematosus (SLE)* and *systemic sclerosis (SSc,* commonly called *scleroderma*). Lupus, or SLE, is a chronic autoimmune disease that occurs primarily in women during their child-bearing years (Ramsey-Goldman, 2001). Medical management can be quite complex, and it is essential that patients be regularly followed by a rheumatologist. Clients may have multiple medical challenges to address, such as coping with kidney dialysis, as well as common signs and symptoms like rashes, fatigue, and joint pain. People with SLE are photosensitive; therefore, sunblock and protective clothing are required to prevent sunburn and exacerbation of skin rashes, even when the sun does not appear to be intense. As with RA and AS, SLE often leads to work disability and difficulties with household work, parenting, and other valued activities (Katz, Morris, Trupin, Yazdany, & Yelin, 2008).

SSc is colloquially described as hardening of the skin, as this is the most apparent feature. Particular occupational performance issues arising as a result of SSc include difficulty eating and managing oral care (secondary to decreased ability to fully open the mouth and difficulty swallowing), and decreased ability to grasp and manipulate objects required in everyday activities (secondary to joint contractures and skin changes in the hands and to Raynaud's symptoms). Like other systemic rheumatic conditions, the pain, fatigue, and physical limitations arising from SSc create challenges to participation in important life roles, such as mother (Poole, Willer, & Mendelson, 2009).

Osteoporosis

Osteoporosis (OP) is a growing public health concern because it affects such a large proportion of the aging population. The risk of osteoporotic fractures is high. Caucasian women over 45 have about a 40% to 50% chance of sustaining an osteoporotic fracture during their lifetime, and the risk of hip fracture doubles for every 5 years of age past 45 (Maricic, 2001). OP is treated with medications aimed at decreasing the rate of bone resorption and also with calcium and vitamin D supplements. Occupational therapy for people with OP addresses fall prevention, increased physical activity (especially weight-bearing activities), and reinforcement of nutritional guidelines (e.g., when assessing and intervening with meal preparation or kitchen safety).

Occupational therapy clients also present with *nonarticular rheumatic conditions*, including *tendinitis* or *tenosynovitis* (tennis elbow; golfer's elbow; or local inflammation of the tendon sheaths surrounding tendons to the fingers and thumbs, such as de Quervain's tenosynovitis), *carpal tunnel syndrome* (impingement of the median nerve affecting sensation in the hand and strength of thenar muscles), and *bursitis* (inflammation of the bursa in joints such as the shoulder and knee). Each of these conditions may result in pain and motor impairment, and thus difficulty managing everyday activities the client needs and wants to do.

Occupational Therapy in Rheumatic Diseases

As in many areas of practice, the role of the occupational therapist is to maintain, restore, and improve clients' abilities to manage their daily activities and enable full participation in life. In rheumatology, some therapy interventions address the underlying pathology of the condition and thus focus on improving body function. Examples include splints to decrease joint pain and inflammation or improve the biomechanics of a specific motion (e.g., carpometacarpal [CMC] splint to stabilize a thumb and improve grasp), as well as interventions that target tasks necessary for effective occupational performance (e.g., strategies to enable note-taking at school).

Adaptive strategies, equipment, and environmental modifications incorporate joint protection and energy conservation principles in order to manage the main symptoms of most rheumatic diseases: pain and fatigue. It is essential that principles be illustrated with practical examples directly applicable to the individual client's roles and occupations; otherwise, routines and behaviors are unlikely to change. See Box 8.1 for brief case examples highlighting an individualized approach.

There is growing evidence to support the effect of occupational therapy in the management of rheumatic diseases. In a systematic review of occupational therapy interventions in managing RA, Steultjens and colleagues (2004) reported that both comprehensive occupational therapy and joint protection education improve functional abilities, that wrist splints decrease pain and improve grip strength, and that there were insufficient data available to evaluate the effect of assistive devices. This rigorous review was based on a research paradigm for which quantitative data collection in controlled clinical trials is fundamental to drawing conclusions. However, compelling support is also found in qualitative reports on the effect of occupational therapy on participation in valued activities—evidence that is not readily captured in controlled trials. Examples are found in a narrative analysis of negotiating life with RA (Stamm et al., 2008), where participants described the use of environmental modifications at home and work, and in a thematic analysis of employment experiences of women with RA, OA, and FM (Crooks, 2007), where participants described job accommodations such as modified duties or work hours or specific physical accommodations such as ergonomic keyboards.

Occupational therapy is part of an interdisciplinary team approach to managing rheumatic diseases (Hennell & Luqmani, 2008). All team members contribute to education and principles of self-management, in addition to discipline-specific interventions, and all aim to help clients manage their illness and minimize its impact on participation in life activities. Patient education programs improve functional status, at least in the short term (Riemsma, Kirwan, Taal, & Rasker, 2002). The Arthritis Self-Management Program, a series of six educational sessions, offered in small groups by trained lay leaders following a standard curriculum, enhances self-efficacy, reduces pain, and decreases the number of physician visits (Brady & Boutaugh, 2006).

The Stanford University Patient Education Research Center Web site (http://patienteducation. stanford.edu) is an excellent resource for instructional materials and outcome measures for arthritis and chronic disease self-management.

Performance Skill Impairments Associated With Rheumatic Diseases

Rheumatic diseases may affect all performance skills, but motor skills are typically most limited. Depending on the specific condition, its severity, and how well it is managed by medications, there may be damage to joint surfaces, cartilage, bone, and the soft tissue surrounding the joint. These changes lead to decreased range of motion, joint instability when ligaments are stretched, or joint stiffness when swelling is profuse or soft tissues contract. Joint biomechanics are compromised; there may be joint deformities or malalignment. Strength, endurance, and hand function may be impaired. Subsequent to pain and periods of inactivity, many people with rheumatic diseases will be deconditioned. Clients may report difficulty with standing, walking, transferring, bending, rising, reaching, grasping, holding, and carrying. Even resting and sleeping become problematic in the presence of pain and difficulty positioning joints and moving in bed.

The central nervous system is not usually involved in most rheumatic diseases, but systemic conditions, especially the connective tissue diseases, may have an impact on central nervous system processing, as revealed by sensory or cognitive problems. Cognitive assessment and intervention may be appropriate for people with SLE, for example. Impaired sensation and parathesia may result if inflammation compresses peripheral nerves passing through soft tissue compartments, as happens with

Box 8.1. Case Illustrations of Meredith and Ray

Meredith, 39, is presently on maternity leave from her work as a museum curator. She's married and has two daughters, a 4-year-old and a 5-month-old infant. She was diagnosed with RA shortly after delivering her older daughter. Tim, her husband, commutes over 90 minutes to the school where he teaches 7th grade. They live in an older, three-storey Victorian home: kitchen, bathroom, living room, and dining room on the main floor; two bedrooms upstairs; and laundry in the basement. They've lived here since Meredith and Tim were married 7 years ago but are building their first home on a lot purchased close to Tim's work. Meredith will likely leave her job once they move. The benefit to building their own home is the opportunity to incorporate design features to accommodate some of Meredith's physical limitations; the challenge has been to figure out concurrently how to incorporate "childproof" with "easy access."

Meredith is very resourceful: She repurposed the dining room with a place for the baby to sleep and a changing table (in addition to the crib upstairs) and a play area for her older daughter. This way, she makes only one trip up and down to the bedroom level each day. She describes alternative ways of doing things to accommodate pain and limited hand dexterity, such as having Tim open/unfasten items she's going to need during the day before he leaves for work. Tim does the laundry and quite a bit of the cooking. Meredith's happy to nurture her eldest daughter during less demanding activities like reading, playing music, and the occasional visit to the local pool, while Tim takes charge of playing soccer and bike riding. Recently, Meredith experienced a flare of her RA and has just started on a new DMARD. Her rheumatologist also referred her to occupational therapy and physical therapy to "update" her ability to manage her arthritis better, since her attention has been focused on her children rather than her health.

After an initial interview, the occupational therapist and Meredith identified two main goals related to managing child care tasks better and designing the kitchen in the new house. After a functional assessment, they noted several active joints (both wrists, two metacarpal phalangeal joints on the right hand and three on the left, two proximal interphalangeal joints on each hand, and right knee), as well as reduced strength and dexterity. In Meredith's words, though, "fatigue is the biggest challenge—I'm exhausted to the point of tears sometimes." After participating in group sessions on joint protection and energy conservation principles, Meredith and her occupational therapist applied those principles to Meredith's daily routine: They identified a baby stroller that would be easy to push, fold, open, and lift in and out of the car; practiced lifting and carrying using proper body mechanics; revised Meredith's weekly schedule to better pace her activities to accommodate her fatigue and incorporate some "me time" to take care of herself; fabricated bilateral wrist splints to stabilize and protect her wrists during activities; and discussed the merits of a cognitive–behavioral self-management group that might advance Meredith's natural ability to problem solve in order to engage in the activities of greatest importance to her.

Ray, 44, lives on reserve in a rural aboriginal community. He is the elected chief of his band council and oversees their business/financial affairs. He has ankylosing spondylitis, a diagnosis that was only recently confirmed. Ray reports a history of aches and pains he attributed to his active lifestyle: plantar fasciitis, heel spurs, and pain and stiffness in his back and neck over the past 7–8 years. About a year ago, his pain became more persistent, and he has lost considerable mobility in his spine and developed a painful hip. He gave up camping and hiking, which he loves, thinking that the dampness was contributing to his pain and stiffness. Ray is single and shares custody of his 12-year-old son. One of his concerns is whether or not his son may also develop AS; Ray knows several men with AS, two of whom became quite disabled and unable to work. The community health nurse (the only health professional living in the community) observes that Ray seems somewhat depressed about his circumstances, which is very unlike him—he is known as an energetic and motivating leader in the community.

Ray's assessment by the traveling occupational therapist was his first encounter with the profession. Together they analyzed his work demands and reviewed applied ergonomics to better match the tasks to his physical capacity and safe work habits. For example, they installed his computer monitor onto an adjustable arm so it could be viewed from both a standing height drafting table and a standard-height desk, allowing him to change position frequently and avoid static postures while working at the computer. Ray had an adjustable task chair, but it was not set up to provide optimal seated posture. An interest inventory was used to identify unexplored leisure interests that he could share with his son. Recommendations for supportive shoes and custom insoles addressed the foot pain that often kept him at home instead of socializing with his friends. The occupational therapist provided some additional suggestions for the community health nurse to incorporate in the future and arranged to follow up during a telehealth conference in 3 months' time to evaluate outcomes and adjust the treatment plan as required to support Ray's occupational performance.

the median nerve in carpal tunnel syndrome. Vasculitis may also impair peripheral sensation.

Emotional and social skills affected include the individual's coping skills—the response to pain and managing the sequelae of pain, fatigue, and motor impairment. It is not unusual to experience changes in mood as a result of rheumatic diseases; depression and anxiety are frequently associated with the loss of valued activities (Katz & Yelin, 2001; Katz et al., 2008; Plach, Heidrich, & Waite, 2003). Dealing with chronic pain and changes in mood may have an impact on concentration and memory. Social support appears to mediate the effects of rheumatic diseases in fulfilling roles such as mother (Backman et al., 2007) and employee (Lacaille et al., 2008). Self-efficacy also appears to be related to effective self-managment (Brady & Boutaugh, 2006). The psychosocial impact of arthritis pain is substantial and typically managed with a range of psychoeducational approaches (Backman, 2006).

Concurrently managing an unpredictable chronic illness and multiple life roles requires considerable cognitive and social skills in order to achieve a sense of balance across occupations. In an exploratory study of the impact of RA on occupational balance, the factors most predictive of one's satisfaction with time use, activities accomplished, and satisfaction with participation in one's primary worker role (whether paid or unpaid work) included good general health status, better social function, perceived enjoyment of and ability to perform self-care and work tasks, and high self-efficacy regarding symptom management and everyday functional demands (Forhan & Backman, 2010).

The performance skill limitations associated with rheumatic diseases may be short term, as in the case of some localized inflammatory conditions, an exacerbation of symptoms, or postoperative. In chronic diseases, limitations may progress over time and lead to increasing levels of disability. Yet many people with apparently severe physical impairments are able to effectively manage their daily activities, whereas others who have relatively mild impairments have great difficulty performing the tasks necessary to their life roles and expectations. It is therefore necessary to continually evaluate the interaction of performance components with the demands of the client's occupations and the context in which the client performs each occupation.

Impact of Rheumatic Diseases on Performance Patterns

First-person accounts of living with arthritis give compelling descriptions of how the illness affects routines, habits, roles, and identity, for example, Lewis's (2006) account of living with SLE or Koehn's (2006) experience with RA (see excerpts in Boxes 8.2 and 8.3). Collectively, rheumatic diseases affect all areas of occupational performance and participation in life. Precise effects vary across and within rheumatic diseases, as well as across individuals. Exacerbations and remissions in RA and JIA, for example, mean that clients are able to manage routines and habits supporting their ADLs, IADLs, work, and school activities on some days but not on others. Systemic effects associated with exacerbations include feelings of general malaise that contribute to fatigue and lack of endurance. This pattern has a subsequent effect on relationships with others, because the course of the illness can be unpredictable.

Limitations in hand strength and dexterity result in problems across many roles, because almost every activity requires that objects be grasped, manipulated, moved, smoothed, or pressed. Consider a typical mother's day and the possible difficulties encountered if arthritis limits her hand strength and dexterity: holding a toothbrush, opening a box of cereal, buttoning clothes, picking up a child, opening doors, reaching for groceries, opening a jar of peanut butter, or doing laundry. Multiple tasks throughout the day may present difficulties that need to be assessed and addressed in occupational therapy to enable her to fulfill her role.

When OA, RA, or JIA affect the hips, the knees, or both, mobility is impaired. Standing, walking, managing stairs, rising from a chair, putting on shoes and socks, getting on and off the toilet, and getting in and out of the bathtub become challenges or disruptions in daily routines. It can be difficult, if not impossible, to get down to the floor to play with children or pick up items; a young child with JIA may not be able to sit on the floor at school for reading circles or other classroom activities. Similar difficulties may be present when AS limits movement in the spine and hips.

Depending on workplace demands, employment may be adversely affected by limitations in mobility. Studies show that joint problems are associated with restrictions in social role participation and that discretionary activities are typically the first occupations people give up. For example, middle-aged and older adults with early hip or knee OA reported problems participating in community activities, active leisure, hobbies, and social relationships (Gignac et al., 2008).

Reconstructive surgery presents the need to prepare for and follow precautions to promote healing, and these have an impact on all occupational performance areas. For example, MCP joint replace-

Box 8.2. Kathleen's Experience With SLE

Kathleen, a nurse, writes about her experiences at the onset of her illness:

I arrived at [work] early to get some things done before a staff meeting. As I rushed about, I began having chest pains. They were like the pains I experienced 3 months earlier. I'd thrown a clot to my lung, spending a week in the hospital and a month out of work.

I called my supervisor to one side. She checked me out and had me call my doctor. It was arranged that another nurse would drive me to the doctor's office after the staff meeting. I left work never to return again.

A perfusion lung scan showed a clot in my left lung exactly at the spot of the previous clot, even though I was taking Coumadin. I felt scared. The next few days were filled with tests. The end result was that the doctors made a diagnosis of exertional asthma.

The diagnosis didn't explain what was happening in my body—chest pain, shortness of breath, fatigue, fever, joint pain, hair loss, and other symptoms that had been evolving over the past 8 years. A month later, in preparing to go on a trip to Hawaii, I got a sun lamp to begin a suntan. A rash developed on my chest. I headed back to the doctor.

My doctor ran more tests. My life was changing rapidly. I had only enough energy to be up for short periods of time. It was difficult to carry out my activities of daily living and roles as mother and wife. I was getting more anxious. At the same time, we were getting ready for our trip.

Later that week, 2 days before we were to leave for Hawaii, I called my doctor to get my lab results. "Kathleen, it looks like you have systemic lupus erythematosus. You need to see a rheumatologist. Be sure you wear sunscreen when you are in the sun." His voice came across the phone like a cannon exploding in my ears and kept ringing in my ears as I drove to pick up my sons at soccer practice. At age 34 with 2 boys (8 and 10 years old), a husband, and a career, life would never be the same.

That day I left the office, I went instantaneously from being employed to being disabled. It took 1½ soul-wrenching years to go through the disability process. People handle retirement best when it's their choice, their health is good, and they have adequate financial resources. I had none of those.... (p. 89).

From: Lewis, K. S. (2006). The patient's experience. In S. J. Bartlett, C. O. Bingham, M. J. Maricic, M. D. Iversen, & V. Ruffing (Eds.), *Clinical care in the rheumatic diseases* (3rd ed., pp. 89–94). Atlanta: Association of Rheumatology Health Professionals.

ment surgery requires use of a splint to maintain the alignment of the fingers, so one-handed techniques are used for basic ADLs for a short time during the postoperative period. Total hip arthroplasty requires that excessive hip flexion and adduction be avoided (possibly in addition to other motions, depending on the surgeon's approach), thus a raised toilet seat, bath bench, and cushion to raise the height of car seats or chairs in the household are some of the typical devices used for a postoperative period of up to 3 months. A long-handled reacher, dressing stick, and sock aid may also enable ADLs while hip flexion is restricted, whether due to surgery or the effects of the disease.

Focus of Occupational Therapy Evaluation

The purpose of the occupational therapy evaluation is to understand the impact of rheumatic disease on everyday living, in order to help clients employ strategies to maintain participation in their chosen activities while managing their condition and overall health. Within today's health care context, it is difficult to find time for comprehen-

sive evaluation of clients with complex conditions. Therefore, an initial interview in occupational therapy seeks to identify the most pressing occupational performance issues or problems for each client. Additional assessment tools may then be selected based on the nature of the priority problems (Backman, Fairleigh, & Kuchta, 2004). For example, the Canadian Occupational Performance Measure (COPM; Law et al., 2005) is a semistructured interview that addresses all areas of occupational performance, and has the additional advantage of a scoring system that will measure the outcome of occupational therapy interventions when readministered at a later date. The Occupational Circumstances Assessment Interview and Rating Scale (OCAIRS; Forsyth et al., 2005) is another semistructured interview to gather information on the client's interests, values, roles, habits, and goals to help establish a treatment plan to support occupational participation. Regardless of the interview format used, it should result in an occupational profile and identify which occupations, tasks, or activities require attention.

Box 8.3. Cheryl Living With Rheumatoid Arthritis and Finding "Normal" Again

When I was a kid, I used to love riding roller coasters with my mother. The bigger and scarier the ride, the better. I was thrilled at the uncertainty of the track's direction—how it would suddenly turn to the right or left, or unexpectedly plunge 100 feet or more, leaving my stomach feeling light and my spine tingly. I still love to ride on roller coasters, but 16 years ago, I go on one that frightened me to the core of my being—the rheumatoid arthritis roller coaster.

Unlike the amusement park version, I quickly learned that the turns, ascents, and drops of the rheumatoid arthritis (RA) roller coaster were significantly more daunting than any I had ever experienced at an amusement park. I also learned how it would profoundly affect every part of my life—work, home, and leisure. The onset of symptoms, a pain in the ball of my foot and an inexplicably swollen index finger one day to 35 affected joints 1 month later, was completely overwhelming. From the day I received my diagnosis and throughout the first year of living with the disease, I struggled even to understand the word *arthritis*. I still remember (as though it were yesterday) the precise moment the rheumatologist spoke the words *rheumatoid arthritis*....I'm 30 years old, I can't have arthritis, I'm too young. I'm a former member of the United States Women's Volleyball team; I'm in excellent health and fit as a fiddle. This diagnosis can't possibly be correct....

After...roughly 10 minutes discussing the findings of the lab tests and physical examination, the rheumatologist and I could not be farther apart in terms of a shared understanding of RA and the early steps I needed to take to deal with it....during the first year I lived with RA, I did not follow the rheumatologist's advice to initiate gold and methotrexate therapy. The only recommendation I followed was to attend a once-monthly appointment to check on my disease's progress. To the rheumatologist's credit, he stuck with me and patiently waited for me to acknowledge and accept that the noninstitutional approach I followed for a year was a failure.... (p. 303)

For me, one of the more frustrating aspects of the earliest years of my disease was the time spent by the rheumatologist and other health care professionals collecting information on my function, pain, medication, side effects, and other physical findings, with little or no time spent talking about the aspects of RA that had as significant an impact on my life as the physical symptoms. Those critical aspects of life with chronic illness include fatigue, ability to sleep and sleep well, intimacy, sexuality, family understanding and support, participation (at home, leisure, and work), emotional and social difficulties, challenges in the workplace, among other topics. These are the things that, when balanced, help make me feel "normal" again.

Finding "normal" again—in my personal relationships, work life, and in society—was not easy....When I look back now, RA made me re-examine every aspect of my life, and it was only because I had the disease that I embarked on the journey. I decided that if I was going to have to live with such a crummy disease, I wanted the other parts of my life, at work, at home, and at leisure, to be as balanced and fulfilling as possible....

I think about my health and assess how well my RA treatment plan is working by looking at outcomes that are meaningful to me. Do I have a fulfilling life with my husband? Am I still able to work out and play tennis? Do I have kind, caring friends? Am I able to travel on my own without assistance? Am I financially independent? These are the outcomes I want to achieve with my well-rounded treatment plan. (p. 304)

Cheryl's experience shows the importance of clarifying expectations and clearly communicating and collaborating on intervention goals and plans in the context of the client's everyday life.

From: Koehn, C. L. (2006). Living with rheumatoid arthritis: Accepting the diagnosis and finding "normal" again. In S. J. Bartlett, C. O. Bingham, M. J. Maricic, M. D. Iversen, & V. Ruffing (Eds.), *Clinical care in the rheumatic diseases*, (3rd ed., pp. 303–305). Atlanta: Association of Rheumatology Health Professionals.

Once priority occupational performance issues are identified, there will be a variety of cues to guide the choice of additional evaluation methods to determine the underlying performance skills or environmental conditions that contribute to the problem (Backman & Medcalf, 2000). Evaluation procedures may include

- Goniometry to measure joint range of motion;
- Manual muscle testing and dynamometry (e.g., grip strength);
- Hands-on evaluation of soft tissue integrity;
- Measurement of hand dexterity (e.g., pegboard tests);
- Measurement of hand function (see Table 8.2),

Table 8.2. Selected Tests of Hand/Upper-Limb Function for Clients With Rheumatic Diseases

Test	Description	Reference
Arthritis Hand Function Test (AHFT)	Performance-based test of hand strength, dexterity, and functional tasks for with adults with RA, OA, and SSc	Backman et al., 1991 Poole et al., 2000
Australian Canadian Osteoarthritis Hand Index (AUSCAN HI)	Self-report questionnaire designed for hand OA, with 3 subscales: pain, stiffness, and function	Bellamy et al., 2002
Cochin Hand Disability Scale	Self-report questionnaire evaluating level of difficulty performing 18 functional tasks	Duruöz et al., 1996
Disabilities of the Arm, Shoulder, and Hand Questionnaire (DASH)	Self-report, 30-item questionnaire evaluating level of pain and difficulty with functional tasks, with optional modules for sports, work, and musicians; for any diagnosis	Beaton et al., 2001 (includes entire questionnaire)
Hand Mobility in Scleroderma Test (HAMIS)	Observational test of functional hand range of motion specific to scleroderma	Sandqvist & Eklund 2000
Michigan Hand Outcomes Questionnaire (MHQ)	Self-report questionnaire evaluating symptoms, function, and esthetics for pre- and postoperative evaluations	Chung et al., 1998 (includes entire questionnaire)
Sequential Occupational Dexterity Test (SODA)	Performance-based assessment of ability to do 12 functional tasks, with difficulty scored by both occupational therapist and client	van Lankveld et al., 1996

Note. RA = rheumatoid arthritis, OA = osteoarthritis, SSc = systematic sclerosis.

- Measurement of symptoms affecting occupational performance, such as pain and fatigue, using the National Institutes of Health Activity Record; (Gerber & Furst, 1992); and
- Specific ADL, IADL, work, or leisure assessments, as indicated by the client's occupational performance goals. Promising tools specific to the effect of arthritis on work participation are the Work Limitations Questionnaire (Lerner et al., 2001), the Work Instability Scale (Gilworth et al., 2003), and the Work Experience Survey–Rheumatic Diseases (Allaire & Keysor, 2009). The Ergonomic Assessment Tool for Arthritis (EATA) involves client self-assessment and an occupational therapist interview guide for identifying ergonomic issues in the workplace (Backman, Village, & Lacaille, 2008).

As part of the interdisciplinary team, the occupational therapist may administer or have access to the results of outcome measures used to track clients' progress and program effectiveness. Examples of commonly used tools are in Table 8.3. An excellent review of a comprehensive range of rheumatology patient outcome measures is available in a special supplement to the journal *Arthritis and Rheumatism (Arthritis Care and Research)*, Volume 49,

Number 5, October 2003. Both pediatric and adult measures are summarized, in the areas of function, pain, quality of life, psychological status and well-being, fatigue and sleep, and disease-specific measures.

The initial administration of outcome measures is a useful screening process for referral to appropriate health professionals. For example, a referral to occupational therapy may be initiated by another health professional based on scores from the Health Assessment Questionairre (HAQ) or Western Ontario and McMaster Universities Osteoarthritis Index (WOMAC). Although many outcome measures have content pertinent to occupational therapy, many do not have enough information to help therapists identify precise occupational performance issues and set goals. A combination of interview, standardized measures, and observation is usually required for a comprehensive evaluation.

Factors to Consider When Recommending Adaptive Strategies, Equipment, or Environmental Modifications

The primary factor to be considered when making recommendations is to be client-centered. Not all strategies, equipment, and modifications work for

Table 8.3. Selected Rheumatology Outcome Measures

Test	Description	Reference
Arthritis Impact Measurement Scales 2 (AIMS–2)	Self-report of mobility, physical, household, and social activities, ADLs, pain, depression, and anxiety	Meenan et al., 1992
Bath Ankylosing Spondylitis Functional Index (BASFI)	Self-report of ability to perform 10 functional activities frequently limited in AS	Calin et al., 1994
Child Health Assessment Questionnaire (CHAQ)	Interview or self-report for children 8 and older with 8 ADL subscales	Singh et al., 1994 Lam et al., 2004
Fibromyalgia Impact Questionnaire	Self-report of physical function, symptoms, and well-being	Burckhardt et al., 1991
Juvenile Arthritis Functional Status Index (JASI)	Self-report of functional activities for children 8-17 yrs. Computer and interview. Ranks 5 priority activities	Wright et al., 1994
Health Assessment Questionnaire (HAQ) Disability Index; HAQ–II	Self-report of difficulties performing in 8 categories of ADLs (20 items). Download tool from http://patienteducation.stanford.edu/research/haq20.html HAQ–II is a shorter (10 items) revised version by different authors	Fries et al., 1980 Wolfe et al., 2004
Western Ontario and McMaster Universities Osteoarthritis Index (WOMAC)	Self-report of pain, stiffness and function for adults with OA affecting hips and/or knees.	Bellamy (1995)

Note. ADLs = activities of daily living, AS = ankylosing spondylitis, OA = osteoarthritis.

all people, even when they have similar joint involvement and similar problems. Collaborative problem solving between occupational therapist and client leads to recommendations that best fit the client's priorities and contextual limitations and opportunities (Law, 1998). Finding the most appropriate solution often involves trial and error; encouragement and perseverance are necessary. Feasibility of recommendations will vary according to context and the anticipated duration of the limitation. A renter in an apartment is less likely to make structural changes to a kitchen or bathroom than a homeowner. The cost of the recommendation is a consideration for most people, and even when insurance is expected to cover the costs, there may be restrictions regarding the circumstances under which devices or modifications are reimbursable. Or, there may be a "lifetime limit" on total rehabilitation expenditures. Large corporate employers may have more resources available than do small businesses to facilitate adjustment at work; some clients may choose to disclose their arthritis to supervisors and coworkers, and others will not. These contextual factors dictate careful planning.

Group support influences the acceptability of many recommendations. For example, in a group session on joint protection and energy conservation principles, Cathy, the occupational therapist, re-

sponded to Alisha's comment about delegating work to others to accommodate fatigue or mobility limitations. "You can ask your children to pick up after themselves," said Cathy. "I don't want my RA to ruin my kids' childhoods," said Alisha, a mother with RA and two young children. "It's not fair that they should have to clean up after themselves just because it's hard for me to do it." "There's nothing unfair about it," interjected Leona, another client in the group. "It's got nothing to do with your arthritis; part of your role as a parent is to teach your kids to be responsible and pick up after themselves."

In this example, Leona had more credibility because she had both RA and children, and Cathy, the occupational therapist, had neither. Alisha asked Leona several more questions and was pleased to hear Leona say that RA did not have a "detrimental" effect on raising her children. Sharing experiences and strategies among people who have similar issues is an important part of planning effective interventions.

Consider involving family members, as appropriate, when negotiating recommendations. Suggesting home modifications, such as adding handrails to staircases or hallways, changing furnishings, installing lever handles on faucets, or raising a toilet seat all affect the entire family. Some clients may be reluctant to adopt such modifications. An open discussion of options with the client's spouse, parents, or children, facilitated by the occupational therapist, may be very useful.

The appearance of assistive devices and modifications is important to some people. Fortunately, increasing attention to universal access and ergonomic tools means that many devices are less identifiable as such, as they are readily available in the general marketplace rather than medical supply stores alone. Examples are the range of cooking utensils in gourmet cooking stores and casual clothing features such as rings or pull tabs on zippers. Some children find neon-colored spiral elastic shoelaces to be a "cool" accessory—that they eliminate the need to tie laces is secondary.

Adaptive Strategies, Equipment, or Environmental Modifications

Joint protection and energy conservation principles guide the recommendation of adaptive strategies and equipment recommendations for all occupational performance areas. To be incorporated into daily routines, it is essential that these principles be applied to relevant examples for individual clients (examples are in Table 8.4). Recent studies suggest that practice applying joint protection principles improves function (Hammond & Freeman, 2001; Steultjens et al., 2004). Splints help stabilize joints, address underlying biomechanics of motion, reduce pain during activity, and improve hand strength and function (Harrell, 2001; Haskett, Backman, Porter, Goyert, & Palejko, 2004). Energy conservation principles involve prioritizing activities; planning and pacing activities over the day, week, or month; and engaging in regular physical activity. Physical activity reduces pain and fatigue regardless of the type of rheumatic disease. It is therefore important to find physical activities that the client will enjoy and maintain.

Self-management strategies also contribute to improved occupational performance. *Self-management* has been defined as "learning and practicing the skills necessary to carry on an active and emotionally satisfying life in the face of chronic illness"

Table 8.4. Joint Protection and Energy Conservation Principles and Sample Techniques

Principle	Sample Techniques or Application
Respect your pain.	Reduce time and/or effort spent on an activity if pain occurs and lasts for more than 2 hours after the activity has been discontinued. Avoid nonessential activities that aggravate your pain.
Balance rest and work.	Take short breaks during your work. For example, take a 5-minute rest at the end of 1 hour of work. Intersperse more active tasks with more passive or quiet work.
Reduce the amount of effort needed to do the job.	Use assistive devices such as a jar opener or lever taps. Slide pots across the counter instead of lifting. Use a trolley to transport heavy items. Use a raised toilet seat and seat cushion to reduce stress on hips, knees, and hands. Use frozen vegetables to minimize peeling and chopping.
Avoid staying in one position for prolonged periods of time.	Change position frequently to avoid joint stiffness and muscle fatigue. For example, take a 30-second range of motion break after 10–20 minutes of typing or holding a tool; after standing for 20 minutes, perch on a stool for the next 20 minutes; walk to the mailroom after 20–30 minutes sitting at your desk.
Avoid activities that cannot be stopped immediately if you experience pain or discomfort.	Plan ahead. Be realistic about your abilities so you don't walk or drive too far or leave all your shopping and errands to a single trip.
Reduce unnecessary stress on your joints while sleeping.	Use a firm mattress for support. Sleep on your back with a pillow to support the curve in your neck. If you prefer to lie on your side, place a pillow between your knees, and lie on the least painful side.
Maintain muscle strength and joint range of motion.	Do your prescribed exercises regularly. Strong muscles will help support your joints. Regular exercise will reduce fatigue.
Use a well-planned work space.	Organize your work space so that work surfaces and materials are at a convenient height for you, to ensure good posture. Place frequently used items within close reach. Reduce clutter by getting rid of unnecessary items, or storing less frequently used items away from the immediate work space.

Source. Occupational Therapy Department, Mary Pack Arthritis Program, Vancouver Coastal Health, Vancouver, BC. Used with permission.

(Lorig, 1993). Helping clients acquire self-management skills requires an interactive approach that focuses on skill development and increasing their confidence and ability to manage their arthritis (Brady & Boutaugh, 2006). Approaches based on cognitive behavioral treatment, self-efficacy theory, and other learning theories include strategies such as goal setting and making contracts, problem-solving discussions, *role modeling* (learning from others in similar circumstances), and experiential learning (practicing techniques).

These strategies, offered in a range of patient education packages, including the *Arthritis Self-Management Program, Fibromylagia Self-Help Course*, and *Bone-up on Arthritis Course*, have been shown to increase knowledge, self-efficacy, self-care behaviors, functional status, and quality of life and to decrease perceived pain, depression, helplessness, and health care utilization in the form of visits to physicians and specialists (Brady & Boutaugh, 2006).

Activities of Daily Living

Morning stiffness may limit one's ability to manage morning ADLs. Laying out clothes the night before, setting timers on appliances like the coffee maker at bedtime, and doing gentle range of motion exercises in bed prior to rising minimize the effect of morning stiffness on task performance. Assistive devices facilitate many personal care activities related to dressing, bathing, grooming, and eating (Mann, 1998; Mann, Tomita, Hurren, & Charvat, 1999). Many devices are attractive as well as functional, but no one device suits all people. Enlarged or curved handles on eating and cooking utensils accommodate limited range of motion and may facilitate optimal anatomical alignment of vulnerable joints. However, some clients will manage better with a smooth, flat utensil that fits more easily into the web space between the thumb and finger or several fingers. The effect of devices on joint biomechanics requires careful attention: In some cases, devices will increase joint stress, require more strength, or make tasks more difficult to perform. The occupational therapist needs to analyze the client's skills and activity demands to recommend appropriate devices or adaptations. Commonly used aids to dressing are the button hook and stocking aids illustrated in Figure 8.1.

Purchasing two long-handled sponges facilitates bathing when one is reserved for hard-to-reach body parts and the second for cleaning the tub. Extended handles on combs and styling aids are useful for hair care when shoulder motion is restricted. Sitting in the bathroom and resting the elbow on the vanity accommodates reduced

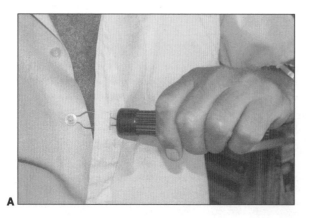
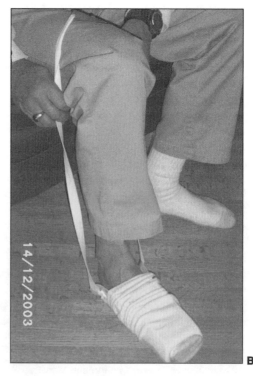

Figure 8.1. A. Button hook to compensate for reduced pinch or in-hand manipulation. Photo: Wendy D. B. Sock aid to accommodate pain or limitations in hip and knee flexion. Photo: C. Parker.

strength and endurance. Mounting the blow dryer on a wall bracket eliminates the need for holding the dryer over the head.

Mobility may be facilitated with the use of a cane or walking stick when hips, knees, and feet are painful or weak. It is important to consider all of the joints when recommending a cane: If hands and wrists are involved, a modified or custom-molded grip on the cane or walking stick may be required. A wheeled walker with a basket for holding parcels and a fold-down seat for waiting in line or taking brief rests may enable people who are otherwise limited to walking very short distances manage errands.

Environmental modifications such as a walk-in shower and installing lever taps can be expensive; some people will incorporate them into home renovations over a number of years. Grab bars to facilitate tub and toilet transfers should be installed by a qualified tradesperson to ensure they are adequately anchored to wall studs and sustain body weight. (Towel racks are designed to hold towels, not people, and are not a safe alternative.)

Limitations in upper-limb ROM and strength may prevent adequate pericare and toilet hygiene. A curved toilet tissue holder is a portable and simple aid; an attachable bidet-style toilet seat that washes and dries the perineal area is a more expensive home-based option. When home renovations are under consideration, applying universal design principles to the bathroom, for example, may ease difficulties with daily hygiene. (See the shower arrangement in Figure 8.2 and additional suggestions in Table 8.5.)

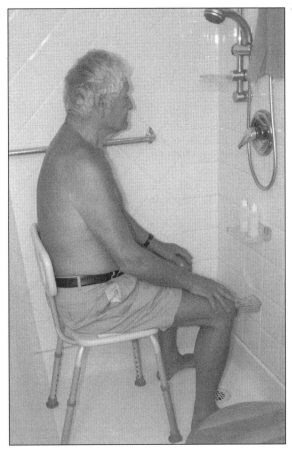

Figure 8.2. Sitting to shower, with fixtures and supplies in easy reach, to reduce risk of falls and/or accommodate pain in weight-bearing joints. Photo: Wendy D.

Instrumental Activities of Daily Living

Shopping can be a tiring experience. One option is to delegate the task to family members or friends in exchange for doing other tasks that can be more easily paced. Shopping by phone or Internet with grocery or parcel delivery is relatively stress-free. If clients prefer to choose their own products, shopping in person but requesting delivery eliminates the need to carry parcels. Grocery stores may provide delivery services for a reduced fee on specific days of the week. These options may be more readily available in urban than rural areas, but exchanging services with friends is sometimes accepted more readily in rural communities.

The huge volume of cookbooks and magazines on the market are full of suggestions for making meal preparation quick and easy. Using one-pot meals or slow cookers or tiered bamboo steamers put the entire meal into one pot, reducing cleanup afterward. Partially prepared ingredients save time and energy, or compensate for weak or painful hand

joints, and include cleaned and chopped salads in a bag, deli-prepared main and side dishes, and frozen meals. While sometimes more expensive, they are nevertheless an option suitable for some clients or as a back up on a "bad day." Cook once, eat twice: Prepare large casseroles, soups, or stews, and freeze leftovers for later use (in individual containers for school or work lunches).

Opening packages and containers can be difficult for people with arthritis affecting the hands. Box openers, jar openers, a sharp knife, nonskid mats, and electric scissors are examples of helpful kitchen equipment. Lightweight pots, sliding pots along counters, or cooking food inside a steamer basket to avoid the need to lift and drain a heavy pot are additional suggestions (Figure 8.3). A pull-out bread board, or two pull-out boards at different work heights, provide multiple height work surfaces in one kitchen, facilitating an effective work posture whether sitting or standing (Figure 8.3). A trolley is useful to transport items when unpacking groceries or setting and clearing the table. For clients who at-

Table 8.5. Sample Difficulties Performing ADLs and Potential Solutions

Task	Underlying Performance Skills	Potential Solutions
Difficulty holding toothbrush	Pain in thumb and finger joints Stiffness and decreased ROM in hand joints	Enlarged handle on standard toothbrush; electric toothbrush with easy-to-manage switch (handle is larger, powered brush does all the work)
Difficulty pinching and managing small objects (e.g., buttons/zippers, foil lids on yogurt and similar containers)	Pain in CMC joint of thumb, together with decreased joint stability and strength	CMC splint/orthosis to stabilize thumb; assistive devices specific to task (e.g., button hook, zipper pull); alternative strategies specific to task (e.g., stab center of foil lid with knife and peel back from center)
Difficulty bathing: transferring to and from tub	Pain and decreased ROM in hips and knees Fear of falling	Bath bench or bath stool and hand-held shower attachment; water-powered bath seat that lowers into tub; walk-in shower and bath seat; bath safety rails/bars; nonskid mat
Difficulty bathing: holding soap and reaching body parts	Limited ROM in multiple joints Decreased grasp	Long-handled sponge/loofa; soap-on-a-rope; nylon "poofy" sponge with wrist strap and bath gel in pump dispenser
Difficulty putting on and removing socks and shoes	Limited ROM in hips and knees	Sock/stocking aid; dressing stick for pushing off shoes and socks; boot jack for pushing off shoes; long-handled shoehorn and elastic laces in shoes

Note. ADLs = activities of daily living; CMC = carpometacarpal; ROM = range of motion.

tribute strong meaning to cooking or value it as a leisure activity, some suggestions may be unacceptable. It is a matter of setting priorities and making choices within the client's entire spectrum of routine and roles. Presenting a few examples often facilitates the problem-solving process, helping the generate additional ideas for managing the tasks most important to them. Other suggestions are listed in Table 8.6.

Work

Many people with rheumatic disease will already have an established career or job at the time they are diagnosed. Depending on the task demands at work and their disease status, they may be able to continue working at the same job with minor modifications and equipment, or it may be necessary to consider changes in employment. One frustration for some workers is the assumption that they need a sedentary job—a misconception, as many sedentary jobs require static postures or repetitive motions that are just as difficult to manage as physically demanding jobs. Vocational rehabilitation services may assist with job retraining or reentry. Self-employment is also an attractive option for those who have a well-defined skill set and the desire for autonomy (Adam, White, & Lacaille, 2007).

In the case of children who have rheumatic diseases, the transition to adulthood and employment presents different issues. Identifying career options, attaining skills through postsecondary education, and seeking and securing employment are concerns to be addressed with the young adult. By young adulthood, some individuals will no longer have active arthritis, some will have residual physical impairments, and some will continue to manage active disease. Occupational therapy may involve enabling task performance specific to the training and employment goals of the individual.

Computer work stations are part of many work and study environments. They should be adjustable and adapted to the needs of the individual client. The occupational therapist may suggest modifications to the typical baseline ergonomic recommendations (designed with population health needs in mind) to accommodate restricted reach, a painful hip or knee, or a stiff neck. For example, if the feet dangle when the office chair is adjusted to optimal height, a footstool is recommended. While a tilted footstool may be adequate support for some people, if there is inflammation or limited ankle dorsiflexion, a flat footstool is more appropriate. A document holder set at eye level accommodates a stiff or painful neck. An angled drafting table may be a better choice of desk for those who read and write rather than use the computer. Other work modifications are in Table 8.7. Figure 8.4 illustrates a trial session using a wrist splint and split keyboard.

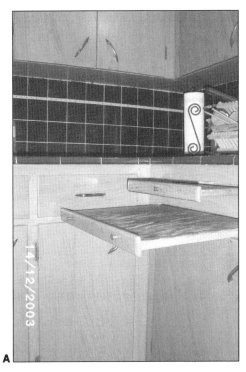

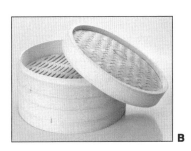

Figure 8.3. A. Work surfaces of varying heights can be integrated into a kitchen with pull-out boards. Photo: C. Parker. B. Steam fish and vegetables quickly in a single pot using a 2- or 3-tiered bamboo steamer. Photo: 123RF.com. Used under license.

Table 8.6. Sample Difficulties With Performing IADLs and Potential Solutions

Task	Underlying Performance Skills	Potential Solutions
Difficulty preparing meals: chopping vegetables, lifting pots	Pain and/or decreased grasp Decreased upper-limb strength Fatigue	Purchase prewashed and chopped vegetables; use lightweight, large-handled utensils, cutting boards with food spikes to stabilize vegetables; food processor; lightweight pots; slide pots on counters; use spray hose from sink to fill pots without lifting
Difficulty turning taps on and off or turning doorknobs	Decreased hand strength	Replace taps/doorknobs with lever fixtures; carry removable tap turner when visiting or traveling; use rubber disk jar opener to improve friction when grasping door knobs or taps
Carrying books, bags, parcels when shopping, going to/from work or school	Pain in hands and/or wrists Decreased hand and wrist strength Desire to protect small joints from strong forces	Backpack, if shoulder ROM permits, with padded shoulder straps; lightweight nylon briefcase with shoulder strap diagonally across trunk; wheeled briefcase, bag, or grocery cart
Difficulty turning keys (car door, ignition, house door)	Decreased pronation and supination Limited hand strength	Key extension, commercial or custom-made; where feasible, change locks to key cards or push-button codes (use eraser end of pencil or dowel rod to push buttons)
Difficulty vacuuming and other heavy housecleaning	Decreased strength Limited reach Fatigue	Delegate some tasks to others in household; use lightweight stick vacuum or carpet sweeper in between heavy cleanings; when feasible, choose hard surface floors and lightweight dustmops; purchase selected services

Note. IADLs = instrumental activities of daily living; ROM = range of motion.

Table 8.7. Sample Occupational Performance Problems at Work and Potential Solutions

Task	Underlying Performance Skills	Potential Solutions
Difficulty managing computer mouse and keyboard at work, exacerbates wrist symptoms	Wrist pain and swelling Limited strength and endurance	Resting splints at night and/or rest periods; ergonomic evaluation and adjustments to work station to maintain optimal posture and arm position; frequent brief pauses to move limbs through full ROM; consider feasibility of arm rests or wrist splints
Talking on phone and taking notes exacerbates neck and back pain	Painful cervical spine and shoulders	Lightweight telephone headset (maintains privacy); speaker phone (less private); explore options available from telephone company
Difficulty writing on blackboard, whiteboard, or flipcharts (teachers, facilitators, consultants)	Decreased grasp Limited hand strength and dexterity Limited shoulder/elbow ROM and strength	Invite students or participants to record information; anticipate key points, and prepare overheads or charts in advance; adapted chalk holder or marker
Difficulty standing for long periods at work	Decreased endurance Foot and ankle pain	Supportive shoes and foot orthoses; antifatigue mats (if standing in single work station); high stool to perch on periodically; footstool or ledge to support one foot for short periods in alternate posture; lie, sit, and stretch during breaks
Unable to read for sustained periods at work or school	Difficulty grasping book Neck pain and upper-limb pain and weakness	Try various bookstands: wire bookholder on stack of books to hold book at eye level; cookbook stand on desk; drafting table in place of desk; lapdesk to support book while seated in easy chair; adjustable music stand in office or study area

Note. ROM = range of motion.

One of the predictors of retaining employment among people with RA or AS is control over the pace of work (Allaire, Anderson, & Meenan, 1996; Chorus, Boonen, Meidema, & van der Linden, 2002). Occupational therapists may review work duties and advise clients on pacing or rotating activities to accommodate arthritis limitations or symptoms. Simple strategies integrated into work habits, such as standing up to answer the phone, reduce static postures that lead to discomfort.

Clients may be reluctant to incorporate suggestions in the workplace, especially if they have not disclosed their arthritis (Lacaille, White, Backman, & Gignac, 2007). The Ergonomic Assessment Tool for Arthritis (EATA) can be used to identify ergonomic solutions without a worksite visit (Backman et al., 2008). Many of these suggestions improve productivity and reduce complaints and absenteeism for all workers.

Clients should be encouraged to share ideas with coworkers and take advantage of occupational health nurses or ergonomists when available, as is the case with some large corporate employers. With the client's consent, the occupational therapist may find an onsite visit the most efficient way to evaluate work duties and make feasible suggestions. Consulting with employers may also facilitate the acquisition of appropriate equipment or modifications. A recently developed program for preventing work loss shows promise: It uses education, group support, and expert consultation with vocational counselors and occupational therapists (Lacaille et al., 2008). It is based on efficacy-enhancing principles such as goal-setting and homework to help participants apply new knowledge to their own work situation.

Up to one-third of people with RA will stop work prematurely, before usual retirement age (Allaire et al., 2008; Lacaille et al., 2004). Exploring alternative activities to make the transition to retirement may be appropriate, such as volunteer work or leisure activities. After many years of managing arthritis, sharing this knowledge with others as a volunteer lay leader for an arthritis education course or as a tele-

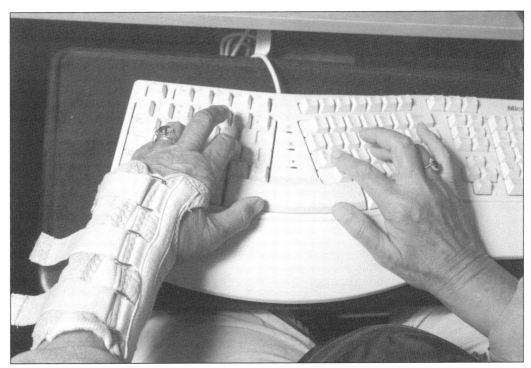

Figure 8.4. A client with RA tries a commercially available wrist splint and split keyboard to encourage a neutral position of the wrist joints. Photo: Wendy D.

phone service volunteer may appeal to some clients. Those who have done so appear to have better health outcomes (Hainsworth & Barlow, 2001). Others may serve as "patient partners" to educate health professional students or as consumer advisors to research projects. The Arthritis Foundation (USA) and The Arthritis Society (Canada) are key resources for these types of volunteer opportunities.

For others, the transition to retirement may present the opportunity for a greater focus on leisure activities. Exploring interests and suggesting community resources encourage people to maintain a physically active lifestyle; gardening, swimming, Tai Chi, and dancing are just a few examples.

School and Play

When children are feeling good, they will participate in the play activities that interest them (Taylor & Erlandson, 2001). When their arthritis is holding them back, they may benefit from specific suggestions to encourage active and quiet play activities at home and school. To protect vulnerable joints, low-impact sports (swimming, bicycle riding) are generally favored over high-impact sports (running) and body contact sports (hockey, football). Summer camps for children with JIA present opportunities to

explore interests and try out new play activities in a supportive environment.

While it may be possible to modify games and school activities to enable the child to participate, they may not wish to stand out among their peers as being different. It is therefore important to involve even the youngest child in problem solving, to find out what is acceptable or "cool" in his or her eyes, and plan accordingly.

For example, there are many "fat pens" on the market; encouraging the child to try a variety of styles and colors to determine the easiest pens to write with, and select a favorite, is likely to be more successful than prescribing a writing aid to accommodate poor grip. Inviting children to choose their favorite color of splint material for orthoses, supportive running shoes, or assistive devices involves them in the process. Obtaining two sets of textbooks, one for home and one for school, minimizes carrying heavy loads and accommodates both fatigue and painful joints.

Consultation with teachers is also useful in helping integrate joint protection principles into the classroom. For example, once the child has established a skill, such as handwriting or solving arithmetic problems, repetitive pencil-and-paper exercises are not necessary. Instead, the child can take a brief period to rest his or her hand joints. Coping with pain affects concentration; mood; and thus, the child's interaction with peers. Finding ways to incorporate short rest periods or minimize activities that exacerbate pain will facilitate overall function (Kuchta & Davidson, 2008).

Leisure

Gardening is a popular leisure activity for which there is a wide range of tools and methods that accommodate limitations secondary to arthritis. Lightweight, flexible hoses with easy-to-manage trigger nozzles decrease the strain of watering. Lightweight, long-handled, wide-handled rakes, trowels, hoes, and shears provide the "right tool for the job" so that garden maintenance is both achievable and enjoyable. Other gardeners, garden shops, clubs, or botanical display gardens are a source of good advice on tools, garden designs, and plant selection for easy care.

It is important to stay involved and connected with family, friends, and community activities. The "inability to perform integrated life activities, such as housework, leisure and recreational activities, or social activities appears to be more closely linked to poor psychological outcomes than does difficulty with performing basic ADL" (Katz & Alfieri, 1997, p. 90). Therefore, it is highly recommended that occupational therapists take time to evaluate the occupations of greatest value to the client and focus on improving participation in those occupations in order to have the greatest impact on health and well-being. Sailing, golf, dancing, crafts, woodworking,

reading for pleasure, and more can all be enjoyed when the "tools of the trade" are adapted to accommodate physical limitations. Sample solutions for commonly encountered difficulties in leisure pursuits are in Table 8.8 and Figures 8.5 and 8.6.

Sources for Assistive Devices

Increasingly, manufacturers are designing products to be user-friendly regardless of one's ability. For example, OXO Good Grips™ produces widely available kitchen tools that are easier and more effective to use. Photographs of the assistive devices commonly used by people with rheumatic diseases can be found at the Arthritis Storefront on the Canadian Arthritis Society's Web site at www.arthritis.ca. Equipment can be ordered worldwide and paid for in Canadian or U.S. dollars through a direct link to Sammons Preston (http://www.sammonspreston.com) on the Arthritis Society's site. The Wright Stuff Arthritis Supplies is a similar site at www.arthritissupplies.com. Hundreds of assistive devices and technologies are described at www.abledata.com. Subscribing to consumer magazines like *Arthritis Today*, through the Arthritis Foundation (AF), or *Arthritis News*, through the Arthritis Society (TAS), also provides ongoing information about useful devices, strategies, and ways to promote health and well-being. The AF and TAS also provide information about community-based self-management and exercise programs. JointHealth™ (http://www.jointhealth. org/), founded by Cheryl Koehn, author of the RA

Table 8.8. Sample Difficulties Performing Leisure Occupations and Potential Solutions

Task	Underlying Performance Skills	Potential Solutions
Inability to maintain garden	Limited ROM prevents reaching to ground Unable to grasp tools Painful knees Fatigue	Explore garden designs like raised beds/terraced gardens, and containers; select low-maintenance plants; long-handled tools for leverage, lightweight tools, and enlarged handles; use knee pads or kneeling bench with handles; pace tasks
Difficulty walking for pleasure	Hip and knee pain and weakness Foot pain	Supportive shoes and orthoses; shock-absorbing insoles; graded exercise program to build up endurance; cane or walking stick to minimize load on hip/knee; knee support or orthosis
Difficulty playing musical instrument	Joint pain and instability Muscle weakness, decreased hand dexterity	Custom-designed orthoses; adapt instruments to compensate limited movement; pace activities; select music to match abilities; create nontraditional fingering pattern

Note. ROM = range of motion.

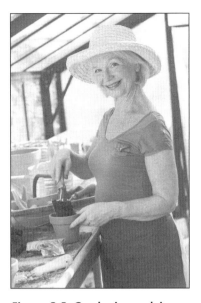

Figure 8.5. Gardening as leisure. Maintain good posture while gardening with potting table at an appropriate height. Photo: 123RF.com. Used under license.

experience shared in Box 8.3, is a source of plain-language, evidence-based, information for managing arthritis.

Summary

There are over 100 rheumatic diseases, many of which have progressive symptoms that lead to impairment of joint motion, muscle strength, endurance, and eventual disability. Occupational therapy offers a range of physical, cognitive, and

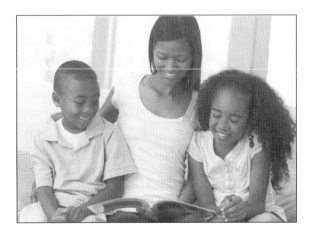

Figure 8.6. Client goals established in occupational therapy may address social roles of importance to individuals, in this case, nurturing children. Photo: 123RF.com. Used under license.

attitudinal strategies, assistive devices, and environmental modifications to enhance occupational performance and overcome many of the limitations caused by arthritis.

The increasing prevalence of arthritis, and the fact it is one of the most frequent causes of long-term pain and disability, led to 2000–2010 being named the Bone and Joint Decade, an initiative endorsed by the United Nations and dozens of organizations worldwide. The goal is to improve the health-related quality of life for people with musculoskeletal disorders throughout the world. Occupational therapy practitioners actively contribute to achieving this goal every time they work to improve the occupational performance of people living with arthritis.

Acknowledgments

The author acknowledges the occupational therapists at the Mary Pack Arthritis Program, Vancouver Coastal Health, in Vancouver, BC. Through collaborations over the years, they have undoubtedly contributed many of the ideas presented in this chapter.

Study Questions

1. Contrast and compare the effects of OA and RA on occupational performance and performance skills.
2. Gary is a 65-year-old man with OA in his right knee, secondary to injuries sustained during his college football years. Jenny is a 67-year-old woman who has had rheumatoid arthritis for 23 years, affecting her wrists, hands, knees, and feet. Both Gary and Jenny are having knee replacement surgery. Anticipate the occupational performance problems for both Gary and Jenny in the 3 months following surgery, and propose strategies and equipment for resolving those problems.
3. List 5 principles of joint protection. Give an example of how each one can be applied to a specific limitation in occupational performance you anticipate might arise for Meredith and Ray (see their case stories in Box 8.1).
4. Write down 3 of the most important tasks you must complete this week. If your metacarpal and wrist joints were painful, your grip strength reduced, and feelings of fatigue made you want to rest just 5 hours after you got out of bed, what impact would this have on your ability to complete those tasks?
5. Propose alternative strategies, assistive devices, or environmental modifications that might assist you to do the tasks you listed in response to Question 4. Critically evaluate each one, and state whether or not you would accept these suggestions. Why or why not?

6. List 3 principles of self-management, and describe how you will reinforce Gary and Jenny's capacity for self-managing their arthritis. Now consider Meredith and Ray, and outline ways to enhance self-management.

References

Adam, P. M., White, M. A., & Lacaille, D. (2007). Arthritis and self-employment: Strategies for success from the self-employment literature and from the experiences of people with arthritis. *Journal of Vocational Rehabilitation, 26,* 141–152.

Allaire, S. H., Anderson, J. J., & Meenan, R. F. (1996). Reducing work disability associated with rheumatoid arthritis: Identification of additional risk factors and persons likely to benefit from intervention. *Arthritis and Rheumatism, 9,* 349–357.

Allaire, S., & Keysor, J. J. (2009). Development of a structured interview tool to help patients identify and solve rheumatic condition-related work barriers. *Arthritis and Rheumatism (Arthritis Care and Research), 61,* 988–995.

Allaire, S., Wolfe, F., Niu, J., & LaValley, M. P. (2008). Contemporary prevalence and incidence of work disability associated with rheumatoid arthritis in the U.S. *Arthritis and Rheumatism (Arthritis Care and Research), 59,* 474–80.

Backman, C. L. (2006). Arthritis and pain. Psychosocial aspects in the management of arthritis pain. *Arthritis Research and Therapy, 8,* 221. Retrieved September 12, 2009, from http:arthritis-research.com/content/8/6/221

Backman, C. L., Del Fabro Smith, L., Smith, S., Montie, P. L., & Suto, M. (2007). The experiences of mothers living with inflammatory arthritis. *Arthritis and Rheumatism (Arthritis Care and Research), 57,* 381–388.

Backman, C. L., Fairleigh, A., & Kuchta, G. (2004). Occupational therapy. In B. Hayes, D. S. Pisetsky, & B. St. Clair (Eds.), *RA: Rheumatoid arthritis* (pp. 431–439). Philadelphia: Lippincott Williams & Wilkins.

Backman, C. L., Kennedy, S. M., Chalmers, A., & Singer, J. (2004). Participation in paid and unpaid work by adults with rheumatoid arthritis. *Journal of Rheumatology, 31,* 47–57.

Backman, C., Mackie, H., & Harris, J. (1991). Arthritis hand function test: Development of a standardized assessment tool. *Occupational Therapy Journal of Research, 11,* 245–256.

Backman, C., & Medcalf, N. (2000). Identifying components and environmental conditions contributing to occupational performance issues. In V. G. Fearing & J. Clark (Eds.), *Individuals in context: A practical guide to client-centered practice* (pp. 55–67). Thorofare, NJ: Slack.

Backman, C. L., Village, J., & Lacaille, D. (2008). The ergonomic assessment tool for arthritis (EATA): Development and pilot testing. *Arthritis and Rheumatism (Arthritis Care and Research), 59,* 1495–1503.

Badley, E., & DesMeules, M. (2003). Introduction. In *Arthritis in Canada: An ongoing challenge* (pp. 1–6). Ottawa, Ontario: Health Canada. (Cat. #H39-4/14-2003E)

Beaton, D. E., Katz, J. N., Fossel, A. H., Wright, J. G., Tarasuk, V., & Bombardier, C. (2001). Measuring the whole or the parts? Validity, reliability, and responsiveness of the disabilities of the arm, shoulder, and hand outcome measure in different regions of the upper extremity. *Journal of Hand Therapy, 14,* 128–146.

Bellamy, N. (1995). *WOMAC Osteoarthritis Index: User's guide.* London, Ontario: University of Western Ontario.

Bellamy, N., Campbell. J., Haraoui, B., Gerecz-Simon, E., Buchbinder, R., Hobby, K., et al. (2002). Clinimetric properties of the AUSCAN Osteoarthritis Hand Index: An evaluation of reliability, validity, and responsiveness. *Osteoarthritis Cartilage, 10,* 863–869.

Brady, T. J., & Boutaugh, M. L. (2006). Self-management education and support. In S. J. Bartlett, C. O. Bingham, M. J. Maricic, M. D. Iversen, & V. Rugging (Eds.), *Clinical care in the rheumatic diseases* (3rd ed., pp. 203–210). Atlanta: Association of Rheumatology Health Professionals.

Burckhardt, C. S., Clark S. R., & Bennett, R. M. (1991). The Fibromyalgia Impact Questionnaire: Development and validation. *Journal of Rheumatology, 18,* 728–734.

Calin, A., Garrett, S., Whitelock, H., Kennedy, L. G., O'Hea, J., Mallorie, P., et al. (1994). A new approach to defining functional ability in ankylosing spondylitis: The development of the Bath ankylosing spondylitis functional index. *Journal of Rheumatology, 21,* 2281–2285.

Cassidy J. T., & Petty, R. E. (2001). *Textbook of pediatric rheumatology* (4th ed.). Philadelphia: W.B. Saunders.

Chorus, A. M. J., Boonen, A., Miedema, H. S., & van der Linden, S. (2002). Employment perspectives of patients with ankylosing spondylitis. *Annals of Rheumatic Diseases, 61,* 693–699.

Chung, K. C., Pillsbury, M. S., Walters, M. R., et al. (1998). Reliability and validity testing of the Michigan Hand Outcomes Questionnaire. *Journal of Hand Surgery, 23,* 575–587.

Crooks, V. A. (2007). Women's experiences of developing musculoskeletal diseases: Employment challenges and policy recommendations. *Disability and Rehabilitation, 29,* 1107–1116.

Duruöz, M. T., Poiraudeau, S., Fermanian, J., Menkes, C., Amor, B., Dougados, M., et al. (1996). Development and validation of a rheumatoid hand functional disability scale that assesses functional handicap. *Journal of Rheumatology, 23,* 1167–1172.

Forhan, M., & Backman, C. L. (2010). Exploring occupational balance (OB) in adults with rheumatoid arthritis (RA). *OTJR: Occupation, Participation and Health.* Available from http://www.otjronline.com/advanced.asp.

Forsyth, K., Deshpande, S., Kielhofner, G., Henriksson, C., Haglund, L., Olson, L., et al. (2005). *The Occupational Circumstances Assessment Interview and Rating Scale (OCAIRS)* (version 4.0). Chicago, IL:

MOHO Clearinghouse. Available from http://www.moho.uic.edu/assess/ocairs.html

Fries, J. F., Spitz, P., Kraines, R. G., & Holman, H. R. (1980). Measurement of patient outcomes in arthritis. *Arthritis and Rheumatism, 23,* 137–145.

Gerber, L. H., & Furst, G. P. (1992). Validation of the NIH activity record: A quantitative measure of life activities. *Arthritis and Rheumatism, 5,* 81–86.

Gignac, M. A. M., Backman, C. L., Davis, A. M., Lacaille, D., Mattison, C. A., Montie, P., et al. (2008). Social role participation: What matters to people with arthritis? *Journal of Rheumatology, 35,* 1655–1663.

Gilworth, G., Chamberlain, M. A., Harvey, A., Woodhouse, A., Smith, J., Smyth, M. G., et al. (2003). Development of a work instability scale for rheumatoid arthritis. *Arthritis and Rheumatism (Arthritis Care and Research), 49,* 349–354.

Hainsworth, J., & Barlow, J. (2001). Volunteers' experiences of becoming arthritis self-management lay leaders: "It's almost as if I've stopped aging and started to get younger!" *Arthritis and Rheumatism (Arthritis Care and Research), 45,* 378–383.

Hammond, A., & Freeman, K. (2001). One-year outcomes of a randomized controlled trial of an educational–behavioural joint protection programme for people with rheumatoid arthritis. *Rheumatology, 40,* 1044–1051.

Hannan, M. T. (2001). Epidemiology of rheumatic diseases. In L. Robbins, C. S. Burckhardt, M. T. Hannan, & R. J. DeHoratius (Eds.), *Clinical care in the rheumatic diseases* (2nd ed., pp. 9–14). Atlanta: Association of Rheumatology Health Professionals.

Harrell, P. B. (2001). Splinting of the hand. In L. Robbins, C. S. Burckhardt, M. T. Hannan, & R. J. DeHoratius (Eds.), *Clinical care in the rheumatic diseases* (2nd ed., pp. 191–196). Atlanta: Association of Rheumatology Health Professionals.

Haskett, S., Backman, C., Porter, B., Goyert, J., & Palejko, G. (2004). A crossover trial of commercial versus custom-made wrist splints in the management of inflammatory polyarthritis. *Arthritis and Rheumatism (Arthritis Care and Research), 51,* 792–799.

Helmick, C. G., Felson, D. T., Lawrence, R. C., Gabriel, S., Hirsch, R., Kwoh, C. K., et al. (2008). Estimates of the prevalence of arthritis and other rheumatic conditions in the United States. *Arthritis and Rheumatism, 58,* 15–25.

Hennell, S., & Luqmani, R. (2008). Developing multidisciplinary guidelines for the management of early rheumatoid arthritis. *Musculoskeletal Care, 6,* 97–107.

Katz, P. P., & Alfieri, W. S. (1997). Satisfaction with abilities and well-being: Development and validation of a questionnaire for use among persons with rheumatoid arthritis. *Arthritis and Rheumatism, 10,* 89–98.

Katz, P., Morris, A., Trupin, L., Yazdany, J., & Yelin, E. (2008). Disability in valued life activities among individuals with systemic lupus erythematosus. *Arthritis and Rheumatism, 59,* 465–473.

Katz, P. P., & Yelin, E. H. (2001). Activity loss and the onset of depressive symptoms: Do some activities matter more than others? *Arthritis and Rheumatism, 44,* 1194–1202.

Khani-Hanjani, A., Lacaille, D., Hoar, D., Chalmers, A., Horsman, D., Anderson, M., et al. (2000). Association between dinucleotide repeat in non-coding region of interferon-gamma gene and susceptibility to, and severity of, rheumatoid arthritis. *Lancet, 356,* 820–825.

Koehn, C. L. (2006). Living with rheumatoid arthritis: Accepting the diagnosis and finding "normal" again. In S. J. Bartlett, C. O. Bingham, M. J. Maricic, M. D. Iversen, & V. Rugging (Eds.), *Clinical care in the rheumatic diseases* (3rd ed., pp. 303–305). Atlanta: Association of Rheumatology Health Professionals.

Kuchta, G., & Davidson, I. (2008). *Occupational and physical therapy for children with rheumatic diseases: A clinical handbook.* Oxford, England: Radcliffe.

Lacaille, D., Anis, A. H., Guh, A. H., & Esdaile, J. M. (2005). Gaps in care for rheumatoid arthritis: A population study. *Arthritis and Rheumatism (Arthritis Care and Research), 53,* 241–248.

Lacaille, D., Sheps, S., Spinelli, J. J., Chalmers, A., & Esdaile, J. M. (2004). Identification of modifiable work-related factors that influence the risk of work disability in rheumatoid arthritis. *Arthritis and Rheumatism (Arthritis Care and Research), 51,* 843–852.

Lacaille, D., White, M. A., Backman, C. L., & Gignac, M. A. M. (2007). New insights gained from understanding people's perspectives on problems faced at work due to inflammatory arthritis. *Arthritis and Rheumatism (Arthritis Care and Research), 57,* 1269–1279.

Lacaille, D., White, M. A., Rogers, P. A., Backman, C. L., Gignac, M. A. M., & Esdaile, J. M. (2008). Employment and arthritis: Making it work—A proof of concept study. *Arthritis and Rheumatism (Arthritis Care and Research), 59,* 1647–1655.

Lagace, C., Perruccio, A., DesMeules, M., & Badley, E. (2003). The impact of arthritis on Canadians. In *Arthritis in Canada: An ongoing challenge* (pp. 1–6). Ottawa, Ontario: Health Canada. (Cat. #H39-4/14-2003E)

Lam, C., Young, N., Marwaha, J., McLimont, M., & Feldman, B. M. (2004). Revised versions of the Childhood Health Assessment Questionnaire (CHAQ) are more sensitive and suffer less from a ceiling effect. *Arthritis and Rheumatism (Arthritis Care and Research), 51,* 881–889.

Law, M. (1998). Does client-centered practice make a difference? In M. Law (Ed.), *Client-centered occupational therapy* (pp. 19–27). Thorofare, NJ: Slack.

Law, M., Baptiste, S., Carswell, A., McColl, M. A., Polatajko, H., & Pollack, N. (2005). *The Canadian Occupational Performance Measure* (4th ed.). Ottawa, Ontario: CAOT.

Lerner, D., Amick, B. C., Rogers, W. H., Malspeis, S., Bungay, K., & Cynn, D. (2001). The Work Limitations Questionnaire. *Medical Care, 39,* 72–85.

Lewis, K. S. (2006). The patient's experience. In S. J. Bartlett, C. O. Bingham, M. J. Maricic, M. D. Iversen, & V. Rugging (Eds.), *Clinical care in the rheumatic diseases* (3rd ed., pp. 89–94). Atlanta: Association of Rheumatology Health Professionals.

Lorig, K. (1993). Self-management of chronic illness: A model for the future. *Generations, 17*(3), 11–14.

Mann, W. (1998). Assistive technology for persons with arthritis. In J. Melvin & G. Jensen (Eds.), *Rheumatologic rehabilitation series. Volume 1: Assessment and management* (pp. 369–392). Bethesda, MD: American Occupational Therapy Association.

Mann, W. C., Tomita, M., Hurren, D., & Charvat, B. (1999). Changes in health, functional, and psychosocial status and coping strategies of home-based older persons with arthritis over three years. *Occupational Therapy Journal of Research, 19*, 126–146.

Manuel, D., Lagace, D., DesMeules, M., Cho, R., & Power, J. D. (2003). Life Expectancy and Health-Adjusted Life Expectancy (HALE). In *Arthritis in Canada: An ongoing challenge* (pp. 40–41). Ottawa, Ontario: Health Canada. (Cat. #H39-4/14-2003E)

Maricic, M. J. (2001). Osteoporosis. In L. Robbins, C. S. Burckhardt, M. T. Hannan, & R. J. DeHoratius (Eds.), *Clinical care in the rheumatic diseases* (2nd ed., pp. 121–126). Atlanta: Association of Rheumatology Health Professionals.

Meenan, R. F., Mason, J. H., Anderson, J. J., Guccione, A. A., & Kazis, L. E. (1992). AIMS2: The content and properties of a revised and expanded arthritis impact measurement scales health status questionnaire. *Arthritis and Rheumatism, 35*, 1–10.

Nell, V. P. K., Machold, K. P., Eberl, G., Stamm, T. A., Uffmann, M., & Smolen, J. S. (2004). Benefit of very early referral and very early therapy with disease-modifying anti-rheumatic drugs in patients with early rheumatoid arthritis. *Rheumatology, 43*, 906–914.

Plach, S. K., Heidrich, S. M., & Waite, R. M. (2003). Relationship of social role quality to psychological well-being in women with rheumatoid arthritis. *Research in Nursing and Health, 26*, 190–202.

Poole, J. L., Gallegos, M., & O'Linc, S. (2000). Reliability and validity of the Arthritis Hand Function Test in adults with systemic sclerosis (scleroderma). *Arthritis and Rheumatism, 13*, 69–73.

Poole, J. L., Willer, K., & Mendelson, C. (2009). Occupation of motherhood: Challenges for mothers with scleroderma. *American Journal of Occupational Therapy, 63*, 214–219.

Ramsey-Goldman, R. (2001). Connective tissue diseases. In L. Robbins, C. S. Burckhardt, M. T. Hannan, & R. J. DeHoratius (Eds.), *Clinical care in the rheumatic diseases* (2nd ed., pp. 97–103). Atlanta: Association of Rheumatology Health Professionals.

Riemsma, R. P., Kirwan, J. R., Taal, E., & Rasker, J. J. (2002). Patient education for adults with rheumatoid arthritis (Cochrane Review). *The Cochrane Library*, Issue 2.

Sandqvist, G., & Eklund, M. (2000). Hand Mobility in Scleroderma (HAMIS) test: The reliability of a novel hand function test. *Arthritis and Rheumatism, 13*, 369–374.

Singh, G., Athreya, B., Fries, J., & Goldsmith, D. (1994). Measurement of health status in children with juvenile rheumatoid arthritis. *Arthritis and Rheumatism, 37*, 1761–1769.

Stamm, T., Lovelock, L., Stew, G., Nell, V., Smolen, J., Jonsson, H., et al. (2008). I have mastered the challenge of living with a chronic disease: Life stories of people with rheumatoid arthritis. *Qualitative Health Research, 18*, 658–669.

Steultjens, E. E. M. J., Dekker, J. J., Bouter, L. M., Schaardenburg, D. D., Kuyk, M. A. M. A. H., & Van den Ende, E. C. H. M. (2004). Occupational therapy for rheumatoid arthritis. *Cochrane Database of Systematic Reviews 2004, Issue 1* (Art. No.: CD003114). doi: 10.1002/14651858.CD003114.pub2

Taylor, J., & Erlandson, D. M. (2001). Pediatric rheumatic diseases. In L. Robbins, C. S. Burckhardt, M. T. Hannan, & R. J. DeHoratius (Eds.), *Clinical care in the rheumatic diseases* (2nd ed., pp. 81–88). Atlanta: Association of Rheumatology Health Professionals.

van Lankveld, W., van't Pad Bosch, P., Bakker, J., et al. (1996). Sequential Occupational Dexterity Assessment (SODA): A new test to measure hand disability. *Journal of Hand Therapy, 9*, 27–32.

Wolfe F., Michaud K., Pincus T. (2004). Development and validation of the Health Assessment Questionnaire II: A revised version of the Health Assessment Questionnaire. *Arthritis and Rheumatism, 50*(10), 3064–3067.

Wright, F. V., Law, M., Crombie, V., & Goldsmith, C. H. (1994). Development of a self-report functional status index for juvenile rheumatoid arthritis. *Journal of Rheumatology, 21*, 536–544.

Yelin, E., Cisternas, M., Foreman, A., Pasta, D., Murphy, L., & Helmick, C. G. (2007). National and state medical expenditures and lost earnings attributable to arthritis and other rheumatic conditions—United States, 2003. *Morbidity and Mortality Weekly Report, 56*(01), 4–7.

Zhang, Y., & Jordan, J. M. (2008). Epidemiology of osteoarthritis. *Rheumatic Diseases Clinics of North America, 34*, 515–529.

Chapter 9

Enabling Performance and Participation Following Spinal Cord Injury

THERESA GREGORIO-TORRES, MA, OTR, ATP; RAFFERTY LAREDO, MA, OTR, ATP; AND SUZANNE KRENEK ANDREWS, MOT, OTR, ATP

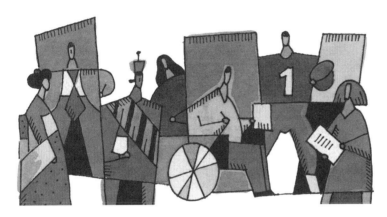

KEY WORDS

ASIA impairment
scale

autonomic
dysreflexia

intermittent
catheterization

paraplegia

pressure ulcer

tenodesis grasp

tetraplegia

HIGHLIGHTS

- The American Spinal Injury Association recommends that therapists use the International Standards for Neurological Classification of Spinal Cord Injury as the standard measure of impairment among people with SCI (Cohen, Sheehan, & Herbison, 1996).

- People with SCI above the T6 level must be familiar with how to manage autonomic dysreflexia and be able to instruct others, such as their family members and caregivers, in what to do should this life-threatening condition occur.

- Once a person gains skill and proficiency in ADLs and IADLs, focus can be turned to returning to productive living in the community.

- Addressing a client's level of participation in managing his or her own bowel and bladder needs plays an important role in increasing quality of life.

- Many types of assistive technology are available to assist clients in communication, computer access, and environmental control.

- People with SCI should be educated on upper-limb complications that they might experience after years of overuse and take measures to preserve their upper extremities.

OBJECTIVES

After reading this material, readers will be able to

- Distinguish between paraplegia and tetraplegia;
- Discuss the prevalence of spinal cord injury (SCI), the potential secondary health complications, and possible innovative treatment strategies;
- Understand how a SCI affects every aspect of a person's daily life;
- Describe the performance limitations experienced by people with various levels of SCI; and
- Describe adaptive strategies, equipment, or environmental modifications for activities of daily living (ADLs), instrumental activities of daily living (IADLs), work, play, and leisure for people with SCI.

The term *spinal cord injury (SCI)* refers to the disruption of the spinal cord secondary to trauma that results in the loss of sensory and motor function below the level of the injury. SCI is a life-altering event that can interfere with every aspect of occupational performance and quality of life. Unlike injuries to the extremities, SCI is complex and often results in an overwhelming loss of function, thereby presenting enormous multidimensional problems and challenges for patients and therapists alike.

Prevalence of Spinal Cord Injuries

Not until the 1940s, following World War II, were rehabilitation programs developed for people with SCI. These represented a new philosophy of care (Clifton, Donovan, & Frankowski, 1985; DeVivo, 2007). Today, more than 259,000 people in the United States live with SCI, and approximately 12,000 new cases are reported every year (National Spinal Cord Injury Statistical Center, 2008). The war veteran population makes up 22% of people with SCI (Weaver, Hammond, Guihan, & Hendricks, 2000).

The most frequent causes of SCI are motor vehicle crashes (42.1%), falls (26.7%), acts of violence (15.1%), and recreational sporting activities (7.65%). SCI occurs most frequently in males (80.9%). As the median age of the general population of the United States has increased since the 1970s, the average age at injury has also steadily increased. Since 2005, the average age at injury is 40.2 years. Among patients injured since 2005, 66.1% are Caucasian, 27.1% are African-American, 8.1% are Hispanic, and 2% are Asian (National Spinal Cord Injury Statistical Center, 2009). Almost half of people with SCI had completed high school, and more than half were unmarried (DeVivo, 2002). More than half (57.4%) of those with SCI admitted to one of the federally funded SCI research centers (Model Systems centers) reported being employed at the time of injury. In the past, the major cause of death was renal failure. Due to improved methods of urological management, the major causes of death for this population are now pneumonia, pulmonary emboli, and septicemia. Other complications that may arise soon after injury—and that can become lifelong problems—are spasticity, fractures, heterotrophic ossification, osteoporosis, pressure ulcers, hypotension, and urinary tract infections (National Spinal Cord Injury Statistical Center, 2008).

Role of Occupational Therapy

The role of occupational therapy in the evaluation and treatment of people with SCI has evolved into a complex array of intervention categories. Occupational therapists assume responsibility for evaluation and training in all aspects of occupational performance, including activities of daily living (ADLs) and instrumental activities of daily living (IADLs). Therapists also design, fabricate, or recommend assistive devices that maximize independence; help the client strengthen innervated muscles, particularly in the arms; explore avocational and vocational interests and skills; facilitate psychosocial adjustment to disability; and apply the latest approaches and technologies that promote maximum independence (Atkins, 2002; Gadberry & Frauenheim-Finke, 1996; Garber, 1985). Therapists primarily focus on helping their SCI clients use adaptive strategies, including equipment and environmental modifications, to enhance ADLs, IADLs, work, education, play, leisure, and social participation.

Rehabilitation of people with SCI involves evaluation and treatment in environmental access, pressure ulcer prevention, mobility, assistive technology use, adaptive skills training, and sexuality (Atkins, 2008; Garber, 1985). New challenges for occupational therapists include the reduced length of hospital stay and being fully informed of the growing community-based vocational rehabilitation and independent living programs for people with SCI (Tate, Henrich, Pasuke, & Anderson, 1998). Over the past decade, use of outpatient or home health occupational therapy services has become essential in helping clients achieve levels of functional independence that were previously achieved during inpatient hospitalization (Atkins, 2008). Consequently, long-term improvements have been seen in social integration, occupational independence, and economic self-sufficiency (DeVivo, 2007). Occupational therapists must be equipped with the requisite knowledge and resources to meet these functional independence needs for their clients with SCI in community settings.

The Functional Independence Measure (now known as The FIM™) is a common assessment used by occupational therapists to document their clients' occupational performance and progress throughout the intervention process. It is often supplemented by other objective scales that provide the sensitivity and detail necessary to document changes in performance of all meaningful occupations (Watson, Kanny, White, & Anson, 1995). The Canadian Occupational Performance Measure (COPM) is another useful interview tool to query clients' performance, participation goals, and priorities for their treatment regime (Atkins, 2008).

This chapter describes the performance challenges in daily living faced by people with SCI. Four major categories, based on level of injury, are considered: (1) High-level tetraplegia C1–C4; (2) Tetraplegia C5–C6, C7–C8; (3) Paraplegia T1–T6; and (4) Paraplegia T7–S5. The neurological levels of the spinal cord form the basis of this chapter. (The cervical spinal cord and its associated muscles and functional levels are described in Table 9.1.)

In addition to describing the neurological levels of the spinal cord, physicians and therapists also determine the neurological completeness of an injury. The American Spinal Injury Association (ASIA) recommends that therapists use the International Standards for Neurological Classification of Spinal Cord Injury as the standard measure of impairment (Cohen et al., 1996). ASIA has adopted the ASIA Motor and Sensory Scale (modified and updated from the Frankel grading system) to define the level of injury. The determination of which segments of the spinal cord have been affected is established by systematically examining the dermatomes and myotomes of the body (ASIA, 2008). The ASIA Scale is described in Table 9.2. The examination components (i.e., motor and sensory testing) are reliable, but confident and competent interpretation of the results requires thorough training and experience.

Among people with SCI, injuries to the cervical spine often result in greater loss of functional performance. Table 9.3 provides an overview of the expected performance outcomes in ADLs for different levels of injury. Not all lesions are complete, however, so the actual abilities and levels of independence achieved by clients with injures at different levels will vary. The client's age, motivation, pre-injury lifestyle, body size and shape, circumstances, and the presence of other injuries all influence rehabilitation outcomes.

Traumatic SCI not only causes sensorimotor impairment but also affects all body systems. Members of the rehabilitation team (physicians, therapists, nurses) assess the client's neurological status in conjunction with comprehensive and systematic assessments of the musculoskeletal, pulmonary, cardiovascular, gastrointestinal, genitourinary (GU), and integumentary systems (James & Cardenas, 2003). Spasticity, bowel and bladder dysfunction, and respiratory and circulatory complications can significantly interfere with rehabilitation, participation in occupational therapy, and overall quality of life. Because people with SCI are living longer than even a decade ago, they are at risk to develop some of the medical conditions that affect the general population, such as diabetes, heart disease, arthritis, musculoskeletal conditions, age-related cognitive decline, and cancer. The frequent medical complications seen in patients who have survived 30 years include pressure ulcers; musculoskeletal conditions; gastrointestinal and cardiovascular problems; GU problems, including urinary tract infections; pneumonia; osteoporosis; and syringomyelia (Cardenas, Burns, & Chan, 2000; Cardenas, Hoffman, Kirshblum, & McKinley, 2004).

People with SCI must be familiar with how to manage autonomic dysreflexia and be able to instruct others, such as their caregivers, in what to do should this condition occur. *Autonomic dysreflexia* (also called *autonomic hyperreflexia*) is a sudden and severe rise in blood pressure. It is a potentially life-threatening condition that affects people with SCI above vertebral level T6. Caused by various noxious stimuli that trigger sympathetic hyperactivity, autonomic dysreflexia can result from bladder or bowel distension, suppository insertion, skin irritation,

Table 9.1. Functional Levels of the Cervical Spinal Cord

Roots	Muscles	Function
C2, C3	Sternocleidomastoid	Neck flexion and head rotation
C3, C4	Trapezius Superior Middle Inferior	 Neck extension and scapular elevation Scapular adduction Scapular adduction and depression
C3, C4, C5	Diaphragm	Respiration
C4, C5	Rhomboids	Scapular medial adduction, retraction, and elevation
C5, C6	Deltoid Anterior Middle Posterior Supraspinatus Infraspinatus Teres minor Subscapularis Teres major Biceps brachii Brachialis Brachioradialis Extensor carpi radialis longus	 Shoulder flexion to 90° Shoulder abduction to 90° Shoulder extension and horizontal abduction Shoulder abduction Shoulder lateral rotation Shoulder medial rotation Elbow flexion and forearm supination Elbow flexion Wrist flexion and abduction
C5, C6, C7	Serratus anterior	Shoulder forward thrust; scapular rotation for shoulder abduction
C5, T1	Pectoralis major Pectoralis minor	Shoulder adduction, flexion, and medial rotation Shoulder forward and downward
C6, C7	Supinator Pronator teres	Forearm supination Forearm pronation
C6, C7, C8	Latissimus dorsi Triceps brachii Extensor digiti communis Extensor digiti minimus	Shoulder medial rotation Elbow extension MCP extension Little finger extension
C7, C8	Extensor indicis proprius Extensor carpi ulnaris Extensor pollicis longus Extensor pollicis brevis Abductor pollicis longus	Index finger MCP extension Wrist extension Thumb IP extension Thumb MCP extension Thumb abduction
C7, C8, T1	Flexor digitorum superficialis Flexor digitorum profundus	IP flexion DIP flexion
C8, T1	Flexor carpi ulnaris Interossei Dorsales Palmares Flexor pollicis longus Flexor pollicis brevis Abductor pollicis Adductor pollicis brevis Opponens pollicis Lumbricales	Wrist flexion and adduction MCP flexion Finger abduction Finger adduction Thumb IP flexion Thumb MCP flexion Thumb abduction Thumb adduction Thumb opposition MCP flexion

Note. DIP = distal interphalangeal; IP = interphalangeal; MCP = metacarpophalangeal.
From *Specialized Occupational Therapy for Persons With High Level Quadriplegia* by S. L. Garber, P. Lathem, and T. L. Gregorio, 1988, Houston: TIRR. Copyright © 1988 by TIRR. Reprinted by permission. There may be some variation among references regarding actual nerve roots and innervated muscles.

Table 9.2. International Standards for Neurological Classification of Spinal Cord Injury (ASIA Impairment Scale)

A = *Complete:* No motor or sensory function is preserved in the sacral segments S4–S5.

B = *Incomplete:* Sensory but not motor function is preserved below the neurological level and includes the sacral segments S4–S5.

C = *Incomplete:* Motor function is preserved below the neurological level, and more than half of key muscles below the neurological level have a muscle grade less than 3.

D = *Incomplete:* Motor function is preserved below the neurological level, and at least half of key muscles below the neurological level have a muscle grade of 3 or more.

E = *Normal:* Motor and sensory function are normal.

clothing or legbag straps that are too tight, or pressure ulcers. It can lead to a cerebrovascular accident or death if not relieved (Consortium for Spinal Cord Medicine, 2001).

Occupational therapists should not overlook cognitive and psychosocial problems associated with SCI. Although cognition usually remains intact unless concomitant brain injury occurred at the time of the spinal injury, standardized assessment tools should be used to determine cognitive status. Depression, adaptation to disability, family dynamics and support, sexuality, and the risk of secondary complications must all be evaluated.

High-Level Tetraplegia: Levels C1–C4

High-level tetraplegia is paralysis resulting from an injury to the spinal cord at any segmental level between the C1 and C4 vertebrae. For the purpose of this chapter, this term describes those individuals with any of the following conditions: a neurological level of C4 or above, (complete motor and sensory deficits bilaterally), total or partial dependence on breathing aids, long-term medical and personal care needs, and limited expected functional recovery (Garber et al., 1988).

Although people with high-level SCI usually are dependent on others for self-care, they learn to verbally instruct others in their care, thereby attaining and maintaining some control in their life. The three major objectives in the rehabilitation of clients with C1 through C4 tetraplegia are (1) education for clients and their caregivers regarding their care, (2) exposure to ADLs and IADLs, and (3) adaptation through the use of assistive technology.

Clients with SCI at the C1 through C2 level are ventilator-dependent and may be candidates for bilateral phrenic nerve stimulator implants and diaphragm pacing. The primary innervated muscle is the sternocleidomastoid, which controls neck flexion and head rotation. At the C4 level, the significant innervated muscles are the diaphragm and the upper trapezius. A client with SCI at this level may need a ventilator at first, but he or she usually can be weaned from the ventilator over time. Active movement includes full neck rotation, neck extension and flexion, and some scapular elevation. Little or no scapular depression exists (Hislop & Montgomery, 2002).

Clients with SCI at the C1 through C4 level need stable head and neck support for safety and comfort when washing or shaving the face, combing hair, or applying makeup. A caretaker must perform those tasks, as well as those related to dressing, feminine hygiene, and bowel/bladder care. Clients with tetraplegia naturally will have preferences regarding how those tasks should be performed. They must be able to give accurate directions to caregivers to ensure that the tasks are completed in the preferred manner and with the necessary care.

Eating

Head position and sitting angle may affect a client's ability to chew and successfully swallow food or medications, especially if the SCI includes any involvement of the brain stem. For both safety and enjoyment, clients must be able to independently direct another person in proper positioning when eating. Sensitive cooperation between the client with high-level tetraplegia and the helper can make mealtimes more enjoyable and satisfying (Martinsen, Harder, & Biering-Sorensen, 2008). Assistive devices with switch access allow clients with high-level SCI to participate in self-feeding. The Winsford Feeder™ (Figure 9.1) allows clients without the use of their arms to operate a mechanical device with a chin control to bring food from their plate to their mouth. Another piece of equipment that is often helpful is a long straw so that the client can drink when he or she desires without having to reach for

Table 9.3. Expected Performance Outcomes for Individuals With Complete Spinal Cord Injury

Location of Injury	Mobility	Orthotic Devices	Community Transport	Communication	Feeding	Grooming	Bathing	Dressing	Toileting
C1–C4	Can use pneumatic, chin/lip control, head array switch, or remote proportional switch power wheelchair with power weight-shifting system	Dorsal cock-up splint, positioning orthosis	Needs assistance of others in accessible van with lift, cannot drive	Can use phone and computer with adapted equipment; mouthstick or EADL device used to turn pages and write	Dependent in feeding or may use electronic feeding device; drinks with long straw after setup	Must rely on personal care assistance	Must rely on personal care assistance	Must rely on personal care assistance	Must rely on personal care assistance
C5	Can use power W/C with WSS indoors and outdoors; short, level distances in manual wheelchair with adapted hand rims on level/unlevelled surfaces	Upper-extremity positioning orthosis, dorsal cock-up splint, MAS	Can drive with specially adapted van	Can use phone, computer, write with adapted equipment	Can feed self with adapted equipment after setup	Will rely on assistance and will use adapted equipment	Must rely on personal care assistance	Requires assistance with U/E dressing; dependent for lower-extremity dressing	Needs personal care assistance and equipment
C6	Can travel short level distances with manual W/C with adaptations; may need assistance on unlevelled surfaces; independent in hand-controlled power W/C	Wrist-driven wrist-hand orthosis, universal cuff, writing devices, built-up handles	Independent driving in adapted van/vehicle; may need assistance with W/C loading	Can use phone, can also use computer and write with adapted equipment; can turn pages without assistance	Can be independent with adapted equipment, can drink from glass	Can be independent with adapted equipment	May require some assistance with upper- and lower-extremity bathing with adapted equipment	Independent with U/E dressing; assistance needed for L/E dressing	Independent for bowel routine; needs assistance with bladder routine and adapted equipment or technique
C7	Can use manual W/C on level/unlevelled surfaces except curbs/stairs	May use short opponens	Independent driving vehicle/adapted van with hand controls; can independently place W/C in vehicle	Independent in use of phone, keyboarding, writing and turning pages	Independent	Independent	Independent with equipment	Independent	Independent
C8–T7	Can use manual W/C on level/unlevelled surfaces	None	As above	Independent	Independent	Independent	Independent with equipment	Independent	Independent
T8–L3	Independent at W/C level; possible ambulation	KAFO with forearm crutches or walker	As above	Independent	Independent	Independent	Independent with equipment	Independent	Independent
L4–S1	Independent	AFO with forearm crutches/or cane	As above	Independent	Independent	Independent	Independent with equipment	Independent	Independent
S2–below	Independent	None	As above	Independent	Independent	Independent	Independent	Independent	Independent

Note. AFO = ankle–foot orthosis, EADL = electronic aids to daily living, KAFO = knee–ankle–foot orthosis, L/E = lower extremity, MAS = mobile arm support orthosis, U/E = upper extremity, W/C = wheelchair, WSS = weight-shifting system.

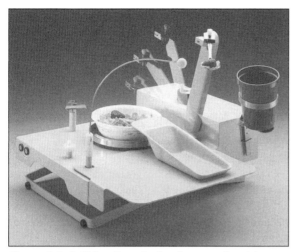

Figure 9.1. Self-feeding device for people with high-level SCI.
Photograph compliments of North Coast Medical Inc., Morgan Hill, CA., USA, www.ncmedical.com.

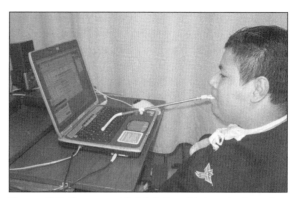

Figure 9.2. Person with high-level tetraplegia using a mouthstick.

the container of liquid. This simple act of taking a drink on their own allows clients to feel empowered and helpful in their care.

Medication Management

All people with SCI should be knowledgeable about the prescribed dosage and frequency of all their medications. Clients with C1 through C4 tetraplegia should be able to identify their medications visually and know the dosage, purpose, and side effects of each so that, in an emergency, they can let others know their medication history. Therapists can provide clients, their families, and caretakers with notebooks that are organized according to the client's current medications. Clients and caregivers not only must keep track of this information but also must commit it to memory; occupational therapists should test them on accuracy of the details.

Dental Care

To brush and floss their teeth, rinse their mouths, use mouthwash, or clean dentures, clients with C1 through C4 tetraplegia must rely on a caretaker. Because people with this level of injury may use a mouthstick to perform certain tasks, dental hygiene is extremely important. The structure and health of teeth and gums can affect their ability and ease in using a mouthstick or other similar device (see Figure 9.2). Clients should be encouraged to obtain dental evaluations at least annually to ensure healthy oral hygiene.

Bathing

Although people with C1 through C4 tetraplegia are totally dependent in bathing, options are available to allow caregivers to accomplish this activity efficiently and effectively. Bathing often takes place in bed because the bathroom is inaccessible or appropriate bathing equipment is not available. Some type of plastic covering can be used under the client to keep the bedding from getting wet, or a commercially available inflatable bathtub can be used on top of the bed to hold water. The inflatable bathtub is portable, which enables bathing while traveling. A basin of water and all necessary items (e.g., soap, washcloth and towels, shampoo, and a razor) should be brought to the bedside before the bath begins to reduce the time the client is exposed to the water and the possibility of cool room air. An inflatable shampoo basin also can be used for washing hair while the client is in bed.

If the bathroom is accessible, a tall-back shower lift sling with head and neck support may be used to support the body while the person sits on a padded tilted or reclined shower/commode chair. The sling helps ensure safe transfers and body support under wet conditions (Consortium for Spinal Cord Medicine, 1999b). A client who uses a ventilator must be protected from the possibility of water entering the trachea and the ventilator should be well protected from coming into contact with any water or moisture.

Dressing/Undressing

Clients with C1 through C4 tetraplegia will depend on others for dressing and undressing, but they can retain control over this task by making daily clothing selections. Considerations should be given to purchasing clothing designs that reduce the effort needed to dress and undress. Some suggestions for clothing choice include loose-fitting garments, stretchable fabrics, touch-fastener closures, slip-on shoes, minimal zippers and buttons, and elastic sleeves and waistbands (Farmer, 1986). V-neck or shirts with lower necklines may also be desirable to avoid interference with placement of a tracheostomy.

Because clients with SCI at C1–C4 have impaired sensation, fabrics should be selected that do not irritate the skin. Breathable materials, such as cotton, are best for air exchange between the atmosphere and the skin. Pants with double-welted seams and studs or rivets should be avoided because they can cause excessive pressure. Removing the rear pockets of pants reduces the risk of pressure from seams. Jewelry should be carefully selected for size because tight bracelets, necklaces, watchbands, and rings can restrict circulation. If swelling occurs, it might be necessary to cut off the jewelry.

The caregiver performs upper-body dressing in one of three ways: overhead, side to side, or around the back. People with C1 through C2 injury will need assistance to extend the neck; people with C3 through C4 injury can assist by flexing the neck forward. Nonrestrictive front access means that bras with front-touch fasteners or hooks will be easier to put on using the around-the-back method. Bras with back closures can be fastened first and then slipped over the head, much as one would put on a t-shirt. Clip-on ties or ties knotted partway are the easiest for a caregiver to put on someone with a C1 through C4 injury.

To undress the person's upper body, the caregiver performs the same technique in reverse. If the client is sitting in a wheelchair, he or she must be well supported during dressing and undressing to maximize trunk balance.

Lower-body dressing presents additional challenges. For example, the thick border seams at the leg openings of brief-style underpants sometimes cause pressure-induced skin breakdown over the ischial tuberosities. The seams of boxer shorts do not fall directly over these sensitive areas, so they may be a safer underwear choice. Excess cloth should be smoothed against the buttocks and upper legs, however, so that the underwear does not become wadded and cause undo pressure. Boxer-brief styles of underwear are also a smart choice, as the material remains smooth over pressure-prone areas.

Dressing technique also makes a difference. If the client is rolled side to side so that the garments can be pulled up over the hips, shearing and friction can occur and damage the skin. A safer technique is to place one leg in both the underwear and pants leg

openings simultaneously and pull up to knee level. Next, the other leg's underwear and pants leg openings are put on and pulled up to knee level. Then, the client is rolled to one side and the underwear and pants leg on that side are pulled up into place. Finally, the client is rolled to the opposite side and underwear and pants leg on that side are pulled into place. This minimizes excessive rolling, decreasing the likelihood of skin shearing and friction to the buttocks.

Loose-fitting socks are much easier to pull over the foot than tight, elasticized socks. Slip-on shoes or shoes with self-fastening closures also are recommended. If thigh-high antithrombolitic stockings are required for edema control or circulation issues, the caregiver must ensure that the top portion of the stockings stay properly in place around the thighs and do not roll down, causing a tourniquet effect around the legs.

Dressing and undressing tasks provide caregivers with convenient opportunities to thoroughly inspect the client's skin. Pressure ulcers or other lesions should be noted carefully and treated promptly.

Bowel and Bladder Care

Clients with C1 through C4 tetraplegia require assistance in all bowel and bladder management and feminine hygiene tasks, except for emptying legbags. Legbags can be emptied using a special electric legbag-emptying device, powered by the electric wheelchair battery. The emptying device is connected to the clamp that surrounds the legbag tubing. The client uses a breath control or lever switch mounted in an accessible place to activate the device. When not activated, the tube is held closed by pressure and does not allow urine to pass. When the electric switch is activated, the pressure is released from the tube, allowing urine to leave the legbag. This device limits a person to emptying the legbag into a floor drain, basin, or outdoors. Nonetheless, particularly for clients who are active in the community, the device can be liberating because it frees them from having to ask others to perform this personal task for them. Urine can be collected into a sealed bag that is attached to either the client's leg or around the abdominal area.

Maintaining a sitting position during a bowel program can assist in bowel evacuation (Consortium for Spinal Cord Medicine, 1998). A padded commode chair with a high back and head positioner is needed to give proper body support during this ADL. If the client needs to perform the bowel program at bed level, it is recommended that the client lie on his or her left side for the most effective evacuation (Consortium for Spinal Cord Medicine, 1999a). A disposable pad should be placed under the client for increased efficiency with cleanup. The caregiver must have adequate access to the rectal area for suppository insertion and completion of the bowel program.

Ovulation and fertility usually are not altered in women with SCI once spinal shock resolves. Women with C1 through C4 tetraplegia are dependent on caregivers to manage menstrual needs and birth control. Therapists and caregivers should respect client's choices in these intimate, personal matters.

Communication

People with C1 and C2 tetraplegia have limited head and neck control; using electronic equipment helps them more successfully complete tasks such as turning pages, computer use, activating audio/video devices, or using a telephone. People with C3 and C4 tetraplegia may use electronic devices or a mouthstick to achieve such tasks (Figure 9.3). People with SCI at this level often also use mouthsticks to participate in leisure and avocational activities, such as board games or games activated by remote control. Other frequently used communication-enhancing equipment includes bookholders; electric page turners; height-adjustable tables; modified work stations; mouthstick holders; computers with modified input devices; electronic aids to daily living (EADLs); keyboard keyguards; voice recognition software; hands-free technology; and phone enhancements like gooseneck supports, cellular phones, phone flippers, and speaker phones (Figure 9.4).

EADLs and computer input devices now operate reliably with voice commands. Access to phone systems may require a combination of mouthstick skills, voice activation, and setup by another individual.

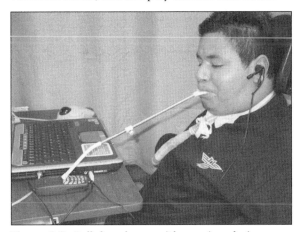

Figure 9.3. Cellular phone with earpiece being used by a person with high-level tetraplegia.

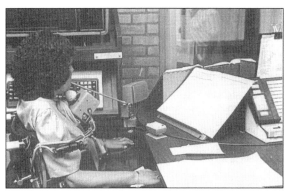

Figure 9.4. Work station modified for the person with high-level tetraplegia.

Meal Preparation

People with C1 through C4 tetraplegia use verbal instruction to fulfill family life roles, such as instructing a child in preparing a simple meal or using household appliances. During rehabilitation, a goal of occupational therapy for clients with C1 through C4 tetraplegia is for the person to learn to effectively direct someone to prepare a simple food item, such as a sandwich, and to use the microwave oven. The therapist's responsibility is to give the client direct feedback regarding the effectiveness of the instructions. Because difficulties with voice volume and word choice can decrease others' willingness to listen to assist the client, these aspects of verbal direction are considered as important as accuracy.

Functional Mobility

Transfers with clients with C1 through C4 tetraplegia can be accomplished in any of the following ways: a mechanical or electric lift transfer, a three-person lift, and a dependent sliding-board transfer. Therapists should take into account the client's size, weight, level of spasticity, and the caretaker's strength, in determining the safest and most effective method. The client must be prepared to verbally direct each step of the transfer using complete and accurate instructions.

Most people with C1 through C4 tetraplegia use a motorized (power) wheelchair for independent mobility. Appropriate driving mechanisms depend on the exact level of injury and may include a sip-and-puff control, chin control, fiberoptic head array, remote proportional joystick, or head control. A manual wheelchair is recommended as a backup to the power wheelchair. The frame style of the manual wheelchair may be upright, tilt, or reclining, depending on the client's needs. A pressure-redistribution seat cushion is required to distribute weight equally across the buttocks and provide pelvic stability while sitting (Consortium for Spinal Cord Medicine, 2000).

To activate the sip-and-puff breath control switch, the operator seals his or her lips around a straw-like tube and either softly or forcefully blows or sucks air into the tube to trigger the motors in the chosen direction. The chin control is operated by moving the jaw to direct a small, remote, proportional-drive joy stick positioned midline and mounted under the person's chin. A mini-joystick may also be used at the client's lips if they prefer this over using their chin. A fiberoptic head array or a remote proportional joystick mounted behind the person's head are additional options. Optimal positioning of the head array or remote proportional joystick is crucial for safe and reliable head placement and control (Figures 9.5 and 9.6). It is imperative that a stop switch be mounted in a reliable accessible location. The stop switch will allow the wheelchair to be stopped should the drive switch that normally is used become dislodged or out of reach of the person in the chair. An attendant control allows the caregiver to operate the power wheelchair when the client is unable to. The attendant control is often a small joystick mounted to the back or side of the wheelchair that can easily be controlled when needed by the caregiver.

A power-tilt or reclining system on a power wheelchair will allow the client to perform independent weight shifting to reduce the risk of pressure ulcers (Consortium for Spinal Cord Medicine, 1999b, 2000). A power-reclining system offers the most effective weight shifting because more body weight is distributed over a larger body surface during the maneuver. For people who experience postural problems from spasticity, changing the hip angle can cause them to sit out of alignment after a weight shift is performed. If spasticity is a significant problem, a power-tilt system would allow for shifting weight 45 degrees to 60 degrees, depending on

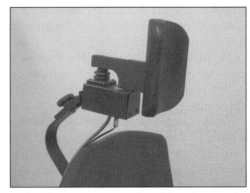

Figure 9.6. Remote proportional head control.

the manufacturer of the system (Cook & Hussey, 2002; Goossens, Snijders, Holscher, Heerens, & Holman, 1997; Lathem, Gregorio, & Garber, 1985). A power-tilt system preserves the hip-to-back angle at a constant position during a weight shift, thus maintaining pelvic positioning (Consortium for Spinal Cord Medicine, 1999b, 2000).

Community Mobility

The client with C1 through C4 tetraplegia will require assistance with all community mobility. The therapist must discuss information about adapted vans with wheelchair lifts and tie-down systems with the client and caregiver. The wheelchair must have adequate positioning devices to support the client's body and to maintain stability while the van is in motion. These devices may include head supports, chest straps, seatbelts, and lateral supports.

Clearance through the van door is important because wheelchair backs with head supports tend to be higher than a conventional van doorway opening. The safest position for securing the wheelchair to the floor is facing forward (Schneider, Manary, Hobson, & Bertocci, 2008). Visual restriction from the van's headliner sometimes is a problem. This may be resolved by raising the van's roof or dropping its floor.

Clients who are unable to afford a modified van for personal transportation need education in how to use public transportation systems. Supervised outings provide the best preparation for clients who are learning how to access public transportation.

Tetraplegia: Levels C5–C6

Individuals with C5 tetraplegia have functional shoulder flexion and abduction and elbow flexion, demonstrating the ability to perform a useful hand-to-mouth pattern. At level C6, radial wrist extension is preserved, allowing for tenodesis grasp. *Tenodesis*

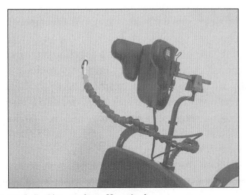

Figure 9.5. Sip-and-puff switch.

refers to opposition of the thumb and index finger with either active or passive wrist extension. Achieving a functional tenodesis grasp is a primary focus of the occupational therapist to optimize functional hand skills for ADL performance. Tenodesis grasp is achieved by employing a range of clinical interventions, including passive wrist and hand range of motion; active and/or resistive wrist extension exercises; short opponens hand splinting; grasp/release training; and graded object manipulation, reach, and functional activity.

People with C5–C6 tetraplegia sometimes undergo tendon transfer surgery to improve hand and arm performance. Upper-extremity tendon transfer surgery can improve clients' quality of life by increasing their independence in performing ADLs (Bryden, Wuolle, Murray, & Peckham, 2004; Wuolle, Bryden, Peckham, Murray, & Keith, 2003).

In tendon transfer surgery, an innervated but nonessential muscle is used to replace a muscle that has lost its function. This type of surgery has been perfected more for the upper extremities than the lower extremities. Typically, it is not considered until a year following the SCI, to allow time for normal return of function (Waters, Sie, Gellman, & Tognella, 1996). People who seek tendon transfer surgery must tolerate several weeks of postoperative immobilization, during which time performance that had been previously gained may be diminished or lost. Family or caregiver availability is crucial during this healing phase. Several weeks of ongoing therapy follow the postoperative phase to retrain the person in the use of the returned muscle function. Successful surgery and retraining may allow the person to discontinue the use of orthotic or assistive devices used to complete specific ADLs. The Freehand system is a neuroprosthesis consisting of an implanted electrical stimulation system that allows people with C5–C6 injuries to open and close the hand by moving the opposite shoulder to activate wrist motion. An external controller interface mounted on the wheelchair controls the device remotely with no connecting wires (Atkins, 2008). Despite the many functional successes experienced by people who have received the device, it has essentially been "orphaned" by the commercializing company because of the small number of people who actually received it (Giszter, 2008).

People with SCI at C5 may have good shoulder control and strong elbow flexion. With SCI injury at this level, however, active elbow extension is absent, which makes overhead activities nearly impossible. The ability to lift the forearm and hand against gravity or reach forward more completely can greatly aid performance of certain self-care activities. Clients with SCI at C5 may benefit from a posterior deltoid-to-triceps tendon transfer to provide for this absent muscle function (Cardenas et al., 2000). Clients also may lack effective lateral pinch and therefore may benefit from a transfer of the brachioradialis to the tendon of the flexor pollicis longus (Hill, 1994). The transfer of the pronator teres to the flexor digitorum profundus may allow for active finger flexion and extension (Gansel, Waters, & Gellman, 1990).

Eating

For clients with SCI at levels C5–C6, self-feeding can be achieved using a variety of techniques and adaptive devices. People with C5 tetraplegia may use a device to position the wrist in a neutral position, and people with C5–C6 tetraplegia may use other types of devices to hold eating utensils or for stability during the task.

The person with SCI at levels C5–C6 may use a universal cuff (an elastic or self-fastening strap attached to a leather pocket) that is easily donned and simply used with a regular utensil inserted into the palmar pocket. The client can pick up a modified cup or glass using a wrist-stabilizing device. A cup or glass can be given a modified handle so the hand can passively lift it to the mouth. Some clients prefer using a long straw so they do not need to lift the cup or glass from the table. For convenience and ease of reach, a straw holder can be used to keep the straw pointed toward the person's face.

If the person is using a ratchet-type orthosis, the orthosis itself can be positioned around the cup or glass for lifting. Once this is done, the client usually can drink independently. A nonbreakable, lightweight cup or glass is safer and gives less stress to arm musculature.

Eating with utensils can be accomplished with a variety of adaptations such as a hand orthosis or wrist-stabilizing splint with the ability to attach a spoon or fork. A ratchet-type orthosis can be used to hold utensils in the conventional way, allowing the client to self-feed independently once set up. A mobile arm support (MAS) or monosuspension feeder can help clients with significantly diminished upper-extremity range of motion and strength to eat independently.

If the client has a difficult time keeping the food on the utensil because of a lack of forearm rotation, swivel utensils may be used. A plate-guard can be used as an border against which food can be scooped so that it does not fall off of the plate. Initially, a client may not have sufficient upper-extremity strength and endurance to self-feed an entire meal. Practice to gain endurance in this task should be encouraged to gain task independence. Cutting food takes much practice, and the person with C5–C6 tetraplegia usually requires minimum to moderate assistance and adapted equipment to complete this task. A client with sufficient shoulder internal rotation may use a rocker knife. A knife with a serrated edge can be used if a sawing motion is used to cut. Some clients with C5–C6 lesions choose to have others cut their food because it is safer and neater. This choice should be respected.

Medication Management

Medications can be placed in an easy-to-open container or a shallow, open cup. A person with C5 tetraplegia may use a ratchet orthosis and a person with C6 tetraplegia may use a wrist-driven, wrist–hand orthosis (WDWHO) to pick up and place medication in his or her mouth (Figure 9.7). A person with stabilized wrists will be able to raise the open cup to the mouth by clasping it between both hands. Safety issues with this method include the consequences of dropped medications and open containers, which could be handled by small children if they are in the home. The client should try different types of containers, requesting that the pharmacist provide containers with simple-to-open flip-top or regular screw-off caps. The most difficult containers are those with "push-and-turn" or "child-proof" caps.

Dental Care

A functional hand-to-mouth pattern is the first prerequisite to brushing teeth. A client with C5 tetraplegia can use various orthoses or assistive devices to stabilize the wrist in a neutral position and a MAS with a proximal elevation arm to lift his or her arm against gravity. To facilitate brushing teeth and rinsing the mouth, the caregiver

- Sets up the toothbrush in a utensil holder;
- Puts toothpaste on the brush; and
- Sets up a cup of water with a straw next to a second, empty cup.

The client first brushes the teeth on one side of the mouth. He or she then turns the toothbrush around in the utensil holder by holding the brush between the teeth and rotating the head or by grasping the brush between the teeth, removing it from the holder, and then reinserting it, facing the opposite direction, into the holder. The client then brushes the teeth on the other side of the mouth, uses the straw to draw rinse water into the mouth, uses the lips to transfer the straw to the empty cup, and allows the rinse water to flow back out of the mouth through the straw.

Clients with adequate muscle strength to move an arm against gravity may be able to use one of the following other orthotic devices to stabilize the hand:

- Ratchet orthosis
- Long opponens splint
- Universal cuff
- Wanchik writer (Figure 9.8)
- Dorsal wrist cock-up splint
- Elastic wrist brace.

These devices usually are reasonably priced. Most people prefer a toothpaste tube with a flip-top cap because it can easily opened by bringing it to the mouth with both hands and using the teeth to open it. As an alternative, a pump tube can be mounted on a fabricated stand to stabilize it while dispensing toothpaste.

Washing the Face and Hands

To be totally independent in washing the face and hands, a person with C5 or C6 tetraplegia must be able to maneuver his or her wheelchair up to a sink. Proximity to sink and faucet handles is crucial to independent performance. Lever handles on the water faucets maximize the client's ability to turn them on and off. If the client uses a D-ring wash mitt, he or she may want to use a stabilizing wrist device under the mitt. Soap can be secured to the sink using a suction pad. Using a MAS, the person can employ a combination of head, neck, and upper-extremity

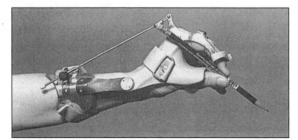

Figure 9.7. Flexor hinge/WDWHO.

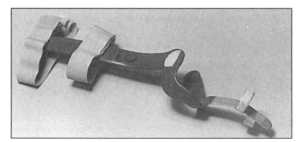

Figure 9.8. Wanchik device for daily living.

movements to reach all areas. Excess water is squeezed out of the wash mitt by pushing it against the side of the sink or between the palms of the hands. A person with C6 tetraplegia may use a regular washcloth, bar soap, or liquid soap dispenser utilizing tenodesis motion for prehension.

Hair Care

Hair washing is performed most easily while showering or bathing. If a roll-in shower stall is unavailable, then hair washing is performed by leaning over a sink. Because it is necessary to stabilize the trunk while leaning forward over a sink, most people with SCI at this level choose to have someone else wash their hair. A commercially available shampoo basin can be used for hair washing when bathing in bed. This type of basin has a drain tube that can be placed in a bucket to collect the used water.

A person with C5 tetraplegia will have difficulty holding a blowdryer up against gravity, so drying hair is most easily achieved by mounting the blowdryer on a gooseneck stand or the wall. Rather than move the blowdryer, the person moves his or her head to catch the warm air generated by the dryer. A person with a C6 SCI may use a modified cuff on a blowdryer (Figure 9.9). If the person is able to stabilize his or her elbow on a countertop, this can enhance stability and endurance during this task.

For a person without innervated triceps, brushing and styling the hair requires creativity and skill in using substitute muscle function. A client with C5 tetraplegia who uses a MAS will not be able to perform this task without maximal assistance. Long-handled brushes are useful to accomplish this task. Using a curling iron or hair curlers also requires maximum assistance. The client may consider adapting by using a permanent wave or a low-maintenance hairstyle.

A client with this level of injury who can move his or her arm against gravity needs to stabilize the wrist. Brushes and combs with extended handles can be stabilized using the previously mentioned orthoses or assistive devices. People with SCI at the C6 level can use a WDWHO or their tenodesis grasp to hold a brush or comb (Figures 9.7 and 9.10). A universal cuff and a phone holder (used as a brush holder) also can help the client perform this task.

Shaving

Shaving can be performed with either an electric razor or a safety razor, depending on the client's personal preference. Some clients prefer electric razors to avoid the cuts and nicks from blades. The therapist should work to support the client in achieving safety and independence in shaving using the selected method. A person using a MAS will need assistance setting up the razor and shaving cream. Some clients also will need assistance with shaving difficult-to-reach contours of the face, neck, and body.

Using a WDWHO, a ratchet orthosis, or a specially adapted cuff permits the client with C5–C6 tetraplegia to hold an electric razor. The razor's weight is a major consideration, because it may give more resistance than the limb can support. Safety razors can be adapted with a variety of low-temperature plastics for ease of handling. If the person can move his or her arm against gravity, a utensil holder can be used to stabilize the razor. Commercially available razor holders must be used in conjunction with a wrist-stabilizing brace for people with C5 SCI. Keeping the razor from falling can be a challenge, but it can be done using a two-handed technique. A commercially available shaving cream dispenser with a long lever handle can assist with this aspect of the activity.

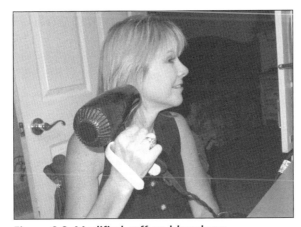

Figure 9.9. Modified cuff on blowdryer.

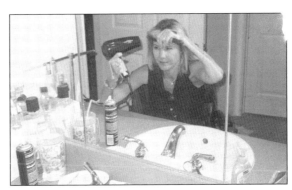

Figure 9.10. Tenodesis grasp for holding a hairbrush.

Most women with C5 tetraplegia require assistance in shaving their underarms and legs because of impaired trunk stability while leaning forward and the need to maintain upright balance using both upper extremities. A woman with C6 tetraplegia may be able to use a WDWHO universal cuff or tenodesis action of her hands to hold the razor to shave her underarms and legs, but she may need the assistance of another person.

Makeup Application

Typically, a woman with SCI at level C5 will need assistance to apply makeup to her face. Hands may be clasped together to hold makeup items when tendodesis is insufficient for coordinated movement. Actions that require fine motor coordination are performed by a caregiver. A woman with injury at the C6 level can use a WDWHO, tenodesis, or adapted handles to grasp makeup brushes, pencils, or wands. Sanding or slightly filing the clasps on makeup compacts makes them easier to open. Makeup containers may be left open and caps left off tubes at all times to allow for ease of manipulation. Small tubes, such as those containing mascara, can be held in the mouth, while using the most dexterous hand to obtain and apply the makeup, allowing greater independence.

Dressing and Undressing

A person with C5 SCI may require minimal to moderate assistance with upper-body dressing for pullover or button-front clothes because of decreased upper-extremity range of motion, lack of fine motor coordination, and lack of trunk stability. The client will need assistance to fasten or unfasten buttons. Pull strings attached to zippers allow manipulation without fine motor finger movement. To put on a front-fastening shirt or jacket, the client can use the around-the-back method, which will require moderate to maximal assistance, or may use a buttonhook–zipper pull device to fasten closures independently. Front-fastening or self-fastening bras can be modified with sewn-in loops through which the thumb can be inserted. Bras also may be put on like a T-shirt. First the caregiver fastens the bra closure, then either the client or the caregiver pulls the bra over the head and down along the upper chest into place. For men who wear ties, options include either the clip-on tie or having the caregiver pre-knot the tie and pull it over the client's head. Either the client or the caregiver will tighten or fasten it in place.

Because people with SCI at the C5 level lack bed mobility, they require assistance in lower-extremity dressing. Slacks and skirts cut longer and slightly larger in the hips are easier to put on and fit a person sitting in a wheelchair with flexed knees more precisely. Independent lower-body dressing begins with long sitting in bed (legs extended toward the foot of the bed with trunk flexed at hips). The pants are positioned with the front facing up and the pants legs over the bottom of the bed. The pants are put in position by tossing them or by using a dressing stick to move the pants legs away from the body. The client lifts one leg by using the opposite wrist or forearm placed under the knee and tunnels the foot into the pants leg. The client may use the thumb of the other hand to hook a belt loop or pocket to hold the top of the pants open. Then the client inserts the other foot. Using the palms of the hands, the client slides the pants legs up along the calves.

Some people find it helpful to wear friction gloves to provide resistance to the pants cloth for improved manipulation. Tenodesis motion or wrists hooked under the waistband inside the pants can be used to pull the pants up over the knees. These motions are continued until the waistband reaches the upper-thigh area. The person then returns to a supine position, where he or she rolls side to side on the bed. Lying on one side, the client hooks the thumb of the top arm in the back belt loops to pull the pants up over the buttocks. The client repeats this process on alternating sides until the pants are in place. Clients can fasten pants using a zipper pull, a loop added to the zipper, or hook-and-loop tab closures. To remove pants, the person reverses these procedures.

The person with C5–C6 SCI can put socks on in a sitting position in bed by crossing first one leg and then the other. If flexibility allows, clients can reach forward, with legs fully extended at the knees and heels over the edge of the bed, to put on socks. Two loops may be sewn on opposite sides of the top of the sock, where the thumbs can be hooked to manipulate the sock onto the foot, or a sock aid may be used to get the sock over the toes if the person is unable to reach his or her feet. Socks are removed by pushing them off with a dressing stick, long shoehorn, or by hooking the thumb in the sock edge (James, 2008).

Modified clothing is commercially available through catalogs such as USA Jeans (www.usajeans.net), Wardrobe Wagon (www.wardrobewagon.com), Adaptations by Adrian's Closet (www.adaptationsbyadrian.com), and Adaptive Clothing Showroom (http://www.adaptiveclothingshowroom.com).

Bowel and Bladder Management

People with SCI at C5 require assistance in bowel and bladder care because of the lack of hand function and inability to position themselves independently. The client should be able to verbally direct the caregiver in this task.

A client with C5 tetraplegia may be able to empty his or her legbag using either a manual pneumatic legbag clamp or an electric legbag emptier. The switch that controls the clamp must be positioned so the client can access it easily. The legbag may be emptied into a floor basin, a cat litter box, or onto grass. The electric legbag emptier must be mounted onto the client's wheelchair. Gravity assists in draining urine from the tubing.

For the person with C6 tetraplegia, clean and safe self-catheterization is a realistic goal. Accurate tenodesis grasp and sufficient hand manipulation skills allow for increased potential success with this task. It also takes a tremendous amount of motivation, patience, and dedication on the part of both the client and occupational therapist. This task is more challenging for females than males because of the difference in genitalia and access to the urethral opening. The entire task includes managing lower extremity clothing, positioning hips and legs, managing the catheter into the urethra to drain the bladder, disposing of the urine, and cleaning all reuseable catheters and supplies as necessary.

Self-catheterization is often easiest for men wearing elastic waist pants and use of a pant holder to access the penis. A button-hook and zipper-pull can also be used to manipulate clothing fasteners. Women are required to remove at least one leg out of pants or shorts and spread their legs wide enough to access the urethra. They may also opt to wear a loose skirt for easier access. Clients will need to learn to position themselves in their wheelchair or bed in a posterior pelvic tilt. Holding the catheter tightly between both wrists, or using adaptive equipment like a WDWHO or commercially available catheter holder, can accomplish adapted grip on the catheter. Urine will need to be collected into a urinal or can be drained directly into the toilet. Often a catheter extension will be required for reaching into toilet, urinal, or other urine collection device. The catheter should be cleaned daily with mild soap and water, air-dried, and placed in a clean container until the it is ready to be reused (Consortium for Spinal Cord Medicine, 2006). To flush water through the catheter, a large syringe connected it is useful. The client can hold the syringe between the wrists, use the teeth to pull the plunger back to suc-tion the water into the syringe, then use pressure against the chin to push the water out through the catheter. The client should be trained to manage self-catheterization at both the bed and the wheelchair level.

Bowel management for the C6 client is also possible with the appropriate skills training. The task includes inserting the suppository, performing digital stimulation, and post-bowel program hygiene. Because the C6 client presents with limited finger dexterity, adaptive devices for suppository insertion and digital stimulation are required. These devices are illustrated in Figure 9.11 and can be custom-modified by the occupational therapist to optimize their use. Modifications may include adjusting the overall length of the device and/or angle of the distal end. Independence with bowel program management is most easily accomplished on a padded rolling shower commode chair (RSCC) with a seat cutout to allow for front or side access. Cleanup is most often performed simultaneously with bathing. Considerations should be made for performance of this task sitting and from the bed level.

For both bladder and bowel management, the client should be able to verbally instruct, in detail, the entire task process. A consistent, routine schedule and proper food and fluid intake help regulate waste elimination. Foods with a proper balance of fiber, nutrients, and liquids aid bladder and bowel regulation.

Occupational therapists have the unique skills required to perform an activity analysis and can be helpful in problem solving for positioning and techniques. The therapist may need to fabricate and modify equipment or provide suggestions for

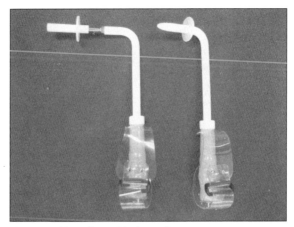

Figure 9.11. Adjustable bowel management devices: suppository inserter and digital stimulator.

greater independence with bowel and bladder routines. Most important, the therapist can provide emotional support and encouragement as the client develops strategies for handling this extremely personal task (Atkins, 2008).

Communication

Initially, assistive devices may be indicated to assist people with SCI at the C5 level in writing. One such assistive device is a MAS in conjunction with a long opponens orthosis (Figure 9.12). Most people will gradually reduce or eliminate the use of MAS but continue to need a wrist-stabilizing orthosis with an adaptation to hold a pen or pencil.

Other assistive devices, such as a Wanchik Writer (see Figure 9.8), a WDWHO (Figure 9.13), or a dorsal wrist cock-up splint with cuff can help the client hold the wrist in a neutral position and position the writing utensil. A Dycem™ nonslip pad is useful for holding the paper in place while writing. As the client's arm control improves, letters and numbers may be attempted. The first attempts at writing may be difficult. Therapists should encourage clients to begin with drawing lines or circles. Asking the client to form letters or numbers early on can lead to disappointment or frustration because of the unrefined arm movement. Practice is the key to improving this skill.

Typing offers a clear visual presentation, but typing may be frustrating to the client if too much skill is called for before arm control is developed. The client's wrists must be stabilized and a typing implement must be attached to depress the keys for typing (Figure 9.14). Use of a standard mouse may prove to be difficult. If so, a trackball mouse may be an alternative. A therapist can use typing as an exercise for MAS training because it requires fine con-

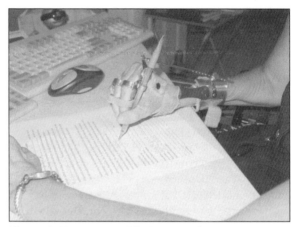

Figure 9.13. Person with C6 tetraplegia using WDWHO for writing.

trol of the arm to select and depress exact keys. Usually the client is asked to type each row of keys individually from right to left, left to right, then up and down, before actually typing words. Once the client has achieved control of arm placement, he or she can type words.

Telephone Use

Accessing a telephone is important for people with SCI at the C5 level. Some clients who may still have traditional base-unit corded telephones can use a gooseneck stand to hold the telephone receiver to ear height and use a phone flipper (an extended lever) to depress the switch hook connector on the phone base. The lever is lifted to obtain a dial tone or to receive a call when the phone rings. Most people using a MAS use this method or choose to use hands-free phone technology because they are unable to hold the receiver to the ear. People who have adequate arm strength and can hold the receiver to

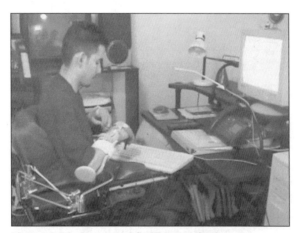

Figure 9.12. Person with C5 tetraplegia using mobile arm orthosis.

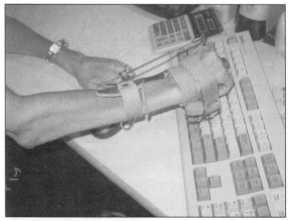

Figure 9.14. Person with C6 tetraplegia typing on the computer.

the ear may use a phone holder for independence with handling. Cordless telephone receivers can generally be held by people with C5 tetraplegia by sustaining pressure against their hand cupping the receiver against the ear. Using telephones with automatic dialing, memory, or redial functions often increases efficiency. A speakerphone decreases necessary hand function but also decreases privacy.

For people with SCI at C6, using a corded or cordless phone can be made easier with an adapted handset, universal cuff, WDWHO used to press the buttons, or other custom adaptations (Figure 9.15). Some clients at this level use tenodesis to handle a corded, cordless, or cellular telephone without any adaptive equipment. In a vocational setting, earphones or a headset can streamline the tasks of simultaneous noted writing and phone use. Cellular telephone technologies now offer more hands-free options, such as remote earpieces and speakerphone capabilities (Figure 9.16). Mainstream services like text messaging, downloading text or data, and wireless transmissions also can benefit people with SCI by allowing more efficient use of their cellular telephones in ADLs.

Bathing

A client with C5 tetraplegia requires moderate to maximum assistance from another person for task completion and safety during bathing. If a person with C5 or C6 tetraplegia has an accessible shower, he or she typically uses a padded, rolling, shower–commode chair in a modified shower stall. Levers versus knobs are recommended, as is water temperature regulation to prevent scalding. Wall-mounted dispensers make accessing liquid soap and shampoo more successful and safer during this task. Chest straps mounted to the shower–commode chair may help stabilize the upper trunk during the activity. The client also may use a D-ring wash mitt to wash the face, neck, anterior chest, upper legs, and perineum region. A person with C6 tetraplegia

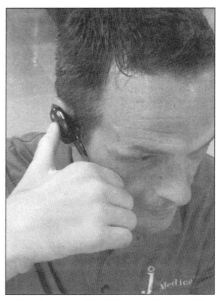

Figure 9.16. Person with C6 tetraplegia utilizing hands-free technology.

may use long-handled brushes to reach the feet, between the toes, and other hard-to-reach body areas. A hand-held showerhead may be useful, but the occupational therapist may need to add an adapted handle to it. The availability of skin protection, postural support, and adapted handles make bathing a more independent and private activity. Bed baths offer an alternative bathing method for people whose homes are not modified or for whom equipment is not yet available.

Meal Preparation and Cleanup

For individuals with C5 tetraplegia, preparing meals may be difficult and time-consuming, so preparation by a caregiver is a frequently used strategy. Assistance with meal preparation for clients with lesions at the C6 level may range from no assistance to maximal assistance. Clients who use a WDWHO find it easier to accomplish more meal preparation tasks than do clients who use passive wrist-stabilizing orthoses. The performance range of clients with SCI at this level varies considerably, partly because of each person's individual functioning but also because of varying levels of motivation to achieve the task, tolerance for problem solving, and accessibility in their kitchens.

Lifting pans safely into and out of the oven poses a major challenge for clients with SCI. A microwave or toaster oven may eliminate this problem and be adequate if the client is preparing meals for just one or two persons. Stove-top cooking is accomplished using over-the-stove mirrors, long-handled pots, shallow fry pans, and long oven mitts to

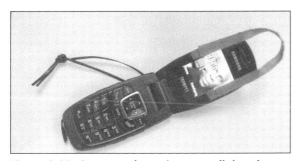

Figure 9.15. Custom adaptations to cellular phone.

prevent burns. A suction stabilizer that holds the pans securely increases safety when preparing hot food. Using adapted utensils or a palm-to-palm method to grasp utensils, the client can accomplish many mealtime tasks. To transport food from one place to another, clients find it easiest to slide the item along the counter or use a lap-tray. Commercially available one-handed can openers with adjustable stands or battery operated one-touch button can openers are difficult for a person with C6 tetraplegia to use, but with practice the technique may be mastered. Using a blender or mixer can conserve the client's energy. Controls should be levers or pushbuttons.

Clients can cut food items using an adapted knife and a cutting board with a stainless or aluminum nail protruding on which to stabilize the food. Suction cups on the bottom of the cutting board provide stability on the countertop, which allows a two-handed cutting method to be used, either palm-to-palm or with one hand securing the food and the other doing the cutting. A table or lower counter can be used to support the client's elbows, thus bringing the objects closer and making them more easily manipulated. Because of a lack of triceps strength and the need for support to maintain trunk balance, the client is most successful when working close to the body. Jars can be opened by holding them with both hands and pushing and turning against an adaptive device that has serrated edges. In general, jar lids should be kept loosely engaged for ease of opening.

Ovens can be difficult to use because of the weight or spring action of the door. Lifting pans into and out of the oven can be hazardous. A toaster oven or a broiler used on a low tabletop offers a safer way to bake. Clients use lever action to open the door and depress buttons. Microwave ovens also are safer than conventional ovens if placed on a table at an accessible height. A button or lever often controls the door, or loops can be added to the door handle to aid in opening. The refrigerator door also can be made easier to open by adding loops to the door handle. Frequently used items should be placed on shelves that are at eye level or lower (Figure 9.17). Food storage containers should be made of lightweight plastic in case they are dropped or slip from the person's grasp.

Cleanup is easier if the sink is accessible. A scrubber with soap in the handle is a useful step saver. Brushes with large open handles that the hand can fit through provide a better grasp. A rubber pad on the bottom of the sink decreases the likelihood of breakage. An adapted scrub brush and a

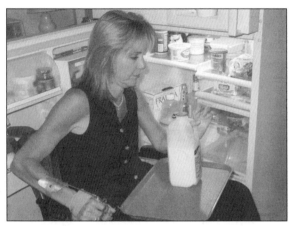

Figure 9.17. Person with C6 tetraplegia removing items from the refrigerator.

liquid soap dispenser, a bottlebrush, a wash mitt, and levers on sink controls can help during dishwashing. The dishes can be dried either in the sink or in a sink rack. Using a dishwasher is feasible but can be difficult given the weight of the door. A loop can be added to the handle to assist in opening it. Some people choose to use their dishwasher to store clean dishes in order to eliminate the step of returning them to kitchen cabinets that may be less accessible to them.

Prepared foods and microwave dishes may be relatively expensive, but they save time and energy and reduce frustration.

Meal preparation presents challenges that may include

- Getting the food out of the pantry, refrigerator, or freezer;
- Reaching the pots and pans;
- Opening plastic, frozen, or metal containers;
- Operating manual and small electric kitchen appliances;
- Setting the table; and
- Using large kitchen appliances.

For the client with SCI, the design of the kitchen environment is important because it can facilitate or complicate tasks related to meal preparation or cleanup. The following elements of design and adaptation can strongly influence client's independence in the kitchen:

- The kitchen area should have adequate room for wheelchair maneuvering to open drawers and doors.
- Cabinet doors should be easy to open, with glides and handles to assist people with limited strength and hand function (or the client may choose to remove cabinet doors altogether).

• Food and cooking items should be placed within reach at wheelchair level as much as possible, noting that clients with SCI likely will use a reacher to access items placed above head level.

• The preferred refrigerator design is a side-by-side style that makes both the freezer and the refrigerator compartments accessible.

Small manual kitchen appliances must be on a work surface at desk height to be operated with little or no adaptation. Manual appliances often require more energy to operate and often are not as effective as electric ones. Many appliances are available to assist in common meal preparation tasks: electric can openers, peelers, and knives as well as food processors, countertop grills, and mixers. Small electric appliances, like electric can openers, may require a supporting base and lever switches or special push buttons for efficient and safe operation (Figure 9.18).

Because of sensory deficits, the person with SCI at this level needs to be careful around sharp items and surfaces with extreme temperatures. For example, safely operating the range or oven requires that switches be within reach, eliminating the need to lean over hot burners. The therapist and client should ensure control knobs are positioned on the front or side of the stovetop to eliminate this safety hazard.

It takes creativity to adapt the kitchen environment, appliances, and utensils to meet the needs of a person with C5–C6 tetraplegia. Preplanning can help save time and increase efficiency in meal preparation. Meals on Wheels or a similar community-based program that delivers prepared meals may be an option for providing one nutritious meal a day for those who qualify for this service.

Functional Mobility

For people with C5–C6 tetraplegia, transferring or moving the body from one surface to another can require a tremendous amount of effort; many choose to have others perform the task for them. In most cases of transfer to and from level surfaces, a person with C5 tetraplegia needs moderate assistance. Transfers between positions of different heights require maximal to total assistance. A transfer board provides a smooth surface to slide across and decreases resistance during the task.

Among people with C6 tetraplegia, performance ability varies greatly, depending on body size, strength, motivation, and age. Some clients may need no assistance and others may need maximal assistance. A sliding board may or may not be necessary. Prefunctional considerations include static and dynamic trunk balance and proximal shoulder stability and use of shoulder depressors for "lift." Moving the head away from the side the hips are moving toward and creating momentum with trunk rotation ease the slide across the board. Clients whose weight or degree of body spasticity impact transfers may find it easier and safer to use a mechanical or electric lift.

Wheelchair Mobility

A person with C5–C6 tetraplegia can move independently over both level and uneven surfaces with a manual wheelchair. The wheelchair must be specifically measured to accommodate the body for proper support and occupational performance (Figure 9.19). The wheelchair's back must be high enough to support the trunk so arm function can be maximized. Vertical-oblique or friction rims are recommended to push the wheelchair forward and re-

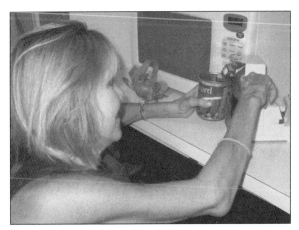

Figure 9.18. Person with C6 tetraplegia operating an electric can opener.

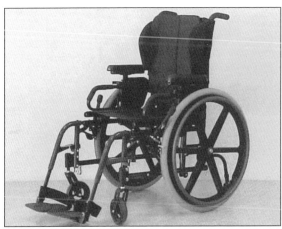

Figure 9.19. Manual wheelchairs for people with C5–C6 tetraplegia.

verse. The scapular stabilizing musculature must be strengthened so as not to overstretch supporting shoulder structures. A wrist-stabilizing splint is used to enhance hand placement of the person with C5 injury. People with SCI at the C5–C6 level can use a folding or rigid manual wheelchair.

A grade aid (or hill climber), a type of secondary braking device, is recommended for propelling the wheelchair up an incline or ramp. The grade aid is mounted under the wheelchair brakes. The device lies on the surface of the tire, allowing the tire to be pushed forward. The client engages the grade aid by pushing a lever handle downward. When the push stroke is completed, the device clutches the tire and prevents it from rolling backward but continues to allow forward motion. When the incline or ramp has been climbed, the client pushes the lever up to disengage the device.

Brake extensions also provide increased lever advantage in operating wheelchair brakes. On ultra-lightweight wheelchairs, anti-tip bars are a safety option that prevents the wheelchair from tipping backward on an uneven surface.

For some people with SCI, propelling the weight of a manual wheelchair takes too much effort, and endurance is compromised. Sometimes the slowness of manual wheelchair propulsion limits the client's functional mobility in the community. Rough terrain, long distances, or shoulder pain can challenge the person's abilities and may necessitate a power wheelchair or manual wheelchair with power assist wheels (Figure 9.20). Using these devices may conserve energy, allow the client greater mobility, and expand the client's opportunities for

school or work. A manual wheelchair usually is purchased to serve as a backup to the power wheelchair.

A power wheelchair with a hand control usually is chosen for people with SCI at C5 and may be selected for people with SCI at C6 (Figure 9.21). A person who uses a MAS needs extensive practice to master driving a hand-controlled power wheelchair. It is important to look for the position of the MAS that provides the greatest mechanical advantage.

Therapists and clients must thoroughly discuss issues related to community mobility to anticipate, prevent, and solve problems. Most motorized wheelchairs do not fold easily for loading into a conventional vehicle. People who use motorized wheelchairs are unable to independently load the wheelchair into a car, sport utility vehicle (SUV), or truck, which limits their independent mobility in the community. Transporting this type of wheelchair requires a modified van with and electric lift.

For safety and efficiency, some clients may need to adapt the wheelchair's hand control with an extended joystick. The wrist is supported with an orthosis and assistive device. A powered recliner or tilt system typically is considered for independent weight shifting if the person is unable to lean side to side or push up independently to reduce peak sitting pressure over sitting surfaces of the pelvis.

Community Mobility

New technology in adapted driving, including modified vans with low- or zero-effort steering and electric lifts, enables some people with SCI at C5 to be independently mobile (Figures 9.22–9.25). A person with an injury at this level usually drives from a motorized wheelchair that is secured to the floor with an electric tie-down system. Evaluation and supervised driver's training are critical to ensure safety. A person who is unable to achieve this level of independence must rely on someone else to drive. A per-

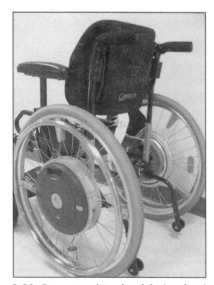

Figure 9.20. Power-assist wheelchair wheels.

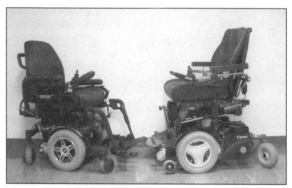

Figure 9.21. Power wheelchair options for people with C5–C6 tetraplegia.

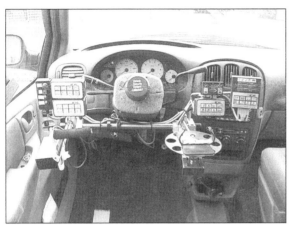

Figure 9.22. Driving controls in an adapted van for person with C5 tetraplegia.

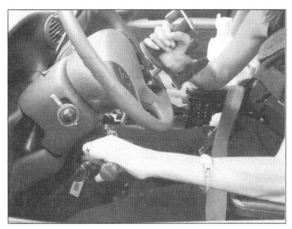

Figure 9.24. Driving control for a person with C6 tetraplegia.

son with C5 tetraplegia can be transferred into the passenger seat of a van or have the wheelchair stabilized to the floor for transport safety. Whenever the van is in motion, both the wheelchair seat belt and the van safety restraint should be fastened. A vehicle ramp or an electric lift can also be used if the person with C6 tetraplegia chooses to drive from the manual wheelchair.

If the person does not own a van, the client with SCI at C5 must be transferred into a car with assistance. The caregiver then loads the wheelchair in the back flooring or in the trunk or rear compartment of the vehicle. Loading a motorized wheelchair is a difficult and time-consuming task because of the necessary dismantling and handling

of the batteries. Power wheelchairs with power-recline or power-tilt systems cannot be dismantled to be loaded into a car and must be transported in an adapted van. A manual wheelchair usually is substituted, which may mean the person with SCI has less functionality once at the destination. The client with SCI at C6 may have the potential for self-loading a manual wheelchair with focused skills training.

Some cities make bus service with modified lifts available. People with impaired trunk balance use a chest strap or wear lateral supports during public transportation. These supports provide stability and ensure upright sitting to counter the force of the motion. Compliance with the Americans with Disabilities Act (ADA) of 1990 has resulted in more widespread use of wheelchair lifts on buses and other public vehicles designed specifically for people with physical disabilities.

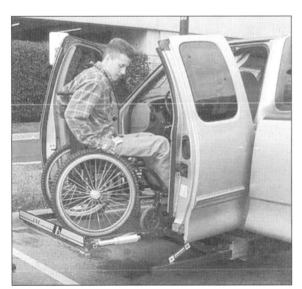

Figure 9.23. Person with C6 tetraplegia entering vehicle with power lift.

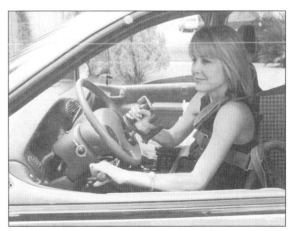

Figure 9.25. Person with C6 tetraplegia driving adapted van.

Tetraplegia: Levels C7–C8

People with C7–C8 have functional triceps and some finger flexor and extensor intrinsic muscles and thumb flexor muscles innervated. They can raise their arms up against gravity and have some hand dexterity. Many such clients can live alone or without assistance with home modifications.

People with SCI at C7–C8 can perform upper-body grooming and hygiene independently, using a sink with few or no adaptive devices. Sink accessibility is important to ensure independence while using the faucets. Lever controls are easier to use, although the client may be able to use some twisting controls. Towels should be placed close to the sink and at a low level for greater independence.

Eating

People with SCI at C7–C8 require minimal assistive devices to eat. They may intertwine utensils between their fingers or use tenodesis action for stability. To cut food, they may use both hands or an adaptation, such as a cuff, to secure the knife. These clients should be able to drink independently from a cup or glass, using a tenodesis grasp or both hands.

Dental Care

People with C7–C8 tetraplegia may secure the toothbrush between their fingers or use a built-up handle to enhance their grip. Some people may choose to use an electric toothbrush. Getting the toothpaste onto the brush may require using the countertop to get enough pressure to push the paste out, or the client may put the toothpaste directly in the mouth before applying the brush. Small, prethreaded dental flossing tools are also helpful.

Dressing and Undressing the Upper and Lower Body

A person with SCI at C7–C8 may dress the upper and lower body independently, using long sitting and leaning over the legs to reach feet or rolling side-to-side method on the bed. Donning and doffing footwear may require assistance if the styles are not slip-on or hook-and-loop tab closure styles. Adaptive shoelaces may help the client put on footwear independently. A buttonhook/zipper pull device may be necessary to fasten buttons or zippers.

Bathing

The person with SCI at C7–C8 needs some adaptations to bathe independently. A padded shower–commode chair in a roll-in shower probably provides the best level of independent functioning. A padded bathtub bench with a back support also can be used to transfer into the tub independently. Assistance may be needed for transfer when the person is wet or if he or she has a high level of spasticity that interferes with movement. A handheld shower allows for greatest independence in showering. If the client finds it difficult to reach the buttocks and lower back for cleansing, long-handled sponges or brushes should allow access as long as the person can maintain his or her balance. Hair washing is best done when the person is supported in the shower or tub. Towels should be placed where they can stay dry but remain within the person's reach. A towel placed on the wheelchair seat will help by soaking up excess water and moisture from the person's body while he or she completes the transfer back into the chair.

Bowel and Bladder Management

People with SCI at levels C7–C8 may need minimal to no assistance managing a regular bowel program. A person at this level of SCI may or may not need adaptive device for task completion because of the amount of preserved finger dexterity. The devices previously shown for bowel management may be used if needed (see Figure 9.11).

Meal Preparation

Meal preparation is a challenge for people with SCI at C7–C8 primarily because of diminished trunk control, weak grasp, and poor kitchen accessibility for wheelchairs. The adaptations listed above for levels C5–C6, such as using toaster ovens and microwaves, may be appropriate. Adapted devices that help stabilize material and assist in opening containers continue to be needed. Kitchens need to be modified for wheelchair accessibility, such as providing lowered work surfaces and space for wheelchair maneuverability. Other modifications are listed in the section on paraplegia function.

Functional Mobility

Clients with SCI at C7–C8 can use a sliding board to transfer to and from the wheelchair. Eventually, they may be able to transfer without using the transfer board. Removable armrests and footrests are essential for safe transfer for both the person and the caregiver or assistant.

People with SCI at this level can be independent in wheelchair mobility using a manual folding or rigid wheelchair (Figure 9.26). Friction-coated hand rims may be used to assist in propulsion. Clients may still have some difficulty pushing up steep inclines or over rough terrain. Clients with SCI at this

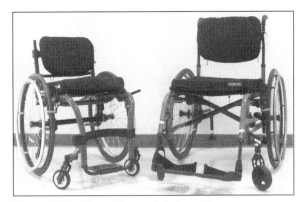

Figure 9.26. Manual wheelchair options.

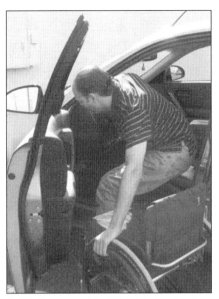

Figure 9.27. Person with C7–C8 tetraplegia transferring into car.

level also will be independent with powered mobility using a joystick. Powered mobility conserves energy, enhancing stamina for other functional tasks, such as dressing and vocational activities.

Community Mobility

People with a C7–C8 injury should be able to drive a modified van or a personal vehicle (car, truck, or SUV) adapted with appropriate controls for community transportation. People with a C7–C8 injury should be able to transfer independently into a passenger vehicle and may be able to independently load their wheelchair. For those who may need assistance with wheelchair loading, car-top loaders or special lifts can assist with this maneuver. They may choose to drive from their wheelchairs in a modified van; doing so will save energy but is a more costly solution (Figures 9.27 and 9.28).

Communication

Writing and typing skills are essential to independent living and handling one's own affairs. Most people with C7–C8 level of SCI can use a simple writing device independently, without help, or use a writing implement with a wider body for better grip. The device selected for writing also can be used for keyboarding. The WDWHO gives dynamic grasp, which is useful for loading paper, computer disks, and peripheral items and for picking up and moving objects. For people with SCI at C7–C8, using the phone can be made easier with a phone holder, universal cuff, or tenodesis motion used to press the buttons. Some people with SCI at this level need no adaptations to use a telephone, type, or write because they have well-developed tenodesis hand skills (Figure 9.29). In a vocational setting, a hands-free earpiece or a headset can streamline requirements for simultaneous note writing and phone use.

Paraplegia: Levels T1–T6

Persons with SCI at T1 through T6 level of injury can independently perform eating, dental care, and hygiene and grooming tasks (e.g., washing face and hands, combing hair, shaving, applying make-up at sink level), provided the bathroom is wheelchair accessible. The muscles of the upper to middle trunk have their roots from T1 to T6. In general, these muscles are responsible for elevation and depression of the ribs during respiration, contraction of the upper abdomen, and upper anterolateral flexion of the

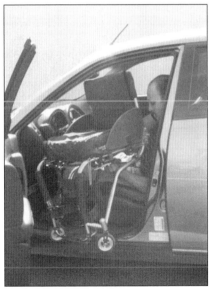

Figure 9.28. Person with C7–C8 tetraplegia loading wheelchair into vehicle.

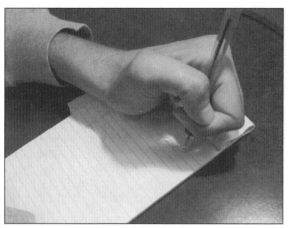

Figure 9.29. Person with C7–C8 tetraplegia using tenodesis for writing.

trunk. People with injury at the T1 level have near-normal hand function yet can present with weakness in hand intrinsic and lumbrical muscles. This may affect fine motor coordination. Wheelchair use is the primary means of mobility; because of extensive trunk muscle paralysis, their ability to maintain upright sitting balance requires external support with adequate wheelchair back-height support. To prevent a loss of trunk balance, people with higher-level paraplegia frequently will stabilize the trunk with one arm while performing an activity with the other.

People with SCI at the T1 through T6 levels have full use of their upper extremities and should be able to live independently in a wheelchair-accessible environment. Although breathing improves at this level, trunk balance is still compromised, and appropriate safety precautions should be implemented. The wheelchair is the primary mode for mobility, although ambulation may be performed for exercise purposes (Hoppenfeld, 1997; Somers, 2001). Static standing using equipment for weight bearing through the lower extremities is considered beneficial in maintaining vital organ capacity (including urinary/bowel functions); in maintaining bone density, circulation, and elongation of muscles about the hips, knees, and ankles; in reducing tone and spasticity, the occurrence of pressure sores, and skeletal deformities; and in enhancing psychosocial well-being (Rehabilitation Engineering and Assistive Technology Society of North America [RESNA], 2007b).

Dressing

People with T1–T6 SCI can dress without personal assistance. Dressing loops, dressing stick, long-handled reacher, and oversized clothing may enhance independence in dressing the lower-body clothing, including shoes and socks, can be put on independently if there is good hip, knee, and ankle range of motion and little interference from trunk or leg spasms while assuming a long sitting position in bed. Applying the clothing over both legs first, then turning side to side to position the clothing, helps minimize the shearing over the skin of the buttocks and conserves energy. A recommendation can be made that clients perform skin inspection during lower-body dressing; the same bed mobility maneuvers are required for both tasks, reducing skin shearing and the need to expend additional energy by repeating these effortful body movements.

These clients do not require assistance in upper-body dressing but may have to use the bed or wheelchair for support to maintain balance.

Bathing

A person with T1–T6 paraplegia may need some adaptations to bath independently. Techniques and equipment described earlier in the C7–C8 tetraplegia section apply to this level of paraplegia, as well.

Bowel, Bladder, and Menstruation Management

Men with SCI T1–T6 are able to apply an external catheter or independently utilize an intermittent catheterization program. Women with SCI at T1–T6 injury can catheterize but may need a mirror and an adaptive device to help position their legs during the task. Initially, both men and women position the body with head and upper body elevated so they may visualize and reach the perineum more effectively. With practice and skill, T1–T6 paraplegia can learn to change/clean their external catheter or perform an intermittent catherization program while sitting upright in a wheelchair or positioned on a toilet or adaptive toilet surface. Bed mobility, body handling, and lower-body dressing skill performance are paramount when attempting to gain independence in personal ADLs. Intermittent catheterization ideally occurs every 4 to 6 hours so that urine volume each time is less than 500 ml, as recommended for kidney and bladder health (Consortium for Spinal Cord Medicine, 2006). This consistent, round-the-clock schedule takes discipline and routine to be successful.

Bowel program management is accomplished independently by using suppositories, digital stimulation, and a consistently followed schedule. Again, positioning may be the one area requiring assistance. If the person has appropriate equipment, such as a padded shower–commode chair, padded bedside commode, or padded raised toilet seat, sitting to perform the bowel evacuation routine is typically more effective. Women can manage pads independently but may need a mirror and an adaptive device to help position their legs when inserting a tampon during menstruation.

Communication

People with SCI at this level are independent in all communication skills, such as keyboarding, writing, and use of the telephone and can easily access computers using a standard keyboard and mouse. An ergonomically sound workstation will decrease musculoskeletal overuse in the upper body. Attending to the height of the computer monitor, keyboard, and mouse in relationship to the body minimizes the effects from extended reach and abnormal postures that sometimes are seen in computer users.

Meal Preparation

People with T1 through T6 SCI have poor trunk control but can prepare meals independently from a wheelchair with or without adaptive devices or modifications, which may include lowered counter tops or work surfaces. A mirror over a standard stove-top is helpful for seeing inside cooking pans and avoiding touching hot areas that are not visible from the wheelchair level. The accessibility of the standard oven, microwave oven, and refrigerator from the wheelchair should be considered. Usually a side approach is best for maintaining balance and securing items from each type of appliance. Dishes, glassware, and cooking pans should be lightweight and are most accessible if located at no higher than shoulder level.

Functional Mobility

People with T1–T6 level of paraplegia have the arm strength to transfer independently with or without a sliding board. However, excessive body weight, medical problems, uneven transfer surfaces, wheelchair position, and general endurance level may compromise transfer independence. Extremes in weight and height, in combination with the poor trunk control, may complicate independent transfer enough for these people to require assistance with this task. Spasticity and muscle tone can help in some instances but compromise transfer safety in others.

People with SCI at this level usually can use a manual wheelchair independently if the wheelchair has been prescribed according to the person's body size and activity level (Consortium for Spinal Cord Medicine, 2000). The wheelchair should be a high-strength, fully customizable, manual wheelchair made of the lightest possible material. An ultra-lightweight wheelchair with a back height below the scapula for optimal propulsion is typically prescribed for this population. This wheelchair may be a folding or a rigid frame model (Figure 9.26). Armrests should be removable to allow for maximal transfer independence. The occupational therapist should consider postural symmetry, stability, and comfort when selecting the type of wheelchair back for trunk balance. Options are standard back upholstery; tension-adjustable back upholstery; or a solid, contoured, padded back used for the preservation of the normal spinal curves. While sitting, a pressure redistributing seat cushion is recommended to reduce excessive pressure over the bony prominences of the buttocks and give pelvic stability (Consortium for Spinal Cord Medicine, 2000; Hobson, 1992; Koo, Mak, & Lee, 1996).

Due to their more impaired trunk control, some people with SCI at T1–T4 may use a power wheelchair rather than a self-propelled (manual) model in order to conserve energy and time expenditure. Because many people with SCI are living longer and have more active lives, musculoskeletal overuse problems are emerging. Those problems must be addressed through the use of different mobility options, which may include a combination of manual and power wheelchair use or powered mobility only (Consortium for Spinal Cord Medicine, 2000).

Community Mobility

People with this level of injury can drive a car, truck, SUV, or van using hand controls, a steering knob, and an emergency brake extension (Figure 9.30). The person's transfer skill, ability to independently load/unload a wheelchair, and overall endurance will determine the decision about the type of vehicle. Transferring independently into a vehicle and loading the wheelchair into the vehicle require a high level of energy, especially if performed frequently throughout the day. Some clients may choose to use a wheelchair-loading device (wheelchair lift, car topper) or to drive an adapted van. If the choice is an adapted van, the client should transfer from the wheelchair to the van's "captain's" seat to drive safely. Information about evaluation requirements and training programs can be obtained from state departments of motor vehicles and local rehabilitation centers. In many states, state vocational rehabilitation services will help fund adaptive driving assessments and equipment procurement.

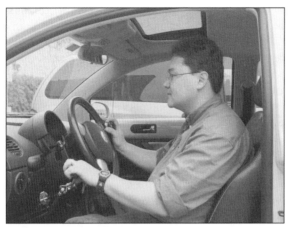

Figure 9.30. Adapted vehicle with hand controls for persons with paraplegia.

Paraplegia: Levels T7–S5

Clients with SCI and resulting paraplegia at levels T7 through S5 have intact upper extremities. T7–L1 have thoracic function intact, which improves trunk stability, wheelchair sitting balance, and transfers. Typically, people with a lower level of paraplegia are able to bend from side to side or forward without losing their balance, allowing them greater proficiency in reaching items out of their immediate, seated reach. People with injuries at L2 have hip flexor use, L3 have knee extensors, L4 have ankle dorsiflexors, L5 have long toe extensors, and S1 have ankle plantar flexor muscles working to provide lower body movement and function. Persons with SCI at T7 through S5 level of injury are independent in eating, dental care, and hygiene and grooming (e.g., washing face and hands, combing hair, shaving, applying make-up) at sink level, provided the bathroom is wheelchair accessible.

Dressing

People with injuries at this level can become independent in upper- and lower-body dressing with or without adaptations. The same lower-body dressing techniques described in the previous section may apply to the T7–L2 level. Persons with injuries below L2 will be able to balance body sitting on the edge of the bed with greater ease and will be able to move legs and feet to apply pants, socks, and shoes in a more typical fashion. Exceptions to this would be persons with a large body size or medical complications such as severe spasticity or range of motion limitations.

Bathing

People with injuries at this level can become independent in bathing using previously described padded shower equipment adaptations. Although people with injuries below S2 may be able to stand and ambulate with only a cane, due to the high risk of falls in a wet environment, it is advised for a shower bench or bottom of the tub be used for a sitting surface for safety.

Bowel, Bladder, and Menstruation Management

Men with SCI T7–S5 are able to apply an external catheter or independently utilize an intermittent catheterization program. Women with SCI at T7–S5 injury can catheterize but may need a mirror and an adaptive device to help position their legs during the task. Women can manage pads and tampons independently for menstruation management. Sacral cord injuries present in myriad ways with bladder and bowel function; management routines may vary widely. Management of these bodily functions is completed with total independence.

Meal Preparation

People with SCI at T7 will use similar meal preparation techniques to those described in the previous section. Those with injuries at T8 and below may be able to pull their body to a standing position and ambulate with the use of orthoses and gait aides during food preparation. This posture may help with access to high shelving or through narrow pantry spaces.

Functional Mobility

All transfers to level and unlevel surfaces are typically performed independently without equipment. A manual folding or rigid wheelchair is the primary means of mobility for people with SCI at this level. Additionally, functional ambulation with knee–ankle–foot orthosis (KAFOs) and forearm crutches is possible below level T8. The paraplegic person with a spinal cord injury at level L4 through S2 can ambulate with ankle–foot orthoses (AFOs) and forearm crutches. People with this level of injury have the potential to be independent ambulators within the home and for limited distances in the community, although most choose wheelchairs for their primary mode of mobility because of the substantial energy requirements of ambulation (Somers, 2001). Those with injuries below S2 may need only a cane for safety during ambulation.

Occupational therapists can help clients who wish to stand and ambulate during ADL/IADL tasks to learn proper body mechanics, energy conservation, and joint protection doing so. Close collaboration with the physical therapist is recommended early in the rehabilitation of persons who are candidates for ambulation so appropriate treatment planning can be determined (Atkins, 2008). It may be necessary (e.g., when a doorway is too narrow for wheelchair access) for some clients to ambulate through home doorways to perform ADLs. Some clients ambulate as a means of weight-bearing exercise for long bone health and others for the psychological benefits of interacting with others at at eye level. These are two among many reasons why integrating ADL performance aspects into a rehabilitation program is important.

Functionally, these individuals are independent in all self-care tasks, mobility, and communication. However, for energy conservation, efficiency, and maximum control, they may use some adapted equipment. A major concern is prevention of secondary complications, such as urinary tract infections and pressure ulcers (Pearman, 1985; Turner, 1985). Although management of these potentially serious problems usually is addressed during initial rehabilitation, once the person returns to the community, family, employment, or school, secondary complications often are ignored or neglected until the situation reaches a negative change in performance patterns. People who return to outpatient clinics at facilities where they originally were rehabilitated are reeducated or updated on advances in medical technology through their follow-up visits.

Community Mobility

People with T7–S1 level can use standard hand controls on vehicles for driving. They may learn to drive cars, trucks, SUVs, or adapted vans depending on their ability to transfer independently and load their wheelchair. Those with injuries S2 and below, with developed strength, endurance, and coordination of ankle–foot muscles, may be safe to drive vehicles without any adaptations. Safe driving ability is determed by each state's department of motor vehicles after passing a real-time driving examination. Ability to independently load a wheelchair into a vehicle is typical of all people at this SCI level.

Ulcer Prevention

Pressure ulcers are serious, costly, and potentially lifelong complications of SCI. Clinical observations and research studies have confirmed staggering costs and human suffering, including a profoundly negative impact on the affected person's general physical health, socialization, financial status, body image, and sense of independence and control

(Langemo, Melland, Hanson, Olson, & Hunter, 2000). Reported prevalence rates range from 25% to 30% in adult populations with SCI (Brem & Lyder, 2004; Fuhrer, Garber, Rintala, Clearman & Hart, 1993; Schryvers, Miroslaw, & Nance, 2000; Walter, et al., 2002).

The financial burden of pressure ulcers does not begin to reflect the personal and social costs experienced by the client and his or her family (Miller & DeLozier, 1994). Those costs include loss of independence and self-esteem, time away from work, school or family, and reduced quality of life. Subsequently, costs of treating and managing SCI-related pressure ulceration place a significant financial burden on the health care system as a whole (Consortium for Spinal Cord Medicine, 2000; Dunn, Carlson, Jackson, & Clark, 2009; Garber & Rintala, 2003).

The major pressure ulcer risk factors for persons with SCI are

- Physical, medical, and SCI-related factors (e.g., level and completeness of SCI, activity, and mobility; bladder, bowel, and moisture control; severe spasticity);
- Pre-existing conditions (e.g., advanced age, smoking, lung and cardiac disease, diabetes and renal disease, impaired cognition, residing in a nursing home);
- Nutrition (e.g., malnutrition, anemia) (Byrne & Salzberg, 1996);
- Demographic factors (e.g., age, gender, ethnicity, marital status, education); and
- Psychological and social factors (e.g., psychological distress, financial problems, cognition, substance abuse, adherence, health beliefs and practices) (Garber, Rintala, Hart, & Fuhrer, 2000).

Additional psychological factors have been associated with the development of pressure ulcers, including a person's unwillingness to take responsibility in skin care, low self-esteem, dissatisfaction with life activities (Anderson & Andberg, 1979), and poor social adjustment (Gordon, Harasymiw, Bellile, Lehman, & Sherman, 1982).

Resolving problems related to pressure ulcers requires a comprehensive evaluation and examination of the client, including

- Medical, SCI, and pressure ulcer history;
- Physical examination, including laboratory tests;
- Psychological health, behavior, cognitive status;

- Social and financial resources, including availability and utilization of personal care assistance; and
- Use of equipment, including positioning and postural support (Garber et al., 2000).

The examination typically is followed by a detailed description of the pressure ulcer itself. Strategies to prevent pressure ulcers are taught to clients and their families both formally and informally during a comprehensive rehabilitation program (Garber et al., 2000). Among these are how to use adapted equipment to inspect the skin (with an adapted mirror) and maintain its integrity, and techniques promoting good hygiene and positioning. The occupational therapist also may instruct clients in turning and repositioning in bed and shifting weight while sitting in the wheelchair. Additionally, the occupational therapist may be directly involved in measuring the client for a wheelchair and evaluating her or him for pressure-redistributing seating systems and padded bath/toilet equipment.

Support surfaces are devices, materials, or systems that redistribute the interface pressure between a person and his or her bed or wheelchair (Bergstrom et al., 1994). They do not heal pressure ulcers; they are prescribed by a clinician, frequently an occupational therapist, and incorporated into a comprehensive pressure ulcer prevention and management program. Static and dynamic mattresses and mattress overlays and specialty beds are examples of support surfaces, as are materials such as foams and gels, alone or in combination, and elements such as air and water, also alone or in combination (see Table 9.4). These are being used across patient care and home environments to reduce the risk of pressure ulcers. Wheelchair cushions and seating systems of various materials and designs, as noted above, can also function as support surfaces. No single product meets all patient needs; clients will be most effectively served by the judgment of an experienced clinician and a choice of products.

Rehabilitation professionals today are challenged to implement high-quality rehabilitation services within the context of limited resources. Fortunately, it is possible to identify people at highest risk for pressure ulcers so that effective prevention strategies can be incorporated into their lifestyles (Garber et al., 2000). Dunn et al. (2009) suggest that the complexity of pressure ulcer progression in real-life contexts dictates that integration of individualized patient care and an educational approach be woven into the fabric of each person's unique, multifaceted life experience. Dunn et al. (2009) suggest that education and individualized patient care be integrated into each person's rehabilitation/prevention program. Interventions may include direct teaching, resource identification, peer-based training and counseling, simulation exercises that address possible life scenarios, and group sharing for problem-solving and learning.

Concomitant Brain Injury and Cognitive Deficits

Paralysis of the body is evident upon observation. What is less visible may be a concomitant brain injury that accompanies a spinal injury. This condition may be overlooked or unattended to during medical care and can have a significant impact upon the rehabilitation process (Zejdlik, 1991). The percentage of patients who sustain concomitant injuries to the brain and spinal cord is 40%–50%. As the injured person has experienced blows to the body great enough to damage the spinal cord—often an automobile accident or a fall—it is apparent that brain injuries can result (Davidoff, Roth, & Richards, 1992). They may be diffuse or focal and range from mild to severe (Zejdlik, 1991).

The occupational therapist must be alert to any observations noted upon initial evaluation, for example, that the client had difficulty with evaluation instructions or seemed unfocused. The therapist should ask the client if he or she has unaccustomed difficulty with memory or detect any differences in thinking. Family and friends can be a good source of information, as they usually know the client's premorbid thinking, behavior, and learning ability.

Other factors that can make assessing brain injury complicated are medication side-effects, fatigue, pain, depression and emotional anxiety, sleep deprivation, and sensory deprivation (Davidoff et al., 1992). In many hospital settings, it has become standard practice to perform a neuropsychological screening on all clients who present with a loss of consciousness at the time of injury. Being proactive in this manner allows the rehabilitation team to be aware of any cognitive learning difficulties so teaching can be tailored to client needs to maximize performance. The therapist may need to take an approach that is more visual or more auditory or may need to teach the client in a quiet, nondistracting environment for better comprehension. When the therapist has made such determinations, written handouts, with illustrations as needed, should be prepared for the client and family with easy-to-follow client care instructions following discharge. Teaching sessions may need to be

Table 9.4. Seat Cushion Types and Their Benefits and Limitations

Cushion Category	Benefits	Limitations
Foams	• Can be shaped to fit the user, for lower pressure and more stable support while sitting • Lightweight • Lower in cost • Available in many forms • Can be flat or contoured	• Wear out relatively fast • Retain heat • Hard to clean • Support features change quickly when exposed to heat or moisture • Become hard in cold weather
Fluid-filled cushions (e.g., water, gel)	• Covered with easy-to-clean material • Effective for many different users • Distribute pressure more evenly • Control skin temperatures better • Gel-filled cushions may reduce shear	• Gel-filled cushions may be better shock absorbers than pressure reducers • May be expensive • Heavier weight
Air	• Lightweight • Easy to clean • Effective for many people • Reduce shear and peak pressures	• Tendency to puncture • Must be checked frequently for proper air pressure and maintenance • Hard to repair • May interfere with balance and posture
Combination*	• Tailored to each person by combining a variety of materials	• Additional individual devices are created by using removable and adjustable parts from cushions with a variety of components such as hip guides, wedges, etc. • May be expensive

*May use foams of different densities or combinations of gel, air, and foam.
Source. Reprinted with permission from the Paralyzed Veterans of America 2002, *Pressure Ulcers: What You Should Know,* Washington, DC: Author. Copyright © 2002, Paralyzed Veterans of America.

videotaped for future reference by the client, their family members, or hired attendants.

It is important to note that cognitive deficits in the SCI population may not be limited to those sustained at the time of injury. Some clients may have sustained a brain injury previously and had premorbid learning or behavioral problems. Learning difficulties or a history of alcohol or drug abuse prior to injury are often present and can affect the client's cognitive functioning (Davidoff et al., 1992). Mild brain injury sequelae may diminish slowly over time, yet more severe effects, such as balance problems or personality changes, may have life-altering consequences.

Upper-Limb Preservation

After a spinal cord injury, clients experience a variety of changes in their anatomical and physiological makeup. For clients with high-level cervical injuries, their bodies may take on changes such as muscle atrophy or ligamentous laxity secondary to nonuse that will result in pain or complications. People with paraplegia are often required to use their upper extremities for tasks that require increased force, repetitive use, or awkward positioning for prolonged periods. Tasks may include using the arms

for mobility by means of a walker, wheelchair, crutches, or other device. Simply sifting or transferring weight turns both of the client's shoulders into weight-bearing joints. Whether atrophy from disuse or stress from unaccustomed use, the anatomical and physiological changes in the client's upper body will frequently lead to complications in the shoulders, elbows, wrists, and hands. The shoulder joint, in particular, in a person with a SCI experience more stress than in the nondisabled population (Ballinger, Rintala & Hart, 2000). Despite advances in rehabilitation, research shows that shoulder pain and functional disability remain among the most significant factors in the CSI population. (Ballinger et al., 2000). Some studies report that 31%–73% of wheelchair users have shoulder pain. Wrist and hand pain is also common, with 49%–73% having carpal tunnel syndrome (Betz, 2007). One of the largest studies on upper limb pain in people with spinal cord injury found that a significant level of pain was present in 59% of individuals with tetraplegia and 41% of individuals with paraplegia (Sie, Waters, Adkins, & Gellman, 1992).

Therapists should consider these potential future complications during the rehabilitation process and address them in their treatment sessions. Education should include anatomy of the upper extremities; mechanisms of injury; possibility of overuse; work simplification; prevention measures; and proper equipment selection, particularly of a wheelchair. Evidenced-based practices confirm the importance of obtaining the best possible wheelchair based on the client's needs and lifestyle and having it set up properly (Cooper, 1998). Some clinical considerations in the selection process include fit, ease of propulsion, ease of transfers, ease of loading into a vehicle, maneuverability, and aesthetics (Cooper, Bonninger, & Rentschler, 1999).

Although the presence of upper-extremity pain and complications in individuals with spinal cord injury is documented in the literature, studies of how to manage the pain or how to prolong function are less prevalent (Consortium for Spinal Cord Medicine, 2005). Clinicians should refer to the information presented in ergonomics literature for the most current evidence-based practice regarding upper limb preservation and function.

The Consortium for Spinal Cord Medicine compiled Clinical Practice Guidelines entitled *The Preservation of Upper-Limb Function Following Spinal Cord Injury* to give health care professionals practical information in a straightforward, concise format that will help them prevent and treat upper-limb pain and injury in their SCI patients (Consortium for Spinal Cord Medicine, 2005). The guidelines cover initial assessment of acute SCI, ergonomics, equipment selection, training and environmental adaptations, exercise, management of acute and subacute upper limb injuries and pain, and treatment of chronic musculoskeletal pain to maintain function. Within each of these areas, the panel of interdisciplinary experts recommends ways clinicians can help their patients preserve upper-limb function. Therapists should be familiar with these concepts and practices and bring them to the attention of clients during ADL and IADL training to reinforce the use of prevention principles.

Leisure

The Rehabilitation Act of 1973 (P.L. 93-112), its amendments of 1986 (P.L. 99-506), and the ADA (P.L. 101-336) created many opportunities for people with physical disabilities to participate in leisure activities in the community. Leisure and recreational pursuits are addressed by the occupational therapist to ensure meaningful social reintegration after spinal cord injury; they have been found to enhance quality of life and personal satisfaction on multiple levels. Engaging in leisure or recreational activities is "viewed as a means of balancing one's lifestyle in order to promote health and life satisfaction through physical, psychosocial, and emotional benefits" (Christiansen, 1991). Often so much energy is exerted in retraining individuals with SCI to perform the basic ADLs that leisure and recreation may be overlooked altogether—but achieving balance in life is a key goal for all people to strive for in everyday performance. Whether one chooses to engage in tabletop games with family, participate in an adaptive sport, or enjoy community activities, engaging in occupations that are relaxing and fun is an important aspect of one's overall well-being. Equally important, involvement also enhances self-worth, improves mental health, and promotes a sense of belonging. Being involved with a leisure pursuit or being a part of the community gives people an "emotional lift"—a feeling of accomplishment.

People who experience SCI face wrenching changes in how they spend their time. Immediately after an injury or upon returning home after rehabilitation, they must redefine what is meaningful to them regarding leisure time or recreation. Many placed great importance on an active lifestyle prior to their injury; returning to their previous activities or identifying new ones that they enjoy are crucial for life satisfaction (Dolhi, 1996). By participating in leisure or recreational activities, people with SCI can enjoy engaging with others in meaningful occupations, can prevent loss of strength and endurance, and experience a sense of success through completing a task.

The occupational therapist has a unique role in initiating and encouraging leisure activities after spinal cord injury. Regardless of the level of injury and physical involvement, all clients can pursue recreational participation, thanks largely to the wide variety of options, adaptive equipment, and resources now available for individuals with disabilities.

The therapist and client together will first determine the client's skills, limitations, and pre- and post-injury leisure interests. This will guide choice of activity; initial education; and ultimately, participation. The therapist can then help the client adapt or learn new leisure or recreational activities (Figure 9.31), perhaps adapting existing game pieces or processes, or using an orthosis or assistive device to manipulate objects, or exploring new activities that interest the client. Considerations include safety of the environment, adaptations for balance and limited hand function, precautions against potential injury (e.g., blisters,

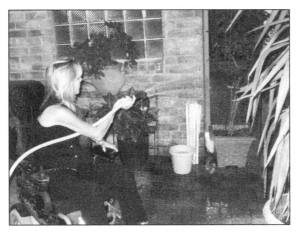

Figure 9.31. Recreational activities.

cuts, pressure ulcers), and identification of appropriate equipment (e.g., sports chairs). Personal issues such as bowel and bladder management, medications, sitting tolerance, and transportation must also be addressed (Blackwell, Krause, Winkler, & Stiens, 2001).

Wheelchair sports, for individual and team competition, have become a popular leisure activity for many people with disabilities, offering physical, psychological, and social benefits to people with SCI (Hanson, Nabavi, & Yuen, 2001). Specialized sports wheelchairs are available, with adaptations such as angled wheels for stability and ease of turning, specialized foot rests for optimal positioning, ultra-lightweight frames, and low backs for maximal upper-body movement.

Belonging to a team gives people with SCI both the warmth of team companionship and an outlet to "blow off steam" in competition. Wheelchair sports also provide invaluable physical exercise and can prevent the effects of deconditioning or disuse of active musculature. Adaptive sports may lead to higher social competence and increased self-esteem. Sporting activities used in the rehabilitation process can help to teach discipline and sportsmanship and assist in accomplishing necessary ADLs.

Work

Once a person gains skill and proficiency in ADLs and IADLs, focus can be directed on returning to productive living in the community. Because people who sustain a SCI tend to be relatively young at the time of injury, returning to paid employment, volunteering, or educational pursuits are common and critical for quality of life.

Factors Affecting Return to Work

It is not unusual for people who have sustained SCI to need to alter their career or life goals significantly. In general, three variables affect a client's return to work: degree of impairment, age, and rehabilitation experiences. People with paraplegia are more likely to return to work than persons with tetraplegia. Within each group, persons with incomplete injuries are more likely to work than those with complete injuries. People injured at a younger age are more likely to return to work. Completion of a vocational rehabilitation program increases the likelihood of returning to work (DeVivo, Rutt, Stover, & Fine, 1987). Findings on employment of people with SCI as reported by Pflaum, McCollister, Strauss, Shavelle, and DeVivo (2006) were

- The more severe the injury, the less likely the person was to be employed.
- Higher education offsets impairment and greatly increases the likelihood of employment.
- People with tetraplegia who had attained less education were particularly unlikely to find employment.
- Being married was associated with a higher likelihood of finding work.
- People with SCI with professional degrees were no less likely to be employed than those without disability of similar educational level.

In looking at vocational and other life roles, researchers have found that access to equipment resources can affect role functioning. Having access to some electronic control devices is associated with increased frequency of participation in educational activities, improved performance in ADLs and increased activity by people with tetraplegia (Efthimiou, Gordon, Sell, & Stratford, 1981). Brown (1983) found that access to a private vehicle increased the probability of being employed up to 50%.

A critical step in returning to paid or volunteer work is independence in community mobility. This step could entail the client learning to drive with vehicle modifications or learning how to use accessible public transportation systems. Occupational therapists can take the lead in educating and training their clients.

In addition to limited body movement, decreased mobility, and decreased independence in daily living skills, people with SCI may face environmental barriers that will physically restrict their ability to access places, materials/objects, and services. Return to work appears to be related to accessing resources (e.g., through personal care assistance, EADLs, and accessible transportation).

Employment following SCI increases slowly but steadily over time. As time elapsed postinjury approaches 5 years, the probability of working increases, after which a plateau is reached and then a fall-off as people approach retirement age. Some explanations of the 5-year mark include completion of education or retraining for new types of jobs that are more consistent with SCI physical functioning and capabilities, the need for psychosocial adjustment to a disability, and the need to overcome barriers and disincentives to work (Pflaum et al., 2006). The percentage of tetraplegic who are employed increases steadily with time from 13.4% at 1 year post-injury to 38.9% at the 25th anniversary of injury. Among paraplegic clients, the percentage employed is only slightly higher, ranging from 13.6% 1 year after injury to 47.1% 20 years after injury.

Most people with SCI maintain full-time jobs rather than part-time jobs, which is probably a reflection of the need for health care insurance coverage (DeVivo, 2002). This pattern indicates that re-entry (or initial entry) into the workplace after SCI is a slow process that may span a decade or more. Significantly, nearly 60% of the overall SCI population appears not to return to a work environment at all. Although people with SCI cannot work at jobs that require manual labor or extensive physical body mobility, many other opportunities exist for them to return to work (Figure 9.32). Many psychological and societal factors, however, discourage people with physical disabilities from doing so. At the psychological level, some people with SCI cannot envision themselves ever being productive at a job again. At the societal level, factors such as Social

Security disincentives, cultural attitudes, and environmental barriers may be barriers to access to the workplace for many. Disincentives weigh heavily against return to work; one major factor is that many people with SCI who return to work may not be able to afford essential services and products that are available through publicly funded programs only to the unemployed.

Occupational Therapy Role

The role of the occupational therapist is to help develop a new set of goals and hopes for the person with SCI, including goals for a return to paid or volunteer work. If the client was previously employed, the therapist should discuss how returning to that employment arena is possible. If the client is entering the workforce for the first time, the therapist should discuss his or her interests and abilities. An occupational therapist may have clients with SCI attempt to perform typical work components to anticipate, evaluate, and solve problems with doing that work. Therapists may establish a simulated work environment so that clients can practice typical work activities.

A therapist can also analyze specific job performance areas that would be practical and determine how they can be adapted. People with SCI who have already re-entered the workplace may be considered "SCI peers" and should be asked to share, if possible, their personal experiences with a newly injured client to help his or her "vision" of possibilities begin to take shape. People with SCI who have returned to work or school may serve as role models in the SCI community, inspiring hopes for a brighter, productive future and a return to a normal life course that was only interrupted—not ended—by the injury.

Volunteer Work

Volunteer work can serve as a proving ground to a client who is re-entering or entering a work setting for the first time following the injury. Volunteer work can enable the client to practice necessary skills, such as completing ADLs in time to meet a work schedule, interacting with co-workers and the public, and accessing transportation. It allows testing of physical endurance and work tolerance in a noncompetitive work environment. Volunteer work frequently can be a springboard to paid employment positions, even if the client is not seeking paid employment. Volunteer work, in and of itself, can give the client the valuable sense that he or she can participate in and contribute to society. Such work is more for psychological than monetary rewards; it

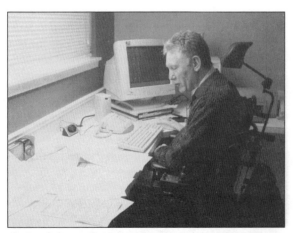

Figure 9.32. Individual with C6 tetraplegia working at home.

can be the initial step to proving to oneself that paid employment can be a feasible goal. It also can prove to reluctant employers that a person with SCI can meet the demands of a job.

Paid Employment

Job seekers with SCI must plan and test specific aspects of their goals:

- Do they need further education to be successful in procuring a particular job?
- Do they have reliable transportation or convenient access to public transportation?
- Can they drive themselves to work, or can family or friends drive them to and from work?
- Does a potential employer have appropriate equipment that will enable the client to efficiently perform the requirements of the job?
- Are they knowledgeable and comfortable discussing with the employer any necessary job accommodations?
- Have they anticipated issues that may arise while on the job, and are they prepared to discuss them and offer possible solutions?

Issues that may arise on the job include situations involving bowel and bladder management or the inability to reach items or access areas of the workplace. Ideally, job seekers will be able to communicate such issues—including suggesting possible solutions—in a manner that does not overwhelm the potential employer. Occupational therapists can help clients anticipate potential problem, generate possible solutions, and practice the communication skills necessary for applying for a job.

People with SCI need to establish what their ability will be to sustain part-time or full-time employment. Beginning conservatively with a part-time position may allow the person to prove his or her ability in the workplace and then advance to a full-time workload. Realistic expectations about energy expenditure are crucial, and they are best assessed by planning and organizing the workday. In addition to the energy necessary to complete work assignments, people with SCI typically expend more energy than those without disabilities in completing ADLs necessary to prepare for and arrive at work. The client's employer must have a good understanding of his or her abilities and limitations so that work expectations can be set realistically. Depending on the worker's level of SCI, job tasks must be broken down into steps that can be analyzed to determine the most efficient and effective way to performed them. The better the communication

between employer and employee, the more successful the work situation typically will be for both parties. It is incumbent on the person with SCI to ask for feedback on job performance and to present questions and concerns to the employer in a professional manner so that problem resolution can be a collaborative effort.

The ADA provided persons with SCI and many other neurological or musculoskeletal conditions opportunities and technology to return to the workplace and gain financial success and a sense of well-being. Published sources cite that after implementation of the ADA, there was a 20% increase in the likelihood of employment post-SCI (Pflaum et al., 2006). Many of the same adaptive methods used to perform ADLs can be used to accomplish work tasks on the job. No prescriptive list exists of jobs that can be performed by people with each level of SCI. Persons with high-level tetraplegia, such as C2–C4, are lawyers and office receptionists. People with C5 tetraplegia are stockbrokers and social workers. People with C6 tetraplegia are secretaries, teachers, or dispatchers. People with C7–C8 tetraplegia are computer system administrators, college professors, and school principles. People with SCI are medical supply sales representatives, theater ticket sales persons, bankers, accountants, actors, business owners, and doctors. Achieving independence and success in the workplace depends on seeking a job that best matches the person's physical and intellectual attributes, personal motivation, and problem-solving creativity.

Sexual Activity and Fertility

Advances in medicine and technology have enhanced sexual functioning and fertility among people with SCI. *Social participation*, as defined by the World Health Organization (WHO), includes engaging in intimate relationships that contribute to quality of life for people with disabilities (WHO, 2001). Although sexuality following SCI has been studied for at least 40 years, it is only within the past 25–30 years that sexual adjustment and function have become part of the occupational therapy intervention process (McAlonan, 1996). Sexuality and sexual function, leading to greater social participation and integration, are an important aspect of holistic occupational therapy treatment in addressing ADL interventions for people with SCI.

Young (2004) describes functional problems associated with sexual functioning following SCI as mobility loss, sensory loss, bowel and bladder problems (including use of catheters), spasticity, erectile dysfunction, and loss of vaginal lubrication in women. In addition to the physical components that contribute to sexual functioning, there are many psychological, social, cultural, and faith belief aspects that determine how a person experiences sexual expression and behaviors. People with SCI may experience orgasm in a different manner than prior to their injury, such as experiencing feelings of pleasure, heightened excitement, or other body reactions such as skin flushing or spasms (Anderson, Borisoff, Johnson, Stiens, & Elliott, 2007; Mooney, Cole, & Chilgren, 1975). SCI does not preclude the ability to achieve orgasm, although it typically takes longer after an injury. People with SCI, armed with this knowledge, can have an open and frank discussion with their partner resulting in enhanced overall satisfaction and understanding of the process (Sipski, Alexander, Gomez-Marin, Spalding, 2007).

For men, erection and ejaculation can be improved with new devices and medical and surgical interventions. Many new options exist for men with SCI; they should be educated on the availability of oral medications for erectile enhancement (Ducharme, 1999). Vacuum constriction devices, intracorporeal injection of vasoactive agents, or penile implants and prostheses can enhance erection. Vibrators or electrical stimulation may be used to induce ejaculation, and retrieval of sperm for insemination can be accomplished through microsurgical techniques if other techniques fail.

Women with SCI may experience inadequate vaginal lubrication or problems achieving orgasm. A water-soluble gel may be used to increase genital lubrication in women and to decrease pressure or friction during sexual activity. A recent review observed that systematic studies are lacking regarding fertility in women following SCI (DeForge et al., 2005). Although the menstrual cycle will be interrupted temporarily for weeks or months following the injury, case reports have widely documented pregnancy and live births in women following SCI. Level of injury does not seem to influence duration of amenorrhea or the occurrence of pregnancy in women with SCI. Successful pregnancies are achievable in women who experience transient amenorrhea after SCI (Bughi, Shaw, Mahmood, Atkins, & Szlachcic, 2008). Pregnancy rates of 51% and a live birth rate of 40% have been noted in recent reviews, qualified with the caveat that the highest success rates have been achieved with the use of advanced fertility treatment (DeForge et al., 2005).

In addition to inadequate lubrication, potential complications of pregnancy among women with SCI include increased medical problems such as urinary tract infections and pressure ulcers, increased spasticity, respiration difficulties, changes in body habitus, and autonomic hyperreflexia (Anderson, Borisoff, Johnson, Stiens, & Elliott, 2006). Autonomic hyperreflexia is considered the most significant potential medical complication that might occur during any stage of pregnancy, labor, delivery, or postpartum (Consortium for Spinal Cord Medicine, 2001).

Role of Occupational Therapy

The role of the occupational therapist in helping clients address limitations in sexual activity has not been well studied. Neistadt (1986) described a four-stage model for occupational therapists to use in sexuality counseling called the PLISSIT model. Neistadt's model involves permission, limited information, specific suggestions, and intensive therapy. According to Neistadt, the first three stages are appropriate for counseling by occupational therapists. In the permission phase, the therapist may mention some aspect of sexuality during ADL skills training, thereby acknowledging legitimate concerns or curiosities of the person. Limited information can be shared that will help to alleviate concerns or counter any misconceptions held. Another consideration is the therapist's comfort level in discussing sexuality with people with SCI. Specific suggestions can be provided by the therapist regarding sexuality or sexual activity if they feel competent to deliver this information. Therapists should not hesitate to refer a client to a counselor trained in providing sexuality counseling to people with SCI.

Therapists need to anticipate a client's concerns and questions about sexual functioning in view of the intimate personal care tasks in which they are

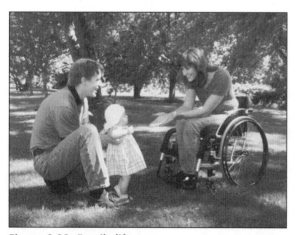

Figure 9.33. Family life.

involved. Clients may consult with the occupational therapist regarding specific performance areas, such as preparation for sexual activity, undressing, bowel and bladder functioning, positioning and body handling, hand functioning, and equipment adaptation. Education of these aspects of sexual performance should be interwoven into a client's ongoing routine therapy sessions for the most natural conveyance of this sometimes sensitive information. Health care providers as a whole can provide effective therapeutic interventions, including discussion of mutual responsibility and education of changes in sexual functioning; facilitating communication between partners; facilitating attitude and behavior change; and recommendation of techniques, aids, and resources (Esmail Esmail, & Munro, 2001).

The psychosocial elements of building relationships, communicating needs and concerns, and satisfaction are as important as physical functioning (Adler, 1996; Esmail et al., 2001; Solet, 2008). Educational and emotional support provided by the occupational therapist can supplement the information people with SCI may receive from other rehabilitation or health care professionals. Sexuality is a sensitive area, however, and the topic should be broached with caution, even though the occupational therapist often is the person with whom the patient feels the most comfortable discussing intimate details because of the therapeutic relationship that develops during treatment (Young, 2004). Therefore, it is incumbent on each therapist to develop a level of basic knowledge, develop a comfort level with imparting that basic knowledge to people who are ready to receive it, and make appropriate referrals as necessary.

Assistive Technology

Advances in technology influence every aspect of daily life, including the quality of life of people with SCI. From the automated teller machines in banks to touch-screen telephone technology and computer systems, technology often provides unique and dynamic solutions to otherwise unsolvable problems. For people with SCI, technology and assistive technology (AT) greatly expand opportunities for independence and productivity.

In the early 1970s, the U.S. government demonstrated its commitment to improving the vocational and self-care goals of people with severe physical impairments through the establishment of rehabilitation engineering centers. The centers combined the efforts of medicine, engineering, and related sciences to identify practical solutions to problems that limited the integration of persons with physical impairments into productive community life (Traub & LeClair, 1975). In 1988, with the passage of the Technology-Related Assistance for Individuals with Disabilities Act (P.L. 100-407), the U.S. government further demonstrated its support for the development and use of technology to enhance rehabilitation outcomes for people with severe physical disabilities. *Assistive technology*—defined as "any item, piece of equipment, or product system, off-the-shelf, modified, or customized that is used to increase, maintain or improve function"—became the byword of the 1990s for consumers and healthcare providers alike. The Individuals with Disabilities Education Act Amendments of 1997 (P.L. 105-117) authorized additional grants for assistive technology that further expanded the use of AT in the schools. The Technology-Related Assistance for Individuals with Disabilities Act was replaced by the Assistive Technology Act of 1998. The Assistive Technology Act as amended (P.L. 108-364) placed AT education and advocacy resources in all 50 states. This led to increased public awareness of the benefits of AT devices and services; helped improve funding, technical assistance, and training; and provided outreach support to community-based organizations to assist individuals in finding and funding AT.

In addition to advanced AT devices, many low-tech devices are still available and widely used today by people with SCI. Among them are

- Reachers and dressing sticks,
- Long-handled shoehorns and sock aids,
- Universal cuffs and built-up handles, and
- Mouthsticks.

AT that is higher-tech includes

- EADLs,
- Computer access systems,
- Augmentative communication devices,
- Cellular phone technologies, and
- Mobility and seating systems.

Some mainstream technologies that are marketed as timesaving or convenience items to the general public may also meet the needs of a person with SCI. These devices include sound-activated (e.g., by hand clapping) light switches, motion detectors, automatic pet feeders, keyless remote controls, and an inexpensive craft tray to transport items.

The appropriate prescription of assistive devices is a major focus of the occupational therapy intervention process during the rehabilitation of people with SCI. Therapists play prominent roles in the AT clinics of public and private rehabilitation facilities. They evaluate each person with SCI for his or her potential to use technology to enhance and expand the skills needed to be more independent in communication, self-care, and return to school or work or to become more socially involved. Working with the AT team, the therapist makes recommendations and trains clients to use technology to achieve their maximum potential (Mann & Lane, 1991). For people with SCI who are being assessed for advanced technology systems for the first time, relying on knowledgeable, credentialed professionals (suppliers or AT practitioners) may ensure a successful fit of equipment with their lifestyle and goals (Minkel, 2002). These specialists are now called *assistive technology professionals,* and are defined by RESNA as a "service provider who analyzes the needs of individuals with disabilities, assists in the selection of the appropriate equipment, and trains the consumer on how to properly use the specific equipment" (RESNA, 2009a).

Occupational therapists have played a leading role in evaluating and recommending EADLs for people with significant disability. These enable a disabled person to access and control objects and devices such as lights, televisions, thermostats, blinds, and audiovideo systems by simple acts such as clapping or moving. People without disabilities frequently use EADLs to automate and facilitate routine household tasks. A familiar EADL is the remote control device for the television or audiovideo equipment. Specialized units that can be accessed through a computer system or voice-activated are also available. The latter are especially useful for people who have impaired motor function of high-level SCI (Swenson, Barnett, Pond, & Schoenberg, 1998).

Although these units are used in hospitals and rehabilitation facilities, they are not widely recommended for use in home settings, primarily because of their high cost and limitations on reimbursement (Holme, Kanny, Guthrie, & Johnson, 1997). As the general public uses these devices more and they become more commonplace, the costs of the commercially available devices are decreasing. Meanwhile, the more common, less sophisticated devices can be found in gift magazines, thrift stores, home solution Web sites, or home improvement stores. Creative use of such devices may provide for more independent performance of a task. It is worth noting that they typically are available at a lower cost than technologies marketed as medical devices (Coppola-Passariello, 2003).

Computers have become essential tools in everyday life for education, employment, communication, shopping, financial transactions, and recreation. Computers and access to the Internet have created education and job opportunities for people with disabilities, including those with SCI. A study by Goodman, Jette, Houlihan, and Williams (2008) demonstrated widespread use of the computer and Internet by persons with SCI. However, access was uneven and related to age, race, and education. Primary uses for this technology documented in the study were communication, shopping, and access to health information. With shorter length of inpatient rehabilitation stays, more people are seeking patient education for online health interventions through the Internet. Use of the Internet for health information offers convenient access, reduction of isolation, and an increase in a sense of control for users (Drainoni et al., 2004).

It is important that people with cervical-level spinal injury gain access to conventional computer systems through alternative methods if the standard way is not feasible or time-efficient. One research study indicated that 19% of computer users have employed some type of assistive device, including voice activation or recognition, modified mouse, typing splint, or head pointer (Goodman et al., 2008). Occupational therapists can assess users for the most appropriate keyboard control. To use a standard computer keyboard, the user must have sufficient upper-extremity range of motion, coordination, and strength to accurately hit target keys, depress the keys, hold down several keys at once, and release keys fast enough to avoid inadvertent repetition of keys. The client must also have access to a computer station that is compatible with his or her wheelchair and set at the appropriate height.

Keyboard adaptations that eliminate the need to hold multiple keys at once can provide stability and slow the repeat rate to avoid unwanted repeats. Alternative keyboards can provide variety in the spacing, size, layout, and activation force of keys. They can also allow for inputting data in ways other than with the hands, such as using a head pointer or mouth stick. Onscreen keyboards represent a virtual keyboard on the computer screen can be used in combination with a mouse input device to eliminate a physical keyboard. Trial versions of this software can generally be found on the Internet for trial prior to purchase. Voice recognition systems allow input using consistent speech. Mouse alternatives can eliminate the need to hold the mouse, vary the movements required to direct the mouse pointer, replace the button with switches that can be activated with alternative actions, and allow pointing with alternative body parts. Trackballs and joysticks are frequently easier to control than a standard mouse. The mouse pointer may also be controlled using head movement, which is tracked with infrared or ultrasound technology. Buttons on some alternative input devices can be programmed to perform a certain feature without the need to hold the button down or double-click. Mouse buttons can also be replaced with sip-and-puff switches or with software that perform the mouse click, double click, and drag by lingering on a target for a predetermined time and then moving the mouse cursor in one of the four directions. Free software or operating systems modifications allow changes to be made to keyboard response by slowing response time, eliminating or slowing key repeat rate, and holding keys used in multiple key depressions when selected sequentially. Miniaturized keyboards accommodate those with limited range of movement or strength (Barker, 2002; Treviranus & Petty, 2002). Mouthstick users also find miniature keyboards easier to use because they decrease the amount of head turning required.

Portable digital assistants (PDAs) and smartphones (phones with PDAs) give people with SCI significant communication functions without the need for fine motor coordination or use of expensive EADLs. A tap on a highlighted hyperlink or a contact saved in a "favorites" file allows for ease in accessing information or audiovideo files or dialing a telephone number; standard software recognizes and hyperlinks telephone numbers on a Web page. Using gross swipes across the touch screen makes selecting functions easy, as compared to the daunting task of pressing small buttons on a standard cellular phone. PDA devices can be synchronized with computers to update contacts, access calendars, music, and a variety of applications. The hugely popular Nintendo Wii® gaming system also has proved useful in in rehabilitation. Clinics use Wii systems to help people with SCI perform movements in need of functional improvement. Wii can proviide continuing benefits if the client chooses to buy the system for his or her home. In the home, it and other gaming systems also create oppportunities for social integration with family and friends.

Body weight–supported (BWS) locomotor training has recently been seen in larger SCI rehabilitation centers to improve over-ground walking ability in individuals with motor-incomplete SCI. Typically, these programs are staffed and run by physical therapy personnel with the focus on gait-related functions. It is important to note that even though the majority of participants in these programs continue to use a wheelchair as their primary means of mobility, many people who have participated in this new approach to report experiencing meaningful differences to their daily function (Field-Fote, Lindley, & Sherman, 2005). These improvements have enabled them to successfully perform activities they were previously unable to do, such as enter an inaccessible bathroom, climb stairs, or perform food preparation or kitchen clean-up while moving around the kitchen using the countertops for support. Occupational therapists should recognize these newly gained mobility skills and offer continued ADL and IADL training to take advantage of further occupational performance improvement.

Two robotic devices that have shown promise are the Assistive Robotic Service Manipulator (ARM) and the MIT Manus for the Upper Limb. These devices provide mechanical assistance for upper-extremity training (i.e., range of motion) and for compensation functional movement after SCI (Harwin, Patton, & Edgerton, 2006; Hesse, Schmidt, Werner, & Bardeleben, 2003). Although neither is widely seen in mainstream rehabilitation clinics, their functional potential may be a springboard for future technologies.

Although robotics and video game technology are not seen in every rehabilitation setting, there is a trend of clinics moving from a more manual operation to a more technology-rich environment

Prostheses for SCI in current use are likely to improve significantly over the next decade. Peripheral nerve stimulation systems have been used for a number of years in SCI rehabilitation for gait assistance and upper-limb activation. A variety of new neuroprostheses, interfacing either with the central or peripheral nervous system, above and below lesion, are currently in research and development. Invasive and noninvasive brain–machine interfaces (BMI) as control signal channels may be seen in the future. Intraspinal stimulation, although requiring significant technical advances, is a potential technology for improving ADL and IADL functioning. The continued work in neuroplasticity with devices, training, and rehabilitation are of paramount therapeutic importance; occupational therapists will be have to understand their clinical applications and help them transition from research lab to clinic, as well as reasonable translation into the clinic (Giszter, 2008; Hesse et al., 2003).

BMI neuroprosthesis is being considered for use by SCI clients (Patil & Turner, 2008). Research focusing on bridging the brain and peripheral motor activity seems promising. Occupational therapists must stay abreast of these advances to optimize care for clients with SCI in the future.

Another AT is the use of service dogs (or assistance dogs) to provide compensatory functions both at home and in the community (Hanebrink & Dillon, 2000). Service dogs can help individuals with SCI achieve greater independence in a variety of performance areas, including ADLs, home management, functional mobility, socialization, emergency alerting, and environmental control (Delta Society, 2009). Service dog ownership has also been shown to have significant psychosocial benefits, such as improved self-esteem, increased social interaction, decreased stress, and greater internal locus of control (Camp, 2001; Valentine, Kiddoo, & LaFleur, 1993). Camp (2001) found that common themes voiced by service dog owners were that their dogs increased their social participation, facilitated their personal skill development, provided an opportunity to care for another living being, and provided an opportunity to achieve greater ADL/IADL independence in their home and community. Service dog training is tailored to meet the specific needs of each individual with an SCI; the particular tasks any dog performs will vary according to circumstance and master. Examples may include picking up a dropped writing pen, moving an obstacle out of the way of the wheelchair, giving money or a credit card to a cashier, dialing 911 or alerting bystander of an emergency, retrieving a ringing telephone, and opening the door for a delivery person (Allen & Blascovich, 1996; Delta Society, 2009; Sunderlin, 1999; see Figure 9.34).

Summary

At the time of injury and throughout the adjustment phase of SCI, the occupational therapist plays a critical role in establishing the framework and resources to ensure a purposeful life after this life-altering event. Although the most obvious signs of disability after SCI are loss of motor and sensory control below the level of injury, the most profound obstacles involve reintegrating back into a meaningful and productive life. The occupational therapist has the unique skills to look at the person, environment, context, and culture of the person with SCI and create an individualized plan to regain a life with purpose. Creativity and holistic understanding become the tools that will bring

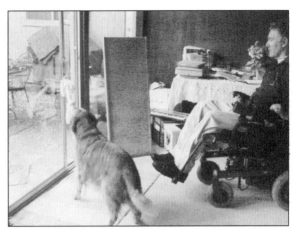

Figure 9.34. Service dog assisting an individual with C6 tetraplegia.

positive outcomes through this journey with the client.

This chapter has provided details of life with SCI, as well as strategies that an occupational therapist can employ to give a client confidence to live life with a disability. Adjustment involves being able to use these strategies, techniques, and adaptations in a variety of settings and situations to face potential obstacles with a sense of security. The expected functional outcome will be improvements in ADLs and IADLs at all levels of SCI and the client's increased self-esteem, well-being, and use of community-based resources and organizations.

Life changes dramatically after SCI. It is a significant event that affects not only the person injured but also the lives he or she is connected with. The initial onset of injury may bring feelings of helplessness, fear of the unknown, and sadness. However, as thousands of persons with SCI demonstrate every day, there is real hope for a full life beyond disability.

> The realization of potential usefulness remaining to any man appears to be entirely apart from muscular weakness...it is an adjustment that repeatedly demonstrates to all of us that success in living is not success in bodily movement...creativity, responsiveness, fraternity, responsibility, and equality are not measured by muscle strength...it is as if the man within the shell of mortal clay unleashes himself from the bonds of muscular might and uses the tiniest strengths for the greatest purposes. (Spencer, 1958, p. 1)

Study Questions

1. Discuss the differences between paraplegia and tetraplegia with respect to social participation. What aspects of social participation are likely to be more difficult for persons with tetraplegia. Why?

2. Describe autonomic dysreflexia and the circumstances that can cause it. What can an occupational therapist recommend to a client to help prevent this?

3. What aspects of basic ADLs are likely to be most problematic for a person with tetraplegia? List an example of an adaptive strategy that can be employed for one or more ADLs.

4. What types of orthoses might be appropriate for a person with a C5 level spinal cord injury? Why?

5. Describe the trade-off between self-reliance and independence and the cost of task completion in terms of energy and time. When should a caregiver be used for ADLs? Why?

6. At what SCI level would an occupational therapist expect a client to have potential for independence with bowel and bladder management, using equipment? What equipment and techniques would be anticipated?

7. List goals for clients who are independent in ADLs from a wheelchair level, including mobility.

References

Adler, C. (1996). Spinal cord injury. In L. W. Pedretti (Ed.), *Occupational therapy practice skills for physical dysfunction* (4th ed., p. 770). St. Louis, MO: Mosby.

Allen, K., & Blascovich, J. (1996). The value of service dogs for people with severe ambulatory disabilities. *JAMA, 275,* 1001–1006.

American Spinal Injury Association. (2008). *International standards for neurological and functional classification of spinal cord injury.* Chicago: Author.

Americans with Disabilities Act of 1990, Pub. L. 101–336, 42 USC § 12101.

Anderson, K. D., Borisoff, J. F., Johnson, R. D., Stiens, S. A., & Elliott S. L. (2006). Spinal cord injury influences psychogenic as well as physical components of female sexual ability. *Spinal Cord, 10,* 1–11.

Anderson, K. D., Borisoff, J. F., Johnson, R. D., Stiens, S. A., & Elliott, S. L. (2007). Long-term effects of spinal cord injury on sexual function in men: Implications for neuroplasticty. *Spinal Cord, 45,* 338–348.

Anderson, T. P., & Andberg, M. M. (1979). Psychosocial factors associated with pressure sores. *Archives of Physical Medicine and Rehabilitation, 60,* 341–46.

Assistive Technology Act of 1998, as amended, Pub. L. 108–364, 29 U.S.C. § 3, 118 Stat. 1707 (2004).

Atkins, M. (2002). Spinal cord injury. In C. Trombly & M. Radomski (Eds.), *Occupational therapy for physical,*

dysfunction (5th ed., pp. 965–999). Philadelphia: Lippincott Williams & Wilkins.

Atkins, M. (2008). Spinal cord injury. In M. V. Radomski & C. A. Trombly-Latham (Eds.), *Occupational therapy for physical dysfunction* (6th ed., 1171–1213). Philadelphia: Lippincott Williams & Wilkins.

Ballinger, D. A., Rintala, D. H., & Hart, K. A. (2000). The relation of shoulder pain and range of motion problems to functional limitations, disability, and perceived health of men with spinal cord injury: A multifaceted longitudinal study. *Archives of Physical Medicine and Rehabilitation, 81,* 1575–1581.

Barker, P. (2002). Technologies for information, communication, and access. In D. A. Olson & F. DeRuyter (Eds.), *Clinician's guide to assistive technology* (pp. 89–90). St. Louis, MO: Mosby.

Bergstrom, N., Allman, R. M., Alvarez, O. M., Bennett, M. A., Carlson, C. E., et al. (1994). *Treatment of pressure ulcers* (Guideline Report No. 15 Pub No. 96-N014). Rockville, MD: U.S. Department of Health and Human Services, Public Health Service, Agency for Health Care Policy and Research.

Betz, K. (2007). Pushing a wheelchair: Simple task or accomplished skill? *Paraplegia News, 61*(3), 30–35.

Blackwell, T. L., Krause, J. S., Winkler, T., & Stiens, S. A. (2001). *Spinal cord injury desk reference: Guidelines for life care planning and case management.* New York: Demos.

Brem, H., & Lyder, C. (2004). Protocol for the successful treatment of pressure ulcers. *American Journal of Surgery, 188*(Suppl. 1A), 9S–17S.

Brown, M. M. (1983). Actual and perceived differences in activity patterns of able-bodied and disabled men. *Dissertation Abstracts International, 43,* 2314B.

Bryden, A. M., Wuolle, K. S., Murray, P. K., & Peckham, P. H. (2004). Perceived outcomes and utilization of upper extremity surgical reconstruction in individuals with tetraplegia at model spinal cord injury systems. *Spinal Cord, 42,* 169–176.

Bughi, S., Shaw, S. J., Mahmood, G., Atkins, R. H., & Szlachcic, Y. (2008). Amenorrhea, pregnancy, and pregnancy outcomes in women following spinal cord injury: A retrospective cross-sectional study. *Endocrine Practice, 14*(4), 437–41.

Byrne, D. W., & Salzberg, C. A. (1996). Major risk factors for pressure ulcers in the spinal cord disabled: A literature review. *Spinal Cord, 34,* 255–263.

Camp, M. M. (2001). The use of service dogs as an adaptive strategy: A qualitative study. *American Journal of Occupational Therapy, 5*(5), 509–517.

Cardenas, D. D., Burns, S. P., & Chan, L. (2000). Rehabilitation of spinal cord injury. In M. Grabois, S. J., Garrison, K. A., Hart, & L. D. Lehmkuhl (Eds.), *Physical medicine and rehabilitation—The Complete approach* (pp. 1305–1324). Malden, MA: Blackwell Science.

Cardenas, D. D., Hoffman, J. M., Kirshblum, S., & McKinley, W. (2004). Etiology and incidence of rehospitalization after traumatic spinal cord injury: A multicenter analysis. *Archives of Physical Medicine and Rehabilitation, 85,* 1757–1763.

Christiansen, C. (1991). Occupational performance assessment. In C. Christiansen & C. Baum, (Eds.), *Occupational therapy: Overcoming human performance deficits* (pp. 343–387). Thorofare, NJ: Slack.

Clifton, G. L., Donovan, W. H., & Frankowski, R. F. (1985). Patterns of care for the patient with spinal cord injury. *Current Concepts in Rehabilitation Medicine, 2,* 14–17.

Cohen, M. E., Sheehan, T. P., & Herbison, G. J. (1996). Content validity and reliability of the International Standards for Neurological Classification of Spinal Cord Injury. *Topics in Spinal Cord Injury Rehabilitation, 1,* 15–31.

Cook, A. M., & Hussey, S. M. (Eds.). (2002). *Assistive technologies: Principles and practice* (2nd ed.). St. Louis, MO: Mosby.

Cooper, R. A. (1998). *Wheelchair selection and configuration.* New York: Demos.

Cooper, R. A., Bonninger, M. L., & Rentschler, A. (1999). Evaluation of selected ultralight manual wheelchairs using ANSI/RESNA standards. *Archives of Physical Medicine and Rehabilitation, 80,* 462–467.

Consortium for Spinal Cord Medicine. (1998). *Neurogenic bowel management in adults with spinal cord injury.* Washington, DC: Paralyzed Veterans of America.

Consortium for Spinal Cord Medicine. (1999a). *Neurogenic bowel: What you should know.* Washington, DC: Paralyzed Veterans of America.

Consortium for Spinal Cord Medicine. (1999b). *Outcomes following traumatic spinal cord injury: Clinical practice guidelines for health-care professionals.* Washington, DC: Paralyzed Veterans of America.

Consortium for Spinal Cord Medicine. (2000). *Pressure ulcer prevention and treatment following spinal cord injury: A clinical practice guideline for health-care professionals.* Washington, DC: Paralyzed Veterans of America.

Consortium for Spinal Cord Medicine. (2001). *Acute management of autonomic dysreflexia: Individuals with spinal cord injury presenting to health-care facilities* (2nd ed.). Washington, DC: Paralyzed Veterans of America.

Consortium for Spinal Cord Medicine. (2005). *Preservation of upper-limb function following spinal cord injury: A clinical practice guideline for health-care professionals.* Washington, DC: Paralyzed Veterans of America.

Consortium for Spinal Cord Medicine. (2006). *Bladder management for adults with spinal cord injury: A clinical practice guideline for health-care professionals.* Washington, DC: Paralyzed Veterans of America.

Coppola-Passariello, T. (2003). Creative (and cheap!) alternatives for assistive technology. *OT Practice, 8,* 21.

Davidoff, G. N., Roth, E. J., & Richards, J. S. (1992). Cognitive deficits in spinal cord injury: Epidemiology and outcome. *Archives of Physical Medicine and Rehabilitation, 73,* 275–284.

DeForge, D., Blackmer, J., Garritty, C., Yazdi, F., Cronin, V., Barrowman, N., et al. (2005). Fertility following spinal cord injury: A systematic review. *Spinal Cord, 43*(12) 693–703.

Delta Society. (2009). *Benefits of a service animal/service dog.* Retrieved November 18, 2003, from http://www.deltasociety.org/Page.aspx?pid=315

DeVivo, M. J. (2002). Epidemiology of traumatic spinal cord injury. In S. Kirshblum, D. Campagnolog,& J. DeLisa (Eds.), *Spinal cord medicine.* Philadelphia: Lippincott Williams & Wilkins.

DeVivo, M. J. (2007). Trends in spinal cord injury rehabilitation outcomes from model systems in the United States: 1973–2006. *Spinal Cord, 45,* 713–721.

DeVivo, M. J., Rutt, R. D., Stover, S. L., & Fine, P. R. (1987). Employment after spinal cord injury. *Archives of Physical Medicine and Rehabilitation, 68,* 494–498.

Dolhi, C. D. (1996). *Occupational therapy practice guidelines for adults with SCI.* Rockville, MD: American Occupational Therapy Association.

Drainoni, M. L., Houlihan, B., Williams, S., Vedrani, M., Esch, D., Lee-Hood, E., et al. (2004). Patterns of Internet use by persons with spinal cord injuries and relationship to health-related quality of life. *Archives of Physical Medicine and Rehabilitation, 85*(11), 1872–1879.

Ducharme, S. (1999). Sexuality and spinal cord injury. In S. Nesathural (Ed.), *The rehabilitation of people with spinal cord injury* (pp. 83–88). Boston: Arbuckle Academic.

Dunn, C. A., Carlson, M., Jackson, J. M., & Clark, F. A. (2009). Response factors surrounding progression of pressure ulcers in community-residing adults with spinal cord injury. *American Journal of Occupational Therapy, 63,* 301–309.

Efthimiou, J., Gordon, W. A., Sell, G. H., & Stratford, C. (1981). Electronic assistive devices: Their impact on quality of life of high-quadriplegic persons. *Archives of Physical Medicine and Rehabilitation, 62,* 131–134.

Esmail, S., Esmail, Y., & Munro, B. (2001). Sexuality and disability: The role of health care professionals in providing options and alternative for couples. *Sexuality and Disability, 19*(4), 267–282.

Farmer, A. R. (1986). Dressing. In J. P. Hill (Ed.), *Spinal cord injury—A guide to functional outcomes in occupational therapy* (pp. 125–143). Rockville, MD: Aspen.

Field-Fote, E. C., Lindley, S. D., & Sherman, A. (2005). Locomotor training approaches for individuals with spinal cord injury: A preliminary report of walking-related outcomes. *Journal of Neurologic Physical Therapy, 29*(3), 127–137.

Fuhrer, M. J., Garber, S. L., Rintala, D. H., Clearman, R., & Hart, K. (1993). Pressure ulcers in community-resident persons with spinal cord injury: Prevalence and risk factors. *Archives of Physical Medicine and Rehabilitation, 74,* 1172–1177.

Gadberry, L., & Frauenheim-Finke, T. (1996). *Motivating life skill modules.* Bethesda, MD: American Occupational Therapy Association.

Gansel, J., Waters, R., & Gellman, H. (1990). Transfer of the pronator teres tendon to the tendons of the flexor digitorum profundus in tetraplegia. *Journal of Bone and Joint Surgery, 72,* 427–32.

Garber, S. L. (1985). New perspectives for the occupational therapist in the treatment of spinal cord-injury individuals. *American Journal of Occupational Therapy, 39,* 703–704.

Garber, S. L., Lathem, P., & Gregorio, T. L. (1988). *Specialized occupational therapy for persons with high-level quadriplegia.* [Monograph funded in part by Grant No. G009300044 from the National Institute on Disability and Rehabilitation Research (NID), U.S. Department of Education, awarded to the Research and Training Center for the Rehabilitation of Persons with Spinal Cord Dysfunction at Baylor College of Medicine and The Institute for Rehabilitation and Research (Washington, DC)].

Garber, S. L., & Rintala, D. H. (2003). Pressure ulcers in veterans with spinal cord injury: A retrospective study. *Journal of Rehabilitation Research Development, 40,* 433–442.

Garber, S. L., Rintala, D. H., Hart, K. A., & Fuhrer, M. J. (2000). Pressure ulcer risk in spinal cord injury: Predictors of ulcer status over 3 years. *Archives of Physical Medicine and Rehabilitation, 81,* 465–71.

Giszter, S. F. (2008). Spinal cord injury: Present and future therapeutic devices and prostheses. *American Society for Experimental NeuroTherapeutics, 5*(1), 147–162.

Goodman, N., Jette, A. M., Houlihan, B., & Williams, S. (2008). Computer and Internet use by persons after traumatic spinal cord injury. *Archives of Physical Medicine and Rehabilitation, 89,* 1492–1498.

Goossens, R. H. M., Snijders, C. J., Holscher, T. G., Heerens, W. C., & Holman, A. E. (1997). Shear stress measured on beds and wheelchairs. *Scandinavian Journal of Rehabilitation Medicine, 29,* 131–6.

Gordon, W. A., Harasymiw S., Bellile, S., Lehman, L., & Sherman, B. (1982). The relationship between pressure sores and psychosocial adjustment in persons with spinal cord injury. *Rehabilitation Psychology, 27,* 185–191.

Hanebrink, S., & Dillon, D. (2000). Service dogs: The ultimate assistive technology. *OT Practice, 5,* 16–19.

Hanson, C. S., Nabavi, D., & Yuen, H. K. (2001). The effects of sports on level of community integration as reported by persons with spinal cord injury. *American Journal of Occupational Therapy, 55,* 332–338.

Harwin, W. S., Patton, J. L., & Edgerton, V. R. (2006). Challenges and opportunities for robot-mediated neurorehabilitation. *Proceedings of the IEEE, 94*(9).

Hesse, S., Schmidth, H., Werner, C., & Bardeleben, A. (2003). Upper and lower extremity robotic devices for rehabilitation and for studying motor control. *Current Opinion in Neurology, 16*(6), 705–710.

Hill, J. (1994). Surgical options after spinal cord injury. In G. M. Yarkony (Ed.), *Spinal cord injury medical management and rehabilitation* (p. 137). Gaithersburg, MD: Aspen.

Hislop, J. J., & Montgomery, J. (Eds.). (2002). *Daniels and Worthingham's testing techniques of manual examination.* Philadelphia: Saunders.

Hobson, D. A. (1992). Comparative effects of posture on pressure and shear at the body-seat interface. *Journal of Rehabilitation Research and Development, 15,* 21–31.

Holme, S. A., Kanny, E. M., Guthrie, M. R., & Johnson, K. L. (1997). The use of environmental control units by occupational therapy practitioners in spinal cord injury and disease services. *American Journal of Occupational Therapy, 51,* 42–48.

Hoppenfeld, S. (1997). *Orthopaedic neurology—A diagnostic guide to neurological levels.* Philadelphia: Lippincott.

Individuals with Disabilities Education Act Amendments of 1997, Pub. L. 105–117, 20 U.S.C. § 1400 *et seq.*

James, A. B. (2008). Restoring the role of independent person. In M. V. Radomski & C. A. Trombly-Latham, (Eds.), *Occupational therapy for physical dysfunction* (6th ed., pp. 774–816). Philadelphia: Lippincott Williams & Wilkins.

James, J. J., & Cardenas, D. D. (2003). Spinal cord injury. In S. J. Garrison (Ed.), *Handbook of physical medicine* (2nd ed., pp. 270–295). Philadelphia: Lippincott Williams & Wilkins.

Koo, T. D. D., Mak, A. F. T., & Lee, Y. L. (1996). Posture effect on seating interface biomechanics: Comparison between two seating systems. *Archives of Physical Medicine and Rehabilitation, 77,* 40–7.

Langemo, D. K., Melland, H., Hanson, D., Olson, B., & Hunter S. (2000). The lived experience of having a pressure ulcer: A qualitative analysis. *Advances in Skin and Wound Care, 13,* 225–235.

Lathem, P., Gregorio, T. L., & Garber, S. L. (1985). High-level quadriplegia: An occupational therapy challenge. *American Journal of Occupational Therapy, 39,* 705–714.

Mann, W. C., & Lane, J. P. (1991). *Assistive technology for persons with disabilities: The role of occupational therapy.* Rockville, MD: American Occupational Therapy Association.

Martinsen, B., Harder, I., & Biering-Sorensen, F. (2008). The meaning of assisted feeding for people living with spinal cord injury: A phenomenological study. *Journal of Advanced Nursing, 62*(5), 533–540.

McAlonan, S. (1996). Improving sexual rehabilitation services: The patient's perspective. *American Journal of Occupational Therapy, 50,* 826–834.

Miller, H., & Delozier J. (1994). *Cost implications of the pressure ulcer treatment guideline.* Columbia, MD: Center for Health Policy Studies.

Minkel, J. L. (2002). Service delivery in assistive technology. In D. A. Olson & F. DeRuyter (Eds.), *Clinician's guide to assistive technology* (p. 65). St. Louis, MO: Mosby.

Mooney, T. O., Cole, T. M., & Chilgren, R. A. (1975). *Sexual options for paraplegics and quadriplegics.* Boston: Little, Brown.

National Spinal Cord Injury Statistical Center. (2008). Spinal cord injury: Facts and figures at a glance. *Journal of Spinal Cord Medicine, 25,* 139–40.

National Spinal Cord Injury Statistical Center. (2009). *Spinal cord injury: Facts and figures at a glance.* Retrieved May 24, 2009, from http://www.spinal cord.uab.edu/show.asp?durki=119513&site=471 6&return=19775

Neistadt, M. E. (1986). Sexuality counseling for adults with disabilities: A module for an occupational therapy curriculum. *American Journal of Occupational Therapy, 40,* 542–545.

Paralyzed Veterans of America. (2002). *Pressure ulcers: What you should know.* Washington, DC: Author.

Patil, P. G., & Turner, D. A. (2008). The development of brain–machine interface neuroprosthetic devices. *Neurotherapeutics, 5*(1), 137–146.

Pearman, J. W. (1985). Prevention and management of infection—The urinary tract. In G. M. Bedbrook (Ed.), *Lifetime care of the paraplegic patient* (pp. 54–65). Edinburgh, Scotland: Churchill Livingstone.

Pflaum, C., McCollister, G., Strauss, D. J., Shavelle, R. M., & DeVivo, M. J. (2006). Worklife after traumatic spinal cord injury. *Journal of Spinal Cord Medicine, 29,* 377–386.

Rehabilitation Act of 1973, Pub. L. 93–112, 29 U.S.C. § 701 et seq.

Rehabilitation Act Amendments of 1986, P.L. 99–506, 29 U.S.C § 701.

Rehabilitation Engineering and Assistive Technology Society of North America. (2009a). *Certification.* Retrieved June 10, 2009, from http://www.resna.org/certification/index.php

Rehabilitation Engineering and Assistive Technology Society of North America. (2009b). *Position on the application of wheelchair standing devices.* Retrieved May 15, 2009, from http://www.rstce.pitt.edu/RSTCE_Resources/Resna_position_on_wheelchair_standers.pdf

Schryvers, O. I., Miroslaw, M. F., & Nance, P. W. (2000). Surgical treatment of pressure ulcers: A 20-year experience. *Archives of Physical Medicine and Rehabilitation, 81,* 1556–1562.

Schneider, L. W., Manary, M. A., Hobson, D. A., & Bertocci, G. E. (2008). Transportation safety standards for wheelchair users: A review of voluntary standards for improved safety, usability, and independence of wheelchair-seated travelers. *Assistive Technology, 20,* 222–233.

Sie, I. H., Waters, R. L., Adkins, R. H., & Gellman, H. (1992). Upper extremity pain in the post rehabilitation spinal cord injured patient. *Archives of Physical Medicine and Rehabilitation, 73,* 44–48.

Sipski, M., Alexander, C., Gomez-Marin, O., & Spalding, J. (2007). The effects of spinal cord injury on psychogenic sexual arousal in males. *Journal of Urology, 177*(1), 247–251.

Solet, J. M. (2008). Optimizing personal and social adaptation. In M. V. Radomski & C. A. Trombly-Latham (Eds.), *Occupational therapy for physical dysfunction* (6th ed., pp. 924–951). Philadelphia: Lippincott Williams & Wilkins.

Somers, M. F. (2001). *Spinal cord injury—Functional rehabilitation* (2nd ed.). Upper Saddle River, NJ: Prentice-Hall.

Spencer, W. A. (1958). A message to persons with disabilities. *Promethean, 8*(2), 1–2.

Swenson, J. R., Barnett, L. L., Pond, B., & Schoenberg, A. A. (1998). Assistive technology for rehabilitation and reduction of disability. In J. A. DeLisa & B. M. Gans (Eds.), *Rehabilitation medicine: Principles and practice* (3rd ed., pp. 745–762). Philadelphia: Lippincott-Raven.

Sunderlin, A. (1999). Dog days. *Paraplegia News, 53,* 13–20.

Tate, D. G., Henrich, R. K., Pasuke, L., & Anderson, D. (1998). Vocational rehabilitation, independent living, and consumerism. In J. A. DeLisa & B. M. Gans (Eds.), *Rehabilitation medicine: Principles and practice* (3rd ed., pp. 1151–1162). Philadelphia: Lippincott-Raven.

Technology-Related Assistance for Individuals with Disabilities Act, Pub. L. 100-407, 20 U.S.C. § 2201.

Traub, J. E., & LeClair, R. R. (1975). The rehabilitation engineering program. *American Rehabilitation, 1,* 3–7.

Treviranus, J., & Petty, L. (2002). Computer access. In D. A. Olson & F. DeRuyter (Eds.), *Clinician's guide to assistive technology* (pp. 91–113). St. Louis, MO: Mosby.

Turner, A. N. (1985). Prevention of tertiary complications and management—Decubiti. In G. M. Bedbrook (Ed.), *Lifetime care of the paraplegic patient* (pp. 54–65). Edinburgh, Scotland: Churchill Livingstone.

Valentine, D., Kiddoo, M., & LaFleur, B. (1993). Psychosocial implications of service dog ownership for people who have mobility or hearing impairments. *Social Work in Health Care, 19,* 109–124.

Walter, J. S., Sacks, J., Othman, R., Rankin, A. Z., Nemchausky, B., Chintam, R., et al. (2002). A database of self-reported secondary medical problems among VA spinal cord injury patients: Its role in clinical care and management. *Journal of Rehabilitation Research and Development, 39*(1), 53–61.

Waters, R. L., Sie, I. H., Gellman, H., & Tognella, M. (1996). Functional hand surgery following tetraplegia. *Archives of Physical Medicine and Rehabilitation, 77,* 86–94.

Watson, A. H., Kanny, E. M., White, D. M., & Anson, D. K. (1995). Use of standardized activities of daily living rating scales in spinal cord injury and disease services. *American Journal of Occupational Therapy, 49,* 229–234.

Weaver, F. M., Hammond, M. C., Guihan, M., & Hendricks, R. D. (2000). Department of Veterans Affairs quality enhancement research initiative for spinal cord injury. *Medical Care, 38*(6 Suppl. 1), 182–191.

World Health Organization. (2001). *International classification of functioning, disability and health.* Geneva, Switzerland: Author.

Wuolle, K. S., Bryden, A. M., Peckham, P. H., Murray, P. K., & Keith, M. (2003). Satisfaction with upper-extremity surgery in individuals with tetraplegia. *Archives of Physical Medicine and Rehabilitation, 84,* 1145–1149.

Young, M. E. (2004). Sexuality and people with physical disabilities. In C. H. Christiansen & K. M. Matuska (Eds.), *Ways of living: Adaptive strategies for special needs* (3rd ed., pp. 385–396). Bethesda, MD: AOTA Press.

Zejdlik, C. P. (1991). *Management of spinal cord injury* (2nd ed.). Boston: Jones & Bartlett.

Chapter 10

Intervention to Increase Performance and Participation Following Stroke

TIMOTHY J. WOLF, OTD, MSCI, OTR/L, AND

REBECCA BIRKENMEIER, MSOT, OTR/L

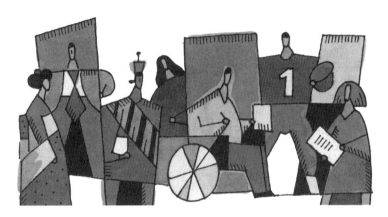

KEY WORDS

aphasia	dysphagia
apraxia	hemianopsia
ataxia	hemiparesis/hemiplesia
dysarthria	neglect

HIGHLIGHTS

- People with stroke present with a wide variety of deficits, including but not limited to motor, speech, cognitive, sensory, perceptual, and psychological, that can influence participation.

- The intensity, duration, and location of rehabilitation are all known to have an effect on functional outcomes following stroke.

- Cognitive deficits following stroke can often go underdetected in the acute care setting; these individuals, therefore, are often discharged prematurely.

- Stroke rehabilitation involves developing an intervention plan based on the client's occupational profile, performance, and goals and on intervention review and outcomes.

- The rehabilitation process needs to incorporate assessment and intervention strategies that focus on the continuum of care across the acute, inpatient, home, and outpatient settings.

OBJECTIVES

After reading this material, readers will be able to

- Describe the two major types of stroke,

- Identify performance components and performance areas to observe during the evaluation of a person with a stroke,

- Describe the challenges to occupational performance experienced by individuals with strokes and how occupational therapy uniquely addresses these issues,

- Define and compare the difference between remediation and compensatory treatment approaches, and

- Describe the common frames of reference used to address motor and cognitive dysfunction following stroke.

Each year approximately 780,000 people experience a new or recurrent stroke. The prevalence of stroke in the United States is now approaching 6 million people. Stroke ranks as the third leading cause of death, behind heart disease and cancer (American Heart Association, 2008).

Stroke is now one of the most prevalent chronic health conditions and is the leading cause of serious, long-term disability in the United States. Each year, the direct and indirect costs of stroke are estimated to be approximately $65.5 billion (American Heart Association, 2008).

Occupational therapy intervention is a vital part of the rehabilitation process. The primary aim of occupational therapy is to facilitate task performance by improving skills or developing and teaching compensatory strategies to overcome lost performance skills and self-manage chronic symptoms of stroke (Weimer et al., 2002). In addition, occupational therapy works to assist with psychosocial adjustment to residual disability. Baum and Christiansen (1997) assert that occupational therapy is unique because it helps people maximize the fit between their capabilities and what they want and need to do.

What Is a Stroke?

A *stroke* is caused from a disruption in blood supply to the brain from blockage or bleeding in the brain that often leads to an infarct (cell death). Diabetes mellitus, high blood cholesterol and other blood lipids, high blood pressure, metabolic syndrome, obesity, physical inactivity, and tobacco use are the main risk factors for stroke (American Heart Association, 2008).

Ischemic stroke is one of the major types of stroke, caused when a plaque fragment or blood clot lodges in an artery and restricts blood flow to the brain. A clot that forms within an artery that supplies the brain is called a *thrombus*. An *embolus* is a plaque fragment or blood clot that travels to the brain from the heart or an artery supplying the brain. Ischemic strokes account for approximately 87% of all cases of stroke (American Heart Association, 2008).

The second major type of stroke is a *hemorrhagic stroke*, which occurs when a blood vessel is ruptured. Although this can happen for a number of different reasons, it is often the result of long-term high blood pressure that weakens blood vessels in the brain and causes them to bulge and eventually burst. When the blood vessel ruptures, blood is spilled into the brain, causing damage to brain cells. Hemorrhagic strokes account for approximately 13% of all cases of stroke (American Heart Association, 2008).

A *transient ischemic attack (TIA)*, sometimes called a *mini-stroke*, occurs when there is a temporary blockage of blood flow to an artery inside the brain or leading to the brain. Symptoms from a TIA are generally temporary, lasting under 24 hours. About 15% of strokes are preceded by a TIA (American Heart Association, 2008).

Impairments

The complexity of the brain and its interconnected networks can lead to considerable variation in the impairments that are seen as a result of a stroke. The most common impairments from stroke are presented in Table 10.1. While some impairments correlate well to specific lesions or infarcts in the brain, such as hemiparesis, others (e.g., cognitive impairment) are not well defined by a lesion in a specific area of the brain. Therefore, although the site of the lesion is important and should be taken into consideration, it should not be used in place of a formal assessment to determine impairments following stroke. The neurological severity of stroke may be just as important in determining the impairments following stroke as the lesion location.

The neurological severity of stroke is determined through a medical evaluation of the extent of injury in the brain. This is determined by two main assessments: neuroimaging and the National Institutes of Health Stroke Scale (NIHSS). Neuroimaging, such as

Table 10.1. Common Impairments Following a Stroke

Impairment	Definition
Hemiparesis	Muscle weakness on one side of the body
Hemianopsia	Loss of vision, usually in half or a portion of the visual field, due to damage to a portion of the visual pathway
Aphasia	Loss of fluent speech and/or the ability to understand spoken or written language
Ataxia	The loss of the ability to coordinate motor movements to accomplish a task
Hemi-attention (neglect)	The inability to attend to one side of the body or visual field
Sensory loss	A loss in the ability of the body to receive a stimulus from the outside world
Apraxia	The loss of the ability to execute a motor plan for an activity
Muscle weakness	Decrease in the ability to generate a muscle contraction
Cognitive deficits tasks	Deficits in one or more thought processes and the ability to perform functional
Dysarthria	Motor deficit of speech
Dysphagia	Difficulty swallowing

CT or MRI scans, is done to obtain a visual picture of the infarct in the brain and to observe for active bleeding that may be occurring from a hemorrhagic stroke. The NIHSS is an assessment that quantifies neurological deficits following stroke; it is widely considered the gold standard stroke scale (Brott et al., 1989). The NIHSS is widely used to evaluate acute stroke status, determine appropriate medical treatment and need for rehabilitation, and often to predict patient outcome. It is a 15-item impairment scale that assesses level of consciousness, extraocular movements, visual fields, facial muscle function, extremity strength, sensory function, coordination, language, speech, and neglect.

Further studies with the NIHSS have established criteria for what is referred to as mild, moderate, and severe neurological impairment following stroke. Using the scores on the NIHSS, mild stroke has been defined as 0–5, moderate as 6–16, and severe as over 16 (Marler et al., 2000). Individuals with mild stroke typically do not display outward signs of impairment and display limited or no motor impairment. Speech is typically fluent, activities of daily living (ADLs) are usually independent on discharge from the acute setting and therefore individuals with mild stroke are not usually seen in rehabilitation. Individuals with moderate to severe stroke are typically the people who are referred to inpatient rehabilitation settings, outpatient rehabilitation, in-home services, skilled nursing facilities, or both.

Prognosis

Following a stroke, individuals can expect to have some degree of neurological recovery. Although the length of time in which neurological recovery may occur will vary from person to person and depend on the amount of damage that was sustained, neurological recovery will typically peak within 3 months post-stroke; may occur at a slower pace for at least 6 months; and for a small percentage of patients, will continue for up to a year (Kwakkel, Kollen, & Lindeman, 2004).

Although neurological recovery has an impact on functional recovery, individuals post-stroke can see functional recovery for a much longer time following stroke—past the point at which neurological recovery peaks. There is strong evidence to support that maximal functional recovery is seen within the first 6 months; however, some studies have observed functional improvement continuing for as long as 5 years post-stroke (Thorsen, Holmqvist, de Pedro-Cuesta, & von Koch, 2005). There is also evidence that the amount and intensity of rehabilitation received following stroke are in large part responsible for the amount of functional recovery achieved (Aichner, Adelwohrer, & Haring, 2002; Kwakkel et al., 2004; Wood-Dauphinee & Kwakkel, 2005).

Studies of functional stroke outcomes found that 80% of stroke survivors were able to attain independence in mobility; 67% attained independence in ADLs (Granger, Hamilton, & Gresham, 1988; Granger, Hamilton, Gresham, & Kramer, 1989). Over 70% of the variance in discharge decisions after stroke rehabilitation is determined by the ability to function independently in bathing, toileting, social interaction, dressing, and eating (Mauthe, Haaf, Hayn, & Krall, 1996). Independence in bowel and bladder control, eating, and grooming have a cumulative influence on predicting the ability of a survivor to live independently following discharge. Although the mastery of ADL and instrumental activities of daily living (IADL) skills may be important following stroke, people who are married or are parents may need the additional skills of caring for others when they return home (Edwards & Christiansen, 2005).

Paid employment, leisure, and self-care occupations are very important to younger people who have had strokes (Edwards & Christiansen, 2005). Similarly, engagement in leisure activities is related to post-stroke well-being (Sveen, Thommessen, Bautz-Holter, Wyller, & Laake, 2004). People also derive life satisfaction from productive work (Hillman & Chapparo, 2002). Although rehabilitation has been successful in helping individuals regain independence in self-care and in the home, it has not been successful in helping them reintegrate back into these more complex adult roles, especially into work (Bendz, 2000, 2003).

A recent study by the Cognitive Rehabilitation Research Group (CRRG) at Washington University School of Medicine assessed all patients being served by Barnes–Jewish Hospital Stroke Service over a 10-year period. The data from the CRRG stroke population ($N = 7,740$) revealed the following three important findings:

1. Forty-five percent of the patients are under the age of 65, and nearly 27% are under the age of 55.
2. Of all the patients who had strokes, 49% had a mild stroke, 32.8% had a moderate stroke, 17.9% had a severe stroke, and 6% died (using definitions from the NIHSS).
3. Of the individuals who had a mild to moderate stroke, 71% were discharged directly home, discharged with home services only, or discharged with outpatient services only. These services have limited focus on work rehabilitation and community reintegration (Wolf, Baum, & Connor, 2009).

All of these findings indicate the need to expand rehabilitation services to include work rehabilitation, as more people who have strokes are of working age, and the majority of the strokes are mild to moderate, making it possible for them to return to work. Yet 36% of people with mild stroke who were working before the stroke, who presented limited to no impairment, and who were not receiving rehabilitation never returned to work. An additional 15% were no longer employed at 6 months—bringing the total unemployment rate to 52% in this population (O'Brien & Wolf, in review). It is important to consider the needs of this changing stroke population in occupational therapy service delivery.

Occupational Therapy Process of Service Delivery

According to the *Occupational Therapy Practice Framework: Domain and Process, 2nd Edition* (hereinafter the *Framework*), occupational therapy service delivery is accomplished in 3 stages: (1) evaluation, (2) intervention, and (3) outcomes (American Occupational Therapy Association [AOTA], 2008).

Evaluation includes an occupational profile and an analysis of the client's occupational performance. *Intervention* is accomplished by developing an intervention plan, implementing the intervention, and then evaluating the client's progress toward goals. Finally, *outcomes* are determined and future plans are made with the client (AOTA, 2008). This chapter will describe the stages of occupational therapy service delivery as they relate to individuals with stroke.

Evaluation

The occupational therapy evaluation begins with gathering information about what the client needs and wants to do and the context in which he or she does them (Coster, 1998). The process begins immediately post-stroke, in the acute care setting. The purpose of evaluation in the acute care setting is to "triage" the individual to determine the need for rehabilitation and the proper discharge location in which to address the need. Evidence on stroke rehabilitation supports that individuals with mild stroke are best treated in an outpatient setting, younger patients with moderate to severe stroke are best treated in an inpatient rehabilitation center, and patients with severe strokes may be best managed in long-term, less intensive rehabilitation units (Teasell & Foley, 2008).

Occupational Profile

The first step in an occupational therapy evaluation is to obtain an occupational profile of the client that provides a summary of the client's occupational history and experiences, patterns of daily living, interests, values, and needs (AOTA, 2008). For individuals with stroke, this stage of the assessment is crucial and will serve as a guide for the rest of the evaluation—rehabilitation will be driven by understanding what is important and meaningful to the client and identifying how his or her impairments will affect the ability to engage in chosen occupations.

The Canadian Occupational Performance Measure (COPM) is an interview assessment that can help create an occupational profile. It typically measures areas of self-care, productivity, and leisure at the level of self-reported performance and satisfaction (Law et al., 1990). The Activity Card Sort (ACS) can be used with the COPM to help clients identify occupations they are having difficulty with. The ACS gathers information on the client's instrumental, leisure, and social activity patterns (Baum & Edwards, 2001, 2008). It lists 80 activities, each of which the client rates as (a) never done, (b) given up since the stroke, (c) continues to participate in since the stroke, (d) participates less in the activity since the stroke, (e) has given up the activity since the stroke (Baum & Edwards, 2001).

Analysis of Occupational Performance

This step of the occupational therapy evaluation is focused on identifying the strengths and limitations following stroke that will support or hinder the client's occupational performance. The occupational therapist may select a specific assessment tool in order to facilitate observation and to focus the evaluation (Moyers, 1999). In the acute care and inpatient setting, this typically begins with assessments of self-care. The Barthel Index and the Functional Independence Measure (FIM™) have been tested extensively in rehabilitation for reliability, validity, and sensitivity and are the most commonly used measures for self-care (Gresham et al., 1995). The FIM is a measure of disability (in terms of burden of care) for clients, regardless of impairments or limitations (Uniform Data Set for Medical Rehabilitation [including the FIM instrument], 1997). It assesses self-care, sphincter control, transfers, locomotion, communication, and social cognition on a seven-level scale. Scoring for the FIM is presented in Table 10.2 below.

Other measures should be used as needed to determine the presence or absence of other common post-stroke impairments. Examples are in Table 10.3. The information gathered in this stage of assessment should be compared with the occupational profile to develop an intervention plan that includes objective goals addressing limitations on occupational performance.

Intervention

Following a thorough evaluation, the occupational therapist and the client develop the intervention plan that addresses deficits following stroke in order to promote independence and participation in meaningful occupations. The client's personal goals, values, and beliefs should be taken into account to ensure interventions are as client-centered as possible. The therapist should take into consideration the deficits resulting from the stroke and the context, environment, and activity demands that will influence a particular task. These should be considered when determining the best current stroke rehabilitation practices. Resulting treatments will be different for each client because of differing occupational roles and needs.

Table 10.2. Description of the Levels of Function and Their Scores—The FIM™

7	**Complete Independence**—All tasks described as making up the activity are typically performed safely, without modification, assistive devices, or aids, and within reasonable time.
6	**Modified Independence**—Activity requires one or more of the following: an assistive device, more than reasonable time, or safety (risk) considerations.
5	**Supervision or Setup**—Subject requires no more help than standby, cueing, or coaxing, without physical contact, or helper sets up needed items or applies orthoses.
4	**Minimal Assistance**—Subject requires no more help than touching and expends 75% or more of the effort.
3	**Moderate Assistance**—Subject requires more help than touching and expends half (50%) or more (up to 75%) of the effort.
2	**Maximal Assistance**—Subject expends less than 50% of the effort, but at least 25%.
1	**Total Assistance**—Subject expends less than 25% of the effort.

Note. From *Uniform Data Set for Medical Rehabilitation* (1997).

Table 10.3. Examples of Occupational Therapy Assessments for the Common Impairments of Stroke

Impairment	Assessment	Reference
Hemiparesis	MMT, Goniometry, Action Research Arm Test (ARAT)	Gutman & Schonfeld, 2003, 2009 Lyle, 1981
Hemianopsia Ataxia	Confrontation testing Finger to nose; finger to finger; finger–nose–finger	Scheiman, 1997 Gutman & Schonfeld, 2003, 2009
Hemi-attention (neglect)	Structured/Unstructured Mesulam; Behavioral Inattention Test (BIT): Star Cancellation Task	Mesulam, 1985 Wilson et al., 1987
Sensory loss	*Light touch:* occlude vision and stroke client's skin with fingertip along dermatome regions; *Pain:* occlude vision and apply sharp end of safety pin or paper clip along dermatome regions; *Temperature:* assess during functional bathing and cooking activities; *Proprioception:* occlude vision, move the upper extremity three times between shoulder flexion and extension. End with shoulder flexion and ask if arm is "up or down"	Gutman & Schonfeld, 2003, 2009
Apraxia	Place everyday items (e.g., toothbrush, comb, clothing, watch, pen) in front of client, and ask client to demonstrate the use of each item	Gutman & Schonfeld, 2003, 2009
Cognitive deficits	Executive Function Performance Test; Test of Everyday Attention; Rivermead Behavioral Memory Test	Baum et. al., 2008 Robertson et al., 1994 Wilson et al., 1985

Setting Goals

Setting treatment goals involves estimating the amount of time it will take for the patient to achieve a specific level of independence. The following factors may determine the length of stay and assist in establishing realistic and attainable goals with the patient and his or her family:

- Funding sources
- Personal financial resources
- Prior level of functioning
- Age
- Lifestyle and role responsibilities
- Family support
- Presence of cognitive and perceptual deficits
- Degree of physical dysfunction
- Discharge disposition.

Goals are written to show the changes in baseline occupational performance and performance skills that are expected to occur as a result of planned intervention (Moyers, 1999). A goal that is well written should suggest a performance outcome and describe the performance improvements expected (Borcherding, 2005). The FIM or other ADL assessments provide useful baseline information that can be used to measure progress but should not be the sole source of baseline information. All measures used to establish a prior level of functioning should be compared to an occupational profile in order to determine the individual's ability to perform his or her chosen occupations. Other improvements in performance may involve increased speed, accuracy, or frequency of performance; baseline measurements of these capabilities are useful. A goal must also specify the timeframe for attaining the goal.

It is critically important that the occupational therapist consider performance measures when writing goals. For example, when writing a goal to improve grip strength, he or she should focus on skills—such as the ability to hold and drink from a glass—not on the number of pounds in grip strength measured by a dynamometer. Consider what specific activity will be affected by improvement of range of motion, coordination, endurance, balance, strength, or cognitive ability.

Other examples would be improving active range of motion so the client is able to retrieve items from a cabinet or groom his or her hair; improving fine motor control to enable him or her to button a front-closure shirt or hook a bra; improving dynamic standing balance so the person can adjust clothing after toileting; and compensating for working memory deficits in order to complete a cooking task. Ponte-Allan and Giles (1999) found that clients who made a functional, independence-focused goal statement when they were admitted to the hospital had significantly higher functional outcomes and a shorter hospital stay than those who did not. They defined a functional, independence-focused goal statement as the desire to perform a specific activity or to be able to resume a specific activity.

Intervention

Remediation Strategies

A variety of treatment approaches can be used, generally in combination to maximize both the level and the quality of occupational performance. It is important to note that component skill training activities should be related to improving the client's ability to perform ADLs. Motor skills practice should not focus on how well a skill can be performed during a single treatment session but on how well it is performed in the context of daily life and how well the skill is retained or remembered (Wishart, Lee, Janzen-Ezekiel, Marley, & Lehto, 2002).

Remediation strategies for clients with stroke are typically focused on improvement or retraining of motor skills. Several factors come into play. Practice of tasks plays a large role in improving movement. Whole tasks should be practiced as much as possible and in a variety of contexts to encourage transfer of skills. Feedback should be given to the client that encourages problem-solving to achieve the desired movement (Schumway-Cook & Woollacott, 2007).

There are relatively few studies on the remediation of attention and other cognitive disorders following stroke. Most often, compensatory strategies are recommended for the rehabilitation of attention and memory deficits (Cicerone, 2002). Limited evidence suggests that computer-aided attention training programs may be beneficial in improving attention deficits (Mazer et al., 2003; Sturm, Willmes, Orgass, & Hartje, 1997). Additionally, it is important to note that most existing research has been done with individuals with traumatic brain injury rather than stroke.

Motor-Learning Theory

Motor-learning theory, as described by Carr and Shepherd (1987), uses a sequential clinical reasoning process. A functional performance problem is identified; the limiting motor components are analyzed; the impaired components are practiced in isolation through visual, verbal, and manual guidance; and finally, the motion is practiced in the context of the functional task with the intent of integrating the components.

Motor-Control Theory

Treatment approaches using contemporary motor-control theory emphasize practice of functional tasks as a way to organize motor behavior (Bass-Haugen, Mathiowetz, & Flinn, 2002). In this approach, the therapist determines and modifies the activity's or environment's demands to allow maximal motor performance given the client's attributes Therapy focuses on practicing the activity in a natural context. For example, if a person has residual weakness on one side and has some difficulty with dressing as a result, the most effective treatment is actually practicing the whole task of dressing with various task and environmental demands rather than practicing components of the activity.

Functional recovery can be predicted following stroke. Exercise and functional training should be directed toward improving strength and motor control, relearning sensorimotor relationships, and improving functional performance. Clients with paresis retain some ability to perform purposeful arm and hand movements and should be encouraged to try to restore functional use of the upper extremity (Barreca, Wolf, Fasoli, & Bohannon, 2003). This can be achieved by performing treatment activities that encourage the use of the affected upper extremity.

Constraint-Induced Movement Therapy and Learned Nonuse

Constraint-induced movement therapy (CIMT) uses principles from motor learning and motor control theories with an emphasis on learned nonuse. Spontaneous recovery of motor function after a stroke occurs to some degree, though many survivors remain chronically impaired, in part because of learned nonuse of the weak extremity (Miltner, Bauder, Sommer, Dettmers, & Taub, 1999). Learned nonuse results from repeated failed attempts to use the impaired limb soon after injury combined with successful use of the unaffected limb. In CIMT aims to counteract learned nonuse by restraining the unimpaired limb, generally in a constraint mitten, for 6 hours a day for a period of 2 weeks. This forces the use of the impaired limb during normal ADLs and during rehabilitation (Wolf, Lecraw, Barton, & Jann, 1989). CIMT has some implications for the treatment of unilateral neglect and may assist in reducing neglect and increasing independence in ADLs (Freeman, 2001).

A similar principle guides approaches to visual field cut. Techniques such as partial visual occlusion, by either patching the non-neglected half field or using hemispatial sunglasses, are thought to force the person to use head-turning and eye movements to scan into the neglected visual field (Freeman, 2001).

Compensatory Strategies

Motor Techniques

Individuals with severe stroke can achieve independence in ADLs by using compensatory techniques focused on using the unaffected upper extremity (Nakayama, Jorgensen, Raaschou, & Olsen, 1994). Compensation through the use of the unaffected side to perform ADLs is common as part of routine stroke care. Therapists should encourage use of the affected extremity when possible; when unable, they should use compensatory strategies with the unaffected arm. There are many one-handed techniques and types of adapted equipment available that allow people with stroke to continue to do the things that are important to them. In cases when the prognosis for functional return of arm use is poor, teaching the client to deal with existing deficits and to use compensatory strategies may be more realistic (Kwakkel, Kollen, VanderGrond, & Prevo, 2003).

Contextual Training

Contextual training involves practicing a task in a specific environment until it becomes learned or habitual. This repetition of specific task sequences has been found to be effective in improving independence in the brain-injured population (Soderback, 1988). Practice is most effective when it is specific to the context in which the task is used and when it is performed in a consistent sequence (Bukowski, Bonavolonta, Keehn, & Morgan, 1996). In addition to the benefit of practicing a familiar activity, contextual training requires the patient to integrate various motor, cognitive, and perceptual skills.

The activity should begin with a low level of challenge and gradually increase in complexity as the client masters each step. Ma and Trombly (2002) recommended using task-specific practice that incorporates strategies of gradually increasing complexity, breaking tasks into simpler steps. An example would include progressing the client from having clothing articles placed within reach or field of vision (setup) to having him or her search a cluttered drawer or a closet for specific articles.

Cognitive Rehabilitation Strategies

Cognitive deficits are prevalent following stroke and can lead to significant problems for stroke survivors and their caregivers. Several studies have found that up to 65% of people experiencing stroke will have some type of cognitive deficit (Mok et al., 2004; Zinn et al., 2004). Moreover, functional recovery is often impaired by cognitive deficits (Mercier, Audet, Hebert, Rochette, & Dubois, 2001). The client may not realize the true benefit of rehabilitation due to problems associated with cognition (Mok et al., 2004).

It is generally accepted that restoration of cognitive function to pre-injury status is not expected as a result of rehabilitation (Geusgens, Winkens, van Heugten, Jolles, & van de Heuvel, 2007). Therefore, cognitive rehabilitation efforts are focused on compensating for deficits through the use of internal or external strategies, or both. Some common internal strategies include self-awareness training (Cicerone, 2002), mnemonics (Kaschel et al., 2002), self-cueing strategies (Robson, Marshall, Pring, & Chiat, 1998), and mental imagery (Niemeier, Cifu, & Kishore, 2001). Common external strategies include memory and planning aids (Wade & Troy, 2001), cueing devices (Boman, Lindstedt, Hemmingsson, & Bartfai, 2004), and developing written plans before performance (Levine et al., 2000).

Specific strategies should be selected based on the individual's deficits, skills, abilities, and the specific activity in which they are trying to re-engage. These cognitive rehabilitation strategies are typically used as part of an intervention frame of reference. The neurofunctional model, the dynamic interactional model of cognition, and the cognitive orientation to daily occupational performance model are examples of these frames of reference.

Neurofunctional Model

The neurofunctional approach is used when a client's cognitive deficits are so severe that there is little expectation of generalization to novel circumstances encountered in everyday life. It develops treatment programs that train an individual in an activity with the goal of developing a habit that can support their daily life function. For example, if a client with a moderate to severe stroke is not able to cross the street safely, the therapist and treatment team would develop a specific cueing system in order to help him or her perform the activity correctly and safely. The goal would be for the client to cross one specific street safely with little to no expectation of generalization based on his or her level of cognitive impairment.

Dynamic Interactional Model of Cognition

The dynamic interactional model of cognition approach uses cues and task alterations to compensate for deficits following neurological injury. This treatment approach focuses on developing internal strategies that increase the client's awareness of his or her deficits and then teaches how to compensate for them (e.g., by changing activities or environments). The approach is based on multidisciplinary literature on how people process, learn, and generalize information (Toglia, 1991; Toglia & Kirk, 2000). This model sees cognition as an ongoing product of the dynamic interaction among the person, activity, and environment—and modifiable, in certain situations (Flavell, Miller, & Miller, 1993). It requires the occupational therapist to present opportunities for the individual to experience different environments and activity demands. For example, if a client is having problems with memory, such strategies as modifying the environment, using internal and external cueing strategies, and compensation techniques may all be used to help the client participate in a chosen environment.

Cognitive Orientation to Daily Occupational Performance

Cognitive orientation to daily occupational performance (CO–OP) is a performance-based, problem-solving framework that enables skill acquisition through a process of developing and using strategies including reinforcement, modeling, shaping, prompting, fading, and chaining techniques (Polatajko & Mandich, 2004, 2005). CO–OP builds on a cognitive view of learning as an active process of acquiring, remembering, and using knowledge in order to perform an activity. The CO–OP problem-solving strategy, "GOAL, PLAN, DO, CHECK," was adopted from Meichenbaum as a general strategy that can be used to guide discovery of domain-specific strategies to support skill acquisition (Meichenbaum, 1977).

The process begins by setting a goal; the therapist then guides the client through the goal–plan–do–check strategy to determine where task performance is breaking down and then to identify strategies that can be used to overcome the breakdown and perform the task. For example, a client wants to prepare a light meal. The therapist teaches her or him to use the global goal–plan–do–check strategy, which the client will use to develop task-specific strategies for preparing a meal. In essence, the client comes up with the strategies necessary to complete the cooking task on his or her own.

Assistive Technology

Prescribing and training clients in the use of assistive devices and adapted equipment is one way occupational therapists try to improve and maintain occupational performance. Activities can be accomplished in more than one way—sometimes simply using equipment that substitutes for a missing skill is all that is required (Moyers, 1999). Lysack and Neufeld found that recommendations for equipment were somewhat more common than recommendations for home modifications and that clients with strokes tended to have slightly more equipment recommended than those in other diagnostic groups (Lysack & Neufeld, 2003). Among the recommendations, commode chairs, wheelchairs, and bathtub benches or chairs were prescribed for more than 50% of clients.

There is no simple formula for recommending equipment based on diagnosis or performance skill deficits. In considering whether or not assistive technology would be appropriate for their clients with strokes, therapists must assess the client's cognitive deficits, his or her willingness to use the recommended equipment, the physical environment in which it will be used, the extent of assistance needed from another person to use it, and the financial feasibility of obtaining it. Even small, inexpensive items (e.g., elastic shoelaces; long-handled bath sponges, combs, and shoehorns) are beyond the financial reach of many clients (Lysack & Neufeld, 2003).

Table 10.4 lists some examples of common performance skill problems associated with limited upper-extremity use following stroke and some frequently used assistive devices to compensate for them. Many items are available in department stores, supermarkets, and hardware stores. Some can also be made using common materials. Pipe insulation, for example, can be applied to eating and grooming utensils to build up handles. A paper clip attached to the hole in a zipper can serve as a zipper pull.

Other Intervention Considerations

Caregiver Training

A caregiver should be trained to help a client who is unable to perform his or her ADLs independently. Some 70%–90% of stroke survivors are cared for in the home (Ozer, Materson, & Caplan, 1994). It can be extremely difficult for one person to be responsible for all aspects of the client's care at home, especially if he or she is also caring for other family members. Hasselkus (1991) reported that caregivers

Table 10.4. Commonly Used Assistive Devices for Individuals With Limited Use of One Extremity Following Stroke

Activity	Common Performance Skill	Assistive Device Equipment
Feeding, grooming	Holding utensils firmly Stabilizing objects Opening containers Performing two-handed tasks Reaching areas on uninvolved side	Universal cuff and built-up utensils/handles Rocker knife Lip plates, plate guard, scoop dish Extended-handle utensils Nonslip mats Wash mitt Hook-and-loop fasteners Suction cup equipment stabilizers
Bathing	Reaching areas on uninvolved side Reaching lower body Getting in and out of the tub or shower Having impaired sitting/standing balance	Same as above Tub bench or shower chair Hand-held shower nozzle Grab bars Non-skid surface
Toileting	Getting up and down from the toilet seat Adjusting clothing Reaching perineal area for cleaning Washing both hands	Raised commode chair (drop arm) Toilet safety frame Grab bars Toilet tissue aid Hook-and-loop fasteners on pants or elastic-waist pants Pump soap dispenser
Dressing	Adjusting clothing closures Reaching lower body	Button aid, elastic shoe laces Long-handle shoe horn Zipper pull Hook-and-loop fasteners Reacher
Cooking and cleaning	Stabilizing pans and dishes Draining liquids Opening jars and cans Washing dishes Carrying items Using nonslip mats	One-handed strainers Pan-handle stabilizers Jar and bottle openers Electric can openers Wheeled cart Apron with front pocket

often experience ethical dilemmas when faced with conflicts between taking good care of a client and meeting other family and personal responsibilities. Evans and colleagues found that clients at risk for less-than-optimal home care had caregivers who were more likely to be depressed, had below-average knowledge of stroke care principles, and had a greater incidence of family dysfunction (Evans, Bishop, & Haselkorn, 1991). See Chapter 20 for more information.

Cardiac Precautions

The occupational therapist must be aware of specific precautions and secondary diagnoses such as hypertension, coronary artery disease, and congestive heart failure that are frequently associated with stroke (Roth, 1988). A careful review of the client's medical chart should be conducted prior to initiating therapy. Physicians may provide parameters for

heart rate, oxygen saturation, and blood pressure for clients whose condition may be unstable. These individuals must be monitored before, during, and after activity to determine whether the activity is too strenuous. Isometric, resistive, and overhead activities increase cardiac stress and should be carefully monitored or avoided in some cases. In addition, community activities in extremely cold or hot weather should be postponed.

Shoulder Pain

Elderly people frequently have some degree of joint damage due to pre-existing conditions such as osteoarthritis. Proper alignment of all joints must be maintained during self-care and passive range of motion to avoid impingement and injury to soft tissues.

The affected shoulder is particularly vulnerable to injury following stroke. When the limb is too weak to resist gravity, placing it in a functional position is essential to avoid deformities, minimize edema, and maintain range of motion (Radomski & Trombly, 2007). The client and caregiver should be taught to position the affected arm correctly during all tasks. All caregivers must be careful to avoid pulling on the affected arm and should mobilize the scapula before attempting overhead movement of a spastic arm. The therapist should be alert for signs of or reflex-sympathetic dystrophy, which include swelling of the hand; trophic changes, including altered skin color, nail appearance, sweating, or hair growth; and pain at rest or upon motion, especially during finger and shoulder flexion, abduction, external rotation, or all three (Eto, Yoshikawa, Ueda, & Hirai, 1980).

Dysphagia

Dysphagia (difficulty swallowing) often accompanies stroke, affecting as many as one-third of stroke patients (Roth, 1988). A speech pathologist may conduct a video-fluoroscopic exam (also called a modified barium swallow exam). In some facilities, this is done by an occupational therapist; in others, the therapist may assist with proper positioning of a patient during the exam. This is the best method for detecting deficits in oral control and swallowing. Food and liquid of various consistencies are mixed with barium, which makes the mixture visible on a video monitor. This mixture is given in small quantities and observed as it moves in the mouth, through the pharynx, and into the esophagus. Any abnormality that suggests risk of aspiration (food caught in the trachea) can readily be detected, and specific recommendations about safe types of food can be made.

In clients with swallowing dysfunction, specific guidelines may include avoiding drinking with a straw, taking one or two sips of liquid followed by solid foods, tilting the head while swallowing, and limiting environmental distractions during eating. During feeding training the occupational therapist should be aware of possible restrictions, such as no oral intake, as well as specifications for texture or consistency of food and beverages. A dietitian should also be consulted to ensure that protein and caloric needs are met and that dehydration is prevented.

Gastrostomy Tube

A client with severe dysphasia may have a gastrostomy tube. The tube must be monitored to avoid disruption during activity. During gastrostomy feedings, the patient must be maintained in an upright position (at least 45 degrees) generally for 1 hour following meals. This prevents back-flow of the feeding, which can lead to aspiration pneumonia. Practi-

tioners should also be aware of the tube's location to avoid pressure from clothing or a gait belt.

Fall Risk

Stroke survivors are more likely to fall than any other population (Vlahov, Myers, & Al-Ibrahim, 1990). From 41% to as many as 83.3% of patients who experienced falls had a prior stroke diagnosis (DeVincenzo & Watkins, 1987; Grant & Hamilton, 1987; Mion et al.,1989; Vlahov et al., 1990). Patients with impaired balance, impaired vision, lower-extremity weakness, impulsivity, confusion, gait disturbances, and perceptual deficits such as depth perception and unilateral neglect are at increased risk for falls. They may require constant or intermittent supervision. Safety belts should be used in wheelchairs and on the toilet if sitting balance or judgment is impaired. A gait belt is recommended when transferring, standing, or walking with a patient.

Evaluating Performance in the Discharge Setting

If the client is in an inpatient rehabilitation unit or center, a therapeutic day pass can be arranged that permits the client to go home for a period of 4 to 6 hours with a caregiver. This can be a useful assessment opportunity for identifying problems that may require specific environmental adaptations or further training. An assessment of actual behavior should take place in the daily living environment where the person performs the tasks (Christiansen, 2004). Reliable friends or family may report how the client performed during a home pass. The report should include information on what kinds of activities were done; any problems they may have encountered such as household ambulation, wheelchair mobility, and kitchen and bathroom mobility; and general accessibility in and around the home. Ask the client's caregiver to note how recommended equipment was used and any barriers encountered when using them.

Home Safety Assessment

Another valuable assessment for discharge planning is the home safety assessment. This generally involves the occupational therapist, physical therapist, the client, and sometimes the caregiver visiting the home. The main purpose is to ensure safety in the home and to determine if sufficient training has taken place for safe movement around the home and participation in important everyday activities. Careful assessment of the client's abilities in his or her home is critical to identifying barriers that can be eliminated or modified in preparation for a successful return home (Lysack & Neufeld, 2003).

The therapist observes if the client is able to generalize to the home setting some of the basic skills learned in the rehabilitation or skilled nursing facility setting: stair climbing, tub and toilet transfers, kitchen mobility, household ambulation, and the like. The advantage of the home safety assessment is that it allows the therapist to see the physical structure of the home and determine if there is adequate space to use recommended equipment. Another benefit of the evaluation may be preventing secondary injuries as a result of falls or other accidents (Lysack & Neufeld, 2003); the therapist can make recommendations specific to the environment.

Driving

Driving is important for maintaining independence in ADLs and social networking (Lee, Lee, & Cameron, 2003). It is generally illegal to drive after a stroke; clients must inform their local driver licensing agency and their insurance company and are not allowed to drive for at least a month (The Stroke Association, 2003). It is recommended that clients seek the advice of their physician before returning to driving.

Occupational therapists play an important role in addressing issues related to the older driver (Hunt et al., 1997). The question of readiness to return to driving following stroke is common in clinical practice; cognitive screening instruments are needed to assess driving competence (Lundqvist, Gerdle, & Ronnberg, 2000). As stated previously, a stroke may affect a person's ability to see, control movement, remember, or concentrate. All are necessary for safe driving, and all must be assessed (The Stroke Association, 2003). Limited research has been done on reliable driving evaluation criteria (Lee et al., 2003). The most common evaluation method has been driving in real traffic. Another method is use of a driving simulator (Lundqvist et al., 2000).

To compensate for hemiplegia, a spinner knob may be attached to the steering wheel. A left-foot accelerator can be used for the person with right-sided weakness or paralysis. The Association for Driver Rehabilitation Specialists (http://www.driver-ed.org/i4a/pages/index.cfm?pageid=1) is a useful resource for vehicle modifications and training. Therapists are advised to check with relevant government bodies to learn about any legal implications of modifying a vehicle.

Intervention Review

Once the intervention plan has been developed and implementation has begun, the process of reviewing the intervention begins immediately. The *Framework* describes the review process as a continuous reevaluation and review of the plan, the effectiveness of its delivery, and the progress toward outcomes (AOTA, 2008). This is accomplished by re-evaluating the plan and how it is implemented relative to achieving outcomes, modifying it as needed, and determining the need for continuing or discontinuing occupational therapy services and for referral to other services.

Outcomes

Outcomes of occupational therapy services should be focused on three overarching domains: health, participation, and engagement in occupation (AOTA, 2008). How these are measured or determined will vary by practice setting; however, determining outcomes of service delivery should incorporate one or more measures within those domains. When a reasonable number of goals have been met or changes in outcomes no longer occur, it may be time for discharge from the rehabilitation unit.

It is generally understood that discharge planning should begin from the day of admission. The occupational therapist, together with the rehabilitation team, the client, and his or her caregivers, must determine whether the client will be able to function in the environment to which he or she is being discharged.

The final concern in discharge planning relates to continuity of care. If therapy should continue, arrangements should be made through home health services, outpatient, day treatment, or a skilled nursing facility. It is important to establish a plan for follow-up care as part of discharge planning. This may be done in collaboration with the client's primary care physician or the rehabilitation physician, or both.

Case Description

Joyce is a 58-year-old woman who had a stroke. Her symptoms in the emergency room were left hemiparesis, slurred speech, impaired sensation on the left side, hemianopsia, and impaired cognitive status. Neuroimaging found multiple infarcts. She scored a 12 on the NIHSS, indicating moderate neurological impairment.

Prior to hospitalization, Joyce was employed as a nurse and lived alone in a single-story home. She was independent in all basic activities of daily living (BADLs) and IADLs. The occupational therapy evaluation during her acute stay revealed that active range of motion was within normal limits in both upper extremities. Her sitting balance was graded as good, but standing balance was graded as poor. She was considered a high risk for falls due to her impulsivity and impaired balance and vision. Joyce required minimal assistance for most self-care tasks. Her score on a cognitive screen indicated moderate impairment. Her rehabilitation stay in the acute setting was 72 hours, and she was transferred to an inpatient rehabilitation unit for 3 weeks. Following her inpatient stay, she was seen for day treatment for an additional 8 weeks.

Inpatient Rehabilitation

Assessment

FIM results at intake to the inpatient rehabilitation unit showed that Joyce still required minimal assistance for most self-care tasks. The inpatient intervention plan was focused on helping Joyce complete all self-care tasks with supervision only. Once Joyce reached this level of independence, she would be discharged home but continue day treatment rehabilitation to address the remaining limitations in her occupational performance.

Intervention

Occupational therapy intervention consisted of scheduled self-care training sessions in Joyce's room. The therapist coordinated with the nursing staff to ensure a consistent arrangement of her meal trays in order to improve her ability to locate food items. It was recommended that she be placed in a private room, as she was severely distracted by environmental stimuli such as conversations between other people, the television, the ringing telephone, and minor changes in the physical arrangement of her room. The structure in Joyce's rehabilitation program allowed her to improve her level of independence in feeding, grooming, and toileting from minimal assistance to independence with modifications.

The following activities were incorporated into the ADL training program:

- *Feeding*. After the meal tray was placed in front of Joyce, she was told what food items were being served. She was then asked to locate all items on the tray. A plate guard and an independence mug with antisplash lid were used to minimize spilling. The plate guard was also used as a guide to locate the left side of her plate.
- *Grooming*. Joyce and her caregiver were instructed to eliminate clutter on the bathroom sink and to keep grooming tools in the same location.

- *Bathing*. Due to impaired balance and low endurance, a tub transfer bench, grab bars, and handheld shower were used. Because she had difficulty holding the bar of soap and wringing out the washcloth, liquid soap and a bathing puff improved her independence.
- *Upper-body dressing*. Joyce had difficulty manipulating small buttons and fasteners. Especially frustrating was hooking her bra. By turning the bra with the hook side up and clipping the left side to her underwear with a clothes pin she was able to fasten it.
- *Lower-body dressing*. Joyce had difficulty putting on her right sock and shoe. She was unable to maintain the position of crossing her right leg over her left, and when she reached down, she would lose her balance. In addition to routine practice and training in donning and doffing of her socks and shoes, the occupational therapist had Joyce sit on the edge of the treatment mat and reach for items just below her knees and eventually on the floor. This helped improve her sitting balance; by discharge, she was able to don and doff both shoes and socks.
- *Leisure*. Joyce was an avid reader prior to the onset of her illness. Although she continued to work on reading during sessions with a speech pathologist, she did not regain proficiency. She experienced some satisfaction with books on tape.

Because there would be times during the day when Joyce would be unsupervised after discharge from the hospital, the occupational therapist worked with her and her caregiver on strategies to store food items so that she would be able to retrieve a cold snack from the refrigerator. Unsupervised cooking was not recommended. Joyce practiced making a sandwich and arranging snacks in a familiar container that she could easily locate. The caregiver participated in several training sessions with the therapist prior to Joyce's discharge from the hospital to ensure follow-through with learned compensatory strategies.

Outcomes

Using the FIM as a measure of participation in self-care tasks, Joyce's outcome goals for inpatient rehabilitation were met. Table 10.5 shows that she was able to complete all self-care with only supervision and setup assistance or less. At this point, the treating therapist recommended discharging Joyce from inpatient services to home, with a referral to a day treatment program to address participation restrictions in her community, work, and leisure roles.

Day Treatment

Assessment

The treating therapist completed the COPM with Joyce on her first visit to day treatment. The results of the COPM yielded three performance goals that Joyce identified, shown in Table 10.6 with her rating of her ability to perform the activity and her satisfaction with her performance. These three activities were the focus of the intervention plan while Joyce was in day treatment.

Intervention

Occupational therapy intervention consisted of seeing Joyce 3 times a week for 1 hour at a time. She was also seen by speech and physical therapists. Each time she came to occupational therapy, the intervention was focused on one of the three activities identified on the COPM. The intervention activities in Joyce's day treatment program included

- Training in internal cueing strategies for her impaired memory; use of external aids for keeping a daily, weekly, and monthly calendar; and homework activities that required her to try using the strategies at home and report back on how they worked;
- Practicing compensation techniques for cooking, given her balance and vision deficits;
- Using verbalization skills and written plans to develop and execute a plan to cook a meal for the day treatment therapists;

- Learning the reasonable accommodation guidelines of the Americans with Disabilities Act of 1990 (P.L. 101–336) and the process for requesting accommodations to return to work;
- Training in energy conservation techniques to help her manage energy for return to work;
- Visiting her job site to evaluate her work environment and determine the essential job functions; and
- Developing a graduated plan for return to work, starting with requesting reasonable accommodations, and developing a modified work schedule to accommodate her residual impairments following her stroke.

Outcomes

The COPM was used as an outcome measure to determine Joyce's ability to perform her chosen activities and her satisfaction with her ability to perform them. Table 10.7 shows that her COPM ratings dramatically increased from intake and were now at a point where she was ready to be discharged from occupational therapy services.

Summary

Occupational therapists frequently are part of the interdisciplinary team that collaborates following stroke to help individuals return to daily living. An occupational therapist is a rehabilitation provider at all stages of recovery, from inpatient rehabilitation to outpatient rehabilitation and finally to community reintegration. The *Occupational Therapy Practice Framework* (AOTA, 2008) views the person and environment as interconnected in influencing an individual's occupational performance. Several

Table 10.5. Joyce's Self-Care FIM Scores

Self-Care	Admission	Discharge
Eating	4	6
Grooming	4	6
Bathing	4	6
Dressing, upper	4	5
Dressing, lower	4	5
Bladder control	4	7
Bowel control	4	6
Bed, chair transfers	4	5
Toilet transfers	4	5
Tub, shower transfers	3	5

Note. Numbers refer to patient's performance scores at admission and discharge on the Functional Independence Measure (FIM); scores range from 0 = *complete dependence* to 10 = *complete independence.*

Table 10.6. Joyce's COPM Ratings on Her First Visit to Day Treatment

Activity	Performance Rating (0–10)	Satisfaction Rating (0–10)
Working as a nurse	1	1
Cooking for herself and friends	2	1
Keeping track of her appointments	4	2

Note. The COPM has caregiver and client ratings scored on a 10-point scale. Caregivers rate the client's performance on the activity (10 = *highest level of performance*) and clients rate their own satisfaction with their performance on activity (10 = *highest level of satisfaction*).

Table 10.7. Joyce's COPM Ratings on Her Discharge From Day Treatment

Activity	Performance Rating (0–10)	Satisfaction Rating (0–10)
Working as a nurse	7	7
Cooking for herself and friends	8	9
Keeping track of her appointments	8	9

Note. The COPM has caregiver and client ratings scored on a 10-point scale. Caregivers rate the client's performance on the activity (10 = *highest level of performance*) and clients rate their own satisfaction with their performance on activity (10 = *highest level of satisfaction*).

deficits may occur following stroke. The occupational therapist can use several compensation techniques and adaptive strategies to improve participation and performance of ADLs throughout the continuum of care.

Acknowledgments

The authors acknowledge with appreciation the contributions to earlier versions of this chapter by Judith A. Jenkins, MA, OTR.

Study Questions

1. How does hemiplegia affect a client's ability to perform ADLs?
2. What are some of the common impairments that result from a stroke?
3. What are the factors that need to be considered when setting goals with a client following stroke?
4. What intervention and compensation strategies may be used when designing an intervention plan for an individual following stroke?
5. What are some techniques or equipment, or both, that may be useful for cooking, cleaning, and driving for an individual who has motor impairment?
6. What are some techniques or equipment, or both, that may be useful for cooking, cleaning, and driving for an individual who has cognitive impairment?

References

Aichner, F., Adelwohrer, C., & Haring, H. P. (2002). Rehabilitation approaches to stroke. *Journal of Neural Transmission, Suppl.* (63), 59–73.

American Heart Association. (2008). *Heart disease and stroke statistics—2008.* Dallas: Author.

American Occupational Therapy Association. (2008). Occupational therapy practice framework: Domain and process (2nd ed.). *American Journal of Occupational Therapy, 62,* 625–683.

Americans with Disabilities Act of 1990, P.L. 101–336, 42 USC § 12101.

Barreca, S., Wolf, S. L., Fasoli, S., & Bohannon, R. (2003). Treatment interventions for the paretic upper limb of stroke survivors: A critical review. *Neurorehabilitation and Neural Repair, 17*(4), 220–226.

Bass-Haugen, J., Mathiowetz, V., & Flinn, N. (2002). Optimizing motor behavior using the occupational therapy task-oriented approach In C. Trombly & M. Radomski (Eds.), *Occupational therapy for physical dysfunction* (5th ed.). New York: Lippincott Williams & Wilkins.

Baum, C., & Christiansen, C. (1997). The occupational therapy context: Philosophy–principles–practice. In C. Christiansen & C. Baum (Eds.), *Occupational therapy enabling function and well-being* (2nd ed.; pp. 26–45). Thorofare, NJ: Slack.

Baum, C. M., & Christiansen, C. H. (2004). Person–environment–occupation–performance: A model for planning interventions for individuals, organizations, and populations. In C. H. Christiansen, C. M. Baum, & J. Bass-Haugen (Eds.), *Occupational therapy: Performance, participation, and well-being* (3rd ed.). Thorofare, NJ: Slack.

Baum, C. M., Connor, L. T., Morrison, T., Hahn, M., Dromerick, A. W., & Edwards, D. F. (2008). Reliability, validity, and clinical utility of the Executive Function Performance Test: A measure of executive function in a sample of people with stroke. *American Journal of Occupational Therapy, 62,* 446–455.

Baum, C., & Edwards, D. (2001). *Activity Card Sort: Test manual.* St. Louis, MO: Program in Occupational Therapy, Washington University School of Medicine.

Baum, C., & Edwards, D. (2008). *Activity Card Sort* (2nd ed.). Bethesda, MD: AOTA Press.

Bendz, M. (2000). Rules of relevance after a stroke. *Social Science and Medicine, 51*, 713–723.

Bendz, M. (2003). The first year of rehabilitation after a stroke—From two perspectives. *Scandinavian Journal of Caring Sciences, 17*(3), 215–222.

Boman, I., Lindstedt, M., Hemmingsson, H., & Bartfai, A. (2004). Cognitive training in home environment. *Brain Injury, 18*, 985–995.

Borcherding, S. (2005). *Documentation manual for writing SOAP notes in occupational therapy* (2nd ed.). Thorofare, NJ: Slack.

Brott, T., Adams, H. P. J., Olinger, C. P., Marler, J. R., Barsan, W. G., Biller, J., et al. (1989). Measurements of acute cerebral infarction: A clinical examination scale. *Stroke, 20*, 864–870.

Bukowski, L., Bonavolonta, M., Keehn, M. T., & Morgan, K. A. (1996). Interdisciplinary roles in stroke care. *Nursing Clinics of North America, 21*(2), 359–374.

Carr, J. H., & Shepherd, R. B. (1987). *A Motor Relearning Programme for Stroke* (2nd ed.). Rockville, MD: Aspen.

Christiansen, C. H. (2004). Assessment and management of basic and extended daily living skills. In J. DeLisa et al. (Eds.), *Rehabilitation medicine: Principles and practice* (pp. 975–1004). Philadelphia: Lippincott Williams & Wilkins.

Cicerone, K. D. (2002). Remediation of "working attention" in mild traumatic brain injury. *Brain Injury, 16*, 185–195.

Coster, W. (1998). Occupation–centered assessment of children. *American Journal of Occupational Therapy, 52*, 337–344.

DeVincenzo, D. K., & Watkins, S. (1987). Accidental falls in a rehabilitation setting. *Rehabilitation Nursing, 12*, 248–252.

Edwards, D., & Christiansen, C. (2005). Occupational development. In C. Christiansen, C. Baum, & J. Bass-Haugen (Eds.), *Occupational therapy: Performance, participation, and well–being* (3rd ed., pp. 42–70). Thorofare, NJ: Slack.

Eto, F., Yoshikawa, M., Ueda, S., & Hirai, S. (1980). Posthemiplegic shoulder–hand syndrome, with special reference to related cerebral localization. *Journal of the American Geriatrics Society, 28*(1), 13–17.

Evans, R. L., Bishop, D. S., & Haselkorn, J. K. (1991). Factors predicting satisfactory home care after stroke. *Archives of Physical Medicine and Rehabilitation, 72*, 144–147.

Flavell, J. H., Miller, P. H., & Miller, S. A. (1993). *Cognitive development* (3rd ed.). Englewood Cliffs, NJ: Prentice-Hall.

Freeman, E. (2001). Unilateral spatial neglect: New treatment approaches with potential application to occupational therapy. *American Journal of Occupational Therapy, 55*(4), 401–408.

Geusgens, C. A., Winkens, I., van Heugten, C. M., Jolles, J., & van de Heuvel, W. J. (2007). Occurrence and measurement of transfer in cognitive rehabilitation: A critical review. *Journal of Rehabilitation Medicine, 39*(6), 425–439.

Granger, C. V., Hamilton, B. B., & Gresham, G. E. (1988). The stroke rehabilitation outcome study: Part I general description. *Archives of Physical Medicine and Rehabilitation, 69*, 506–509.

Granger, C. V., Hamilton, B. B., Gresham, G. E., & Kramer, A. A. (1989). The stroke rehabilitation outcome study: Part II. Relative merits of the Total Barthel Index Score and a four-item subscore in predicting patient outcomes. *Archives of Physical Medicine and Rehabilitation, 70*, 100–103.

Grant, J., & Hamilton, S. (1987). Falls in a rehabilitation center: A retrospective and comparative analysis. *Rehabilitation Nursing, 12*, 74–76.

Gresham, G. E., Duncan, P. W., Stason, W. B., Adams, H. P., Jr., Adelman, A. M., Alexander, D. N., et al. (1995). *Post-stroke rehabilitation clinical practice guideline* (No. 16). Rockville, MD: U.S. Department of Health and Human Services, Public Health Service, Agency for Health Care Policy and Research.

Gutman, S., & Schonfeld, A. (2003). *Screening adult neurologic populations: A step-by-step instruction manual.* Bethesda, MD: AOTA Press.

Gutman, S., & Schonfeld, A. (2009). *Screening adult neurologic populations: A step-by-step instruction manual* (2nd ed.). Bethesda, MD: AOTA Press.

Hasselkus, B. (1991). Ethical dilemmas in family caregiving for the elderly: Implications for occupational therapy. *American Journal of Occupational Therapy, 45*, 206–212.

Hillman, A., & Chapparo, C. J. (2002). The role of work in the lives of retired men following stroke. *WORK, 19*(3), 303–313.

Hunt, L. A., Murphy, G. F., Carr, D., Duchek, J. M., Buckles, V., & Morris, J. C. (1997). Reliability of the Washington University Road Test: A performance-based assessment for drivers with dementia of the Alzheimer's type. *Archives of Neurology, 54*, 707–712.

Kaschel, R., Della Salla, S., Cantagallo, A., Fahlbock, A., Laaksonen, R., & Kazen, M. (2002). Imagery mnemonics for the rehabilitation of memory: A randomized group controlled trial. *Neuropsychology Rehabilitation, 12*, 127–153.

Kwakkel, G., Kollen, B., & Lindeman, E. (2004). Understanding the pattern of functional recovery after stroke: Facts and theories. *Restorative Neurology and Neuroscience, 22*(3–5), 281–299.

Kwakkel, G., Kollen, B. J., VanderGrond, J., & Prevo, A. J. (2003). Probability of regaining dexterity in the flaccid upper limb. *Stroke, 34*(9), 2181–2186.

Law, M., Baptiste, S., McColl, M., Opzoomer, A., Polatajko, H., & Pollock, N. (1990). The Canadian Occupational Performance Measure: An outcome measure for occupational therapy. *Canadian Journal of Occupational Therapy, 57*(2), 82–87.

Lee, H. C., Lee, A. H., & Cameron, D. (2003). Validation of a driving simulator by measuring the visual attention skill of older adult drivers. *American Journal of Occupational Therapy, 57*(3), 324–328.

Levine, B., Robertson, I. H., Clare, L., Carter, G., Hong, J., Wilson, B. A., et al. (2000). Rehabilitation of executive functioning: An experimental–clinical validation of goal management training. *Journal of the International Neuropsychological Society, 6,* 299–312.

Lundqvist, A., Gerdle, B., & Ronnberg, J. (2000). Neuropsychological aspects of driving after a stroke-in the simulator and on the road. *Applied Cognitive Psychology, 14,* 135–150.

Lyle, R. C. (1981). A performance test for assessment of upper limb function in physical rehabilitation treatment and research. *International Journal of Rehabilitation Research, 4,* 483–492.

Lysack, C. L., & Neufeld, S. (2003). Occupational therapist home evaluations: Inequalities, but doing the best we can? *American Journal of Occupational Therapy, 57*(4), 369–379.

Ma, H., & Trombly, C. A. (2002). A synthesis of the effects of occupational therapy for persons with stroke, part II: Remediation of impairments. *American Journal of Occupational Therapy, 56*(3), 260–274.

Marler, J. R., Tilley, B. C., Lu, M., Brott, T. G., Lyden, P. C., Grotta, J. C., et al. (2000). Early stroke treatment associated with better outcome: The NINDS rt–PA stroke study. *Neurology, 55,* 1649–1655.

Mauthe, R., Haaf, D., Hayn, P., & Krall, J. (1996). Predicting discharge destination of stroke patients using a mathematical model based on six items from the Functional Independence Measure. *Archives of Physical Medicine and Rehabilitation, 77,* 10–30.

Mazer, B., Sofer, S., Korner-Bitensky, N., Gelinas, I., Hanley, J., & Wood-Dauphinee, S. (2003). Effectiveness of a visual attention retraining program on the driving performance of clients with stroke. *Archives of Physical Medicine and Rehabilitation, 84*(4), 541–550.

Meichenbaum, D. (1977). *Cognitive behavioral modification: An integrative approach.* New York: Plenum Press.

Mercier, L., Audet, T., Hebert, R., Rochette, A., & Dubois, M. (2001). Impact of motor, cognitive, and perceptual disorders on ability to perform activities of daily living after stroke. *Stroke, 32,* 2602–2608.

Mesulam, M. M. (1985). *Principles of behavioural neurology.* Philadelphia: F. A. Davis.

Miltner, W. H. R., Bauder, H., Sommer, M., Dettmers, C., & Taub, E. (1999). Effects of constraint-induced movement therapy on patients with chronic motor deficits after stroke: A replication. *Stroke, 30,* 586–592.

Mion, L. C., Gregor, S., Buettner, M., Chwurchak, D., Lee, O., & Paras, W. (1989). Falls in the rehabilitation setting: Incidence and characteristics. *Rehabilitation Nursing, 14,* 17–21.

Mok, V., Wong, A., Lam, W., Fan, Y., Tang, W., Kwok, T., et al. (2004). Cognitive impairment and functional outcome after stroke associated with small vessel disease. *Journal of Neurology, Neurosurgery, and Psychiatry, 75,* 560–566.

Moyers, P. A. (1999). The guide to occupational therapy practice. *American Journal of Occupational Therapy, 53*(3), 247–322.

Nakayama, H., Jorgensen, H., Raaschou, H., & Olsen, T. (1994). Compensation in recovery of upper

extremity function after stroke: The Copenhagen Stroke Study. *Archives of Physical Medicine and Rehabilitation, 75,* 852–857.

Niemeier, J. P., Cifu, D. X., & Kishore, R. (2001). The lighthouse strategy: Improving the functional status of patients with unilateral neglect after stroke and brain injury using a visual imagery intervention. *Top Stroke Rehabilitation, 8,* 10–18.

O'Brien, A., & Wolf, T. (in review). Determining work outcomes of mild to moderate stroke survivors. *WORK.*

Ozer, M. N., Materson, R. S., & Caplan, L. R. (1994). *Management of persons with stroke.* St. Louis, MO: Mosby.

Polatajko, H., & Mandich, A. (2004). *Enabling occupation in children: The cognitive orientation to daily occupational performance (CO-OP) approach.* Ottawa, Ontario: CAOT Publications ACE.

Polatajko, H. J., & Mandich, A. (2005). Cognitive orientation to daily occupational performance with children with developmental coordination disorders. In N. Katz (Ed.), *Cognition and occupation across the life span: Models for intervention in occupational therapy* (pp. 237–259). Bethesda, MD: AOTA Press.

Ponte-Allan, M., & Giles, G. (1999). Goal setting and functional outcomes in rehabilitation. *American Journal of Occupational Therapy, 53*(6), 646–649.

Radomski, M., & Trombly, C. (2007). *Occupational therapy for physical dysfunction* (6th ed.). Philadelphia: Lippincott Williams & Wilkins.

Robertson, I. H., Ward, T., Ridgeway, V., & Nimmo-Smith, I. (1994). *The Test of Everyday Attention Manual.* Suffolk, UK: Thames Valley Test Company.

Robson, J., Marshall, J., Pring, T., & Chiat, S. (1998). Phonological naming therapy in jargon aphasia: Positive but paradoxal effects. *Journal of the International Neuropsychological Society, 4,* 675–686.

Roth, E. J. (1988). The elderly stroke patient: Principles and practices of rehabilitation management. *Topics in Geriatric Rehabilitation, 3*(4), 27–61.

Scheiman, M. (1997). *Understanding and managing vision deficits.* Thorofare, NJ: Slack.

Schumway-Cook, A., & Woollacott, M. (2007). *Motor control: Translating research into clinical practice* (3rd ed.). Philadelphia: Lippincott Williams & Wilkins.

Schunk, D. (2000). *Learning theories: An educational perspective* (3rd ed.). Upper Saddle River, NJ: Prentice-Hall.

Soderback, I. (1988). The effectiveness of training intellectual functions in adults with acquired brain damage. *Scandinavian Journal of Rehabilitation Medicine, 20,* 47–56.

Sturm, W., Willmes, K., Orgass, B., & Hartje, W. (1997). Do specific attention deficits need specific training? *Neuropsychological Rehabilitation, 7,* 81–103.

Sveen, U., Thommessen, B., Bautz-Holter, E., Wyller, T. B., & Laake, K. (2004). Well-being and instrumental activities of daily living after stroke. *Clinical Rehabilitation, 18*(3), 267–274.

Teasell, R., & Foley, N. (2008). Module 4—Managing the stroke rehabilitation triage process. In R. Teasell et al. (Eds.), *Evidence-based review of stroke rehabilitation* (12th ed.). Retrieved June 2009, from http://www.ebrsr.com/uploads/Module_4_triage _final.pdf

The Stroke Association. (2003). *Driving after a stroke*. Retrieved October 2003, from http://stroke.org .uk/noticeboard/Driving.htm

Thorsen, A.-M., Holmqvist, L. W., de Pedro-Cuesta, J., & von Koch, L. (2005). A randomized controlled trial of early supported discharge and continued rehabilitation at home after stroke: Five-year follow-up of patient outcome. *Stroke, 36*(2), 297–303.

Toglia, J. P. (1991). Generalization of treatment: A multi-contextual approach to cognitive perceptual impairment in the brain-injured adult. *American Journal of Occupational Therapy, 45*, 505–516.

Toglia, J., & Kirk, U. (2000). Understanding awareness deficits following brain injury. *Neurorehabilitation and Neural Repair, 15*, 57–70.

Uniform Data System for Medical Rehabilitation. (1997). *Guide for the Uniform Data Set for Medical Rehabilitation* (including the FIM™ instrument) (version 5.1.) Buffalo, NY: Author.

Vlahov, D., Myers, A. H., & Al-Ibrahim, M. S. (1990). Epidemiology of falls among patients in a rehabilitation hospital. *Archives of Physical Medicine and Rehabilitation, 71*, 8–12.

Wade, T. K., & Troy, J. C. (2001). Mobile phones as a new memory aid: A preliminary investigation using case studies. *Brain Injury, 15*, 305–320.

Weimer, C., Kurth, T., Kraywinkel, K., Wagner, M., Busse, O., Haberl, R. L., et al. (2002). Assessment of functioning and disability after ischemic stroke. *Stroke, 33*(8), 2053–2059.

Wilson, B., Cockburn, J., & Baddeley, A. (1985). *The Rivermead Behavioral Memory Test*. Reading, England: Thames Valley Test Company.

Wilson, B. A., Cockburn, J., & Halligan, P. (1987). Development of a behavioral test of visuospatial neglect. *Archives of Physical Medicine and Rehabilitation, 68*, 98–102.

Wishart, L. R., Lee, T. D., Janzen-Ezekiel, H., Marley, T. L., & Lehto, N. K. (2002). Application of motor learning principles: The physiotherapy client as a problem-solver. I. concepts. *Physiotherapy Canada, 52*(3), 229–232.

Wolf, S. L., Lecraw, D. E., Barton, L. A., & Jann, B. B. (1989). Forced use of hemiplegic upper extremities to reverse the effect of learned nonuse among chronic stroke and head-injured patients. *Experimental Neurology, 104*(2), 125–132.

Wolf, T., Baum, C., & Connor, L. (2009). Changing face of stroke: Implications for occupational therapy practice. *American Journal of Occupational Therapy, 63*, 621–625.

Wood-Dauphinee, S., & Kwakkel, G. (2005). The impact of rehabilitation on stroke outcomes: What is the evidence? In M. Barnes, B. Dobkin, & J. Bogousslavsky (Eds.), *Recovery after stroke*. Cambridge, England: Cambridge University Press.

Zinn, S., Dudley, T., Bosworth, H., Hoenig, H., Duncan, P., & Horner, R. (2004). The effect of poststroke cognitive impairment on rehabilitation process and functional outcome. *Archives of Physical Medicine and Rehabilitation, 85*, 1084–1090.

Chapter 11

Enabling Performance and Participation for Persons With Movement Disorders

JANET L. POOLE, PHD, OTR/L, FAOTA

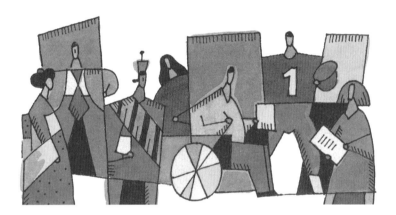

KEY WORDS

adaptive
  strategies
assistive devices
augmentative and
  alternative
  communication
  (ACC)

dysphagia
energy conservation
independent
  living movement
routines

HIGHLIGHTS

- People with movement disorders are faced with too much or too little movement and with difficulties with mental, sensory, and voice and speech functions.

- Adaptive strategies are preferred over remediation for persons with movement disorders because of the complex involvement of many client factors and the progressive nature of the disorders.

- Highly specialized equipment and assistive devices help people with movement disorders manage their environments, socialize and communicate, and perform activities of daily living and instrumental activities of daily living; however, the occupational therapist should consider the expense and the client's adaptability to meet changing capacities and requirements.

- Fatigue management strategies are essential for independence, safety, and postural stability.

- Social supports are important for persons with movement disorders to accomplish tasks; occupational therapy practitioners can foster the development of these supports by exploring the types of support available and the client's and the support-givers' needs.

OBJECTIVES

After reading this material, readers will be able to

- Identify the difference between occupational therapy aimed at remediation of performance skills and occupational therapy aimed at independent living;

- Describe factors to consider when recommending adaptive strategies for individuals with movement disorders;

- Describe adaptive strategies for these individuals using equipment and techniques for feeding, meal management and shopping, community mobility, and communication;

- Describe adaptive strategies using routines and social support for communication, feeding, and meal management for individuals with movement disorders; and

- Identify ways in which routines and social supports can be facilitated.

This chapter presents anecdotal accounts of how adults with movement disorders view and manage daily occupations. Principles for problem solving from the perspectives of the client and the occupational therapist are drawn from case examples. Emphasis is given to the individual's perspective and experience of self within the context of his or her social and physical environments as they relate to occupational performance. The therapist's role in helping the individual develop adaptive strategies is also described. A framework is used that considers techniques, equipment, routines, and social supports as categories of adaptive strategies that help individuals with movement disorders compensate for the lack or excess of movement with which they contend.

Occupational Performance Challenges for Individuals With Movement Disorders

Individuals with movement disorders face the challenge of living with too much or too little movement, associated with some degree of paralysis or weakness. For people with these disorders, actions are frequently difficult to start, stop, or control. Many conditions carry with them a progressive component, often rapid, and some create a disturbance in mental functioning, sometimes affecting memory, concentration, and an ability to organize and sequence events. Sensory abilities, including *proprioception* (knowledge of the body's posture, movement, and position in space), may be impaired. Problems performing daily occupations are often intensified by stress as well as the aging process, even if the medical condition itself is stable (Finlayson, Impey, Nicolle, & Edwards, 1998; Watts & Koller, 2004). Many individuals with movement disorders experience pain; constant fatigue and low energy; poor balance; and difficulties with most areas of occupations, including communication, mobility, eating, dressing, toileting, bathing, and grooming (Finlayson et al., 1998; Shah & Nolen, 2006).

The scope of this chapter includes people with movement disorders including amyotrophic lateral sclerosis (ALS), cerebral palsy, dystonia, Huntington's chorea, multiple sclerosis, muscular dystrophy, Parkinson's disease, tardive dyskinesia, and Tourette's syndrome. This list provides examples of conditions of both hyper- and hypokinetic movement disorders, but it is not exhaustive (Francisco, Kithari, Schiess, & Kaldis, 2005). A list of supplementary reading provides sources for detailed descriptions of the medical conditions under discussion. Table 11.1 provides common definitions of frequently used terms. Table 11.2 describes features and problems of selected movement disorders.

Framework for Identifying Problems in Occupational Performance

A person's environment can support or inhibit independence. Social supports, cultural beliefs and values, environmental designs and furnishings, and the availability of structures and tools are all significant factors in an individual's engagement in daily occupations. For this reason, when addressing problems with the performance of everyday occupations, it is important to evaluate and to intervene within the context of the individual's social, cultural, and physical environments (Christiansen, 2004).

Problems related to accomplishing the necessary activities for daily living (ADLs) are often addressed through adaptive strategies within the domains of techniques and equipment, routines, and social supports. In this chapter, case studies describe specific

Table 11.1. Movement Disorder Terms and Examples of Associated Conditions

Term	Description	Example
Ataxia	Movement, usually of the extremities, that is reduced in speed and distorted in terms of timing and direction	Multiple sclerosis; Charcot–Marie–Tooth
Athetosis	Slow sinuous movement with fluctuations in tone and most commonly found in the distal extremities; more rhythmic and slower than choreiform movements; exacerbated by anxiety and attempted voluntary movements	Cerebral palsy; tardive dyskinesia
Bradykinesia	Slowness of movement resulting in a person "freezing"; often misinterpreted as depression and withdrawal; presents as a loss of spontaneity	Parkinson's disease
Chorea	Usually describes a random pattern of rapid, irregular, unpredictable, and involuntary contractions of a group of muscles; resulting clinical picture may be one of a "dancing" or "clownish" gait with the distal extremities more involved than the proximal ones; movements attenuated during sleep, exacerbated with stress and attempts at action	Huntington's chorea; tardive dyskinesia
Dystonia	Although often found as a clinical descriptor, is in fact used to describe a neurological syndrome in which there is an abnormality of tone; affects muscle groups in the trunk, neck, face, and proximal limbs; presents with slow, sustained, involuntary twisting movement patterns that may be generalized, segmental, or focal; confused with athetosis when slow, and chorea when rapid	
Hyperkinesia and hypokinesia	An excess and a paucity of movement, respectively; difficulty with initiation and enactment of a normal speed of movement	All movement disorders, with exception of amyotrophic lateral sclerosis
Spasticity	Extreme or excessive muscle tone; presents as resistance to passive movement; a constant cocontraction of muscle groups inhibiting relaxation pulls the body into abnormal patterns, rendering it vulnerable to deformities; exacerbated by effort	Cerebral palsy; multiple sclerosis
Rigidity	Resistance of proximal and axial muscles to passive movement; frequently experienced as stiffness and associated with pain	Parkinson's disease
Tremor	Simple, involuntary, rhythmic movement, frequently starting in the hands; difficult to differentiate from generalized shivering or shaking; frequently found at rest but disappears in sleep; most pronounced under stress	Parkinson's disease; multiple sclerosis

daily occupations within these categories. The emphasis of this approach differs from the traditional presentation of problems according to disability and solutions in terms of physical performance by the individual with the disorder. In other words, accomplishing the occupation is the focus, even if it is accomplished through adaptation or substitution; the focus is not on the client performing the occupation physically or independently, and not, as has been traditional, on medical rehabilitation that eliminates the impairment (Christiansen, 2004).

Consistent with the themes expressed elsewhere in this book, this chapter focuses on the process of an individual's adaptation to his or her physical and social environments. Its objective is to show that occupation-related needs can be met despite movement disorders and without emphasizing remediation of physical performance skills. The importance of an individual's social and physical contexts is highlighted as a critical consideration in the assessment and intervention of occupation problems (AOTA, 2008).

The occupational therapist's role in working with adults with movement disorders is to be knowl-

Table 11.2. Summary Data of Major Motor Control Disorders: Manifestations and Presenting Problems

Condition	Features	Movement Problems
Amyotrophic lateral sclerosis	Motor neuron disease of rapid onset; more prevalent in men over 30; affects central and peripheral motor neurons	Progressive muscle weakness and atrophy distally, then proximally; fatigue
Cerebral palsy	Motor disorder resulting from a nonprogressive lesion in the developing brain, resulting in abnormal and fluctuating muscle tone and reflexes	Ataxia; athetosis; flaccidity; spasticity; or mixed pattern of movement affecting the limbs, trunk, head, and neck
Charcot–Marie–Tooth	Inherited, progressive, sensorimotor disorder of nervous system; included mild loss of sensation	Progressive muscle weakness starting in extremities, resulting in loss of balance and tripping
Duchenne muscular dystrophy	Hereditary and progressive disease of the muscles; onset in males ages 2 to 6 years; marked wasting of proximal muscle groups; moves distally	Rapidly progressive muscle weakness, initially affecting pelvic and pectoral groups; fatigue
Huntington's chorea	Hereditary, progressive disorder of the basal ganglia; characterized by abnormal, involuntary choreiform movements; amplified by progressive cognitive impairment	Abrupt, involuntary choreiform movements; exacerbated by stress and effort
Multiple sclerosis	Lesions in the central nervous system; demyelination results in a series of exacerbations and remissions; progressive weakness; sensory disturbances; cognitive damage	Progressive muscle weakness and spasticity; tremors, ataxia, and fatigue
Parkinson's disease	Degeneration of the basal ganglia; progressive; found most frequently in men and women older than 50 years of age; results in muscle rigidity, postural changes, dementia, loss of autonomic reflexes	Slowness in motor planning; difficulty initiating movement; tremors at rest and with intention; shuffling gait; slurred speech; symptoms exacerbated by fatigue and stress
Tourette's syndrome	Involuntary movement disorder; onset 2–5 years of age, primarily males; includes sensory disturbances, impulsivity, compulsive and ritualistic behaviors, with possible attention deficits	Recurrent involuntary, repetitive, rapid movements; hyperactivity; symptoms increase with stress

edgeable about the context of an individual's life and to be committed to supporting his or her perspective, using approaches reflecting principles of the independent living movement. This framework requires therapists to support an individual's acquisition of skills and capabilities for self-direction and to acknowledge his or her ability to be a manager who can communicate effectively, identify and use resources, make choices and decisions, set priorities, and make sound judgments (AOTA, 2008).

Principles for Enabling ADLs Despite Movement Disorders

This chapter is organized according to techniques and equipment, routines, and social supports that enable performance despite the functional limitations imposed by movement disorders. *Techniques*

and equipment refer to the actions or assistive devices an individual uses to accomplish certain tasks, which in turn address the necessary routines constituting everyday life. *Routines* refer to established sequences and patterns used to perform occupations. Social supports include the availability and expectations of significant individuals. Within these domains of adaptive strategies, we describe areas of occupation such as eating, communicating, mobility, and preparing a meal and discuss strategies for occupational therapy intervention (see Case Study 11.1).

An individual's choice of a specific adaptive strategy is not based on performance alone (Lyons & Tickle-Degnen, 2003; McCuaig & Frank, 1991). Deciding how to accomplish a task is highly dependent on values that determine the importance and order of potential actions. The decision to choose

Case Study 11.1. Adaptive Strategies Used by a Woman With Huntington's Disease

Contributed by Kerry Trautwein, OTR/L

M.H. is a 61-year-old, married female who was diagnosed with Huntington's disease (HD) 6 years ago. HD in her family history includes her father (now deceased) and one sister affected. M.H. has another sister who has not been diagnosed with HD but who reportedly has an "essential tremor." She has no biological children and lives with her husband, who is very supportive.

M.H. initially presented to the multidisciplinary HD clinic 4 years ago. Her husband reported that she was exhibiting decreased interest in her work (she worked as an accomplished artist with clay). Her husband also noticed that she had some trouble initiating tasks and was lethargic at times.

At her first visit, M.H. presented with chorea which was present in smaller athetoid involuntary movements. She demonstrated decreased balance and righting reactions but was ambulatory without an assistive device and was not falling at that time. She was independent with mobility and basic ADLs, and her strength and joint motion in all four extremities was within normal limits.

Over the past 4 years, M.H. has shown a slow but progressive decline in balance and cognitive abilities. She has always presented with *anosognosia,* a lack of awareness of physical symptoms, due to brain changes. Despite being presented with evidence to the contrary (i.e., falls), she consistently maintains that she is fine, independent, and has none of the balance problems/physical symptoms of HD, and thus no need for adaptive equipment, assistive devices to ambulate, or therapy services.

As M.H.'s chorea has become more pronounced and voluntary movements have become more impaired, she has needed some assistance with ADLs. She has adamantly refused the occupational therapist's suggestions of a tub bench and grab bars, making life very stressful for her husband, who fears she will fall in the shower. Since M.H. will accept assistance from her husband, the therapist suggested an adaptive routine for bathing: M.H. now showers with her husband; she is able to stand in the shower while he bathes her. This arrangement not only also alleviates her husband's fears but also addresses M.H.'s lack of initiation for hygiene. M.H. also agreed to dressing adaptations suggested by the therapist, including wearing loose-fitting t-shirts, elastic-waistband pants, and hook-and-loop fastener shoes and also sitting on the bed to put her pants, shoes, and socks.

one piece of equipment or one technique or routine rather than another is based on the occupational profile of the individual (his or her history, values, and interests), the context of an activity, possibilities, and the requirements of the situation.

Living with a movement disorder involves more than learning a number of techniques in a clinical setting or choosing a particular piece of equipment. Physical and social supports and limitations, as well as individual constraints and beliefs, strongly influence behavior and adaptation (Lyons & Tickle-Degnen, 2003). An individual's choice of action or adaptive strategy will be shaped by temporal factors, personal values, and beliefs about the activity, self, and environment (Law, 2002; Lyons & Tickle-Degnen, 2003).

Meghan, a woman with cerebral palsy, has personal criteria for choosing her adaptive strategies in self-care activities. These include being viewed as mentally competent, physically able, and socially acceptable (McCuaig & Frank, 1991). To carry out her activities, she chooses from a variety and combination of strategies that include techniques and equipment, routines, and social resources. As might be expected, Meghan's choice of strategy is frequently based not on functional efficiency but on *self-presentation,* or how she wishes to appear to others. The techniques, equipment, routines, and people supporting her identity as a competent, socially and physically able individual are preferred as adaptive strategies.

Meghan's athetosis, physical deformities, and inability to speak affect her ability to function. Therefore, if she makes tea for her sister, whom she believes views her as incompetent and dependent, she completes every step herself, from boiling the water to pouring the cream in the cups and serving the food. When she is with those whom she feels acknowledge her as a competent individual, her desire to present a social self and to communicate are more important than her physical abilities. Under these circumstances, she will ask her guest to fix and serve the tea. This leaves her free to use her hands for pointing to her communication system to "chat" with her visitors. Meghan directs the activity, indicating which dishes to use, noting where the items are located and where tea will be served. Thus, she has a repertoire of strategies for "making tea" and chooses one based on the context of the event. Who is present and how she is perceived are more important than simply getting the tea from the kettle into the cups. The important larger principle is that an individual's desired identity is a key factor in the choice of adaptive strategy (Christiansen, 1999).

Adaptive Strategies Using Equipment and Techniques

Adaptive strategies to address engagement in occupations for people with movement disorders often include methods or techniques involving either specialized or commonplace equipment. See Table 11.3 for factors to consider when making recommendations.

Equipment

Highly specialized equipment used by people with movement disorders might include powered wheelchairs for those unable to walk (discussed later in the chapter) and environmental control systems. With environmental control units or electronic aids to daily living, stereo sound systems, telephones, apartment intercoms, lights, fans, and televisions can be accessed through a wide variety of switching devices. Individuals lacking the dexterity, coordination, or strength to turn knobs or push buttons directly have easy access to many functions within their living environments through the use of such controls (Cook & Polgar, 2008). Moreover, the Internet has become a means for persons with movement disorders to complete instrumental tasks of daily living such as banking, bill paying, shopping, and socialization, as well as a source of leisure (Buning, 2008; Cook & Polgar, 2008). As people without

Table 11.3. Factors to Consider When Recommending Adaptive Strategies

- What is important to the individual about the task?

- Is the strategy viewed as compatible with the particular social context?

- Does the strategy enhance the person's sense of personal control?

- Does the strategy minimize effort?

- Does the strategy interfere with social opportunities or diminish the presentation of self?

- Is the recommended strategy temporally realistic, given the context?

- Does the strategy provide for safety?

dysfunctions also use these approaches, using them provides a transparent, "equalizing" context that can reduce the stigma of disability or difference.

Other equipment may be equally transparent and not readily identifiable as an adaptive device. There are several important advantages to commercially available equipment, including cost, availability, and service and maintenance warranties. (Manufacturers should be contacted before making modifications to ensure that such adaptations will not jeopardize the item's warranty.) Examples of transparent adaptive equipment include a keyboard with widely spaced keys for someone who lacks the coordination and dexterity to type; felt-tipped pens for an individual too weak to exert pressure to write; and front-opening, lightweight clothing to make dressing easier for someone with excess movement. Wall-mounted grab bars are becoming common in many apartment dwellings and provide stability for someone transferring to the toilet. Many individuals with movement disorders use commercially available nonskid mats and adhesive strips for bathtubs and showers. Several models of pagers and cellular phones have features that meet the needs of persons with movement disorders (Barker, 2002; Nguyen, Garrett, Downing, Walker, & Hobbs, 2007).

Assessment, prescription, and adaptation of equipment are familiar activities for occupational therapists. Wielandt, McKenna, Tooth, and Strong (2006) have noted the general absence of consumer-based criteria for the evaluation of equipment. Criteria formulated by consumers could benefit designers, manufacturers, funding agencies, occupational therapists, and ultimately the consumers themselves in the process of choosing appropriate equipment. Wielandt et al. (2006) cite research showing that in addition to identifying the need for the equipment, important criteria from the consumers' perspective include effectiveness, affordability, operability, and dependability. It is also interesting to note that criteria ranking changed according to equipment function. Acceptability (the aesthetics, or psychological "fit") was a high priority for something as personal as a powered wheelchair but of little consequence in an environmental control unit to operate a stereo.

Criteria for equipment specifically to be used by people with movement disorders include an ability to withstand unusual physical force or stress, including falls and inadvertent, uncoordinated hitting. Equipment often needs to be both lightweight to compensate for weakness and durable to withstand being dropped or struck through excess movement. If an individual has involuntary movement, safety factors such as stability, absence of sharp edges, and flexibility must be considered. Equipment may need extra padding, bolts may need to be covered, and raw edges may need to be smoothed or sanded. If the individual has difficulty initiating and sustaining movement, then sensitivity to touch and the use of lightweight material are important features of equipment. If the individual's condition is deteriorating, the equipment must be flexible and easily adaptable with little expense to meet changing requirements.

Techniques

Techniques refer to the methods an individual uses to accomplish a task and often include equipment. Adults frequently use methods that have evolved over the years, often by trial and error, through family intervention, persistence, and experimentation. Often techniques that appear to be awkward, uncoordinated, and precarious are, in fact, finely honed and efficacious elements of a highly integrated system (see the example of Meghan below).

The occupational therapist's role in teaching adaptive techniques to people with movement disorders is to observe closely and assess the individuals within their normal environments and to give attention to the larger and potentially fragile system of movement. Techniques designed for individuals with movement disorders require observation of timing and an understanding of people's adaptive use of their physical abilities and limitations. Body postures that decrease excessive movements and provide trunk support and proximal stability need to be taught and developed (see, e.g., Gillen, 2002). For those with decreased movement as in Parkinson's disease, finding the body part that provides consistent, voluntarily controlled movement and does not fatigue easily is important. Auditory and visual cues may be necessary to facilitate initiation and speed of movement in individuals with movement disorders. Several studies have shown that visual (lines on the floor) and auditory (the sound of a metronome) cues increased functional ambulation speed in persons with Parkinson's disease (Thaut et al., 1996; Willem et al., 2006).

Energy Conservation Strategies

Teaching strategies that minimize fatigue, conserve energy, enhance safety, and foster adequate stability (particularly postural) are essential for managing ADLs for people with movement disorders (Baker & Tickle-Degnen, 2001; Gauthier, Dalziel, & Gauthier, 1987; Gillen, 2002; Mathiowetz, Finlayson, Matuska, Chen, & Luo, 2005; Zinzi et al., 2007). A person who fatigues easily through the course of

the day may need to have at least three strategies for getting to the toilet: one using bars on the wall, one using a sliding transfer board, and one requiring the presence of another person for physical support. The choice of strategy will depend on the individual's energy level, resources available, urgency, and timing. To save energy, persons with movement disorders pre-plan occupations, pace themselves, and prioritize their occupations. Energy conservation education courses have been shown to be beneficial for persons with multiple sclerosis (Mathiowetz et al., 2005; Vanage, Gilbertson, & Mathiowetz, 2003). Providing postural stability using lateral supports and a tilt-in-space wheelchair resulted in more upper-extremity control in a man with multiple sclerosis, which allowed him to propel his wheelchair independently using a joystick (Gillen, 2002).

Adaptations Used in Specific Performance Areas

Feeding

Occupational therapists have paid considerable attention to the development of equipment and specialized techniques for self-feeding. Very sophisticated feeding devices for adults with cerebral palsy, such as the Winsford Feeder™ and Beesons Feeder (Cook & Polgar, 2008), move food from the plate to the mouth by means of a spoon set in motion with an electronic switch (see Figure 11.1).

In other instances, highly individualized devices are fabricated, such as a feeding harness developed for a man with ALS, reported by Takai (1986). Stability for people with movement disorders is often enhanced by the use of nonskid mats, plate

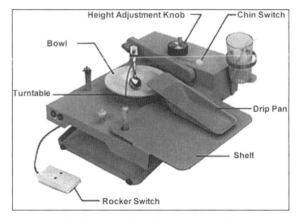

Figure 11.1. Model 5 Winsford Feeder.™ Chin or rocker switch operated. (Available from Winsford Products, Inc., 179 Pennington-Harbourton Road, Pennington, NJ 08534; 609-737-3311).

guards, weighted utensils, and utensil holders, such as the universal cuff (Foti & Kanazawa, 2006). People with poor coordination may use commonplace equipment, such as straws and heavy mugs. However, while weights have been shown to reduce the amplitude of tremors in persons with cerebellar tremors (McGruder, Cors, Tiernan, & Tomlin, 2003), one study reported that using weighted utensils or weight cuffs did not reduce tremors in persons with Parkinson's disease (Meshack & Norman, 2002). Cold temperature also has been shown to decrease essential tremor (Feys et al., 2005) but not tremors from Parkinson's disease (Cooper et al., 2000).

Dysphagia, or difficulty swallowing, frequently occurs in individuals with movement disorders, particularly those with ALS, cerebral palsy, Huntington's disease, multiple sclerosis, or Parkinson's disease. This condition is potentially life-threatening because of the possibility of aspiration and inadequate nutrition. Weakness of the tongue and palate leads to food retention in the mouth and throat and difficulty maneuvering food in the mouth, such that food may slip into the airway. Poor lip closure may result in drooling. Often, correct evaluation and diagnosis, coupled with simple intervention, help normalize oral food intake. Occupational therapy intervention for individuals with dysphagia has been described elsewhere and is well documented (Avery, 2008; Jenks & Smith, 2006).

Returning to the example of Meghan, a woman with athetoid cerebral palsy, provides examples of how techniques and equipment can be part of an adaptive strategy for meal management. Meghan, who has deformities in her trunk and limbs and an inability to communicate verbally, uses her body as a tool to compensate for the changes in muscle tone that make her movements difficult to predict and control (McCuaig & Frank, 1991; see Figure 11.2).

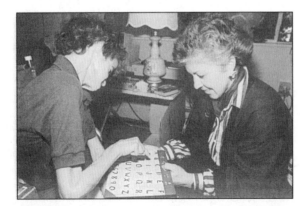

Figure 11.2. Meghan communicating through her letter board.

She holds a fork woven unconventionally in and out of the fingers of her right hand. She spears the food with her fork, and, balancing on her forearm and elbow, brings the food to her mouth. Her chin rests on her chest with her neck rotated so that her left ear is almost touching her shoulder. This seemingly contorted body position provides the balance she lacks when sitting erect and decreases the effects of the excess movements in her arms when her elbow is not stabilized. A colorful, plastic-coated mat stabilizes her dishes, countering the excess movement in her hands. Meghan is not set apart as different from her mealtime partners by her use of "adapted" equipment—she uses ordinary utensils in extraordinary ways.

Equipment and techniques address only the functional aspect of moving food from the plate to the mouth. Of equal or greater importance for Meghan was the social context of meal management and eating. Although Meghan often invited people for tea or lunch, she rarely ate at these functions. The physical stress of eating, the ensuing fatigue, and the fact that when she was eating she could not use her hands to access her communication systems, had led to her decision not to eat with others. She explained her decision in the following comment: "The reason I very often don't eat with people is I feel I can eat after they go, but I won't be able to talk [after they are gone]." Like most of us, Meghan used the occasion of tea or a meal for social purposes. Occupational therapists who emphasize the functional and nutritional aspects of mealtime management have sometimes overlooked this important social aspect of these moments. It might be argued that, for many, meals are as important for social interaction as they are for sustenance.

Thus, important considerations for therapists in recommending equipment and techniques may be the extent to which they permit social interaction and whether independence in meal management is important to the individual. Is eating viewed as a social occasion? Is eating "independently" with equipment more important than the length of time or the physical effort it takes to finish a meal? Is appearance important, and, if so, are the utensils attractive and pleasant to hold to the tongue and lips? Does the plate guard blend with the plate? Does the color of the nonskid mat clash with that of the table? Do the techniques, such as sliding rather than lifting, minimize effort? Does the independent use of the equipment detract from the potential social opportunities available when a person is fed by another (Einset, Deitz, Billingsley,

& Harris, 1989)? What are the time considerations and the fatigue factors? Would several smaller meals a day be more manageable than the traditional three main meals? These are some of the questions that may be important to determine appropriate adaptive strategies for mealtimes. Further suggestions for adaptive strategies for feeding are described in the section "Adaptive Strategies Using Routines and Social Supports."

Mobility

Another factor identified as central for adults with movement disorders is independent mobility, both within and outside the individual's dwelling (Reid, Laliberte-Rudman, & Hebert, 2002). The physical control a person has over the environment and the ease and freedom with which he or she can move within it influence feelings of independence, dignity, and competence. Physical control also helps to conserve energy. Equipment recommended for mobility must be considered from perspectives other than function (Reid et al., 2002). Stronger than the desire to be mobile may be the need to maintain a view of an able self, which may not include using a wheelchair.

Individuals with movement disorders may have substantial changes in ability and endurance over time, even during the course of a day. Accordingly, they may require highly flexible mobility systems. For example, a person with multiple sclerosis may wish to use a manual wheelchair for exercise in the morning, and a powered chair for transportation as the day and ensuing fatigue progress. A person with ALS may need to plan for two chairs over the course of the disease: a lightweight manual chair to give more independence and accessibility in the early stages and a power wheelchair with supports for the neck, arms, trunk, and legs in the later stages (Trail, Nelson, Van, Appel, & Lai, 2001).

Particular concerns for occupational therapists in addressing powered mobility for people with movement disorders are physical and cognitive control, flexibility, and safety. Positioning for maximum stability is critical and may require special seating, with trunk and head supports. Proximal joints and limbs must be stabilized and extraneous movements controlled to enhance distal control. In general, individuals with severe movement disorders involving abnormal or fluctuating muscle tone require customized seating systems. Typically, these include carefully fabricated seating surfaces. Cook and Polgar (2008) provide a useful overview of the issues of seating and positioning for clients with varying levels of need.

Once the most reliable, consistent, voluntarily controlled body movement and location have been determined, the powered wheelchair's control mechanism (usually a joystick) can be adapted to compensate for almost any degree of excess or lack of movement. Wheelchair control mechanisms can be mounted easily in various places on the chair—on the right, the left, centrally, under the chin, or at the back or side of the head. *Latching*, or "cruise control," is an option for individuals who fatigue easily. Tremor dampening is a mechanical means of adjusting the sensitivity of switches so unintentional movement does not activate them. With this feature, switches can be adjusted to work appropriately with almost any degree of excess movement. The speed at which the braking system engages can also be adjusted for someone with a startle reflex. Particular safety points for powered mobility systems include replacing square-headed bolts with round ones, padding sharp edges, removing heel loops if necessary, and using safety belts and anti-tipping devices.

Meghan used a conventional powered wheelchair with a joystick and with the footrests removed. This chair, along with ramped sidewalks, paved roads, and an accessible apartment gave her the independence she required to get about in her home environment, go to her appointments, do her shopping, and visit friends who were within commuting distance. She could approach and leave clerks, friends, store displays, and buildings with the same timing, speed, and grace as the general public. She moved across busy streets during the prescribed "walk" interval.

Meghan's ability to extend her body image to include the wheelchair appeared to be an important adaptation in her mastery of techniques and the use of equipment. A straight cloth sack made by a friend hung over her wheelchair handles, allowing Meghan to carry items in the same manner in which a person might use a backpack or a tote bag over a shoulder. She hung her purse on the right side of the chair, which she had personalized with a sticker saying "Writers have the last word." When looking at Meghan, one had the sense not of a person confined in a wheelchair, but of an individual unit, a "goodness of fit."

Community Mobility

Careful assessment of driving potential is needed for persons with movement disorders because possible perceptual and cognitive involvement may make it difficult to compensate for changes in speed and direction needed for safe motor vehicle operation. Decisions must be made regarding vehicle selection and access. In addition, seating and positioning must be considered if the person is going to use the wheelchair to sit in when driving.

There are numerous options for hand controls for braking, accelerating, steering, and gripping. If an evaluation determines that driving is not an option, transportation via personal and public means is becoming more accessible to persons with movement disorders. Cook and Polgar (2008) state that users of personal and public transportation need to be concerned with wheelchair tie-downs, occupant restraint systems, and the seating system of the wheelchair. They and Babirad (2002) provide criteria for decision making in regard to driving assessment and technology for driving and transportation

Communication

Individuals engage in different modes of communication. Conversation, commonly a brief, temporal, and often spontaneous verbal exchange, is usually thought of as the most common. These verbal exchanges include changes in intonation and timing and are accompanied by facial expressions, gestures, and body language. Conversation takes place in face-to-face situations, over the telephone, or simultaneously with an activity. Messaging, another mode of communication, is the delayed presentation of previously prepared information. Common tools for messaging include pens or pencils, typewriters, fax machines, telephone answering devices, computers, and smart phones.

When an individual is unable to use the conventional modes and tools of communication for conversation or sending messages, the dynamics and quality of the interaction are affected. *Augmentative and alternative communication (ACC)* includes any personal or technical system that enhances a person's present communication abilities. These devices may produce speech, a visual display, or a written message. Body parts, such as a hand, the head, or eyes are used to access them directly or indirectly (Cook & Polgar, 2008). Mobile telecommunication devices now provide many features and options for persons with movement disorders. However, as Nguyen et al. (2007) noted, many people are not aware of all the options. Assessment and training in all the features contribute to successful use of these devices.

Meghan had a wide variety of universal or commonplace communication devices, including felt-tipped pens, an electric typewriter with widely spaced keys, a computer, and a telephone. She also used specialized equipment: an 8" x 11" letter board indicating the letters of the alphabet, to which she pointed to spell her message; a small, portable, battery-operated communication device with keys that she presses to produce a ticker-tape-printed message; and a device attached to her telephone producing synthesized sounds in the form of letters that enabled her to spell messages to her caller. Meghan also used her voice, facial expressions, and gestures to convey a message. She had a repertoire of equipment and techniques from which to choose, based on the context of the communication taking place.

Meghan's decision regarding which piece of equipment to use was based not only on wanting to present an able self but on her perceptions of the demands of the situation and on her expectations of the exchange. If Meghan was having a conversation with a friend, she liked to sit close to that person with the letter board on her lap, point to the letters to spell out her message, and have her friend repeat the letters and say the resulting words. Although this method is slow (approximately 12 words per minute) it allows Meghan to make frequent eye contact and to stay engaged with her partner. She can use her other hand to gesture, and she can use her face and body to express feelings. The "voice" is personal and not synthesized.

When Meghan was in a place like the drug store, a situation that has fewer personal communication expectations, she used her electronic communicator, a device resembling a small pocket calculator, that looked attractive, produced a written message that was easy to see, and was understood by all who could read. Previously, she had attempted to use her letter board in public but found that people reacted as though she were mentally inferior. She found that people are interested in her communication device and that it serves as a conversational icebreaker for people who were not familiar with her methods. When interacting with a store clerk, Meghan needed only to deliver a message to get the items she required. Her desire to present a sophisticated and capable image was supported by her use of her communication device in public. Although technology has become more sophisticated, Meghan still prefers her electronic communicator, which she considers "more dependable."

In evaluation and intervention for communication needs, occupational therapists work closely with speech and language pathologists to identify and prescribe appropriate equipment s suitable to the requirements of the social and physical environment. For people with movement disorders, specific recommendations for communication needs include enlarged pencils, writing aids that hold a pen or pencil, and felt-tipped pens. For people who can use typewriters, computers, or electronic communicators, key guards that prevent more than one key from being pressed at the same time can help those with poor coordination. Enlarged keyboards for computers are useful for people who lack the fine motor skills to access a standard-size keyboard. Mini-keyboards are available for people who lack range and muscle strength in their upper extremities (Cook & Polgar, 2008).

Often a person has sufficient control of the head and neck to permit the use of mouthsticks or head wands for operating ACC devices (see Jasch, 2002, for a review of mouthstick types and uses). Mouthsticks made of lightweight doweling or arrow shafts with rubber tubing on the end may be useful for people with adequate neck and jaw control and movement. Adequate attention must be given to the potential problems of improperly fitted mouthsticks (Smith, 1989). In addition to oral problems, fatigue, gagging, and temporal mandibular joint dysfunction are known consequences of improperly fitting mouthpiece components. Therapists are urged to consider the techniques described by Duncan and Puckett (1993) when prescribing or fabricating mouthsticks. Head pointers and eye gaze systems offer another option for using ACC devices, and these can be custom-made or obtained commercially.

Other important considerations when determining appropriate equipment and techniques for communication are the speed of message transmission, the portability of the system, the device's reliability and flexibility, whether it can be used spontaneously, and the system's potential for communicating the message completely (i.e., not just the words, but the intended meaning and tone). An augmentative system should require as little expenditure of energy as possible, for both the sender and receiver of the message. It must enhance an individual's personal abilities and, wherever possible, encourage physical gestures and expressions of sound. The equipment must also meet the requirements of the physical and social environment.

Adaptive Strategies Using Routines and Social Supports

Behaviors, repeated over time and organized into patterns and habits, form *routines*. Routines and the use of social supports can be considered adaptive strategies for people with movement disorders because they compensate for the inability to perform certain activities, the extended length of time and energy required to accomplish them, and limited co-

ordination and strength. Frequently, an individual's strategy for accomplishing a task employs a unique combination of equipment, techniques, routines, and social supports. These social supports may take the form of family and friends, casual acquaintances, formal and informal organizations, or health care workers within and without institutions.

The use of adaptive strategies employing routines and social supports is often dependent on specific factors. The individual needs to know that a certain activity or interaction is going to take place and what the requirements of the situation will be. He or she must also have time to plan, have a well-developed ability to organize personal and environmental resources, have the perception of how long an activity will take, understand what the specific steps will involve, and know how much energy will be needed. Routines generally have a sense of predictability and familiarity, in that they have usually been used successfully in the past under similar, if not exact, conditions. Social supports need to be initiated, nurtured, and developed.

Communication

Emma, a woman who has ALS and lives in a long-term-care unit, uses a variety of techniques and pieces of equipment for communication to adapt to her inability to speak and her lack of movement in her limbs. She has a letter and word board to which she can point with hand movements that are slow and difficult. She also has a computerized message system, which she operates with a microswitch in her palm, and a system of eye-blinking, which she uses in conjunction with the communication partner's verbal spelling. In addition, Emma has established routines for communication that are considered adaptive because of their premeditated, compensatory nature.

Emma, like Meghan, determines which strategy to use after considering outcome, context, and values. She decides in advance the purpose of the communication, the intended recipient of the message, what she expects from the exchange, and what is important for her to achieve. Emma decides, ahead of time, whether it is more important to save the other person time by having information ready, or whether the conversation process and the elements of the interaction are of greater significance than the message itself. One of her routines for communicating is to provide her communication partner with information in the form of a printout from her computer. This routine requires Emma's knowledge of the visit before it occurs, adequate time to compose her thoughts and messages at the computer, and the ability of her communication partner to read. She is very aware of the importance of her social support system and consciously works at sustaining these networks. It requires much more of Emma's time, but significantly less of her partner's, if she puts her thoughts on paper before the interaction. It also provides the partner with something to read, and on which to focus. Emma can work at her own pace at her computer when she has the energy, and can take rest periods, which in conversation would be awkward and possibly stressful for the partner.

Many people with movement disorders that include loss of speech struggle with the assumption that one disability signals the presence of another (Pentland, Gray, Riddle, & Pitcairn, 1988). An inability to speak is frequently equated with an inability to think. The strategy Emma has developed for communicating with people through a prepared note helps to dispel any misconceptions the partner might have of her cognitive abilities. The notes contain witticisms, inquiries about the partner's well-being, social comments about the news or weather, descriptions of her sons' activities, and her feelings about events on the ward. Emma presents herself as a socially competent woman, full of ideas and feelings, and actively engaged in life.

Meal Preparation and Shopping

The following incident demonstrates the use of routines and social supports as an adaptive strategy for meal preparation and shopping. Lee has Parkinson's disease, with resulting intention tremor in her upper extremities, head, and neck; a slow and shuffling gait; rigidity in her trunk; and slurred speech. She shares a home with her elderly husband. Having friends in for tea once a week is an important social event for her. When her guests arrive, the cups and saucers are out on a cart, along with the cream, sugar, napkins, and a cake. During the tea, Lee plays the host, directing the event. She manages everything, deciding when to hold the tea, what to serve, and who will pour. She has a keen sense of timing, is extremely gracious and social in her requests, is well organized, and gives clear directions.

In order for Lee to execute this very ordinary but important occasion she must invest considerable planning time and effort. She needs to travel in her scooter to the local mall to buy the cake and other grocery items, and transport them safely home. She has to have her cups clean and arranged on the tray ahead of time. Her problems with strength, balance, manipulation, and coordination make an apparently easy task one that requires considerable orchestration.

Eating

For many individuals with movement disorders, eating can be an exhausting and undignified experience, whether managing food independently or being fed. The physical and emotional strain of getting the food on the utensil, bringing it safely to the lips, keeping it in the mouth, chewing adequately, swallowing smoothly, and maintaining a comfortable posture can be great. Weighted handles, nonskid mats, plate guards, and even automatic feeding devices are often not adequate to support a person's nutritional, social, and personal needs related to eating. As with other ADLs, function alone is not sufficient for a satisfying experience at mealtime. While being fed brings its own set of problems, it is often the strategy of choice for people unable to manage a meal in a reasonable amount of time and with a minimum of effort.

Catherine, a young woman with cerebral palsy living in an extended-care facility, prefers to be fed rather than feed herself. She has spent countless hours practicing, trying different pieces of equipment and physical positions. The combination of her severe athetoid movements, poor head control, and general weakness makes eating independently an unpleasant chore. She now prefers to spend her energy writing at her computer, visiting with friends, and going to school.

To make her mealtime pleasant, she has asked to be fed in her room and to invite one other person who also needs to be fed to join her and the aide who is feeding her. When she orders her meal she includes an extra tea and biscuit for the aide. This is a treat for the aide, and adds to the feeling of the meal being more of a shared and social experience. Catherine also has the television turned on to her favorite soap opera at noon and to the news in the evening. This, too, is a treat for the aide, and gives them something on which to focus and to discuss. The conversation, the tea, and the company promote a relaxed atmosphere and reduce the possibility that the aide will be bored and, therefore, stressed.

When occupational therapists plan mealtime interventions, they should always consider how to create an environment that promotes eating as an enjoyable social event rather than simply a nutritional exercise. At its best, eating is an intimate affair; at its worst, it is traumatic. Wherever possible, the physical environment should promote relaxation and comfort. Attention should be given to room temperature, noise level, and visual stimulation, particularly if the individual has a sensitive startle reaction. A quiet room may suit one person, whereas another person might prefer company. Individuals who need to be fed can be taught how to engage the interest and attention of the person feeding them. They can be encouraged to take control of choices, determining what food to eat and when, how quickly items are presented, and in what order. They can also help identify any elements of the mealtime event that are stressful and collaborate with practitioners in addressing them.

Sexuality

Sexuality is another important concern of persons with movement disorders. With some of the movement disorders, physical impairments such as tone, contractures, and loss of mobility; fatigue; medications; and in some cases, actual sexual dysfunction, may affect sexuality (Burton, 2006). Primary dysfunction, such as erectile dysfunction and decreased vaginal lubrication, can be managed with medications. Tone, contractures, and loss of mobility can be managed by using pillows to support body parts, experimenting with different positions, and promoting problem solving by the person and the partner. Energy conservation techniques, such as engaging in sexual relations when the person with the movement disorder has the most energy and assuming positions that use less energy, are helpful in managing fatigue (Burton, 2006; Sipski & Alexander, 1997).

Facilitating the Development of Routines and Social Supports

Research on several movement disorders, including multiple sclerosis (Somerset, Peters, Sharp, & Campbell, 2003), Parkinson's disease (Karlsen, Tandberg, Arsland, & Larsen, 2000), and ALS (Young & McNicoll, 1998), has suggested that social psychological variables are the most important explanatory models of adjustment to the diseases. In particular, integrating the realities of the diseases into the lifestyle, and depending on strong social support networks, have each been identified as important variables for people with these progressive, episodic, and debilitating neuromotor conditions. Development of adaptive routines and social supports is thus an effective therapeutic strategy.

Therapists can help individuals with all types of movement disorders develop strategies that use routines and social supports. Assistance takes the form of facilitating a person's repeated action beyond basic problem solving until a routine is established and acceptable to the individual and those in his or her environment. The routines developed should minimize stress and conserve energy—they require planning and organization to allow people to do the most important activities when they have the most energy, maximizing both safety and enjoyment.

Therapy sessions can be planned to support a person's shift from focusing on the physical to the cognitive domain. A person who is no longer able to execute an activity physically may need to learn to organize and plan in order to direct care. Overvaluing the concept of independence may lead to goals that require too much energy. Assistance with personal care may be preferable to independence in ADLs if the physical and mental costs of attaining independence interfere with social interaction or life satisfaction (Gillette, 1991). Social supports must be sought out, developed, nurtured, and maintained. Attention must be given to ways in which the distress, enormous effort, and tedium of living with and of supporting someone with a physical disability can be managed so that important social supports can be maintained as integral components of a person's adaptive strategies. Addressing the needs and occupational performance issues of caregivers is included in the scope of occupational therapy practice (AOTA, 2008). Several intervention programs for caregivers have been developed by occupational therapists (Bradford et al., 2001; Finlayson, Garcia, & Preissner, 2008).

Summary

Strategies that minimize fatigue, enhance safety, and reduce stress are important. Attention to organization, pacing, timing, and energy conservation are also important in managing self-care by people with movement disorders (Mathiowetz et al., 2005; Zinzi et al., 2007). A philosophy of independent living that emphasizes the importance of an individual's acquisition of skills and capabilities for self-direction in managing physical and social resources has been embraced. However, this philosophy also acknowledges that a person can exhibit an independent spirit while accepting assistance from others and that all adaptive strategies must be considered in terms of their contribution to overall well-being and life satisfaction. In working with individuals with movement disorders, the role of the therapist is to identify, in conjunction with clients, an array of adaptive strategies that can be used comfortably within the context of the client's daily life.

Acknowledgment

Margaret McCuaig made important contributions to earlier versions of this chapter, especially the case study of Meghan. The author is indebted to her for her support.

Study Questions

1. What is energy conservation, and how is it used for individuals with movement disorders?

2. What types of adaptive strategies or equipment are useful for communication, mobility, meal preparation, and feeding?

3. What are two examples of adaptive strategies for communication, mobility, meal preparation, and feeding?

4. What are important factors to consider when recommending equipment for individuals with movement disorders?

5. How can routines and social supports be facilitated?

References

American Occupational Therapy Association. (2008). Occupational therapy practice framework: Domain and process (2nd ed.). *American Journal of Occupational Therapy, 62*(6), 625–683.

Avery, W. (2008). Dysphagia. In M. V. Radomski & & C. A. Trombly Latham (Eds.), *Occupational therapy for physical dysfunction* (6th ed., pp. 1321–1344). Baltimore: Lippincott Williams & Wilkins.

Babirad, J. (2002). Driver evaluation and vehicle modification. In D. A. Olson & F. DeRuyter (Eds.), *Clinician's guide to assistive technology* (pp. 351–386). St. Louis, MO: Mosby.

Baker, N. A., & Tickle-Degnen, L. (2001). The effectiveness of physical, psychological, and functional interventions in treating clients with multiple sclerosis: A meta-analysis. *American Journal of Occupational Therapy, 55,* 324–331.

Barker, P. (2002). Information technology. In D. A. Olson & F. DeRuyter (Eds.), *Clinician's guide to assistive technology* (pp. 115–164). St. Louis, MO: Mosby.

Bradford, M., Kratz, M., Brown, R., Emick, K., Rnack, J., Wilkins, R., et al. (2001). Stroke survivor caregiver education: Methods and effectiveness. *Physical and Occupational Therapy in Geriatrics, 19,* 37–51.

Buning, M. E. (2008). High-technology adaptations to compensate for disability. In M. V. Radomski & C. A. Trombly Latham (Eds.), *Occupational therapy for physical dysfunction* (6th ed., pp. 510–541). Baltimore: Lippincott Williams & Wilkins.

Burton, G. U. (2006). Sexuality and physical dysfunction. In H. M. Pendleton & W. Schultz-Krohn (Eds.), *Pedretti's occupational therapy: Practice skills for physical dysfunction* (6th ed., pp. 248–263). St. Louis, MO: Mosby.

Christiansen, C. H. (1999). Defining lives: Occupation as identity: An essay on competence, coherence, and the creation of meaning. *American Journal of Occupational Therapy, 53,* 547–558.

Christiansen, C. H. (2004). Evaluation and management of basic and extended activities of daily living. In J. Delisa et al. (Eds.), *Rehabilitation medicine: Principles and practice* (4th ed., pp. 137–165). Philadelphia: Lippincott Williams & Wilkins.

Cook, A. M., & Polgar, J. M. (2008). *Cook and Hussey's assistive technologies: Principles and practice* (3rd ed.). St. Louis, MO: Mosby.

Cooper, C., Evidente, V. G. H., Hentz, J. G., Adler, C. H., Caviness, J. N., & Gwinn-Hardy, K. (2000). The effect of temperature on hand function in patients with tremor. *Journal of Hand Therapy, 13,* 276–288.

Duncan, J. D., & Puckett, A. D., Jr. (1993). A one-appointment mouthstick appliance. *Journal of Prosthodontics, 2,* 196–198.

Einset, K., Deitz, J., Billingsley, F., & Harris, S. R. (1989). The electric feeder: An efficacy study. *Occupational Therapy Journal of Research, 9,* 38–52.

Feys., P., Helsen, W., Liu, X., Morren, D., Albrecht, H., Nuttin, B., et al. (2005). Effects of peripheral cooling on intention tremor in multiple sclerosis. *Journal of Neurology, Neurosurgery, and Psychiatry, 76,* 373–379.

Finlayson, M., Garcia, J. D., & Preissner, K. (2008). Development of an educational programme for caregivers of people aging with multiple sclerosis. *Occupational Therapy International, 15,* 4–17.

Finlayson, M., Impey, M. W., Nicolle, C., & Edwards, J. (1998). Self-care, productivity and leisure limitations of people with multiple sclerosis in Manitoba. *Canadian Journal of Occupational Therapy, 65,* 299–308.

Foti, D., & Kanazawa, L. M. (2006). Activities of daily living. In H. M. Pendleton & W. Schultz-Krohn (Eds.), *Pedretti's occupational therapy: Practice skills for physical dysfunction* (6th ed., pp. 146–194). St. Louis, MO: Mosby.

Francisco, G.E., Kithari, S., Schiess, M.C., & Kaldis, T. (2005). Rehabilitation of Persons with Parkinson's disease and other movement disorders. In J. DeLisa B. Gans, N. Walsh, et al. (Eds.), *Rehabilitation medicine: Principles and practice* (4th ed., pp. 809–828) Philadelphia: Lippincott Williams & Wilkins.

Gauthier, L., Dalziel, S., & Gauthier, S. (1987). The benefits of group occupational therapy for patients with Parkinson's disease. *American Journal of Occupational Therapy, 41,* 360–365.

Gillette, N. (1991). The challenge of research in occupational therapy. *American Journal of Occupational Therapy, 45,* 660–662.

Gillen, G. (2002). Improving mobility and community access in an adult with ataxia. *American Journal of Occupational Therapy, 56,* 462–466.

Jasch, C. R. (2002). Adaptive aids for self-care and child care at home. In D. A. Olson & F. DeRuyter

(Eds.), *Clinician's guide to assistive technology* (pp. 405–423). St. Louis, MO: Mosby.

Jenks, K. N., & Smith, G. (2006). Dysphagia: Evaluation and treatment. In H. M. Pendleton & W. Schultz-Krohn (Eds.), *Pedretti's occupational therapy: Practice skills for physical dysfunction* (6th ed., pp. 610–645). St. Louis, MO: Mosby.

Karlsen, K. H., Tandberg, E., Arsland, D., & Larsen, J. P. (2000). Health-related quality of life in Parkinson's disease: A prospective longitudinal study. *Journal of Neurology, Neurosurgery, and Psychiatry, 69,* 584–589.

Law, M. (2002). Participation in the occupations of everyday life. *American Journal of Occupational Therapy, 56,* 640–649.

Lyons, K. D., & Tickle-Degnen, L. (2003). Dramaturgical challenges of Parkinson's disease. *Occupational Therapy Journal of Research, 23,* 27–34.

Mathiowetz, V., Finlayson, M. L., Matuska, K. M., Chen, H. Y., & Luo, P. (2005). Randomized controlled trial of an energy conservation course for persons with multiple sclerosis. *Multiple Sclerosis, 11,* 592–601.

McCuaig, M., & Frank, G. (1991). The able self: Adaptive patterns and choices in independent living for a person with cerebral palsy. *American Journal of Occupational Therapy, 45,* 224–243.

McGruder, J., Cors, D., Tiernan, A. M., & Tomlin, G. (2003). Weighted wrist cuffs for tremor reduction during eating in adults with static brain lesions. *American Journal of Occupational Therapy, 57,* 507–516.

Meshack, R. P., & Norman, K. E. (2002). A randomized controlled trial of the effects of weights on amplitude and frequency of postural hand tremor in people with Parkinson's disease. *Clinical Rehabilitation, 16,* 481–492.

Nguyen, T., Garrett, R., Downing, A., Walker, L., & Hobbs, D. (2007). Research into telecommunications options for people with physical disabilities. *Assistive Technology, 19,* 78–93

Pentland, B., Gray, J. M., Riddle, W. J. R., & Pitcairn, T. K. (1988). The effects of reduced non-verbal communication in Parkinson's disease. *British Journal of Disorders of Communication, 23,* 31–34.

Reid, D., Laliberte-Rudman, D., & Hebert, D. (2002). Impact of wheeled seated mobility devices on adults users' and their caregivers' occupational performance: A critical literature review. *Canadian Journal of Occupational Therapy, 69,* 261–280.

Shah, S., & Nolen, A. (2006). Movement deficits in Parkinson's disease and restorative occupational therapy. *New Zealand Journal of Occupational Therapy, 53*(2), 12–19.

Sipski, M., & Alexander, C. (1997). *Sexual function in people with disability and chronic illness.* Gaithersburg, MD: Aspen.

Smith, R. (1989). Mouthstick design for the client with spinal cord injury. *American Journal of Occupational Therapy, 43,* 251–255.

Somerset, M., Peters, T. J., Sharp, D. J., & Campbell, R. (2003). Factors that contribute to quality of life outcomes prioritized by people with multiple sclerosis. *Quality of Life Research, 12,* 21–29.

Takai, V. L. (1986). Case Report—The development of a feeding harness for an ALS patient. *American Journal of Occupational Therapy, 40,* 359–361.

Thaut, M. H., McIntosh, G. C., Rice, R. R, Miller, R. A., Rathbun, J., & Brault, J. M. (1996). Rhythmic auditory stimulation in gait training for Parkinson's disease patients. *Movement Disorders, 11*(2), 193–200.

Trail, M., Nelson, N., Van, J. N., Appel, S. H., & Lai, E. C. (2001). Wheelchair use by patients with amyotrophic lateral sclerosis: A survey of user characteristics and selection preferences. *Archives of Physical Medicine and Rehabilitation, 82,* 98–102.

Vanage, S. M., Gilbertson, K. K., & Mathiowetz, V. (2003). Effects of an energy conservation course on fatigue impact for persons with progressive multiple sclerosis. *American Journal of Occupational Therapy, 56,* 462–466.

Watts, R. L., & Koller, W. C. (2004). *Movement disorders: Neurologic principles and practice* (2nd ed.). New York: McGraw-Hill.

Wielandt, T., McKenna K., Tooth, L., & Strong, J. (2006). Factors that predict the post-discharge use of recommended assistive technology (AT). *Disability and Rehabilitation: Assistive Technology, 1,* 29–40.

Willem, A. M., Nieuwboer, A., Chavret, F., Desloovere, K., Dom, R., Rochester, L., et al. (2006). The use of rhythmic auditory cues to influence gait in patients with Parkinson's disease, the differential effect for freezers and non-freezers, an explorative study. *Disability and Rehabilitation, 28,* 721–728.

Young, J. M., & McNicoll, P. (1998). Against all odds: Positive life experiences of people with advanced amyotrophic lateral sclerosis. *Health and Social Work, 23,* 35–43.

Zinzi, P., Salmaso, D., De Grandis, R., Graziani, G., Maceroni, S., Bentivoglio, A., et al. (2007). Effects of an intensive rehabilitation programme on patients with Huntington's disease: A pilot study. *Clinical Rehabilitation, 21,* 603–613.

Chapter 12

Managing Daily Activities in Adults With Upper-Extremity Amputations

SANDRA FLETCHALL, OTR/L, CHT, MPA, FAOTA, AND

DIANE J. ATKINS, OTR, FISPO

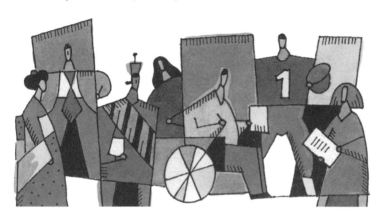

KEY WORDS

biscapular abduction

body-powered
  prosthesis

disarticulation

electronic prosthesis

greifer

humeral flexion

hybrid prosthesis

manual edema
  mobilization (MEM)

myoelectric
  prosthesis

specialized amputee
  team/clinic

targeted muscle
  reinnervation (TMR)

terminal device

transhumeral
  amputation

transradial
  amputation

HIGHLIGHTS

- The timeframe for initiation of a preprosthetic program can influence long-term functional performance.

- Minimizing or preventing problem development in the residual limb facilitates a faster progression to prosthetic training.

- A prosthetic training program should begin immediately after delivery of the prosthesis.

- A thorough assessment of the client's abilities and activities will assist in determining the type of body-powered or myoelectric terminal device used.

- The style of prosthesis used—body-powered, myoelectric, or electronic—is determined by the client's activities, physical and cognitive abilities, and funding. A specialized team, knowledgeable in upper-limb amputations, prosthesis, and components, is an important factor for successful prosthetic long-term use.

OBJECTIVES

After reading this material, readers will be able to

- Identify some assessments appropriate in determining if an individual is a candidate for a prosthesis;

- Identify when a preprosthetic program can begin;

- Describe general goals of the preprosthetic program;

- Describe the components of success that lead to incorporation of the prosthesis into daily life; and

- Describe the differences among body-powered, myoelectric, and electronic prostheses.

"We are often enriched by the personal aura and spirit of persons who manage life with disabilities, each in his individual special way." (Marquardt, 1989, p. 242)

As those who work in amputee health care agree, there is much more to rehabilitation than fitting an amputee with the appropriate device. Achieving the optimum outcome for the patient requires teamwork, commitment, and a willingness to develop solutions uniquely tailored for each individual (Fletchall, 2005, p. 28). Upper-extremity amputation presents a complex loss for the patient. The hand functions in prehensile activities as a sensory organ and as a means of communication. Any loss will interfere with the patient's productivity and feeling of completeness, as well as alter his or her interactions with his or her environment (Bennett & Alexander, 1989, p. 1).

In the nonmilitary adult population, trauma is the most frequent cause of upper-limb amputations, followed by infection, gangrene, and malignancy (National Limb Loss Information Center, 2008). Upper-limb amputations occur most frequently the working-age group aged 18–50 years, with men sustaining loss more frequently than women (Kelly et al., 2009, p. 1).

Upper-limb amputations comprise a small percentage of the total amputations performed in the United States. Their low numbers mean there are relatively few medical personnel specializing and experienced in managing, rehabilitating, and following up on individuals with this diagnosis (Lake & Dodson, 2006).

Amputations associated with chronic conditions (e.g., diabetes, peripheral vascular disease) may be anticipated or planned. Those resulting from trauma occur suddenly, producing a drastic change in function, body image, and psychological state. Loss of the hand and portion of the arm results in decreased manipulation, stabilization, and holding of objects and in reduction in sensory and visual feedback to the somatosensory cortex. Loss of hands, which are frequently used to assist in emotional expression and social interaction, can affect the patient's emotional responses and reactions.

Independence in self-care, work, and leisure activities is frequently attributed to the performance of the upper extremities. For the individual with upper-limb loss, the occupational therapist develops an intervention plan to assist in reestablishing independence in preamputation activities. Each treatment plan is unique and is based on the assessments of sensory and motor skills, process and communication skills, coping mechanisms, learning styles, and cultural and social environments and influences.

Treatment is focused on residual limb function; total body interaction; and fostering an improvement in self-care skills, body image, and self-confidence, with the goal of returning to preamputation activities. With appropriate intervention from a specialized and knowledgeable team, most individuals with upper-extremity amputation can resume independence in activities of daily living (ADLs) and instrumental activities of daily living (IADLs) and return to work or education environments. Individuals with amputations of bilateral short transhumeral or bilateral shoulder disarticulations may have difficulty achieving independence in all areas of daily living; however, performance in selected ADLs and IADLs and return to work or school environments are feasible.

Through the program developed by the occupational therapist, the prosthesis becomes incorporated into the body image and scheme and integrated into the individual's activities and daily occupations. Therapy gives the individual the opportunity to use the prosthesis in everyday life, but the final decision to wear and use the device is made by the individual.

This chapter will focus on the process of preprosthetic and prosthetic training. Case studies will illustrate the concepts and demonstrate the outcomes that can be achieved in programs the occupational therapist develops.

Preprosthetic Therapy Program

In some instances, if the experienced occupational therapist is closely associated with surgeons who perform upper-extremity amputations, the preprosthetic program can begin from within a few hours of the surgery to within 2 to 3 weeks after surgery. Early intervention can involve wound care (see Figure 12.1), edema control, residual limb shaping, and assessment of the client's desired areas of future performance in ADLs, IADLs, leisure, work, or school.

Educating nursing staff regarding potential accomplishments of individuals with amputations can create an environment of hope and opportunity. Currently, an inpatient stay following an uncomplicated upper-extremity amputation can range from 1 to 5 days. Therefore, many individuals may receive occupational therapy intervention on an outpatient basis. For those with bilateral upper-extremity amputations, the stay for inpatient rehabilitation may be brief; the majority of treatment will occur in an outpatient setting.

Regardless of the client's unique social, cultural, or physical contexts, the preprosthetic therapy program's general goals are to

- Provide residual limb edema control and shaping;
- Maintain or acquire normal joint range of motion;
- Increase muscle strength and endurance of the total body and residual limb;
- Minimize or prevent development of potential problems (e.g., pain, contractures, excessive scarring);
- Promote residual limb tolerance to sensory stimuli;
- Initiate an assessment of client's voluntary motor control of the residual limb(s), as voluntary motor responses are needed if myoelectric prosthetic components are prescribed (Atkins, 1989c, p. 12; Fletchall, 1998, p. 6);
- Provide an assessment of learning style and visual motor skills;
- Provide education regarding residual limb hygiene;
- Initiate an assessment of client's pre-injury and postinjury performance roles;
- Initiate training to acquire independence in selected basic ADLs; and
- Initiate education regarding prosthetic options appropriate for client.

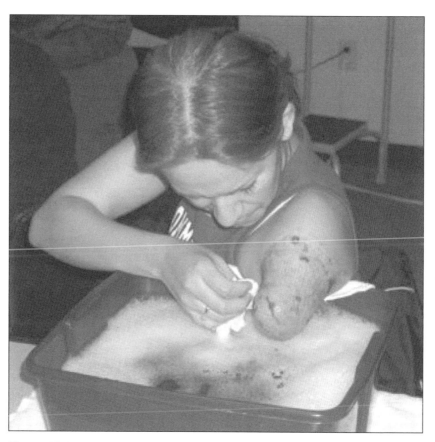

Figure 12.1. Learning to clean the wounds on the residual limb.

The preprosthetic program can begin immediately following surgery, with portions continuing after the prosthesis is received. The length of the preprosthetic program prior to receiving a prosthesis depends on the medical condition of the residual limbs (e.g., type and number of wounds present, fractures, need to return to surgery). The overall medical and physical condition of the individual will also influence the length of the program. For individuals with uncomplicated unilateral upper-limb amputations, the preprosthetic program length may average 4–8 weeks.

Assessments of muscle, skin condition, nerve function, motion, and motor movement should include the residual limb and total body. Assessments of cognitive skills and visual–motor function and of the individual's roles, responsibilities, and funding sources also contribute to the development of a treatment program. Establishment of the occupational therapy program should be based upon the client's goals or desired outcome in activity performance.

Visual inspection of the residual limb provides information related to edema, wounds, scars, adhesions, and muscle tone. For many individuals, removal of wraps or bandages provides the first opportunity to view and touch the residual limb. Education and support must be provided to help the individual acknowledge and begin to integrate the limb into their body image. Visual inspection of the residual limb is an ongoing process, with instruction and education provided to the individual to develop this into a lifelong routine

Once staples/stitches are removed and wounds are healed, education and instruction are provided relating to general skin care of the residual limb, which frequently includes use of mild soap and water with thorough drying. For individuals with several skin creases and folds, extra attention to good hygiene is important to maintain good skin condition. Residual limbs with loss of muscle or fascia or both, or with skin grafts or flaps, frequently have impaired or absent sensation, requiring the individual to obtain instruction in the development of an ongoing program of skin inspection and hygiene care. For use of the prosthesis, residual limb skin must be free of wounds and excess moisture.

Reduction of residual limb edema can also assist with pain reduction. Following a medical history assessment, it may be determined that the person is a candidate for manual edema mobilization techniques (MEM). When MEM is incorporated into the occupational therapy program, a reduction in muscle tone in the upper quadrant is noted and a reduction in anxiety may occur. Initially, the occupational therapy practitioner will perform MEM techniques

on the individual. If positive effects of MEM are obtained, many individuals can be instructed in a modified home program of MEM. Individuals with unilateral upper-limb loss may be instructed in MEM techniques, while the support persons for the individual with bilateral upper-limb loss may be taught techniques appropriate for their home program.

To assist with residual limb edema reduction, application of pressure is frequently used and elastic compression wrap can be implemented. Elastic compression wraps are recommended while the grafts, flaps, or surgical closure cannot tolerate the shear force produced from a compression sleeve known as a residual limb shrinker. Application of the wrap must be done from distal to proximal of the limb and may be done in either a figure eight or a spiral wrap. Many individuals can be taught appropriate wrapping, with success dependent on visual–motor skills and the function of the intact upper limb.

The shape of the residual limb can enhance comfort by proper fit in the prosthetic socket, which will also minimize skin problems. For transradial and transhumeral amputations, a conical shape is the goal, without creating distal bone irritation of the residual limb. The shape is influenced by using ace wraps, and later, a residual limb shrinker a compression arm stocking that applies gradient pressure from distal to proximal to the soft tissue structures (Figure 12.2).

Most individuals with unilateral limb loss can learn to become independent in application of the ace wrap or shrinker. Those with bilateral upper-limb loss can be taught to provide instruction to others for the donning and doffing of the ace wraps or shrinkers. Pressure facilitates scar tissue pliability, reduces internal residual limb edema, and can minimize light tactile stimuli to neuromas. Scar tissue maturity is frequently obtained 12–18 months following wound closure; therefore, it is recommended to maintain application of pressure until scar maturity is obtained. (Staley & Richard, 1994, Chapter 14). Therefore, the residual limb shrinker should be used, whenever the individual is not wearing the prosthesis, for several months.

The experienced occupational therapist will initiate techniques to minimize scar adhesions and improve scar pliability. Scar tissue, if not mobilized, will develop firmness with the potential to adhere to underlying structures. Firm, nonpliable scar tissue can create skin breakdowns and wounds due to the decreased ability to tolerate shear force (Figure 12.3). It can also result in abnormal sensory responses that can result in the withdrawal of the residual limb(s) when attempting to participate in activities. Scar tissue pliability can be improved

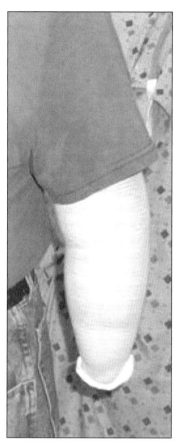

Figure 12.2. Residual limb shrinker used to assist with edema control and shaping.

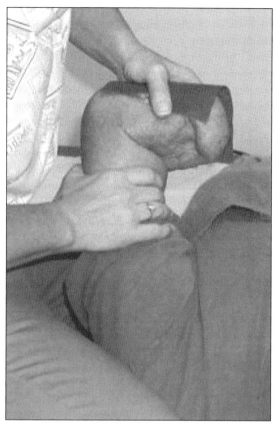

Figure 12.3. Therapist uses dycem on the residual limb to minimize skin shearing during range of motion.

through scar massage, application of pressure, and active movement of the residual limb in all planes.

Immediately following the trauma-related amputation, the individual will experience a significant decrease in activity level and spontaneous active movement of the residual limb(s). Decreased body movement can lead to potential shortening of muscle/tendon units, joint stiffness or both. Decreased activity levels can also result in increased body weight, decreased muscle endurance, poor posture, and a sense of helplessness. Decreased range of motion and poor posture require greater physical efforts by the individual to participate in ADLs. Successful use of an upper-limb prosthesis is dependent upon individuals obtaining maximal motion of the residual limb(s) and body. The occupational therapist will initiate activities to increase these motions, and establish an appropriate cardiovascular program. Initially, an individual's program may focus on residual limb movement, then progress to scapula and trunk motions. If possible, progression to either a stationary bike, walking, or a water program will assist with cardiovascular performance and provide for increased active motion.

Individuals who have sustained bilateral upper-limb loss may benefit from a total body motion program to enhance flexibility of the trunk, hips, knees, neck, and shoulders. The occupational therapist must respect physiological aging changes to eliminate joint stresses or pain in the development of such a program, as well as the individual's lifestyle and interests. Some individuals will respond positively to an elongation and flexibility program with the use of their body or Theraband® or both; others may respond to group programs such as yoga, tai chi, or pilates (Figure 12.4).

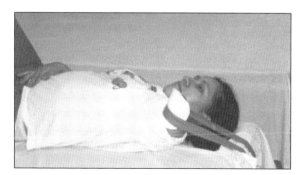

Figure 12.4. Theraband used to assist patient with short transhumeral amputation in gaining motion.

319

A thorough assessment of motor and sensory function can determine if an injury was sustained to a nerve or a joint, and if a muscle, if it has abnormal tone. If any of these problems are present, the specialist team must determine if the individual is a prosthetic candidate and determine the most appropriate prosthetic components to maximize performance of the prosthesis. The occupational therapist must develop a program to eliminate or minimize joint or soft-tissue motion limitations that may occur when active muscle control is lost. Once the limitations of motion are identified, such as soft-tissue tightness, scar adhesions, or ligament tightness, the therapist establishes the technique to enhance passive and active motion. Methods to increase motion may include elongation of soft tissue, joint mobilization, specific massage techniques, or all three (Figure 12.5).

Identification of voluntary muscle function during the preprosthetic phase will foster active muscle contraction and performance for potential myoelectric prosthesis. Additionally, active use of the muscles of the residual limb may be a method to assist with reduction of edema and/or residual limb pain. A home program focused on residual limb isolated muscle contractions must be graded to respect the deconditioning of the body and residual limb. Through observation and assessment, the occupational therapist can identify the individual's motor planning skills. If the individual has apraxia, the therapist needs to modify the program to ensure successful outcomes in self-care and then prosthetic use. Ataxic movements will also require program modifications to ensure the individual returns to pre-amputation independence levels. Kline's studies identified difficulties with motor planning when the dominant right upper limb, versus the nondominant left limb, is amputated (Kline et al., 2009). The occupational therapy program must account for increased treatment time for training in both the preprosthetic and the prosthetic program when the dominant upper limb is involved or motor-planning difficulties are noted.

During the preprosthetic phase, information is obtained related to the individual's phantom limb sensation, phantom limb pain, and residual limb sensation and pain. Client education can begin immediately to reduce pain. Residual limb pain as the result of wounds may be minimized with the use of silver impregnated dressings. These reduce the frequency of wound dressing changes. If residual limb pain is the result of muscle irritation, sprain, or spasm, these problems may be minimized by traditional therapy techniques.

Phantom limb awareness is a nonpainful sensation that the amputated portion of the residual limb is "still there." The sensation is described as tingling, itching, pressure, movement, warmth, or cold in the amputated portion of the limb (Woodhouse, 2005). The sensation does not often interfere with future prosthetic use. Education can ease the anxiety of individuals who experience this sensation such that they will incorporate phantom limb awareness into the prosthetic device (Hunter, Katz, & Davis, 2008; Mayer, Kudar, Bretz, & Tihanyi, 2008).

Phantom limb pain, on the other hand, is a neuropathic pain that can be persistent or episodic. It is present in the postamputation phase and in some cases, throughout life. Phantom limb pain can interfere with purposeful use of the residual limb, including the application or use of a prosthesis. This chronic type of pain can result in decreased attention span and concentration and interfere with particiciaption in IADLs and other important or meaningful occupations.

The amputee team may implement medications, but use of narcotics alone does not resolve phantom limb pain. The occupational therapist may choose use of pressure points or other traditional pain management techniques to minimize the response; use of

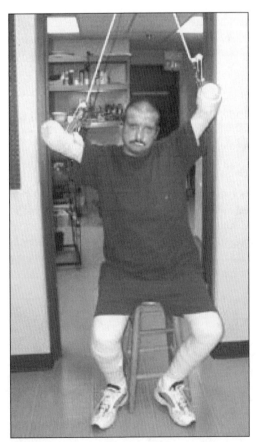

Figure 12.5. Using overhead pulley to assist with shoulder, scapula motion.

mirror visual feedback (MVF) also has been helpful for some individuals (Ramachandran & Alschuler, 2009; Ramachandran & Roger-Ramachandran, 1996). This technique utilizes a box with the top and the side closest to the patient removed. In the center of the box, a mirror is placed vertically. The box has two holes for insertion, one for the amputated upper limb, the other for the noninvolved hand and upper limb. The noninvolved hand and upper limb are viewed in the mirror, creating an image of an intact amputated upper limb. As motor movements are made by the noninvolved hand/upper limb, the patient "sees" movement of the phantom limb. Phantom pain, such as experiencing clenched fists or painful positioning of the phantom limb, can be reduced by this technique, as the noninvolved upper extremity provides the sensation of phantom limb movement. Some patients report less pain and a sensation of freedom of movement in the phantom limb replacing a sensation of fixed position (Ramachandran & Alschuler, 2009; Ramachandran & Roger-Ramachandran, 1996). Phantom limb pain has been seen to occur more frequently when the individual had uncontrolled pain in the limb prior to the amputation (Hunter et al., 2008).

Without use of a prosthesis, an individual with loss of one upper limb can obtain independence in self-care and most IADLs. Some individuals with loss of both upper limbs may be able to complete several self-care tasks independently without prostheses. However, their ability to increase independence and participation in activities will be enhanced by the appropriate prosthesis, components, and training. Therefore, the preprosthetic program may choose to emphasize only basic self-care training, such as cutting food, self-feeding, and bathing. Prosthetic training should expand the focus to to all areas of self-care, enhancing integration of the device into body image and schema. During the preprosthetic phase, the occupational therapist will begin educating the individual regarding styles of prosthesis and components that would assist in achieving the goals established. The opportunity to communicate with other individuals with similar amputations can provide hope for return to function. A peer who has received some guidance or training, such as through the certified peer program with the Amputee Coalition of America, understands the role of a "peer supporter" and can enhance the amputee team's program.

Prosthetic Training Program

Ideally, by the time the prosthesis is fabricated and delivered, the individual has been actively involved in the preprosthetic program. Several authors acknowledge the individual's acceptance and use of the prosthesis is improved by such a program. (Atkins, 1989a; Fletchall, 2005a, 2005b; Fletchall & Hickerson, 1991; Malone et al., 1984; Pezzin, Dillingham, Mackenzie, Ephraim, & Rossbach, 2004; Smurr, Gulick, Yancosek, & Ganz, 2008).

The prosthetic training program must continue to focus on the individual's goals, with a specific timeframe for completion of selected activities and goals. The program is considered effective or successful if it leads to the client's acceptance of the prosthesis as a tool to improve performance. (Atkins, 1989a; Fletchall & Hickerson, 1991).

Body-Powered, Myoelectric, and Electronic Prosthetic Prescription

Prosthetic type, such as body-powered, myoelectric, electronic, or hybrid (combination of two or more styles) must be determined for each client, regardless of the length of amputation.

The advantages of a body-powered prosthesis are

- Lighter-weight, cost-efficient, and durable;
- Shape does not need to be definitive;
- Provides sensory feedback; and
- Hook terminal device allows easy visibility of objects.

The disadvantages are

- Need for a harness;
- Discomfort caused by the axillary loop; and
- Unattractive appearance of the hook terminal device.

It is important to note that individuals with multiple types of prosthesis who perform rigorous or outdoor activities will frequently wear the body-powered prosthesis the majority of the time.

Whether the amputation is transradial or transhumeral, operation of the terminal device on a body-powered prosthesis is through tension on a cable by biscapular abduction or humeral flexion. Without proper training, the client's use of the terminal device may be limited to an area between the chest and knees and within the frontal span of the body. Individuals with transhumeral amputation using a body-powered prosthesis operate the elbow component through the same cable for terminal device function. The occupational therapist teaches the client to activate the prosthetic elbow movement through shoulder abduction, depression, and extension, without operating the terminal device. This allows the individual to be much more proficient in using the prosthesis in a variety of positions and activities.

Myoelectric

A client with a myoelectric prosthesis operates the terminal device or other components from surface electrodes placed over muscles in the residual limb. In a transradial amputation, the residual forearm muscles, under voluntary control, are be used to generate the myoelectric signal. An electronic prosthesis functions by toggle or pull switch, which may be built into the harness or suspension. With operation of the pull switch or toggle to activate, the prosthetic motor units of the terminal device and/or elbow become functional. To be successful in operating either type of prosthesis consistently and daily, the individual must have the cognitive abilities to comprehend the maintenance, care, use of the prosthesis, and battery-charging procedure. Occupational therapists will verify this as part of their ongoing evaluation.

The advantages of the myoelectric or electronic prosthesis are

- Less body movement is required to operate the components.
- Terminal device prehension power is higher than the body-powered prehension.
- Terminal device opening is larger than the body-powered opening.

For the individual with transradial amputation, myoelectric prosthesis can be operated with minimal or no harness, thus creating a greater envelope of range of function. The disadvantages of the myoelectric or electronic prosthesis are

- The weight on the residual limb is greater than with the body-powered prosthesis.
- Transradial or transhumeral residual limb shape and size must be stable.
- It is more expensive—battery costs can be very high for selected myoelectric or electronic prostheses.
- It requires more maintenance by the user.

A specialized amputee team can effectively guide the individual with amputation(s) into the right prosthesis with the most appropriate components. The team can provide the documentation for the recommended prosthesis that is necessary for reimbursement from health care providers. The costs of a unilateral prosthesis can range from $15,000 to more than $80,000. For individuals with complex upper-extremity amputations or bilateral amputations, the costs will be greater. The team members can provide creative options to the client with complex amputations that will help him or her return to satisfactory performance of everyday activities.

When deciding whether a myoelectric prosthesis is the team's recommendation, residual limb shape and size, total residual limb length, strength and endurance, ability to maintain the device, and funding will all be considered. For individuals using a body-powered prosthesis, a recommendation for a myoelectric or electronic prosthesis will be based on

- Client activities that cannot be performed with the current device,
- Potential for development of overuse syndrome(s) with the current device,
- Residual limb issues, and
- Availability of funding.

Terminal Devices

Body-powered hook terminal devices can be voluntary opening or voluntary closing. A voluntary opening device is held closed by bands that open when force creates cable movement. A voluntary closing device closes when force is applied to the cable. Most body-powered terminal devices are voluntary opening, based on the activities to be performed by the individual. Body-powered prosthesis with body-powered terminal devices can be best operated by individuals with transradial or up to mid-level transhumeral amputation.

Bands are used to provide prehensor force to the fingers of the body-powered hook terminal device. One band requires approximately 1.5–2 pounds of muscle force to move the cable to create operation of the device. More bands result in greater prehensor force and of course require more muscle force from the individual.

With an adult body-powered prosthesis, the most common types of terminal devices include, 5X, 5X A, 6, 7, and hand (Figure 12.6). The fingers (inside

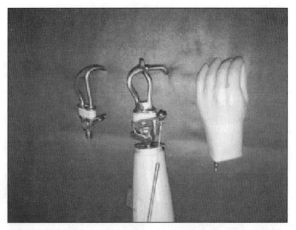

Figure 12.6. Body-powered terminal devices from left to right: 5X, number 6, and number 7.

of the hooks) of the 5X are lined with neoprene, minimizing abrasions to surfaces/objects. This terminal device is canted with symmetrical hooks in a "C" shape. The 5X A is constructed from aluminum, which reduces the weight of the terminal device by 50%. Most active bilateral upper-limb amputees using body-powered prosthesis use the 5X. The inside of the fingers of the 6 and 7 are serrated, and the design is similar to an "L" shape. This terminal device has a large opening diameter facilitating placement of handles, meal preparation utensils, yard tools, and selected hand tools. With the fingers in the closed position, handles on buckets can be lifted and carried.

The difference between the 6 and 7 is that the 6 has the ability to lock in the closed position, thus minimizing the requirement for large number of bands to provide force for prehension or closure. Many active individuals using the 6 terminal device can perform their activities and tasks with use of 5 or 6 bands. The hook style terminal device is lightweight and shaped so the individual can easily view objects for improved manipulation and grasp.

The weight of a body-powered hand terminal device is greater than that of the hook style device. Body-powered hand prehensor force is limited to approximately 3 pounds, with digits forming a three-jaw chuck prehension. With appropriate components, the hook terminal device can be interchanged with the hand device by the individual or family. Because of the limited prehension and the extra weight of the hand terminal device, this may have limited use with manual tasks. Many individuals, however, find it more appropriate for social events.

Except for hand terminal devices, most body-powered terminal devices can have an additional component of a wrist flexion unit. With the use of

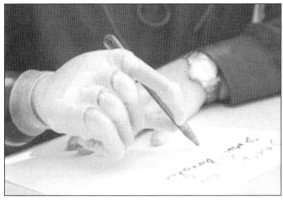

Figure 12.8. i-Limb™ terminal device with tip prehension.

wrist flexion components, the ability of the terminal device to reach midline of the body, without use of abnormal trunk or shoulder motions, is significantly improved. Performance of several self-care tasks (e.g., feeding self, grooming, hygiene) requires placement of the terminal device at midline of the body.

Myoelectric or Electronic Terminal Devices

Any level of upper-limb amputation may be a candidate for myoelectric or electronic prosthesis. For individuals with high transhumeral, shoulder disarticulation, or forequarter amputations, the most successful prosthetic use will be obtained from an electronic or myoelectric prosthesis, or a combination of the two.

Myoelectric or electronic terminal devices may include hand, Greifer, ETD, and i-LIMB™ devices (see Figures 12.7, 12.8, and 12.9). Most devices can be combined with wrist flexion and forearm rotation components that foster nearly normal posturing and

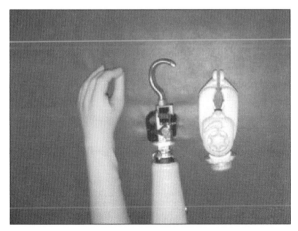

Figure 12.7. Powered terminal devices from left to right: hand, ETD, and Griefer.

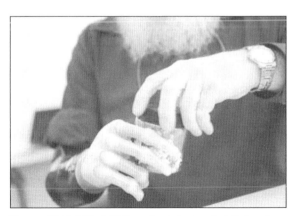

Figure 12.9. i-Limb™ terminal device in bilateral hand task.

body movements during activity performance. Most electronic or myoelectric components have some water resistance, but the individual must be taught to avoid active participation in activities with high levels of moisture or water.

A traditional powered hand has more prehensor force than a body-powered hand, with a three-jaw chuck prehension pattern. This type of device is frequently used for light ADLs but is not recommended for heavy manual tasks. The Greifer (Otto Bock product) and ETD (Motion Control product) have hook-type prehensors and can generate up to 30–32 pounds of force, making them acceptable for several manual tasks. With appropriate components, these devices can be interchanged with a powered hand, giving the prosthesis multiple functional uses.

The i-LIMB™ is another powered terminal device and (Touch Bionics, www.touchbionics.com) and has a rotatable thumb with the ability to obtain key, tip, three-jaw chuck prehension and cylindrical, spherical, and hook grasp. The i-LIMB can generate up to 22 pounds of force with the cylinder grasp and up to 4.4 pounds with the key prehension. This terminal device is appropriate for most self-care and light ADLs but is not recommended for heavy manual activities.

The cost for electronic/myoelectric prosthesis is significantly greater than for a body-powered prosthesis. Documentation by the amputee team can help obtain funding for the most appropriate prosthetic style.

Prosthetic Training

Initial training sessions should familiarize the client with prosthetic components and terminology and should take place in a quiet environment (Atkins, 1989b; 1994).

During this session, training should be directed towards donning and doffing procedures for the prosthesis that vary depending on the style of harness. The design of the harness or suspension should be based upon team collaboration of the occupational therapist, prosthetist, and physician. The harness style or suspension is influenced by the client's physical abilities, prosthetic components, and goals to be achieved.

Daily use of the prosthesis can be highly influenced by the ease of donning and doffing the prosthesis, along with fit and cosmetic appearance (Atkins, 1994).

When using a prosthesis with figure 8 harness, donning is usually done with an overhead method, as in donning a pullover garment (Figure 12.10). Individuals with bilateral high upper-extremity ampu-

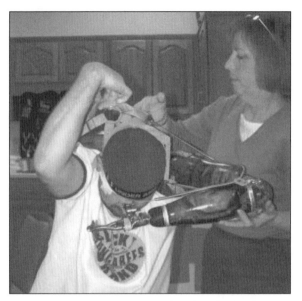

Figure 12.10. Learning to don body-powered prosthesis with figure 8 harness.

tations may require innovative or creative techniques to achieve independence in donning and doffing their prosthesis. Many individuals with such amputations may require fabrication of a customized prosthetic tree that allows placement of the prosthesis, with specific location of straps, such that the individual can maneuver into the device. Some individuals who don their prostheses through use of a prosthetic tree may need to squat, bend, or stand on one lower extremity to do so, making assessment of their total body motion and function very important.

Training should progress to body motions appropriate for operation of the terminal device, elbow, or shoulder components. For an individual with transradial or transhumeral amputation and using the body-powered prosthesis, muscle force is generated through biscapular movement or slight humeral flexion that creates tension on the cable that operates the terminal device. Myoelectric/electronic prostheses operate through surface electrodes over the skin of muscle(s). Muscle contraction produces an electric signal that is captured by the electrode and transmitted to the motor of the prosthesis. Myoelectric/electronic prosthetic use is dependent on the occupational therapist or certified prosthetist or both identifying the appropriate muscle(s) for electrode placement. The occupational therapist will initiate the training program to determine appropriate muscle endurance and signal transmission to activate the electrodes for operation of the terminal device, elbow, and other prosthetic components.

Training in the use of the terminal device is a prolonged stage of the training process. The success or failure of the individual's incorporation and use of the prosthesis depends on his or her motivation, the comprehensiveness and quality of the tasks and activities practiced, and the (critically important) experience and enthusiasm of the occupational therapist. The functional training experience "is most effective if the same therapist remains with the client throughout the process" (Atkins, 1989a, p. 45).

Prepositioning of the terminal device, elbow, or shoulder is important to efficiently incorporate the prosthesis into tasks. Appropriate instruction and training in prepositioning can minimize irritation of the noninvolved extremity secondary to abnormal posturing. One method of instructing the client to preposition the prosthesis is to position it to resemble a noninvolved extremity when participating in a task (Atkins, 1989a).

Training should begin with operation of the terminal device through simple grasp and release of items before progressing to operation of the other components. Performance of activities at tabletop height requires less motor response from the client because the trunk, lower extremities, and noninvolved limb are not moving. Progression of training activities into bilateral upper extremity use should be performed sitting and standing, just as the client would perform basic ADLs in his or her environment.

Providing activities that lead to success will further reinforce the value of the prosthesis. The occupational therapist can grade the difficulty of activities progressing from simple grasp and release of objects to use of the prosthesis in self-care and IADLs. The clinic provides an environment to perform bilateral upper-extremity tasks such as cutting food, opening jars, tying shoes, performing meal preparation, driving, and using hand and power tools. Incorporation of the prosthesis into leisure activities chosen by the client should also be explored, taking care to identify procedures for safety.

Treatment in a clinic with other individuals with amputations also reinforces the functional value of the prosthesis, assists with psychological acceptance of the amputation and injury, and reinforces the accomplishment of established goals (see Figure 12.11; Fletchall & Torres, 1992, p. 6).

Although training is individualized, there are a few general concepts in training that typically apply to everyone with a prosthesis, for example, the

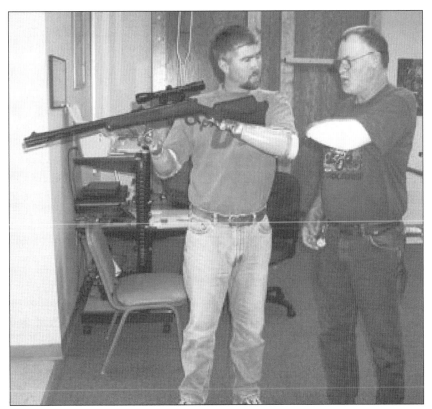

Figure 12.11. Specialized clinic provides environment for peer support and goal completion.

prosthesis will function as the nonpreferred extremity and will act to stabilize objects; dress the prosthesis first, undress it last; and when cutting meat with the prosthesis, the fork is placed between the hook fingers and behind the prosthetic thumb, and the knife is held by the noninvolved extremity.

Individuals with amputations frequently identify prosthetic success as daily wear and incorporation of the device into the majority of their tasks. Inconsistent prosthetic use with high-level amputations is a function of the number of components needed and by the perceived heavy feel of the device secondary to the short residual limb. The prosthesis appears to be incorporated into body image for either unilateral or bilateral amputations when

- Posttraumatic intervention occurs early,
- An experienced team provides intervention,
- A client-centered approach is used in the assessment and treatment,
- The client is provided ongoing education, and
- The client is placed into structured followup (Atkins, 1989a; Fletchall & Torres, 1992).

Functional Outcomes at Various Levels of Amputation

For individuals with a unilateral amputation, most IADLs, work, and leisure activities can be accomplished independently with the use of the noninvolved extremity. Early intervention, with prosthetic fitting within 30 days of the last surgical procedure on the amputated extremity, can foster daily prosthetic wear and use. (Fletchall & Torres, 1992, p. 7). When the individual also sustains a significant injury to the nonamputated extremity, early prosthetic fitting and training can assist in resuming independent performance in IADLs.

Long-term use of the prosthesis has been correlated with early intervention by a knowledgeable and specialized team on upper-limb amputations and prosthetics and participation in a coordinated preprosthetic and prosthetic occupational therapy program (Fletchall, 2005b; Malone et al., 1984; Smurr et al., 2008).

Achieving Sucessful Amputee Rehabilitation

Successful amputee rehabilitation is achieved when a client is able to participate independently and satisfactorily in valued daily activities and roles. Successful prosthetic training is achieved when the individual is able to wear and use the prosthesis daily for a minimum of 8 hours a day. Achieving successful prosthetic wear and use is also dependent on involving the client early in the rehabilitation process. Discussion with the individual of his or her

strengths and weaknesses and development of a timeframe for achieving goals encourage the client to regain control over his or her life. Providing information about different prosthetic styles and components and relating those to the individual's lifestyle can also foster greater goal achievement (Fletchall, 1998; Myers, 1999).

Additional success can be attributed to the specialized team's consideration and accommodation, from the outset, of the individual's social, physical, and emotional states as they consider and make recommendations regarding prosthetic type and components.

At this stage in the process, it falls on the occupational therapist to consider home assessments and perhaps onsite work assessments, as individuals with a higher-level upper-limb amputation may achieve increased safety and independence with selected small environmental modifications. Both home and work assessments must consider how tasks can be performed if the individual has a problem and the prosthesis cannot be worn and used for a period of time.

Unilateral Upper-Limb Transradial Amputation

With the loss of the hand, the most desired length is a medium or long transradial amputation because forearm rotation is preserved. Wrist disarticulation or elbow disarticulation will cause future problems of bone irritation secondary to atrophy of the soft tissue. The shape with either wrist or elbow disarticulation may not be appropriate for comfortable donning of the socket. The desired shape with a medium or long transradial amputation is conical.

Before initiating functional prosthetic training, the prosthesis should fit well and the client should be able to operate all components correctly. Frequent communication between the occupational therapist and prosthetist will determine the style and type of components and can quickly identify need for changes. After completion of the therapy program, the individual with unilateral upper-limb transradial amputation should return to a clinic specializing in amputations and prosthetics regularly to assure proper fit and use.

Bilateral Upper-Limb Amputations

While a basic level of self-care independence may be achieved without prosthesis, individuals with bilateral upper-limb loss can increase their performance and efficiency in activities with appropriate prosthetis. The majority of those with bilateral transradial amputations, and some with bilateral transhumeral amputations, can become independent in IADLs, including living alone, using prosthetic components and styles determined by the amputee team. Prostheses can help most with bilateral shoulder disarticulation or higher achieve independence in ADLs, driving, and performing selected household tasks. Depending on the individual's education or work history and his or her ability to return to a higher educational system, the prosthetic training program should include return-to-work issues. Individuals with bilateral upper-limb loss will benefit from an experienced occupational therapist recommending environmental changes to enhance independence and safety in the home and work environment. However, the ability of the individual to achieve a high level of independence is dependent on the occupational therapist's and the prosthetist's knowledge and experience and on the individual's own problem-solving skills.

In all cases of an active individual with a prosthesis, a second prosthesis should be considered to minimize lifestyle disruption in the event of mechanical wear and breakdown. The minimum of two prostheses per extremity can minimize dependence in ADLs or time away from work and family duties by preventing downtime during prosthetic maintenance or repair.

Individuals with bilateral high-level upper-limb amputation such as shoulder disarticulation may be candidates for targeted muscle reinnervation (TMR) and may progress to a specialized prosthetic system with multiple surface electrodes for activation of shoulder, elbow, forearm, wrist, and hand/terminal device components. The TMR is a surgical procedure transferring the nerves in the residual amputation site to alternative muscle sites. The alternative muscle sites are frequently larger trunk muscles, with a portion of the muscle controlled via the original nerve and a portion controlled via the newly transferred nerve. (Kuiken et al., 2009). TMR can be used for any level of amputation; however, focus has been on the individual with high bilateral upper-limb amputations. The surgery must be performed by an upper-limb amputations specialist who works closely with the amputee team. The occupational therapist will work with the individual to develop control of the portion of the muscle that will be used to activate the highly specialized prosthesis. Funding sources must be considered for this process, as the cost is high. The team must provide communication and documentation regarding the rationale for and benefits of the training, surgery, and prosthesis.

For those individuals using a dexterous hand terminal device such as the i-LIMB use of the Touch Bionics Upper-Extremity Functional Activity Assess-ment could be used (Atkins, 2009). Prosthetic assessments should be done at each scheduled followup. Addition of specific activities associated with that client's lifestyle can be included. Other assessments that should be considered in the routine scheduled followup include vehicle and home, work and avocational. Assessments can provide information to the specialized team to assist the individual with performing new activities, need for referral to other specialists, and/or need for change of prosthetic style or components to enhance performance of activities, especially as one ages.

Reasons for Continued Prosthetic Use

Early interaction with knowledgeable and specialized members of an amputee team was identified as a critical factor in sustained functional use of upper-limb prosthesis (Atkins, 1989a; Fletchall, 2005a, 2005b; Fletchall & Hickerson, 1991; Lake & Dodson, 2006; Malone et al., 1984; Pezzin et al., 2004; Smurr et al., 2008). At the 2005 American Academy of Orthotics and Prosthetics Symposium, Fletchall provided a 10-year review of the outcome differences between individuals with upper-limb amputations and rehabilitation with a specialized amputee team and individuals with upper-limb amputations but without rehabilitation with a specialized team. Two groups were identified and labeled, similar in gender compostion (more males than females) and age. All members of both groups sustained upper-limb amputation secondary to trauma, and all were employed at the time of the amputations.

The initial group averaged 24 hours before referral and interaction with an amputee team, and the secondary group averaged 8.94 months. The average time from date of injury to prosthetic fit in the initial group was 7.16 weeks, and in the secondary group, 41.04 weeks. The outcomes, obtained 1 year after completing an occupational therapy prosthetic training program, were

- Both groups had sustained 100% independence in ADLs.
- Ninety-six percent of the initial group remained prosthetic users, and 56% of the secondary group remained prosthetic users.
- Seventy-four percent of the initial group had returned to work or school, compared to 56% of the secondary group.

Prior to interaction with the amputee team, the secondary group had not received education, training, or treatment from a specialized amputee team. Complaints including poor prosthetic fit, "It doesn't work right," "It's heavy," "It's hot," "I'm uncomfortable with the appearance," and "No prosthetic training" were frequently heard from those in the secondary group who received a prosthesis prior to interaction with the amputee team.

A consequential further finding was that, although the hook terminal device does not resemble the human hand, the individuals in the initial group, having been treated, educated, and trained in its use by the specialized team, focused on how the device enabled activity participation rather than on its appearance. In the secondary group, which received no training or education, the hook terminal device and prosthesis were frequently rejected.

This finding is consistent with others on the high rejection rate of upper-extremity prostheses, which can often be attributed to the following reasons (Burrough & Brook, 1985, p. 41; Fletchall, 2005a, p. 32; Malone et al., 1984, p. 37; Pezzin et al., 2004, p. 728):

- Development of one-handedness, which removes the functional need for the prosthesis;
- Lack of sufficient training or skill in operating the prosthesis;
- Uncomfortable or poorly made prosthesis;
- Unnatural look or profile of the prosthesis;
- Reactions of other people;
- Timeframe from date of amputation to prosthetic fit and training;
- Inconsistent performance due to mechanical or electronic breakdowns; and
- Lack of or poor clinic-scheduled followup over the life of the individual.

Fletchall's and the above-cited studies supported findings of other authors who found that higher levels of functional outcome and greater prosthetic use were associated with early referral and interaction with the amputee team. Malone et al. (1984) identified a "Golden Period" of prosthetic fit and training for sustained prosthetic use at between 4 and 8 weeks following the upper-limb amputation as critical for initiating prosthetic fit and training. His followup found that individuals with early prosthetic fit and training retained purposeful use of the device for the completion of ADLs, home, and leisure activities. In addition, more individuals returning to the work environment were seen among those using upper limb prosthesis.

Potential Problems

Any individual with an amputation may develop any of several problems that can interfere with independent performance of daily activities.

- As the residual limb ages, atrophy occurs, which results in bone irritation or poor socket fit. Poor socket fit frequently results in skin or bone irritation or skin breakdown, resulting in turn to inability to operate the prosthesis. (Total body weight loss or gain can also influence the socket fit in the same way.) To accommodate "normal" atrophy, the individual will require frequent socket modifications and new sockets. The greatest change in the residual limb frequently occurs during the first 12 to 18 months with the possibility of the individual requiring 3–6 adjustments and socket replacement within the first year (Pezzin et al., 2004, p. 728). Structured followup through an amputee clinic will determine the need and timeframe for socket adjustments and new sockets and provide documentation for funding.
- Different types of pain sensation or abnormal sensation can interfere with performance in activities and prosthetic use. Early intervention and education will frequently minimize phantom pain sensation, which can interfere with prosthetic use.
- Neuromas, which develop following nerve laceration, occur in amputations. Light tactile stimuli to the neuroma can increase the abnormal sensation and may result in the limb withdrawing from the activity. Neuroma irritation can be minimized through placement of the nerve endings into padded soft tissue at the time of amputation and with the use of pressure wraps and a proper fitting socket. When traditional methods have not decreased neuroma irritation, the individual may require surgery to relocate the neuroma. Prosthetic use may resume 2–4 weeks after surgical relocation of the neuroma. The amputee team will determine if a new socket must be fabricated to enhance return to prosthetic use.
- Immediately following amputation, the individual must be monitored to minimize the development of hematomas, deep vein thrombus, or infection. Close inspection of the residual limb, which may be required daily for some individuals, can facilitate a more rapid progression to prosthetic fit.
- The development of bone overgrowth or heterotrophic ossification [HO] can occur in individuals who sustained multiple soft-tissue or bone injuries. Surgical removal of the HO or overgrowth occurs when the new bone is

mature, at approximately 6 months. The experienced occupational therapist monitoring the individual will notice specific edema, with unrelenting pain with active or passive joint motion, indicating development of HO. The therapist should attempt to immobilize the joint in the most functional position, which will minimize pain and allow the individual to continue to progress in the treatment program. The elbow joint is a common site for development of HO; placement with immobilization of the elbow into 70 to 90 degrees of flexion will allow functional use of a prosthesis. Development of contractures will decrease the functional performance in tasks, even if using a prosthesis. During the preprosthetic program, the occupational therapist must strive to eliminate soft-tissue tightness, and eliminate the development of contractures. In transradial amputations, the elbow has a potential to develop flexion contracture; transhumeral amputation may develop shoulder contractures and scapula immobility. Some individuals may benefit from instruction on self-ranging to enhance muscle performance and joint mobility.

• An additional potential problem is the development of overuse syndrome. Fletchall's presentation in 2006 at the American Academy of Orthotics and Prosthetists noted that overuse issues were reported by individuals with all types of upper-limb amputation, whether unilateral or bilateral. Overuse problems identified by individuals with upper-limb loss included shoulder pain, cervical neck pain, and low back pain. Those with transradial amputations exhibited hand cramping, carpal tunnel syndrome, and lateral epicondylitis. The overuse syndrome for unilateral amputations involved the nonamputated extremity, while bilateral amputations exhibited trunk and neck pain or discomfort. The specialized occupational therapy program must be designed to minimize the development of overuse syndromes. Educating the individual regarding potential development of such will minimize pain and minimize time away from work. In the scheduled followup with the amputee team, individuals are monitored to prevent or minimize the development of overuse syndrome. For some individuals, as the aging process occurs, the amputee team will make recommendations to change the style of the prosthesis or selected components to decrease overuse syndrome (Fletchall, 2006).

Additional medical problems, such as cardiac conditions or diabetes, may require consideration of alternative prosthetic components or prosthetic styles. As individuals age, participation in activities may change, which can influence prosthetic design or needs.

Unilateral Transhumeral Amputation

Transhumeral amputation results in less extremity length and greater loss of movement. Without a prosthesis, the ability of the residual limb to provide stabilization to the noninvolved extremity may be limited secondary to the length. Attempting to perform a bilateral upper-extremity activity with the transhumeral residual limb stabilizing an item on the table frequently results in neck flexion and forward cervical posturing, which may lead to pain.

Consideration of a prosthesis in this situation requires thorough assessment of total body function, residual limb shoulder function, and desired occupational activities. Shaping and edema control of the residual limb remain vital to achieving an appropriate socket fit. At minimum, mobility, endurance, and strength of the shoulder must be adequate to tolerate the weight of the prosthesis, as well as have the ability to reposition the prosthesis in relationship to the body, such as during donning of clothing.

If the individual is strong or can regain good muscle strength, performance of activities can be accomplished with a body-powered prosthesis. When the individual has limited endurance or strength, consideration should be given to hybrid, myoelectric, or electronic prosthesis. Amputee team members will analyze all factors to make the most appropriate prosthetic recommendations.

The individual with transhumeral amputation and no physical involvement of the remaining extremity should be able to achieve independence in most daily activities with the use of the body-powered, myoelectric, or electronic prosthesis.

Bilateral Transradial Amputation

Trauma leading to loss of both hands can significantly affect performance in activities. A sense of helplessness and depression can be minimized if early intervention is initiated to allow the individual to return to participation in selected activities. Depending on the type of trauma sustained, an individual may require a treatment program ensuring good flexibility and endurance and strength of the

Case Study 12.1. D.F.

D.F. is a 46-year-old man who sustained a partial hand amputation while at work stacking containers for ships and trucks. D.F.'s hand was trapped in the pinlocking mechanism for stacking the overseas containers, resulting in crush injury with partial hand amputation at the site. Following attempts to stabilize several fractures in the partial hand, D.F. requested an amputation. As his was an elective procedure, education was provided regarding the value of a prosthesis in terms of his life activities and work environment. He was given ongoing exposure to other individuals with upper-extremity amputations, where he observed the functional performance abilities of the body-powered prosthesis.

Within 1 day of the transradial amputation, he began outpatient occupational therapy. Initially, the program focused on edema control, residual limb shaping, range of motion, and residual limb and total body strengthening.

Within 30 days of the primary closure transradial amputation, D.F. was fitted with a body-powered prosthesis. Functional prosthetic training focused on independence in bilateral IADLs, work simulation, and leisure activities (Figures 12.12 and 12.13). After residual limb shape and size had stabilized, he was fitted with a myoelectric device with an interchangeable terminal device consisting of a Greifer and hand. He returned to his former employer, performing his previous job, within 4 months after the transradial amputation. He uses both types of prosthesis, preferring the body-powered when performing outdoor activities.

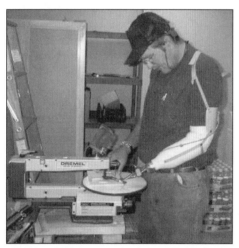

Figure 12.12. Using saw with transradial body powered prosthesis.

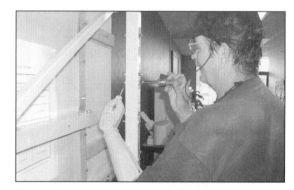

Figure 12.13. Using transradial myoelectric to handle small hand tools.

upper trunk, quadrant, and extremities. Evaluation and upgrade of lower-extremity skills can enhance the individual's ability to return to complete independence in ADLs. With the creativity of the client and therapist, many clients sustaining a bilateral transradial amputation can obtain some independence in selected activities while undergoing a traditional physical rehabilitation program. Upper-extremity movement across the midline, above the head, and to the back can be fostered through use of adaptive techniques and equipment to perform basic self-care independence such as self-feeding, washing the face, and donning upper-extremity garments. Adaptive techniques for toileting must be taught for use with and without the prosthesis. The adaptive toileting techniques are individualized to each client and depend on balance, lower-extremity skills, trunk

flexibility, and midline positioning of the upper extremity's prosthesis (Leonard & Meier, 1998).

Due to the changes in the residual limb and the initial loss of endurance and strength, it is usually preferable to fit the individual with transradial amputation with a body-powered prosthesis. The hook terminal device is lighter than hand or Greifer devices and provides greater visual feedback when interacting with objects. With the body-powered prosthesis, the harness and socket will provide the individual with kinesthetic feedback during performance of activities. Wrist flexion units will provide easier access to midline activities, such as feeding self and managing clothing. Automatic wrist rotators may be added to the prosthesis to position the terminal device, provided consideration is given to the added weight and stress borne by the residual limb.

Case Study 12.2. R.V.

R.V. is a 25-year-old woman who sustained a short transhumeral amputation at the work site. While working for a frozen food company, the nondominant extremity came into contact with the conveyor system producing rotary torque forces, resulting in a crushing injury and amputation. She required circumferential skin graft to the short residual limb. Even though she began the outpatient occupational therapy within 2 weeks of the skin graft, her initial attending surgeon was not supportive of an aggressive preprosthetic program and was not familiar with the benefits of a prosthesis. Following education of the client and case manager on the benefits and cost-effectiveness for the insurance payer of doing so, R.V. was referred to an amputee team.

Her initial program included edema control, residual limb shaping, wound care to areas where the skin graft had failed, shoulder and upper-quadrant range of motion, and scar tissue elongation, followed by residual limb muscle endurance and strengthening. Training was provided in how to independently perform self-care and selected household tasks. As a mother of three children, with one in diapers, instruction in adaptive techniques for managing child care with the non-involved extremity was provided. Until she had received training with the prosthesis, she was instructed in safe techniques for bathing the small child, changing diapers, and physically managing items needed when in the community with the infant. Once R.V.'s wounds had healed and shoulder motion had im-

proved, the occupational therapist fabricated an "extendoarm" from low-temperature thermoplastic that provided additional length to the residual limb, which facilitates use of the extremity in bilateral midline activities, reinforcing shoulder and scapular muscle skills until delivery of the prosthesis (Figure 12.14).

R.V. was given information on the prosthesis and components most appropriate for her strength, motion, and endurance and for helping her accomplish several activities bilaterally. She was initially fitted with a hybrid prosthesis with an electronic hand, passive counterswing elbow, and passive humeral rotation plate. Achieving control of the terminal device, positioning the elbow, and prepositioning the hand were achieved prior to training in functional tasks. Initial functional prosthetic training focused on cutting food and opening packets, and progressed to meal preparation and homemaking tasks (Figure 12.15). Following occupational therapy, R.V. resumed her role as mother and homemaker and returned to competitive employment. She is followed routinely in the amputee clinic, where her residual limb change, appearance, and daily activities are reassessed to determine ongoing prosthetic needs.

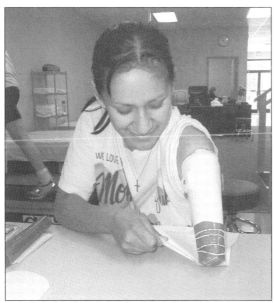

Figure 12.14. "Extendoarm" assists individual with transhumeral amputation in bilateral tasks.

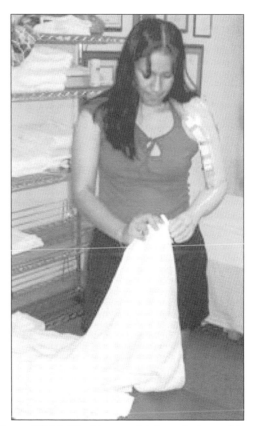

Figure 12.15. Working on folding clothes with hybrid transhumera prosthesis.

331

Case Study 12.3. J.C.

J.C. is a 31-year-old man who sustained 89% total body surface burns, with more than 50% third degree. Injuries were from a thermal explosion while at work. Burn injuries were sustained to all parts of the body except from the ankles distally, genital area, and the very top of the head. As a result of the deep burns to both hands, he required bilateral transradial amputations. Immediately following his discharge from a burn center, he began an intense daily outpatient program of up to 6 hours a day. The treatment program initially focused on multiple problems associated with burn injuries and amputations, as simultaneous burn and amputation rehabilitation programs minimize or prevent potential problems of contracture development, residual limb edema, and shoulder and scapular weakness (Fletchall & Hickerson, 1991, 1995).

During his first day of treatment, adaptive equipment allowed J.C. to feed himself, a task he had not performed for 8 weeks (see Figure 12.16).

While receiving traditional burn rehabilitation treatment, he was also involved in a preprosthetic program. Burns to the back can interfere with shoulder horizontal adduction, which can limit functional use of the prostheses. Therefore, before receiving prostheses, activities and tasks fostering use of upper extremities to midline were implemented to increase J.C.'s performance of the prosthesis in dressing and hygiene tasks (see Figure 12.17).

Due to heterotophic ossification of the right elbow, J.C. was initially placed to a left unilateral body-

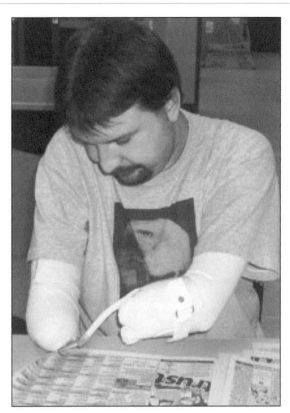

Figure 12.17. Midline activities can improve prosthetic control.

powered prosthesis with hook prehensor and wrist flexion unit. His initial prosthetic program focused on independence with one prosthesis, while continuing to improve the function of the remaining upper extremity. He achieved independence in donning and doffing the prosthetic socks and prosthesis, in feeding self, basic meal preparation, dressing with selected fasteners, bathing, and managing household tasks such as telephone and keys (see Figure 12.18). With an improvement in strength, he progressed to driving with minimal adaptation of a removable amputee driving ring (Figure 12.19).

Following surgery for removal of the heterotophic ossification in the elbow, J.C. was placed into bilateral body-powered prostheses with hook prehensors and wrist flexion units. Return to outpatient therapy provided for prosthetic training with the new prosthesis and an upgrade of his skills in all areas of IADLs.

Muscle assessment of the forearms was performed by the occupational therapist and revealed peripheral nerve loss to flexors and extensors of the forearm in his previously dominant extremity. Myoelectric/electronic forearm muscle training was initiated with the one residual limb that exhibited voluntary control of the

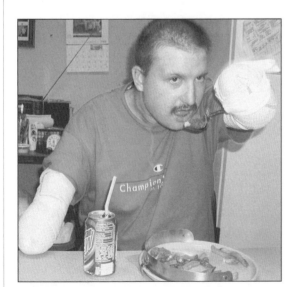

Figure 12.16. Prior to prosthesis, adaptive techniques are used to provide some independence.

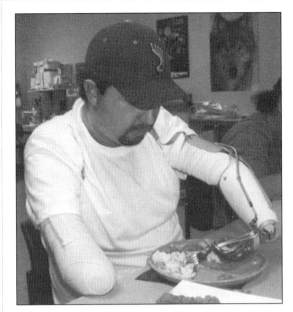

Figure 12.18. With bilateral transradial amputation, prosthetic training can begin with one device.

forearm muscles. Per J.C's request and through his routine scheduled appointments in amputee clinic, the stronger residual limb progressed to myoelectric/electronic prosthesis, with Greifer and hand, with the other extremity placed into unilateral body-powered pros-

thesis. He returned to the occupational therapy clinic for training in functional activities with the myoelectric/electronic prosthesis.

Even though this client has achieved a high level of ADL and IADL independence, including driving, living alone, preparing meals, and assisting his father in the operation of a heavy equipment business, his ability to use other prehensors and styles of prosthesis can influence the amount of daily energy he exerts to perform activities. Different styles of prosthesis require different amount of trunk muscle exertion. A body-powered prosthesis requires more scapula, trunk, and humeral motion than a myoelectric prosthesis. The myoelectric requires forearm muscle function, with "normal" use of the shoulder as one would move the hand through space.

Following appropriate pre- and postprosthetic training, individuals with transradial amputations who have good muscle function, mobility, and cognitive skills can achieve a high level of independence and resume many preinjury activities, including competitive employment (Figure 12.20).

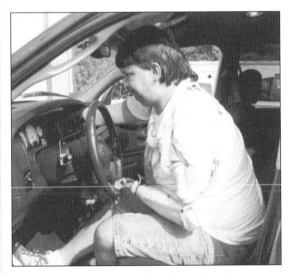

Figure 12.19. Driving with adaptations increases independence with bilateral transradial amputation.

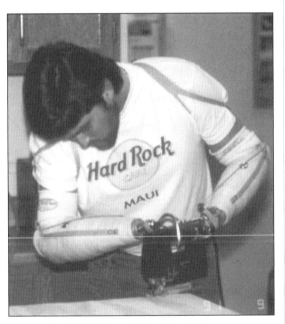

Figure 12.20. With specialized training, power tool use is possible with bilateral transradial amputations.

Case Study 12.4. G.H.

G.H. is a 44-year-old man who sustained bilateral transhumeral amputations in a high-voltage electrical burn injury. In addition to the transhumeral amputations, he sustained loss of both biceps and presented with deep burn wounds to both axillas. He was entered in a burn/amputee program from the day of injury, where the treatment program focused simultaneously on both catastrophic injures. Prior to obtaining wound closure, shoulder motion, and strength, the preprosthetic program focused on independence in selected self-care activities such as self-feeding (Figure 12.21). Initially, he was fitted with bilateral prosthesis with myoelectric/electronic elbows and hooks. Prosthetic training with the myoelectric/electronic prosthesis focused on self-care and ability to be alone for several hours in the home environment. As total body strength and endurance improved, he returned to the clinic for additional prosthetic training with bilateral body-powered elbows and hooks.

G.H. chose to use the bilateral body-powered prosthesis because of the reliability of the components and the speed at which he could operate the elbow and hooks. He resumed independence in many self-care activities with and without the prostheses, drove, and participated in leisure activities with the prostheses. His return to employment required work assessment by amputee clinic staff, who also designed and fabricated custom adaptive equipment for stabilizing items while working outside of the office. G.H. returned to employment within 54 weeks from the date of injury and retired 14 years later (see Figures 12.22 and 12.23).

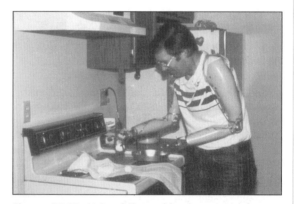

Figure 12.22. Using bilateral body-powered prostheses, client works on meal preparation.

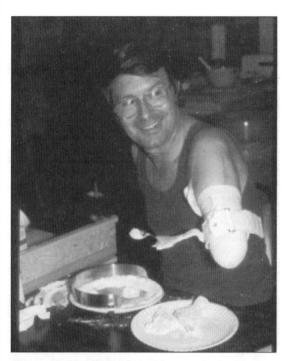

Figure 12.21. Bilateral transhumeral uses adaptive techniques to feed self.

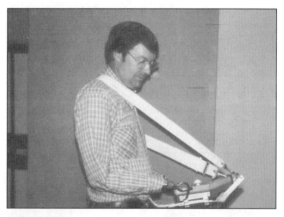

Figure 12.23. Equipment modification assisted with return to work with bilateral transhumeral amputation.

Prosthetic training for the individual with bilateral transradial amputations is similar to what has been previously described. Training focused on terminal device operation and prepositioning can influence time performance in activities. Use of the prosthesis in writing, feeding self, hygiene, toileting, and dressing reinforces daily use. Achieving independence with the prosthesis in basic self-care facilitates accomplishing pre-injury leisure activities. A thorough understanding of the individual, the

Case Study 12.5. V.B.

V.B. is a 30-year-old man who sustained a high-voltage electrical injury while at work. The depth of electrical injury resulted in physical loss of several muscles in the posterior neck, loss of axillary nerve and interosseous branch of the median nerve of the nonamputated extremity, and left shoulder disarticulation.

Following his initial burn care, he received over 9 months of treatment as an inpatient, and later as an outpatient, in a rehabilitation center. His referral to an amputee center came 13 months after the date of injury. V.B was totally dependent in all ADLs, including feeding himself. Through the rehabilitation center, he had been fitted with a prosthesis with a body-powered hook and elbow components. Efforts had not been directed toward achieving soft-tissue and scar-tissue elongation of the neck, right shoulder, or hand. Emotionally, he was distraught and depressed; however, he verbalized goals of achieving independence in ADLs and IADLs, including driving and fishing.

V.B. began a conditioning program geared toward improving total body endurance, motion, and strength. Use of selected tasks incorporated neck flexion, with progression of hand prehension and strength skills for the right upper extremity. Follow-ing a thorough assessment by the clinic, the previous body-powered prosthesis was discontinued, and he was placed into a hybrid myoelectric/electronic prosthesis with chest expansion pull switch that activated elbow and terminal device operation. Prosthetic frame construction respected skin grafts and scar-tissue areas, especially at the shoulder disarticulation site.

Functional prosthetic training began within 1 week of receiving the hybrid prosthesis. He progressed to achieving independence in all areas of self-care. The clinic completed a home assessment that provided recommendations for architectural modifications to accommodate for V.B's inability to achieve right shoulder flexion secondary to loss of axillary nerve. Vehicle modifications, including use of mirrors, were minimal once neck motion increased.

After 3 months in the program, V.B. achieved total independence in IADLs and driving and returned to employment. He lives alone, remains employed full-time, and has participated and placed in several competitive fishing tournaments. Due to his active lifestyle and physical limitations of the right upper extremity, he has two electronic hybrid prostheses. He returns to the amputee clinic yearly for reassessment of prosthetic needs.

---

prosthetic components, and their style is necessary to help the individual return to competitive employment or an educational system. For some individuals, vocational rehabilitation services may provide funding for retraining or education.

Individuals with bilateral transradial amputations can achieve a high level of or complete independence in IADLs. Once strength is achieved and appropriate prosthetic training has been completed, few of the individuals require adaptive devices for performance of everyday tasks. For many individuals, the prostheses tend to become an essential part of life and body image (Atkins, 1994, p. 295).

Bilateral Transhumeral Amputation

In a bilateral transhumeral amputation, the loss of both elbows requires that the prosthesis provide motion at the elbow, wrist, and terminal device. In addition, the residual limb length is shorter than with transradial amputation, placing further demands on the structures of the shoulder and cervical and upper-torso mobility.

Prosthetic components can provide for elbow flexion and extension, but the individual must use more energy to position the prosthesis and operate the terminal device. The ability to construct a lightweight, extremely durable elbow component remains a challenge to manufacturers. For most individuals with bilateral transhumeral amputations, the preferred elbow unit is body-powered. The body-powered elbow is lighter, more dependable, durable, and cost efficient and it requires less maintenance.

Prosthetic training will be influenced by the individual's tolerance for new information, technology, and and his or her available family support, in addition to the previously mentioned emotional and physical components. The ability to achieve independence in basic self-care will require creativity from the therapist and motivation from the client and should be explored with and without the use of prostheses. It may be appropriate to provide staged treatment sessions, allowing the client to practice levels of skills in the clinic, then within the home environment, returning to the clinic to learn additional activities.

Shoulder Disarticulation

Prosthetic components for shoulder disarticulation are frequently myoelectric or electronic, with a pull switch or toggle switch to operate the elbow and terminal device. Chest expansion movements can be used to operate a pull switch.

Self-care training should be focused on achieving independence with and without prosthesis. Prosthetic training must focus on operation of the prosthesis without exaggerated trunk motions and without unintended prosthetic activation during activities of ambulation, coming to standing, and reaching with the noninvolved extremity. Some of the training should use the prosthesis to provide stabilization to items while the noninvolved extremity performs the detail work. Providing instruction in use of the prosthesis in everyday activities, including work duties, can minimize likelihood of overuse of the noninvolved extremity.

Upper-Limb Amputations With Complications

Burns

When an amputation is the result of a burn, the residual limb may have significant fascia and soft-tissue loss. The occupational therapist will initiate motion, shaping, and edema reduction of the residual limb without creating additional skin problems. The fabrication of the socket requires good fit to avoid bone irritations, shearing, or pressure.

H.T., a 31-year-old man, sustained 63% total body surface burns, with third-degree burns to the left nondominant extremity. The extremity required skin grafts for wound closure. A short transradial amputation was performed within 2 weeks of his admission to a burn center. However, within 4 hours after the amputation, unrelenting pain required return to the operating room. During the second surgery, several muscles and fascia in the residual limb were noted to be necrotic secondary to severe artery spasm. The necrotic tissue was removed and the client resumed the burn/amputee program within 24 hours after surgery. The short transradial length resulted in approximately 1 inch of forearm surface to tolerate and support the socket of the prosthesis (Figure 12.24). The loss of fascia and several muscles resulted in low tolerance to pressure or shearing to the distal radius and medial and lateral epicondyes. The construction of the socket had to eliminate pressure points and shearing to the identified bony areas, while distributing the weight of the prosthesis over the one surface area of the forearm.

H.T. was initially fitted with a body-powered prosthesis with manual forearm supination, wrist flexion, and number 7 terminal device.

To minimize skin irritations as he ages, H.T. progressed from the number 7 to the number 6 terminal device. With the number 6 device, he was able to obtain firm closure pressure for terminal device closure with use of only 6 or 7 bands; up to 15 bands had been used with the number 7 device. Fewer bands meant less stress on the right shoulder, and minimized pressure, or shearing, to the bony areas of the residual limb. With the change in prehension power of the body-powered terminal device, he found it less stressful to perform heavy manual tasks.

During his body-powered prosthetic training program, H.T.'s occupational therapist worked with isolated forearm muscle contractions to progress the client to myoelectric with a Greifer and hand, and later to the ETD terminal device (Figure 12.25). In his scheduled followup, he presented several overuse syndromes: right shoulder joint irritation, lateral epicondylitis, and carpal tunnel syndrome. These required two different surgical procedures to the nonamputated extremity. With three different

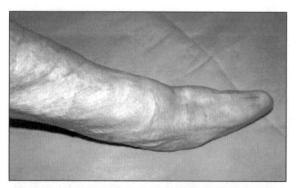

Figure 12.24. Burns resulted in loss of fascia and muscles in short transradial amputation.

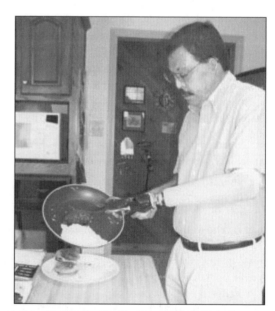

Figure 12.25. ETD with myoelectric prosthesis facilitates bilateral tasks for meal preparation.

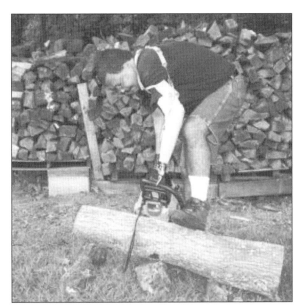

Figure 12.26. With specialized training, large power tools can be safely managed with short transradial amputation.

powered terminal devices for the myoelectric/electronic prosthesis, he was able to continue with several activities during the recovery phase following surgeries.

The occupational therapist helped refer H.T. to a vocational rehabilitation service, where he earned a bachelor's degree in industrial technology. He remains functional in IADLs, work, and leisure activities (Figure 12.26). He is followed a minimum of once a year in the amputee clinic.

Upper- and Lower-Limb Amputations

When an individual sustains amputations to upper and lower limbs, the amputee team must consider the most appropriate prosthetic components and styles to enhance return to functional activities.

E. M., a 38-year-old man, sustained left transhumeral and left hip disarticulation amputation when an large forklift fell on him at a construction site. Loss of muscle and fascia at the left hip occurred, leaving bony prominence of the hip; he also required a colostomy and ileostomy. E.M. entered an amputee program 9 months after the injury, fitted with two body-powered prostheses. Poor socket fit and inappropriate component selection did not foster successful prosthetic use. He was dependent upon a manual wheelchair for mobility and remained dependent in basic self-care. Upon referral to the amputee program, he was also referred to the amputee clinic and team.

After being fitted with different, more appropriate body-powered prosthesis and components, E.M. progressed quickly to integration of the device into IADLs. As his strength improved, he progressed to ambulation with a walker. The only special modification required for the walker was leather padding to minimize the number 6 terminal device cutting into the frame. He was fitted with and trained for lower-extremity prosthesis, progressing to use of a cane for long distances. Within his work environment at a rehabilitation clinic, where his job duties included managing the laundry, stocking water and soft drinks in the refrigerator, cleaning floors, and emptying trash, he prefers the walker to lower-extremity prosthesis (Figures 12.27, 12.28, and 12.29); lower-extremity prosthesis is used for social activities. Following a work assessment, the occupational therapist recommended equipment and modifications of task performance to improve E.M.'s productivity and safety in the work environment. To safely manage the walker with the body-powered upper-limb prosthesis, the harness alignment is nonstandard.

E.M. is independent in all IADLs, driving, and working. He has a minimum of two body-powered prosthesis with number 6 terminal device and wrist flexion units. Progression to alternative styles of prostheses has been limited secondary to the applied forces on the walker from the prosthesis and

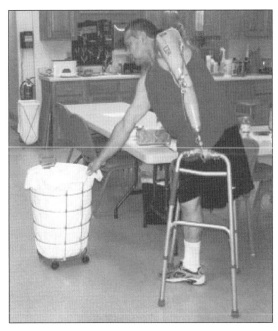

Figure 12.27. Wheels on laundry basket foster safety and independence with transhumeral and hip disarticulation amputation.

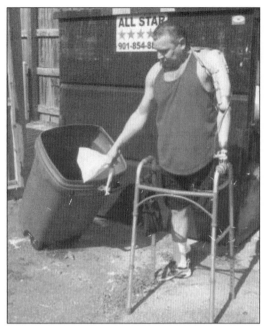

Figure 12.28. Wheeled trash can be moved with use of pull cord.

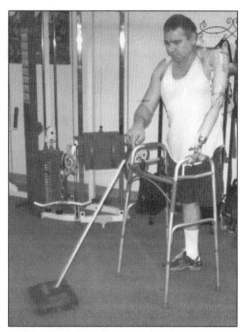

Figure 12.29. Recommendations for floor sweeper improved work safety and performance.

the need to lift items of up to 5 pounds. He is followed a minimum of once a year in the amputee clinic.

Four-Limb Amputation

When an individual sustains amputations of four limbs, a sense of helplessness and dependence occurs rapidly. The individual's program should include trunk, neck flexibility, and motion of any joint remaining in any extremity. Many individuals with quad amputations will require housing modifications and caregiver or attendant care for selected hours of the day. With motivation and appropriate prosthetic components and training, the individual can progress into school or selected employment.

D.H., a 26-year-old man, sustained bilateral short transfemoral amputations and bilateral transradial amputations following medication reaction. Skin and soft-tissue loss was sustained to the ears, nose, and back of the head.

D.H. entered an amputee program 13 months after the trauma. He was noted to have bilateral HO in the elbows, severe bilateral hip flexion contractures, and tightness of trunk and bilateral shoulder muscles. The amputee team focused on the client's goals of achieving independence and becoming eligible for prostheses. Prior to removal of HO from the upper limbs, the program focused on decreasing hip flexion contractures; increase in muscle endurance;

and strength of trunk, scapula, and shoulder muscles. While awaiting removal of HO, D.H. achieved independence in feeding self and brushing teeth with devices specially designed by the occupational therapist (Figure 12.30). He also progressed to independence in transferring from the wheelchair to bed and commode.

As he progressed in selected self-care independence, D.H. received education and instruction in

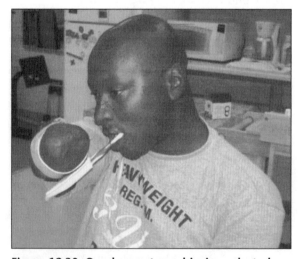

Figure 12.30. Quad amputee achieving selected self-care independence prior to receiving prostheses.

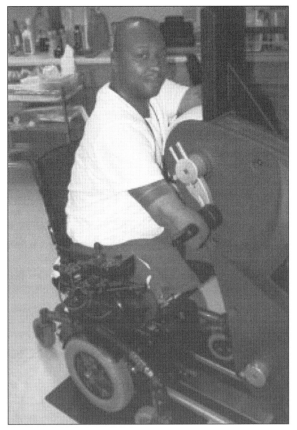

Figure 12.31. Bilateral transradial and transfemoral amputee participating in cardiovascular program.

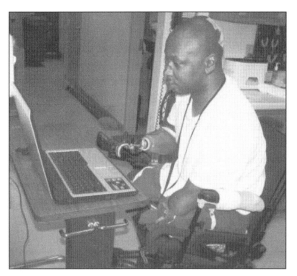

Figure 12.32. Using ETD with myoelectric prosthesis for computer work.

the importance of a cardiovascular program (Figure 12.31). The occupational therapist helped identify the type he could independently perform in his home environment.

Four months after HO removal from the right upper limb, D.H. began training with a myoelectric/electronic prosthesis with ETD. He progressed to using it for feeding himself, selected hygiene, computer keyboard use, writing, basic meal preparation, and leisure activities (Figures 12.32 and 12.33).

The occupational therapist assisted with referral to community agencies for Meals on Wheels, community handicap transportation, caregiver services, housing for handicapped individuals, and vocational rehabilitation services. D.H. had progressed from dependence on a family member to planning and implementing his daily schedule and "being on my own" with some assistance from a paid caregiver for limited hours each day.

Future of Amputations and Prosthetics

The immediate future of prosthetics will see lighter-weight, highly durable materials. The ability

to design an upper-limb prosthesis to duplicate the range of movement of the extremity, while providing stability and reliability, remains a challenge. The other challenging problem is the development of a method or mechanism to provide consistent, reliable sensory feedback.

Current prosthetic work is exploring the use of other body functions to operate the prosthesis. Use of the foot, through footpad electrodes, is being explored to control multijoint, high-level prosthetics. In other areas, laboratory work is focusing on the use of a brain–computer interface (BCI). Through BCI technology, nonpenetrating electrodes can be

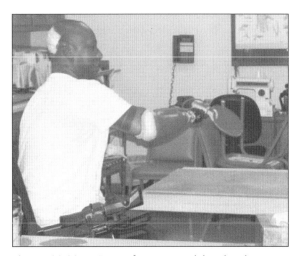

Figure 12.33. ETD use fosters participation in leisure activities.

placed on the brain surface, allowing control of limb prosthetics through purposeful brain-wave activity. Other studies have explored the sensitivity of the tongue, with its highly innervated surface, to provide sensory feedback for prosthetic use. These and other high-level technology advances require the occupational therapist to keep abreast of new ways to use neurofunctions to help people achieve their goals.

The future also promises advances in specialized surgical procedures. For example, new techniques have have resulted in over 50 hand transplants worldwide in the past decade (Shores, Brandacher, Schneeberger, Gorantla, & Lee, 2010). There remain, however, some limitations on on these procedures, including the lack of immunomodulating protocols and the need for careful oversight and screening procedures. Because of the risks inherent in the surgery, there are ethical concerns because the techniques are not required as a life-saving procedure. However, individuals are accepting the inherent risks as a trade-off for improved quality of life.

The difficulties currently facing immunosuppressive regimens may become less problematic as new developments minimize post-transplant lymphoproliferative disease. In facilities specializing in microsurgical reconstruction of upper-limb transplants, occupational therapists keep abreast of solutions to complex hand and arm problems while continuing to foster patient goal achievement.

Other medical advances such as tissue engineering and cell technology may facilitate new approaches to upper-limb regeneration. The issues associated with these technologies, and whether they may be used to help an individual with an amputation, may include the reason for the amputation (e.g., gangrene secondary to diabetic neuropathy versus trauma) and the individual's age, as these factors can influence the quality of the tissue and cells and increase the risks of surgery to the patient.

Manufacturers are developing terminal devices to replicate digit movements of the hand. As improvements are made in materials of the dexterous hands, they will be able to generate grasp and prehension force that will enhance their use in numerous activities.

Remaining focused on team participation, education, and knowledge of multiple medical procedures and technologies is vital for occupational therapists to provide the highest level of quality rehabilitation for individuals with upper-limb amputations.

Summary

Thorough evaluation by the occupational therapist can provide information to develop a program to achieve the client's intended goals. An individual sustaining loss of an upper extremity can achieve success in many preinjury activities when treatment is initiated early and by professionals who specialize in amputations and prosthetics. The degree of independence regained and the level of daily prosthetic use depend on the prosthetic style, components, training, and followup. Specialized amputee team members play a profound role in educating and encouraging the individual in what prosthesis can and cannot do. Early intervention by professionals specializing in amputations and prosthetics can minimize costs and maximize positive outcomes by identifying appropriate components and providing insightful, compassionate training.

Study Questions

1. What are the benefits of involving patients in a pre-prosthetic program?
2. What are the advantages and disadvantages of a body-powered hook terminal device and a hand terminal device?
3. What are the differences between receiving therapy and prosthesis soon after amputation versus several months later?
4. What components determine if a patient is a prosthetic candidate?
5. What are the elements that facilitate successful prosthetic use?
6. Why do patients with upper-limb amputations develop complications?
7. What are the advantages or disadvantages of a structured clinic followup?

References

Atkins, D. J. (1989a). Adult upper-limb prosthetic training. In D. J. Atkins & R. H. Meier (Eds.), *Comprehensive management of the upper limb amputee* (pp. 39–59). New York: Springer-Verlag.

Atkins, D. J. (1989b). Functional skills training with body powered and externally powered prostheses. In D. J. Atkins & R. H. Meier (Eds.), *Comprehensive management of the upper limb amputee* (pp. 145–149). New York: Springer-Verlag.

Atkins, D. J. (1989c). Postoperative therapy programs. In D. J. Atkins & R. H. Meier (Eds.), *Comprehensive management of the upper limb amputee* (pp. 11–15). New York: Springer-Verlag.

Atkins, D. J. (1994). Managing self-care in adults with upper extremity amputations. In C. H. Christiansen (Ed.), *Ways of living* (pp. 277–304). Bethesda, MD: American Occupational Therapy Association.

Atkins, D. (2009). *i-LIMB^TM hand training protocol for therapists*. Hilliard, OH: Touch Bionics and Touch EMAS.

Bennett, J. B., & Alexander, C. B. (1989). Amputation levels and surgical techniques. In D. J. Atkins & R. H. Meier (Eds.), *Comprehensive management of the upper limb amputee* (pp. 1–10). New York: Springer-Verlag.

Burrough, S., & Brook, J. (1985). Patterns of acceptance and rejection of upper limb prostheses. *Orthotics and Prosthetics, 39,* 40–47.

Fletchall, S. (1998). Using professional experience to lead people with recent amputations to success. *Capabilities, 7*(4), 6–7.

Fletchall, S. (2005, March). *Value of specialized rehabilitation with trauma and amputations*. Paper presented at American Academy of Orthotists and Prosthetists Annual Symposium, Orlando, FL.

Fletchall, S. (2005a). Occupational Therapy from the Onset. *InMotion 16*(5), 34–38.

Fletchall, S. (2005b). Returning upper-extremity amputees to work. *The O&P Edge, 4*(8), 28–33.

Fletchall, S. (2006, March). *Upper-extremity amputation overuse syndrome-types and incidence*. Paper presented at American Academy of Orthotists and Prosthetists Annual Symposium, Chicago.

Fletchall, S., & Hickerson, W. L. (1991). Early upper-extremity prosthetic fit in patients with burns. *Burn Care and Rehabilitation Journal, 12*(3), 234–236.

Fletchall, S., & Hickerson, W. L. (1995). Quality burn rehabilitation: Cost-effective approach. *Journal of Burn Care and Rehabilitation, 16*(5), 539–542.

Fletchall, S., & Torres, H. (1992). Benefits of early upper extremity prosthetic training. *Capabilities, 2*(2), 6–8.

Hunter, J. P., Katz, J., & Davis, K. D. (2008). Stability of phantom limb phenomena after upper limb amputation: A longitudinal study. *Neuroscience, 156,* 939–949.

Kelly, B. M., Pangilinan, Jr., P. H., Rodriguez, G. M., Mipro Jr., R. C., & Bodeau, V. S. (2009). *Upper limb prosthetics*. Retrieved September 29, 2009, from http://emedicine.medscape.com/article

Kline, J. E., Clark, A. M., Chan, B., McAuliffe, C. L., Heilman, K. M., & Tsao, J. W. (2009). Normalization of horizontal pseudoneglect following right, but not left, upper limb amputation. *Neuropsychologia, 47,* 1204–1207.

Kuiken, T. A., Li, G., Lock, B. A., Lipschutz, R. D., Miller, L. A., Stubblefield, K. A., et al. (2009). Targeted muscle reinnervation for real-time myoelectric control of multifunction artificial arms. *JAMA, 301*(6), 619–633.

Lake, C., & Dodson, R. (2006). Progressive upper limb prosthetics. *Physical Medicine and Rehabilitation Clinics of North America, 17,* 49–72.

Leonard, J. A., Jr., & Meier, R. H. III. (1998). Upper- and lower-extremity prosthetics. In J. A. DeLisa & B. M. Gans (Eds.), *Rehabilitation medicine: Principles and practice* (pp. 669–696). Philadelphia: Lippincott-Raven.

Malone, J. M., Fleming, L. L., Roberson, J., Leal, J. M., Poole, J. U., & Grodin, R. (1984). Immediate, early and late postsurgical management of upper-limb amputation. *Journal of Rehabilitation Research and Development, 21*(1), 33–41.

Marquardt, E. (1989). The Heidelberg experience. In D. J. Atkins & R. H. Meier (Eds.), *Comprehensive management of the upper limb amputee* (pp. 240–252). New York: Springer-Verlag.

Mayer, A., Kudar, K., Bretz, K., & Tihanyi, J. (2008). Body schema and body awareness of amputees. *Prosthetics and Orthotics International, 32*(3), 363–382.

Myers, C. (1999 December/January). A one-woman show. *Rehab Management*, pp. 74–77.

Pezzin, L. E., Dillingham, T. R., MacKenzie, E. J., Ephraim, P., & Rossbach, P. (2004). Use and satisfaction with prosthetic limb device and related services. *Archives of Physical Medicine and Rehabilitation, 85,* 723–729.

Ramachandran, V. S., & Alschuler, E. L. (2009). The use of visual feedback, in particular mirror visual feedback, in restoring brain function. *Brain, Journal of Neurology, 132,* 1693–1710.

Ramachandran, V. S., & Roger-Ramachandran, D. (1996). Synaesthesia in phantom limbs induced with mirror. *Proceedings of the Royal Society of London 262,* 377–386.

Shores J. T., Brandacher, G., Schneeberger, S., Gorantla, V. S., & Lee, W. P. (2010). Composite tissue allotransplantation: Hand transplantation and beyond. *Journal of the American Academy of Orthopaedic Surgery, 18*(3), 127–131.

Staley, M. J., & Richard, R. L. (1994). Scar management. In R. L. Richard and M. J. Staley (Eds.), *Burn care and rehabilitation principles and practice* (pp. 380–418). Philadelphia: F.A. Davis.

Smurr, L. M., Gulick, K., Yancosek, K., & Ganz, O. (2008). Managing the upper extremity amputee: A protocol for success. *Journal of Hand Therapy, 21,* 2160–2175.

Woodhouse, A. (2005). Phantom limb sensation. *Clinical and Experimental Pharmacology and Physiology, 32,* 132–134.

Appendix 12.A. Functional Activity Assessment

Patient Name

FUNCTIONAL ACTIVITY ASSESSMENT
RATING SCALE   0=Impossible
                        1=Accomplished with strain and awkward movements
                        2=Accomplished with some labored and awkward movements
                        3=Accomplished, smooth, minimal delay

Activity	ACTIVITY RATING					Notes
	BASELINE w/current prosthesis	POST i-LIMB Hand TRAINING w/ i-LIMB Hand TD	1-MONTH FOLLOW-UP w/i-LIMB Hand TD	6-MONTH FOLLOW-UP w/i-LIMB Hand TD	12-MONTH FOLLOW-UP w/i-LIMB Hand TD	
Date						
Prosthetic Management						
Understands how to don prosthesis						
Open/close terminal device						
Understands how to change batteries						
Understands how to care for prosthesis						
Understands how to doff prosthesis						
Dressing						
Buttons						
Zippers						
Hooks						
Snaps						
Tie shoelaces						
Don/doff socks						
Don/doff shoes						
Don/doff shirt						
Don/doff pants						
Tie necktie						
Fasten belt buckle						
Don/doff jacket or coat						
Grooming						
Brush/comb hair						
Shave						
Squeeze toothpaste on brush						
Brush teeth						
Apply makeup						

Patient Name

FUNCTIONAL ACTIVITY ASSESSMENT

RATING SCALE   0=Impossible
1=Accomplished with strain and awkward movements
2=Accomplished with some labored and awkward movements
3=Accomplished, smooth, minimal delay

Activity	ACTIVITY RATING					Notes
	BASELINE w/current prosthesis	POST i-LIMB Hand TRAINING w/ i-LIMB Hand TD	1-MONTH FOLLOW-UP w/i-LIMB Hand TD	6-MONTH FOLLOW-UP w/i-LIMB Hand TD	12-MONTH FOLLOW-UP w/i-LIMB Hand TD	
Date						
Feeding/Meal Preparation	UNILATERAL ACTIVITIES					
Pick up utensils						
Eat with fork						
Eat with spoon						
Drink from glass/cup						
Eat potato chips						
Drink from bottle						
Pour liquid						
	BILATERAL ACTIVITIES					
Cut with knife/fork						
Eat sandwich						
Peel banana						
Peel orange						
Peel vegetables						
Spread butter on bread						
Cut vegetables						
Open bottle lid (screw)						
Use bottle opener						
Carry a tray						
Open condiment packs						
Open snack boxes						
Open chip bag						
Use can opener (manual)						
Use microwave						
Use oven						
Open fridge/obtain items						
Use stove						
Manipulate hot pots						
Use colander/strainer						

Patient Name

FUNCTIONAL ACTIVITY ASSESSMENT
RATING SCALE   0=Impossible
                          1=Accomplished with strain and awkward movements
                          2=Accomplished with some labored and awkward movements
                          3=Accomplished, smooth, minimal delay

Activity	ACTIVITY RATING					Notes
	BASELINE w/current prosthesis	POST i-LIMB Hand TRAINING w/ i-LIMB Hand TD	1-MONTH FOLLOW-UP w/i-LIMB Hand TD	6-MONTH FOLLOW-UP w/i-LIMB Hand TD	12-MONTH FOLLOW-UP w/i-LIMB Hand TD	
Date						
Feeding/Meal Preparation	BILATERAL ACTIVITIES					
Crack eggs						
Use measuring cups						
Mix ingredients (mixer/spoon)						
Pass dishes						
Use salt/pepper shaker						
Open pop-top						
Use Ziploc baggies						
Wrap/unwrap food in foil						
Use Saran Wrap						
Household Management						
Load/unload dishwasher						
Wash dishes in sink/dry						
Put dishes in overhead cabinet						
Mop floor						
Sweep floor/use dustpan						
Use vacuum cleaner						
Set up ironing board						
Iron clothes						
Load/unload washer, dryer						
Sort laundry						
Fold laundry						
Make bed						
Place pillow in pillow case						
Thread needle						
Sew on buttons						
Put on gloves						

Patient Name

FUNCTIONAL ACTIVITY ASSESSMENT
RATING SCALE   0=Impossible
                          1=Accomplished with strain and awkward movements
                          2=Accomplished with some labored and awkward movements
                          3=Accomplished, smooth, minimal delay

Activity	ACTIVITY RATING					Notes
	BASELINE w/current prosthesis	POST i-LIMB Hand TRAINING w/ i-LIMB Hand TD	1-MONTH FOLLOW-UP w/i-LIMB Hand TD	6-MONTH FOLLOW-UP w/i-LIMB Hand TD	12-MONTH FOLLOW-UP w/i-LIMB Hand TD	
Date						
Desk/Office Procedures	**BILATERAL ACTIVITIES**					
Use phone/take notes						
Use eraser						
Use ruler – draw straight edge						
Tear paper from pad						
Use scissors						
Fold paper, place in envelope						
Open sealed envelope						
Use paper clip						
Use stapler						
Use tape dispenser						
Open mailbox/deposit letter						
Use computer						
File paper						
Trace shapes						
General Procedures						
Money management (bills)						
Money management (coins)						
Use key in lock						
Ring door bell						
Lights (switch/dimmer)						
Use door knob						
Turn on outside faucet						
Open/close window						
Use remote control for TV						
Use CD/DVD/VHS player						

Patient Name

FUNCTIONAL ACTIVITY ASSESSMENT

RATING SCALE 0=Impossible
1=Accomplished with strain and awkward movements
2=Accomplished with some labored and awkward movements
3=Accomplished, smooth, minimal delay

Activity	ACTIVITY RATING					Notes
	BASELINE w/current prosthesis	POST i-LIMB Hand TRAINING w/ i-LIMB Hand TD	1-MONTH FOLLOW-UP w/i-LIMB Hand TD	6-MONTH FOLLOW-UP w/i-LIMB Hand TD	12-MONTH FOLLOW-UP w/i-LIMB Hand TD	
Date						
General Procedures	BILATERAL ACTIVITIES					
Play cards/shuffle						
Light a match						
Wrap/unwrap a package						
Use umbrella						
Carry a tray						
Take a picture						
Operate a video camera						
Change a light bulb						
Change air conditioning filter						
Hang a picture						
Carry a suitcase/groceries						
Gardening						
Water lawn/use hose						
Use a lawnmower						
Use of Tools						
Hammer nail into wall						
Saw						
Screwdriver						
Wrench						

Patient Name

FUNCTIONAL ACTIVITY ASSESSMENT
RATING SCALE   0=Impossible
                    1=Accomplished with strain and awkward movements
                    2=Accomplished with some labored and awkward movements
                    3=Accomplished, smooth, minimal delay

Activity	ACTIVITY RATING					Notes
	BASELINE w/current prosthesis	POST i-LIMB Hand TRAINING w/ i-LIMB Hand TD	1-MONTH FOLLOW-UP w/i-LIMB Hand TD	6-MONTH FOLLOW-UP w/i-LIMB Hand TD	12-MONTH FOLLOW-UP w/i-LIMB Hand TD	
Date						
Car Procedures	**BILATERAL ACTIVITIES**					
Manipulate steering wheel						
Raise hood						
Use a jack						
Change a tire						
Use signals/wipers						
Manipulate mirrors						
Open car door						
Fasten seat belt						
Start ignition						
Advanced Activities						
Prepare a simple meal						
Complete a small woodworking project						
Simple repair/home fix-it project						
Grocery shopping						
Visit a mall/shop/ negotiate food court						
Other:						
Recreation/Hobbies						

Therapists Name

Prosthetist Name

Chapter 13

Enabling Life Roles After Severe Burns

MARK PROCHAZKA, OTR/L, MHA; SYDNEY THORNTON, OTR/L; AND HEATHER SCHULTHEIS DODD, MS, OTR/L

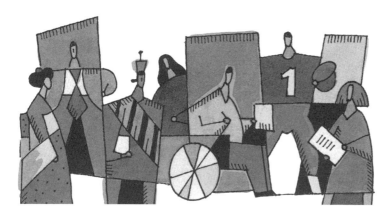

KEY WORDS

autograft

boutonnière deformity

boutonnière precautions

donor site

ectropion

eschar

full-thickness burn

heterotopic ossification

hyperpigmentation

hypertrophic scar

hypopigmentation

keloid scar

microstomia

partial-thickness burn

scar maturation

split-thickness skin graft

total body surface area (TBSA)

HIGHLIGHTS

- Burn injuries require consistent and focused treatment and therapies.

- A multidisciplinary, team-driven approach is required to return patients to functional, productive, and engaged lives.

- Patients, their families, and their occupational roles and activity levels are all affected by a major burn.

- Timely initial treatment after a burn can often prevent contractures and decreased functional capacity.

- Care of burn patients and their need for positive coping strategies can last a lifetime.

OBJECTIVES

After reading this material, readers will be able to

- Recognize and understand the characteristics of the different depths of burn injury;
- Describe the phases of recovery and the focus of occupational therapy intervention for each phase;
- Identify factors that increase the potential of scar hypertrophy or contractures;
- Understand how early patient and caregiver education and their active involvement in establishing occupational therapy goals will influence long-term compliance with the treatment program;
- Understand the rationale and benefits of early involvement of burn patients in their self-care;
- Recognize the impact that a severe burn has on a person's life roles, self-image, values, and occupational performance; and
- Describe factors to consider when recommending adaptive techniques, equipment, or environmental modifications for individuals with burns.

Role of Occupational Therapy in Burn Care

The primary purpose of occupational therapy intervention with burn patients is to return them to their pre-injury level of occupational performance. Occupational therapists should have a basic understanding of burn treatment and their role within the burn population. It is the role of the therapist to interpret the benefit of occupational therapy for their clients and to apply the basic tenets of therapy in an acute care medical setting.

The *Occupational Therapy Practice Framework* describes areas of occupation as activities of daily living (ADLs), instrumental activities of daily living (IADLs), rest and sleep, education, work, play, leisure, and social participation (American Occupational Therapy Association [AOTA], 2008a). Burn victims' injuries affect all of these daily occupations because the injuries are complex and dynamic and must be considered in a holistic manner. The severe trauma of such injuries requires a continuum of care lasting months to years for victims and their families.

Performing ADLs is often complex for burn patients. Simple activities such as bathing and showering require careful dressing of wounds, temperature precautions, wearing of compression garments, and decisions about the type of soap products and lotions to use. Dressing requires consideration of weather, sun exposure, and donning and doffing of compression garments to maximize healing potential. Eating may be complicated by *microstomia* (a scarring of the mouth orifice), preventing patients from opening their mouths enough to take in food. Patients may need to manipulate utensils and the upper extremities in order to feed independently. Scarring, heterotrophic ossification of elbow joints, dressings, nerve injuries, and amputation all require therapeutic interventions and adaptations for feeding activities.

To achieve functional mobility, patients often require lower-extremity compression dressings, splints, management of low endurance through energy conservation, and functional range of motion (ROM) and daily stretching regimens. Mobility places the lower extremities in a dependent position, requiring compression garments to be appropriately donned before mobility.

Personal device care takes on a new level of complexity as clothing, reusable compression garments, splints, and prosthetic devices require proper cleaning daily to reduce risk of infection, as wounds may remain open for weeks or months. Personal hygiene and grooming require manual dexterity often compromised from severe burns. This is critical in the burn population as 70%–80% of all burn patients have injuries to their hands. Sexual activity is often a long-term psychosocial issue for severe burn survivors, resulting from severe deformity and post-traumatic stress.

IADLs are often affected because they require a higher level of planning, endurance, and complexity than basic self-care. Caring for oneself initially predominates a burn patient's life. Caring for pets, children, and others often becomes the responsibility of the patients' families, friends, and caregivers. Engagement in these IADLs is part of role fulfillment that contributes to a positive identity. Giving up these occupations, even temporarily, after a severe burn injury is difficult for patients and their families. Communication also can be an issue because patients with large burns require prolonged sedation and intubation. Patients awake lethargic and unable to vocalize over the ventilator or past their tracheotomy intubation. Patients initially require augmented communication devices such as communication boards or switch buttons.

Communication issues may subside after extubation or may continue as a result of deformities of the face and jaw or injury to vocal cords from repeated intubations. Community mobility is affected because patients must be wary of prolonged exposure to sunlight, maintain elevation of burned extremities, and may suffer fatigue from severe muscle atrophy as a result of inactivity in an intensive care unit (ICU) and a hypermetabolic state. Financial management often becomes overwhelming, as implications of sustaining resources after a severe burn can be devastating to families and patients. Severe burns may require significant personal and community financial resources for continued care and can disrupt family roles and careers.

Health management and maintenance are required for supplemental strengthening and nutrition programs because of the devastating extent of burns and prolonged ICU stays. Home establishment and management are complex because physical limitation and modifications are needed after hospital discharge. Home environments may be destroyed or damaged by fire, and burn patients may need to take precautions against exposure to the sun, caustic cleaning agents, extreme heat, and so forth. Meal preparation and cleanup may be complicated by a post-trauma fear of exposure to fire. Other complications involve exposure to heat, planning a high-protein meal to facilitate healing, and managing underlying health issues.

Religious observance is offered to patients and families at the time of admission to the hospital because patient and family belief systems are vital for them to cope with such a traumatic event. Safety and emergency maintenance for patients as they discharge from medical settings to communities with fewer resources requires planning and follow-up. Families undergo training and education by staff and are connected to resources within the community. Shopping and purchasing proper, nutritious foods require coordination with caregivers. Driving to the stores may be prohibited due to narcotic pain medication use, and limited finances may prohibit purchasing recommended foods. Rest and sleep are often disrupted because of itching, nervousness, sleeplessness, pain, nightmares, or fears related to the event leading to injury. Rest and sleep are essential for healing, strengthening, and maintaining focus during treatment. Patients' sleep is often disturbed for months to years after the initial injury. Occupational therapists work to resolve symptoms through pressure support garments, massage, adaptation, stretching, and elevation but should also advocate for medications or other remedies as needed through the assistance of the medical team.

Returning to school requires the resolution of many physical problems. Students must be able to mentally focus, which requires reducing their medications for pain and itching. They must to sit for prolonged periods of time, putting their lower extremities in dependent positions that cause swelling and increased pain. Younger students with open wounds are often not allowed back into the classroom because of school policy. Deformities and the appearance of scar tissue change the self-image of students returning to school and add stress and anxiety to the situation. Occupational therapists and the burn team often engage in school reentry programs to help students understand how to relate to their classmates' questions and stares.

Returning to work after a severe burn is a complex social activity. It can include fear of being fired because of performance issues related to decreased endurance and strength and worries about self-image and whether or not the employer will provide reasonable accommodations to address disability concerns. Understandably, patients' employment and finances dominate their focus as they heal and obligations to pay medical and utility bills become a reality.

Play for children remains as important as work for adults. Occupational therapists teach families of children with severe burns to facilitate safe play that is graded to the child's ability. Play should not threaten wound integrity or contribute to scarring or deformity. Goals for children are active engagement in activities that create challenging, enjoyable environments, allowing them to develop the social and physical skills necessary for their healthy growth.

Leisure and social participation are stressed and encouraged for patients with burns and their families to reengage in society and normalizing activities. Leisure exploration or continuation can be hampered by precautions related to burn management, such as managing sun exposure and other environmental risks. Patients need encouragement and support to grade their level of participation in leisure activities to re-engage in activities that are meaningful to them. Returning to community activities with scarring, pigment loss, amputations, or deformity can be difficult to manage, resulting in social anxiety and a tendency to become reclusive and fearful. Sometimes it also involves dealing with the loss of family members or loved ones.

Burn centers employing occupational therapists provide interdisciplinary, specialized medical teams whose primary focus is the management of patients with burns ranging from benign to life-threatening. The American College of Surgeons (ACS; 2006) defined a *burn therapist* as "a physical or occupational therapist who has a commitment to the care of burn patients and is responsible for providing rehabilitation services in the burn center." Each discipline brings unique skills and perspectives to the treatment of burn patients.

Patients suffering severe burns (20% or greater total body surface area [TBSA]) have performance areas that are affected across the *Occupational Therapy Practice Framework* (AOTA, 2008a) spectrum. Functional performance is diminished when pain affects behavior, judgment, sleep cycles, and motivation. Patients often suffer disfiguring scars, contractures, and amputations, resulting in years of reconstructive surgeries and diminished body images. They also go through significant mental health counseling. Additionally, the pre-existing environments burn patients had known as "home" may be forever altered; homes may be burned, workplaces exploded, and families suffering terrible losses. Trauma related to burn injuries is physical, psychological, and spiritual, affecting patient engagement in occupations that supported health, well-being, and positive identities.

The occupational therapist's role begins as patients enter the burn center setting. The focus is on functional recovery. Verified burn centers require occupational therapy evaluations within 24 hours of patient admittance (American Burn Association, 2007). The roles of genetics, pharmacology, and rehabilitation are still not fully understood (Helm, Herndon, & deLateur, 2007), but keeping patients engaged in activity and movement is considered the best course of treatment during rehabilitation. Within this rehabilitation activity regimen, occupational therapists advocate for patients' needs and full resumption of meaningful and rewarding lives.

People with burn injuries typically have such highly complex medical issues that it is sometimes difficult to know where to begin occupational therapy intervention. Using clinical reasoning and multiple frames of reference (e.g., the Model of Human Occupation [MOHO], Occupational Adaptation [OA] Model, Model of Human Ecology [MHE], and Person–Environment–Occupation Performance Model [PEOP]), experienced therapists can begin to chart an intervention plan. Occupational therapists in burn care need to find ways to provide client-centered intervention in a high-paced acute care environment where facility demands must also be considered (Addy, 2006). Flexibility in approaches is important because the diversity of patients and injuries requires constant adjustment of intervention approaches and grading of activities. These approaches must consider the aggressive physiological response to wound healing. Non–burn-specific treatment programs have shown a 67% increase in hypertrophic scarring and an average hospital length of stay 4 days longer than patients undergoing burn-specific rehabilitation programs (Okhovatian & Zoubine, 2006).

Clinical practice in burn care can be overwhelming, requiring facility-developed competencies and mentorship. Burn-related therapies require an understanding of physiology, wound-healing processes, scar management, the vascular system, and splinting, as well as the ability to work with a diverse range of ages. Burn therapy should be guided by senior clinicians, evidence-based practice, and research. Burn-related therapies continue to grow with evidence from qualitative case studies, use of standardized evaluation tools, and multicenter studies (Edgar, 2009).

Factors That Influence Burn Injury Outcomes

Burn team members consider many factors when developing goals and treatment plans for specific patients. Those factors include the depth of the burn; the mechanism of injury; the percentage of total body surface area burned (% TBSA); and the severity of the burns, including their location and subsequent quality of wound healing. A patient's age, preinjury health and emotional stability, motivation, and engagement in treatment, as well as family member support, are other factors that can have a direct affect on the recovery process.

Burn Depth

Prediction of the potential for long-term activity impairment begins with an evaluation of burn depth. Burn injuries are labeled *superficial, superficial partial-thickness, deep partial-thickness, full-thickness,* or *subdermal*. The period required for healing and the risk for scarring are directly related to the depth of the burn and the time the wound requires to close, which are estimated from clinical evaluation of the wounds appearance, vascularity, sensitivity, and pliability (Table 13.1).

Superficial burns heal without surgical intervention, like a sunburn, whereas deep partial-thickness burns may require surgery. Surgeries range in severity and complexity. Once wounds are healed, they tend to be excessively dry, itchy, and vulnerable to injury from trauma and shearing forces often caused by rubbing or scratching. These shearing forces result

Table 13.1. Burn Wound Characteristics

Burn Depth	Tissue Depth	Clinical Findings	Healing Time	Common Causes	Scar Potential
Superficial (first degree)	Epidermis	Erythema, dry, no blisters Moderate pain	3–7 days	Sunburn, brief flash burns, brief exposure to hot liquids or chemicals	No potential for hypertrophic scarring or contractures
Superficial partial-thickness (superficial second degree) and donor sites	Epidermis, upper dermis	Erythema, wet, blisters Significant pain	Less than 2 weeks	Severe sunburn or radiation burns, prolonged exposure to hot liquids, brief contact with hot metal surfaces	Minimal potential for hypertrophic scarring or contractures unless secondary infection or trauma delays healing for longer than 2 weeks or if the patient has a genetic predisposition for scarring
Deep partial-thickness (deep second degree) and traumatized or infected donor sites	Epidermis and deeper dermis, but skin appendages survive, from which skin may regenerate	Erythema; usually broken blisters (but palms and soles of feet have large, possibly intact blisters over beefy red dermis) Severe pain to touch Hypersensitivity to heat	More than 2 weeks May convert to full thickness with onset of infection or repeated trauma	Flames; firm or prolonged contact with hot metal objects; prolonged contact with hot, viscous liquids	High potential for hypertrophic scarring and contractures across joints, web spaces, skin cleavages, and facial contours; high risk for boutonnière deformities if dorsal fingers are involved
Full thickness	Epidermis and dermis; skin appendages and nerve endings are nonviable	Pale, nonblanching, dry, coagulated capillaries may be seen No sensation to light touch except at deep partial-thickness borders	Large areas require surgical intervention for wound closure; small areas may heal in from the borders over an extended period of time	Extreme heat or prolonged exposure to heat, hot objects, or chemical agents	Very high potential for hypertrophic scarring and contractures, depending on the method used for wound closure and period required for wound healing
Subdermal	Full-thickness burn with damage to underlying tissues	Nonviable surface; may be charred or with exposed fat, tendons, muscle, or bone Electrical injuries may have small external wounds but significant subdermal tissue damage and peripheral nerve damage	Requires surgical intervention for wound closure May require amputation or significant reconstruction	Electrical burns and severe long-duration burns (e.g., house fires, motor vehicle accidents with passenger entrapment inside the burning vehicle or under the hot exhaust system, smoking in bed, or alcohol-related burns)	Similar to full-thickness burn, except when amputation removes the burn site and the borders of the surgery are closed primarily without grafting

in separation of the newly healed skin layers and consequential blister formation. With repeated injury, the skin's integrity is further compromised, and potential for scarring increases.

Partial-thickness and full-thickness burns usually result in uneven pigmentation, with combinations of hypopigmentation and hyperpigmentation of the healed skin tissue. Deep-partial and full-thickness burns also have greater potential for developing thick, hypertrophic scarring and contracture formation because of the prolonged healing period and resulting collagen overgrowth. This potential is higher with partial-thickness burns that convert to full-thickness as a result of infection or repeated trauma.

To obtain prompt wound closure, larger full-thickness wounds require surgical intervention such as skin grafting. The longer a full-thickness burn is allowed to heal independently without surgery intervention, the greater the potential for scarring. Skin graft donor sites usually have healing timeframes of 1–2 weeks and end results similar to those of superficial partial-thickness burns, with less scarring but sometimes uneven pigmentation. However, if healing is delayed by trauma or infection, then a donor site has the same scarring potential as a deep partial-thickness burn.

Mechanism of Injury

The mechanism of a burn injury and the duration and intensity of exposure to the damage-causing agents are also determinants of severity. Superficial partial-thickness burns typically occur after a brief contact with hot liquids, heated surfaces, or flash flames. Deep partial-thickness burns are caused by longer-duration exposure to intense heat, such as with hot water immersion scalds or prolonged exposure to flaming materials and hot surfaces. Full-thickness and subdermal burns usually result from electrical currents, prolonged contact with viscous liquids or adhesive melted substances (e.g., hot grease, tar, melted plastics), contact with caustic chemical agents such as battery acid, extended exposure to flames, or high-temperature immersion scalds. Chemical burns may be deceptive in appearance and should be considered full-thickness until they are proven otherwise (Herndon, 2007). Chemical burns may result in complex, neuropathic, long-term symptoms that may remain for years.

Percentage of Total Body Surface Area Involved

The severity of a burn injury is measured by estimating the proportion of the body's skin that has been affected. The percentage of TBSA is estimated by using the "rule of nines" and the Lund and Browder Chart (Herndon, 2007). The rule of nines method is simple and quick and may be useful for fast estimates in the emergency department, but it is relatively inaccurate. It divides the body surface into areas comprising 9%, or multiples of 9%, with the perineum or neck making up the final 1%. The head area is 9%, each upper extremity is 9%, each leg is 18%, and the front and back of the trunk are each 18%. The rule of nine applies only to adults, however; body proportions vary in children, especially in the head, neck, and legs, depending on their age (Herndon, 2007).

The Lund and Browder Chart (Lund & Browder, 1944), which is used in most burn centers, provides a more accurate estimate of the total percentage of TBSA. Lund and Browder designed the original template on which many mapping evaluation tools are based today. It assigns a percentage of surface area to body segments, with adjusted calculations for different age groups. For smaller percentage of TBSA injuries, the therapist can get a quick estimate using size of the patient's palm (hand excluding the fingers), which equals approximately 1% of the person's total body surface area.

Severity of Injury

The percentage of TBSA and the depth of the burn together serve as the primary determinants of burn injury severity. A deep partial-thickness or full-thickness burn to more than 20% TBSA is often the determining factor for admission to a burn ICU. Depending on the patient's age and preinjury health, smaller partial-thickness or full-thickness burn wounds of less than 20% TBSA can still be considered severe burn injuries. For most adults, a deep partial-thickness and full-thickness burn of greater than 40% of total body surface area is considered severe. Children younger than 5 years of age and adults older than 50 years of age are considered to be at greater risk of death from large burns, so a 20% burn is considered severe for these populations. The presence of associated injuries such as inhalation injury, fractures, or other trauma contributes to severity.

Burns to specific body areas also influence severity, even though the percentage of TBSA is relatively small. Patient referrals to verified burn centers often are determined by the severity of burn. The guidelines set forth for referral to a burn center by the ACS (2006) are

- Partial-thickness burns of greater than 10% of the total body surface area;
- Burns that involve the face, hands, feet, genitalia, perineum, or major joints;
- Third-degree burns in any age group;

- Electrical burns, including lightning injury;
- Chemical burns;
- Inhalation injury;
- Burn injury with pre-existing medical disorders that could complicate management, prolong recovery, or affect mortality;
- Burns and concomitant trauma (e.g., fractures) in which the burn injury poses the greatest risk of morbidity or mortality (in such cases, if the trauma poses the greater immediate risk, the patient's condition may be stabilized initially in a trauma center before transfer to a burn center; physician judgment will be necessary in such situations and should be in concert with the regional medical control plan and triage protocols);
- Burned children in hospitals without qualified personnel or equipment for the care of children; and
- Burn injury in patients who will require special social, emotional, or rehabilitative intervention.

Burns of the face, eyes, and neck often interfere with respiration, vision, and feeding and may result in long-term functional and cosmetic impairment. Bilateral hand burns may initially limit the person's self-care ability and can result in permanent impairment of occupational performance if not properly managed from the onset of treatment.

Wound Care and Surgical Intervention

Most burn wounds are treated with some form of antibacterial agent that reduces the potential for wound infections (Richard & Stanley, 1994). If the wound is relatively clean, a biological dressing may be used as a temporary wound covering. Types of biological dressings include *homografts*, which are processed cadaver skin; *cultured epithelial autografts*, which are autograft grown in labs from skin biopsies of the patient; *xenografts*, which are processed pig skin; and *synthetic products* or *artificial skin substitutes*.

The extent and depth of the burn wound determine the need for surgical treatment. When it appears that a deep partial-thickness burn will take more than 2 weeks to heal, surgery may accelerate wound healing, shorten hospital length of stay, and reduce the potential for hypertrophic scarring. The most common form of surgical intervention for serious burn wounds is the use of split-thickness skin autografting. In this procedure, the dead burned tissue, or *eschar*, is surgically debrided. Then the top

layer of skin is harvested from an unburned donor site and applied over the debrided burn site. In 3–7 days the transplanted split-thickness skin graft is revascularized and permanently adhered. During this period the graft site is kept immobilized, often with thermoplastic splints, to keep the skin graft from being dislodged or sheared. The donor site has the appearance and discomfort of a severe abrasion and usually heals in 7–10 days.

If adequate donor sites for autografting are not available, or when burn depth or infections create conditions such that the grafted tissue will not survive, temporary xenograft, cadaver, or synthetic biological dressings may be used over the burns until the site is ready for autografting. The use of these temporary biological dressing helps to control pain, decrease infection, and prevent evaporative loss. Full-thickness skin grafts may be used for areas such as around facial features or over an area of chronic skin breakdown; such areas require greater flexibility and durability and have a lower potential for scar contraction than what a split-thickness graft could provide. This type of autografting usually involves excising a full-thickness fold or flap of unburned skin and transplanting it to an open area created where a tight scar or eschar has been released. The full-thickness donor site is then closed primarily or split-thickness skin grafted to repair the defect.

Scar Formation

According to recent surveys of the professional burn community, nearly one-third of all respondents identified burn scarring as an area needing further research and investigation (Richard et al., 2009). Scar formation and severity are difficult to predict and objectively evaluate, which leads to competing opinions and treatment approaches. After initial healing, some scars rise above the original level of the skin surface and become thick and rigid, remaining erythemic in appearance. These are referred to as *hypertrophic scars*. Hypertrophic scarring is the burn injury complication that most often limits independence with daily activities. The longer a wound remains open and a scar stays inflamed, the higher the potential for excessive scarring. Scarring has been shown to have profound rehabilitation consequences, including loss of function, impairment, disability, and difficulty pursuing recreational and vocational pursuits (Engrav, Garner, & Tredget, 2007).

Hypertrophic scars usually begin developing during the first few months after a deep-partial or full-thickness burn heals. Secondary trauma and infection can impede healing and prolong the inflammatory response, resulting in collagen overgrowth and the development of hypertrophic scar tissue. A hypertrophic scar that not only rises above the original skin surface but also expands horizontally beyond the original borders of the scar is referred to as a *keloid scar.*

A scar's functional and cosmetic significance depend on its anatomical location. Joint motion is limited when a scar complex develops across a joint surface and contracts, creating a restrictive band of scar tissue. This is known as a *scar contracture.* When tight or hypertrophic scars develop on the face, they distort facial features and interfere with eating, eye closure, and facial expression.

Regardless of the wound care methods used and the time taken for wound closure, scar maturation differs with each person. As a scar matures it becomes metabolically inactive and no longer attempts to contract. The erythema fades, the texture softens, and the scar becomes more pliable and elastic. Superficial partial-thickness, nonhypertrophic scars can mature in 5–8 weeks. However, hypertrophic scars can take 18–24 months to mature, and keloid scars take even longer. Surgical scars from reconstruction procedures may mature faster, depending on the length of time to heal. Once scars are mature, compression therapy, massage, and other scar management interventions may be discontinued, although some skin care precautions will continue lifelong.

Although it is sometimes possible to anticipate outcomes from the depth and location of the wound, other factors can also affect the final results. Genetic predisposition for scarring, age, and preexisting health problems, for example, also influence healing and scar formation. Elderly patients may heal more slowly and with less incidence of collagen overgrowth. Small children tend to heal quickly but have a much higher potential for hypertrophic scarring. Patients with diabetes, peripheral vascular disease, or other conditions that restrict circulation may heal more slowly and be at greater risk for secondary infection.

Special Consideration for Hand Burns

Hand burns are often prevalent in patients because of their attempts to defend themselves from fire, escape burning structures, manage flammable materials, or put out fires. Hands support our ability to engage within the environment and are visible as we interact within the community. "Despite the fact that the surface area of the hand represents 1/40th of an individual's TBSA, an isolated hand burn is an indication alone for referral to a burn center for care" (Richard et al., 2009, p. 543). Because the hands are a tool of independence, it is important to address the burn wound promptly. A quarter of all patients in a study of 985 patients had burns resulting in contractures and, of those, an average of 10 contractures were noted in the hand (Schneider et al., 2008). Deep full-thickness burns are the most severe and are estimated to make up 5% or less of all hand burns (Kowalske, Greenhalgh, & Ward, 2007). The rare occurrence of these hand burns may lead to mismanagement of the burns and to contractures that place clients at risk for deformity and long-term dysfunction.

Pediatric hand burns are particularly common because it is the natural curiosity of children to touch and feel their surroundings without fear of hot surfaces (Figure 13.1). "Dorsal burns are frequently scald injuries from hot liquids, whereas burns to the palm usually result from direct contact with a radiator or iron" (Feldman, Evans, & O, 2008, p. 942). Though the severity of the burn may be in question, it is always suggested that a child with a hand burn

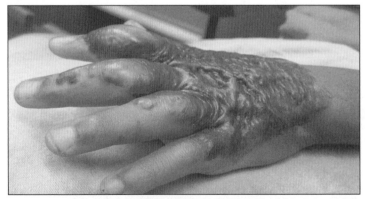

Figure 13.1. Hypertrophic scarring to the dorsum of a child's hand.
Photo Credit: Beth Bale, 2009.

be evaluated by a burn center where appropriate resources and education can be provided to prevent potential scar contracture formation, as recommended be the American Burn Association (Feldman et al., 2008, p. 943).

Burn Patients in the Intensive Care Unit

Occupational therapists should provide services even when patients are sedated and intubated in order to facilitate proper healing and keep them positioned to maximize function when they recover. During periods of medically induced comas, patients will receive continuous and repetitive hours of therapy, including splinting, ROM, positioning, family and caregiver education, and advocacy to the medical team on the progress of the patient.

Families and caregivers often develop strong relationships with therapists while their family member or loved one is sedated. Those relationships assist the therapist in gaining the trust of their patients once they are awake. Even before sedation is weaned and patients are able to engage, therapists can begin to interpret their patients' stories: who they are, their roles, and the occupations that were meaningful to them. Bedside ICU care can often last for months, requiring the team of occupational therapists and occupational therapy assistants to use all the resources available to them to maximize the patient's functional outcomes.

ICUs are highly technical, and occupational therapists should be aware of precautions for all the medical lines and leads that provide fluid, pain relief, and antibiotics. Burn patients have a high risk of infection and require continuous central line changes. Occupational therapists must assume that precautions my change quickly and day to day. The primary registered nurse should be consulted, and an in-depth review of the patient's daily status should be addressed before the occupational therapist begins to work with him or her. Infections prevalent in burn centers are often multidrug-resistant strains, which cause sepsis and further compromise patients. Therapists are required to wear protective gowns and gloves and follow strict hand hygiene and cleaning practices when disinfecting clinical surfaces.

Phases of Recovery

Burn rehabilitation can be divided into early, intermediate, and long-term phases of recovery (Richard et al., 2008). Occupational therapists play a vital role through all phases.

Early Rehabilitation Phase

The *early rehabilitation phase* begins immediately after injury and usually continues until extensive wound care needs are minimal, wounds are 50% closed, or grafting has been initiated (Richard et al., 2008). During the first few days of this phase, the focus of the burn team members is on the survival of the patient. During this time there is a severe fluid shift into the interstitial tissues and generalized swelling, and burn team members must work to reduce edema while ensuring that circulatory fluid resuscitation is accomplished. Fluid loss resulting from severe burns can cause burn shock and subsequent failure of the kidneys if not managed carefully. Smoke and heat inhalation injuries often accompany burns and result in the need for mechanical ventilation or a tracheostomy to protect the patient's airway.

As the medical team members work to stabilize the patient, the occupational therapist should be anticipating and planning for the patient's rehabilitation needs. This initial evaluation should involve the total patient, not just the burn wound, which means that the occupational therapist should learn as much as possible about the patient's pre-injury personality, performance patterns, and life context. Many patients with severe burns arrive intubated at the time of admission, and the occupational therapist may need to interview family and friends for pertinent information.

As the patient becomes medically stable, prevention of deformity and preservation of function become more significant. A more extensive evaluation of ROM, sensation, general strength, cognition, and overall abilities is performed. The therapist then develops and initiates a customized intervention program designed to minimize or prevent long-term loss of occupational performance.

Intermediate Rehabilitation Phase

When a burn patient enters the *intermediate rehabilitation phase* of recovery, preserving independent function and prevention of disability and deformity become the central themes of intervention. Wound care continues, with increasing active participation by the patient and family members. Emphasis in this phase is placed on general reconditioning (e.g., strength, flexibility, endurance), scar management, improving performance with self-care activities (e.g., self-feeding, wound skin care, personal hygiene and grooming skills, dressing), and social reintegration.

Long-Term Rehabilitation Phase

The *long-term rehabilitation phase* is identified as beginning at the time of wound closure or discharge from the hospital setting. The focus of care continues to center on minimizing hypertrophic scar and contracture formation; improving flexibility, strength, and endurance; assuring proper skin and scar care techniques; and promoting independence in normal daily activities, including self-care and social and recreational pursuits. Community reintegration and socialization issues become more important. A primary objective is to help the patient adjust physically and emotionally to residual effects of the injury. This phase of rehabilitation may include reconstructive surgeries and lifelong services for contractures being exacerbated by patients' growth and aging. Vascular support compression garments, splints, and ADLs may require updating and adjustments as well as adaptations.

Most burn patients discontinue routine outpatient rehabilitation services when they achieve the skills needed to perform ADLs independently at home and can return to school or work full-time. The time a burn patient requires before returning to work is dependent on the TBSA, depth of burn, and whether hands were involved (Richard et al., 2008). Before discharge from the hospital, follow-up visits to a burn outpatient clinic should be scheduled to monitor scar maturation, pain levels, and wound healing.

Role of Occupational Therapy

The role of occupational therapy in intervention with patients who have severe burns is multifaceted and changes as the patient moves through the phases of recovery. It is necessary to preserve ROM, strength, and endurance so the patient is capable of performing ADLs in the future. Fatigue is almost universally reported by patients with burns who are working to become independent in ADLs and return to work (Helm et al., 2007). Dynamic conceptual models of occupational therapy are useful for understanding the effect of a serious burn injury on the life of a patient (Baum & Christiansen, 1997; Kielhofner, 1995; Law et al., 1996). Such models suggest that restrictions in the ability to move and perform tasks reduce the patient's ability to accomplish necessary roles, which in turn influences his or her view of self as a competent person. Over time, diminished self-perception can affect interests and values and reduce motivation, resulting in adverse physical, social, and emotional consequences.

When people sustain severe burn injuries, they are initially unable to complete self-care activities. Reasons for this include the severity and location of the wounds, scarring, weakness, restrictive dressings, medication, hospital routines, pain, and anxiety.

Impaired physical abilities, changed appearance, isolation, and dramatic changes in one's usual daily routines seriously alter the patient's previous roles.

Changes in motivation may occur at the time of injury and can continue for many years after discharge. Values can change, and self-esteem and confidence may be adversely affected because of negative body-image issues. Social and personal interests may diminish, particularly if the injury occurred during a specific social activity or was connected to a tragedy that resulted in loss of a loved one.

By viewing the patient within a dynamic conceptual model, rehabilitation focuses on the relationship between the injury and the patient as a multifaceted being. Within this context, both evaluation and intervention strategies should be planned to initially address the patient's personal, emotional, social, cultural, and spiritual priorities as well as the easily identified physical and performance skill deficits.

Acute Rehabilitation Phase: Evaluation

Whenever possible, patients are evaluated by an occupational therapist within the first 24 hours after admission to the hospital. A pre-assessment review of the medical record is pertinent for obtaining information regarding the mechanism of injury; the percentage of TBSA affected; the depth of the burn; the presence of associated injuries such as inhalation injury or fractures; and previous medical history, social history, and living situation (Figure 13.2). This information should be confirmed and supplemented by communication with the patient and family members.

Ideally, at least part of the initial occupational therapy evaluation should take place when wound dressings are removed, when the patient has had pain medications, and when the depth and exact location of the burns can be viewed directly and documented in detail. Distinctions should be made between superficial and deep partial-thickness burns, as well as full-thickness burns, by appearance and quality of sensation. The therapist needs to view the wounds as soon as possible after the injury. Burn eschar develops quickly, making accurate evaluation of burn depth difficult by causing deep partial-thickness burns to closely resemble full-thickness burns in appearance and sensitivity. Attention should also be directed to burns involving joint surface areas and the presence of any circumferential burns.

The extremities should be screened for possible peripheral nerve damage by checking for the presence and quality of sensation. This is especially important with electrical or multiple trauma injuries. The dorsum of the hands should be checked for

Burn Estimation Chart

Date of Admission_____

Date of Injury_____Time of injury:_____

Age:_____Sex:_____

Type of Injury:
      Flame   _____
      Electrical   _____
      Scald   _____
      Chemical   _____
      Inhalation   _____

Height (cm):   _____

Weight (kg):   _____

Body Surace (m2):   _____

Date completed: _____

Completed by: _____
                     Name
             _____
              ID# (Required)

BURN ESTIMATE - AGE VS AREA

Area	Birth-1 year	1-4 years	5-9 years	10-14 years	15 years	Adult	2°	3°	TBSA %
Head	19	17	13	11	9	7			
Neck	2	2	2	2	2	2			
Anterior trunk	13	13	13	13	13	13			
Posterior trunk	13	13	13	13	13	13			
Right Buttock	2.5	2.5	2.5	2.5	2.5	2.5			
Left Buttock	2.5	2.5	2.5	2.5	2.5	2.5			
Genitalia	1	1	1	1	1	1			
Right upper arm	4	4	4	4	4	4			
Left upper arm	4	4	4	4	4	4			
Right lower arm	3	3	3	3	3	3			
Left lower arm	3	3	3	3	3	3			
Right hand	2.5	2.5	2.5	2.5	2.5	2.5			
Left hand	2.5	2.5	2.5	2.5	2.5	2.5			
Right thigh	5.5	6.5	8	8.5	9	9.5			
Left thigh	5.5	6.5	8	8.5	9	9.5			
Right leg	5	5	5.5	6	6.5	7			
Left leg	5	5	5.5	6	6.5	7			
Right foot	3.5	3.5	3.5	3.5	3.5	3.5			
Left foot	3.5	3.5	3.5	3.5	3.5	3.5			
					TOTAL				

Figure 13.2. Burn estimation chart.
Source. NC Jaycee Burn Center: UNC Healthcare. Used with permission.

deep burns, especially over the proximal interphalangeal joints, which could indicate the need to initiate boutonnière deformity precautions or hand splints. In addition, an active or active–assistive ROM assessment should be done to evaluate joint mobility and general strength before restrictive dressings are applied or significant edema develops.

Once the dressings are in place and nursing care is completed, a more comprehensive occupational therapy evaluation can be performed. An in-depth history is needed from the patient and/or family members to establish the patient's preburn level of occupational performance, including physical, cognitive, and social skills and previous performance patterns (habits, routines, and roles). This history would include information about the patient's home environment and responsibilities, occupational background and work skills, educational level, hand dominance, and any pre-existing conditions (physical, psychological, or social) that would affect the patient's occupational performance. Understanding the patient's pre-injury performance patterns and life context is important for setting realistic treatment goals and also for establishing a therapeutic relationship with the patient and family members. Patient and caregiver education should be initiated on this first contact and continued as an essential part of therapy throughout the stages of recovery.

During the first 24–72 hours postburn, acute, generalized edema develops, limiting the end ranges of joints, weighing down extremities, and impairing active ROM. For this reason, formal joint goniometry may not be practical. However, the therapist should note any developing joint stiffness not explained by pre-existing conditions such as old injuries, congenital abnormalities, or age-related joint disease. Edema may mask acute related orthopedic issues from the time of injury. If injuries are suspected, treatment should be held, and X-rays may be recommended. Acute edema in the extremities can be monitored by taking circumferential measurements over established anatomical landmarks or by using a finger impression method. The impression method measures pitting edema by documenting, in millimeters, the depth of the impression a fingertip will make if pressed over a bony prominence for 5 seconds.

During the initial 24- to-72-hour period, patients should be properly positioned with upper extremities or lower extremities elevated above heart level to prevent conversion of wounds resulting from fluid congestion in burned extremities. Often swelling of the extremities can lead to deformity, which occupational therapists must monitor and prevent. As wounds over joints close, the scarring may lead to joint contractures and deformities. Splints should be placed on patients who are sedated and not able to participate actively in therapy to prevent burn scar contractures and to maintain functional positioning. Unstable joints from burn-related trauma may require splints to promote functional position and improve joint stability. Splints stabilize deformity and decrease contractures of the skin, while stretching and ROM activities progress the function.

If active ROM is not promptly regained as acute edema decreases, then goniometric measurements should be used to formally document changes in joint mobility. When possible, goniometer measurements should be compared between involved and uninvolved joints to assist in establishing the patient's personal norms. The extent and the causes of limitations in motion should be determined from both the physical and psychological perspectives. A comparison of active and active–assistive ROM is preferred, but a patient may resist assistive or passive motion because of apprehension, pain, or confusion. If the patient is unresponsive or unable to participate, the therapist should evaluate joint mobility using nonaggressive–passive ROM.

An initial screening of gross strength is performed by a manual test of major muscle groups, such as by using a dynamometer for measuring a patient's grip strength. Because the burn does not initially affect muscle strength, this test can help identify any associated injuries, peripheral nerve damage, or preexisting conditions. However, assessment of muscle strength several days postinjury can be adversely affected by pain, medications, and edema. Actual performance of daily skills should be assessed beginning in the acute phase and continued throughout the phases of recovery. Observation of eating, grooming, and basic self-care skills is important in determining whether appropriate or compensatory actions are being used. To overcome interference from dressings, edema, or pain, patients often demonstrate resourcefulness by initiating adaptive methods on their own. However, some compensatory motions may also be associated with abnormal posturing, which may lead to additional problems in the future and will need to be addressed in discharge planning.

Acute Rehabilitation Phase: Intervention

During the acute rehabilitation phase, pain is a primary issue with patients. Most patients with a severe burn injury naturally respond to pain by resisting painful motions or activities. Therapists should be supportive, explaining beforehand what is to be done in terms the patient can comprehend. Involving the patient and family in goal setting and offering choices when establishing schedules is a way to offer more control to the patient, which is often helpful in promoting his or her commitment to treatment. Patients have to develop rapport with their therapists and understand the rehabilitation process in order to maximize their outcomes.

The patient is usually more interested in whether a procedure will be painful or how long it will last than in the logistical information. Coordinating treatments with the nursing staff for scheduled pain medications is often helpful and highly recommended, especially if active participation is needed. Relaxation techniques, such as breathing exercises and guided imagery, may be helpful with motivated patients. These practices are often taught by recreational therapists. However, if a patient's anxiety or pain is disproportionate to the treatment, anti-anxiety medication may be indicated both to relieve anxiety and to increase the effectiveness of pain medication. Time limits on painful treatment sessions should be predetermined with all patients who are cognizant and capable of participation. These limits should be consistently adhered to by the therapist to foster trust and a sense of control for the patient. Depending on the presence of associated conditions or complications, the patient may be disoriented or unable to follow verbal cueing and thus require passive ROM exercise. In these circumstances, it is still important to continue to attempt full ROM using verbal encouragement, and smooth, rhythmic patterns of movement with nonaggressive, sustained end-range stretches. Individual joint ROM may be needed for problem areas, but in most cases, combined joint stretches are more effective when stretching large surface area burns. This also decreases the length of time spent in painful therapy for the patient.

Positioning

Positioning and splinting recommendations should be made based on the need to reduce edema, preserve joint mobility and structural integrity, and protect trauma or surgical sites. The general rule for positioning is to keep the head and extremities elevated above the heart and all joints positioned in the antideformity position—when the specific body area (e.g., extremity, trunk, neck, facial feature) is positioned with the healing skin stretched opposite to the line of pull of any anticipated contracture (Reeves, 2001). This is accomplished by elevating the head of the bed, propping extremities up on pillows, and using commercial or custom-fabricated positioning devices and splints. Active; active–assistive;

and, if necessary, passive ROM exercises should be initiated promptly for all joints that develop stiffness due to edema or that are showing evidence of skin tightness.

During the transition from dependence on others to self-reliance, patients frequently demonstrate abnormal posturing during exercise or self-care activities. This protective self-positioning usually begins as a guarding response to avoid pain and discomfort, and usually in a flexed position. For example, a patient with a burned axilla may hold the extremity close to his or her side, giving in to the pull of tight scars. This results in a progressive loss of active motion that eventually leads to difficulty performing activities such as dressing and bathing. This protective self-positioning has often been referred to as the "position of comfort." Unfortunately, this position is often the "position of deformity" as well. For this reason, preventive positioning and corrective splinting may be needed to preserve long-term joint mobility.

Splinting

Splinting in burn-patient care is an art (and a skill) that maximizes the functional outcomes of patients (see Figures 13.3–13.6). Occupational therapists build on skills developed through their graduate and clinical studies to become proficient in fabricating splints to oppose and stretch active hypertrophic tissue. Burn centers differ in how and when they use splinting, whether during the acute rehabilitation phase, post-operatively, or during the intermediate rehabilitation phase. The use of splints to manage and prevent hypertrophic scar contractures remains ubiquitous throughout the burn care community in terms of effectiveness. As noted in the *Journal of Burn Care and Rehabilitation Research* (Richard & Ward, 2005), there is controversy about splinting in burn care because of the lack of valid evidence; there appears to be anectdotal support for the theoretical foundation of splinting and its success in achieving the desired outcomes, but validity and outcome research is needed.

Splints are generally used to maintain the extremities in the antideformity position, often applied within the first day of admission. However, a splint may not always fit properly and may become constrictive if applied the first day postinjury, when the patient is undergoing fluid resuscitation and swelling is increasing. Exposed tendons can quickly become denatured and may rupture if not kept moist and splinted to prevent tension or stretching. Another situation requiring early splinting is when the patient is at risk of boutonnière deformities.

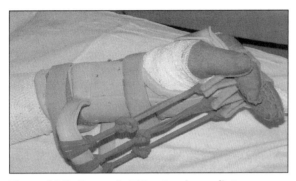

Figure 13.3. Dynamic MP extension splint. Photo Credit: Beth Bale, 2009.

When deep burns occur to the dorsal proximal interphalangeal (PIP) joints, the fingers are at risk of extensor hood disruption and subsequent boutonnière deformities. When disruption occurs, the PIP joint protrudes up through the extensor tendon mechanism, and all attempts to actively extend the finger result in flexion of the PIP joint and hyperextension of the distal interphalangeal (DIP) joint. If the PIP joints of a hand with deep dorsal burns are passively or forcefully flexed, the risk for dorsal hood disruption increases significantly. When exercising a finger under boutonnière precautions, the PIP joint is passively extended but never flexed by either the patient or the practitioner. The adjacent (DIP) and metacarpophalangeal (MP) joints can be individually flexed only with the remaining two joints of the finger held in full extension. The finger should be kept in a digit extension splint ("gutter splint") to maintain full extension of the PIP and the dorsal hood in a slacked position, and removed only to exercise the DIP. Immobilization of the PIP will allow the PIP to heal if ruptured. The stability of the joint should be reevaluated upon every treatment. The

resulting stiff PIP joint will later respond to exercise, whereas a ruptured extensor hood mechanism results in permanent loss of joint mobility and hand disfigurement.

Most splinting can be divided into three categories—*preventive, protective,* and *corrective.* Preventive splints are static, used to keep the functional position of the extremities, neck, or mouth from losing mobility due to skin tightness or contractures. The affected area is immobilized in the antideformity position, or the position that holds the skin and underlying tissues at maximum safe, tolerable stretch. Preventive splints are usually worn at night or during rest. Volar antideformity hand splints and elbow or knee extension conformers are examples of preventive splints. Protective splints are also static splints that immobilize an area to prevent motion that could compromise damaged subcutaneous structures or disrupt recently placed skin grafts or surgically reconstructed tissues. Positioning for these splints varies with the surgical procedure performed, not necessarily in the antideformity or functional positions. Corrective splinting includes dynamic or serial static splints that exert a force to stretch out tight tissues or correct a contracture. Depending on the setting, occupational therapists may splint any part of the body with the underlying

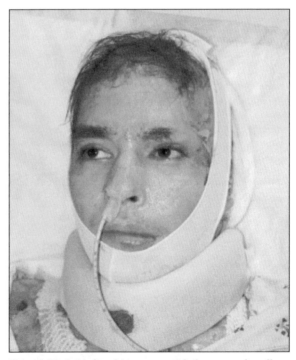

Figure 13.5. Light chin strap with foam neck collar for improved neck and lip ROM. Photo Credit: Beth Bale, 2009.

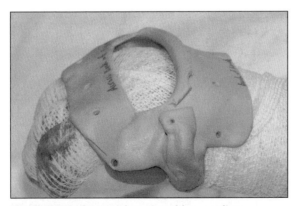

Figure 13.4. Custom functional burn splint. Photo Credit: Beth Bale, 2009.

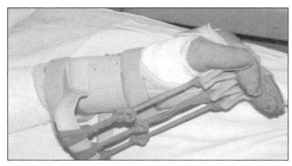

Figure 13.6. Dynamic MP flexion splint.
Photo Credit: Beth Bale, 2009.

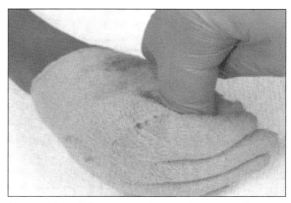

Figure 13.7. Coban wrapping to decrease edema.
Photo Credit: Beth Bale, 2009.

purpose of maximizing function and integrity of movement. Splints may include hand, wrist, elbow, axilla, foot, knee, mouth, and neck, in a static splint or with a dynamic component.

If the patient is able to participate, an active ROM exercise program should be initiated and taught to the patient and family members. Active exercise programs should be simple, easy to remember, and follow functional patterns of movement. Positioning recommendations, precautions, and splint wear schedules and instructions for exercises should be documented in the medical record and provided to the patient and family when appropriate. They should also be posted bedside in the form of simple drawings that can be easily seen from a distance by the staff, patient, and family members.

Edema

Managing edema of the extremities continues as an acute care objective (Figure 13.7). Many of the positioning techniques established initially will be continued throughout recovery. Legs should be elevated in bed or when sitting. If a patient has hand burns, the upper extremity should be elevated on a pillow with the elbow(s) above the heart and the hand(s) above the elbow. For persistent edema, external compression, through use of pressure wraps, compression garments, or treatment with intermittent compression devices, may be indicated. Patients should be expected to exercise their hands independently, especially using the intrinsic muscles. They should also be encouraged to use their hands for eating, grooming, and other functional activities as much as possible, using adapted aids as needed. The combination of active exercise, performance of self-care activities, elevation, and external compression not only helps to decrease hand edema but also promotes recovery of strength and coordination.

Self-Care Activities

Regardless of burn severity, education, or emotional support provided, some patients may perceive their injury as a permanent disability. They experience decreased self-confidence and become increasingly dependent on staff and family members. When asked to perform an ADL task, their immediate response is to anticipate failure and refuse to even try. Rather than labeling the patient "uncooperative" or "unmotivated," the therapist should grade and carefully select tasks to promote success and increase self-confidence. Self-feeding is one of the first ADL tasks learned as a child, and the inability to do so carries much significance for a person's self-esteem. Therefore, as soon as a patient is allowed any oral intake, self-feeding should be introduced, regardless of the assistance required (Figure 13.8). Early involvement in basic self-care activities, however limited, promotes a sense of efficacy by engaging the patient in goal-directed tasks that focus attention on accomplishment instead of impairment.

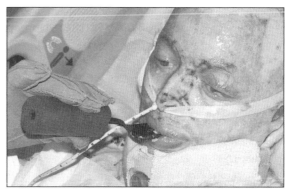

Figure 13.8. Modified cylindrical foam handle for self-feeding.
Photo Credit: Beth Bale, 2009.

When first attempting ADLs, the focus should be on accomplishing simple skills, such as holding a spoon with an enlarged handle or bringing a cup to the mouth. Initially, self-care tasks should be simplified with adapted aids, as needed, to ensure patient participation and success, which will provide a sense of efficacy and control.

As the patient progresses with ROM, strength, and endurance goals, use of adapted aids should be reduced as more challenging and complex tasks are introduced into the patient's routine. Although considerable time and patience may be involved when using this approach, the patient's general endurance and confidence both will be enhanced for later attempts with more complex IADL tasks.

Activities as Exercise

The need for immobilization after surgical procedures will periodically limit activity participation and independence. Before surgery, the patient should be informed that a defined period of immobilization will follow the procedure, but that under supervision, certain rehabilitation activities will continue. For example, if a patient's hands and forearm burns are surgically excised and grafted, the therapist may still provide shoulder activities at the patient's bedside during the postoperative immobilization period. When a patient's hands are in postoperative dressings, self-feeding may be possible only with adaptive equipment. If adaptations are used to enhance postoperative participation in activities, the patient should understand that they are only temporary.

Loss of strength and endurance, and the resulting decrease in daily activity, are frequently a consequence of prolonged bed rest. Severe burns also increase metabolism, placing further demands on the body's general physical condition. To prevent deconditioning, acute burn patients should be involved in active exercise, structured activities, and ambulation throughout the day (Figure 13.9). A combination of active–assistive ROM, composite and individual joint stretching, and purposeful activities should be used. A therapist should communicate daily with the burn team members to help determine when to increase or decrease the patient's activity schedule. If the patient is confined to bed due to lower-extremity grafts, a modified exercise program and ADLs, such as self-feeding, simple hygiene tasks, or upper-body grooming, should still be performed. Bedside activities that require a variety of fine and gross motor skills can promote upper-extremity flexibility and general strength plus provide opportunities for socialization. Whenever

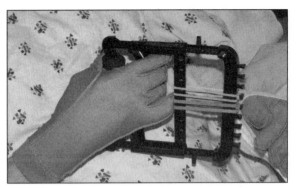

Figure 13.9. Bedside therapeutic hand exerciser. Photo Credit: Beth Bale, 2009.

possible, these activities should include current leisure interests or previous pastimes of the patient.

When a patient is medically cleared to ambulate, the intervention program should be adjusted to include out-of-bed exercise and activity. Walking or standing to do exercises, sitting up in a chair for all meals, and standing at a sink for grooming tasks help promote general conditioning. Patients often complain of fatigue during this phase of increased activity. They will need ongoing support and encouragement to ambulate, perform their exercise program, and complete their self-care tasks independently.

During acute care, a formal schedule may be needed to provide structure, support appropriate patient behaviors, and emphasize treatment objectives. The schedule should include morning and afternoon therapy sessions; dressing changes and nursing procedures; periods for ADLs, including ambulation, grooming, eating, and dressing; and highly valued free time for visitors and rest. The schedule should be developed in agreement with the patient and should be adhered to by the entire burn team. Defining daily expectations in advance will help give the patient a sense of control, reduce anxiety, and foster active involvement in the rehabilitation process.

Intermediate Rehabilitation Phase: Evaluation

During inpatient and outpatient rehabilitation phases, the therapist continuously reevaluates ROM, strength, activity tolerance, self-care abilities, work skills, skin and scar condition, and social and emotional adaptation. Goniometric measurements should be done weekly, biweekly, or as needed, depending on the frequency of treatment or need to document noted changes. Muscle strength, dexterity, and endurance can be evaluated by manual muscle testing and other evaluative tools or by using treatment modalities such as a Baltimore Therapeutic Equipment (BTE) Work Simulator. When the patient has hand burns, dynamometer recordings of grip strength and pinch gauge measures of pinch strength should be documented at regular intervals. Chronic edema of the hands can be documented using circumferential and volumetric measurements. If a volumeter is inappropriate due to open wounds or dressings on the hand, a figure-eight hand edema measurement can be taken, measuring volume changes in the dorsal compartment of the hand (Dewey et al., 2007).

Improvement in general endurance and activity tolerance should also be documented. The therapist should quantify the patient's activity tolerance during self-care activities by monitoring and recording the

- Position in which the task is performed;
- Grade or level of physical exertion the task demands;
- Amount of assistance needed (using language described by the FIM™);
- Adaptations or assistive devices required to complete the task;
- Duration of participation prior to signs of fatigue;
- Frequency and the length of needed rest breaks or percentage of the total treatment session spent resting; and
- Amount of pain noted during treatment on a scale from 1–10; if pain exceeds 4, an action in response must be documented.

Hypertrophic scars and contractures require close monitoring during this phase because they often affect the patient's ability to maintain mobility to perform everyday tasks. When assessing a scar, it is important to notice changes in appearance, texture, flexibility, and the location of any scars that restrict end-range movement in single or combined joint motions. Tight or thick scars near joints restrict mobility and cause discomfort as the patient tries to stretch to the end-ranges of the involved joint's motion. Scarring on the face often result in facial distortion, incomplete eye closure, or constriction of nasal and oral passages that impair breathing and eating abilities.

Early recognition and therapeutic intervention can often stretch out developing contractures and help reduce the likelihood of surgical intervention (Figure 13.10). However, some scar bands may be unstable and may break down during exercise, which would result in prolonged inflammation with further scarring and progressive loss of mobility.

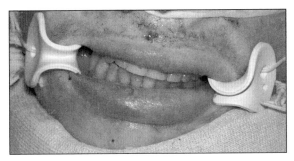

Figure 13.10. Mouth splint.
Photo Credit: Beth Bale, 2009.

Patients with tight, unstable scar bands should be referred to the surgeon for possible release of the scar band and repair of the defect with more durable grafted skin.

Continual reevaluation of a burn patient's occupational performance is an ongoing responsibility of the occupational therapist. The patient should be observed during self-care activities and watched for unnecessary exertion or use of abnormal posturing and movements. Therapy intervention should include instruction in energy conservation techniques and demonstration of methods for performing the task in normal movement patterns. For example, a patient with burns involving the trunk and extremities may become frustrated and fatigued during upper-body dressing activities and feel incapable of correctly completing the task without excessive posturing or unnecessary assistance. The patient's ability to integrate correct motions for the activity should be closely monitored while encouraging the patient's creativity in problem solving for task accomplishment.

Awareness of the patient's emotional status is important throughout recovery. Because of pain, fatigue, frustration, and other difficulties encountered with rehabilitation activities, patients may experience extreme anxiety and emotional distress, especially during painful procedures or exercises. The therapist should be aware of a patient's coping abilities and report noticeable declines in affect to the team members. As appropriate, the patient should be encouraged to discuss problems with the burn team's social worker, psychiatrist, or chaplain.

Intermediate Rehabilitation Phase: Intervention

During the inpatient intermediate rehabilitation phase, the patient's role in self-care increases as the need for wound care and nursing procedures decreases. The goal is for the patient to complete self-care activities (e.g., feeding, grooming, toileting, dressing) as independently and with as little adaptation as possible (Figure 13.11). Continued patient education stresses the importance of resuming preinjury activities, emphasizing the daily routines and habits that will give the patient more control over his or her care. However, decreased ROM, flexibility, strength, and activity tolerance may interfere with performance of more demanding ADLs, such as bathing or dressing in regular street clothes. Decreased dexterity may interfere with the completion of fine motor tasks, such as fastening clothing, and decreased sensation may put the patient at increased risk of reinjury. Poor strength and decreased activity tolerance and endurance may prevent the patient from performing repetitive activities or completing ADL tasks within acceptable time limits.

Physical Reconditioning

Exercise and ROM programs are essential; it has been shown that early intervention, begun during the acute treatment phase, has long-term implications for restoration of function (Helm et al., 2007). A burn exercise program should include stretching and flexibility exercises for the face, neck, trunk, and all extremities, as well as strengthening activities. When possible, exercises should be performed in front of a mirror so patients can self-monitor their posture and progress. Stretching should be performed slowly and prolonged at the point where the scar blanches. For scars that extend over more than one joint, the extremity should be involved in a multijoint stretch to elongate the scar fully. Active ROM should progress to resistive ROM as early as tolerated.

Independent exercise programs may include use of soft hand exercise sponges progressing to

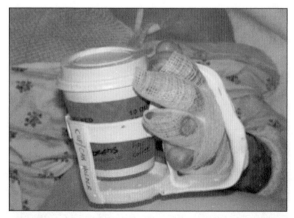

Figure 13.11. Modified cup holder for participation in ADLs.
Photo Credit: Beth Bale, 2009.

therapy putty, dynamic resistive exercises, hand grippers, pulleys, and free weights. When establishing an independent exercise program, special attention should be given to the proximal shoulder and hip muscle groups, which are often weaker from disuse or immobilization postsurgery.

Scarring, decreased sensitivity, and muscle atrophy can impair fine motor skills and hand coordination. Hand dexterity and sensitivity can be monitored and improved with tasks that require manipulation of small items of various sizes and textures. Fine motor activities of personal interest should be incorporated into the patient's independent exercise program, such as playing cards or board games; completing jigsaw puzzles, needlework, or other previous hobby interests; doing crossword puzzles; and corresponding with family to improve writing dexterity.

Aerobic activities should be incorporated into the patient's comprehensive exercise program to enhance the cardiovascular system and gain general endurance. Ideally, the patients should be able to tolerate at least 20 minutes of exercise or rhythmic activity at 60% of maximum heart rate at least 3 times a week by discharge (Breines, 2001). Endurance can be promoted by encouraging the patient to participate in independent strengthening activities such as progressively paced ambulation activities around the hospital, riding a stationary bike or using an upper-body ergometer, climbing stairs, and standing at the sink for hygiene tasks. Equipment such as a BTE Work Simulator can imitate functional motions to increase upper-body ROM, strength, and endurance, as well as provide printed results to monitor patient performance. A comprehensive circuit training program that includes stretching, strengthening, endurance, and work-hardening activities in a gym setting promotes patient independence in his or her exercise program in preparation for discharge. Occupational therapists often team with physical therapists and recreational therapists in addressing and creating strengthening and endurance program for patients.

Modalities

Therapists using modalities with patients need to have the required demonstrated training and experience outlined by AOTA and state licensing agencies. These modalities can be used as a preparation for, or concurrently with, purposeful and occupation-based activities or interventions that ultimately enhance engagement in occupation (AOTA, 2008b). Certain modalities may be beneficial in the treatment of burn scars, but due to compromised vascularity and sensitivity in the burn sites, special care must be taken when using modalities with burn patients. Cold modalities, such as ice massage or ice packs, are contraindicated, as the accompanying vasoconstriction makes the scars less pliable and may compromise skin circulation.

Heat modalities may be of benefit but should be used with close supervision. Hypertrophic scars, which already have decreased sensation, may dissipate heat more slowly and therefore be at risk for reinjury. Hot packs should have additional towel layers, and ultrasound settings should be set at a lower intensity. Paraffin used at a low temperature works well to heat and relax collagen fibers, and the mineral oil in it lubricates and softens the scars for stretching. Gauze can be dipped into the paraffin and layered onto any scar band; this modality is an effective heat treatment with areas that require sustained, low-load stretching of contractures. Some patients continue using paraffin as part of their home therapy program after discharge.

Skin Care

Newly healed skin is fragile and prone to breakdown. Problems include hypersensitivity, blisters, bruising, or excoriation resulting from friction or even minor trauma. Reduced numbers of oil and sweat glands leads to excessive dryness and possible potential damage to the skin if stretched too aggressively. Skin-conditioning education and activities should be initiated as soon as wounds are well healed, addressing the use of massage, frequent application of appropriate moisturizing products, and safe donning of intermediate and custom-made pressure garments.

Massage

Patients should be taught to massage their healed burns, graft sites, and donor site scars with a moisturizing lotion at least 3 times a day. Massage should only be performed with lotion, to prevent shearing friction, and just firm enough to cause blanching of the skin. Ideally, scars should be massaged and moisturized prior to and during stretching exercises and whenever the scars feel dry or itchy. Keeping the scars well-moisturized helps prevent spontaneous skin tears that may occur in dry scars during exercise or activity. The mechanical action of massage helps to soften the scars by promoting collagen remodeling and reducing hypersensitivity. In addition to the physical response, massage can provide psychological and emotional benefits by decreasing distress during dressing changes, as well as decreasing pain sensitivity and

depression from the initial injury (Morien, Garrison, & Keeney Smith, 2008).

Addressing Vascular Symptoms

Early compression therapy should be used to provide continuous external vascular support. Poor venous return in burned extremities is evident by the presence of edema in the limb and vascular pooling (as evidenced by erythemic skin color), and patients may report "throbbing," "itching," "stinging," and "pain." Edema can increase in dependent extremities without external venous support, especially when the patient is inactive. Vascular stockings or elastic wraps should be applied to the feet and legs to aid venous return whenever the patient is out of bed or ambulating. Because the hands and feet are especially prone to edema and contractures, they should always be elevated when at rest. Compression wraps should be applied as soon as initial healing occurs and sometimes earlier if extremities are significantly edematous.

Early compression therapy is provided with a variety of transitional compression techniques and products. For the torso and extremities, these products include elastic bandages such as Ace wraps, tubular compression sleeves, and stockings of a light compression. For the hands and digits, compression can be provided using light compression gloves such as Isotoners, digit-sized tubular support bandages, or self-adherent elastic dressings. All flexion creases, web spaces, skin cleavages, and other skin surface concavities should be padded under the wraps to insure adequate pressure.

After most wounds are healed and the patient's areas of edema have stabilized, the patient can be measured for long-term, high-compression garments, typically 20 mm Hg to 40 mm Hg pressure. Most compression garments are lightweight, 60% porous, and provide a more graded, therapeutic level of compression than temporary compression techniques.

Custom garments will require underlying conformers to equalize pressure over concavities and to increase pressure over areas of heavy scarring. Conformers can be made from a variety of materials including foam strap padding; silicone or hydrogel gel sheets; or custom molded of silicone and prosthetic foam combinations, silicone putty, or any number of products. However, even with the conformers, custom garments are less bulky than pressure wraps or temporary compression techniques and allow the patient to move more freely. Wearing personal clothing over the scar compression garments should be encouraged to promote a feeling of normalcy and to give the patient practice in donning both compression garments and street clothes. Many sunproof nylon clothing products are available that provide patients with critical protection from the sun on burned as well as grafted skin.

Activities of Daily Living

Independent performance of daily life tasks is the ultimate goal of occupational therapy. It may require regaining physical skills or adaptations to the patient's environment or routines. Some of the adaptations may be temporary, but in the case of permanent loss of physical ability, the needed adaptations may mean changes in the lifestyle and roles of the patient. Uncontrolled scarring or noncompliance with exercise programs often result in contractures, which impair motion and skin flexibility. When this occurs, previous performance patterns cannot be completed without compensatory techniques or adaptive equipment. Impaired trunk or hip mobility may prevent a patient from donning pants, underwear, socks, and shoes unless a dressing stick, sock aid, or long-handled shoehorn is provided. Impaired shoulder or elbow mobility will make donning and doffing shirts difficult, and adapted techniques or modified clothing styles with special fasteners may be needed.

For patients with contractures of the hands and fingers, feeding utensils or drinking cups with easy-to-grip handles may be needed, as well as adapted writing implements, button aids, adapted zippers, or elastic shoe laces. As soon as the patient is able to attempt basic self-care tasks, family members should be asked to bring the patient's own clothes and personal grooming items from home so that these items can be modified if needed.

Despite the extra time and effort it may take, patients should be encouraged to first attempt self-care activities with minimal reliance on compensatory motions or use of adaptive equipment. However, recognizing that motivation cannot be maintained without successful task completion, the occupational therapist should intervene and modify the task before the patient becomes too frustrated or fatigued. Otherwise, the patient may lose motivation and refuse further attempts.

As in the acute phase, the therapist should encourage self-care tasks that promote both independence and self-confidence. Attempting a task using only adapted techniques before providing adapted devices allows the patient to have an active part in the problem-solving process. This provides the patient with the empowering experience of overcoming difficulties through learning new skills rather than providing potentially unnecessary devices that send a visual message of continuing disability.

When an adaptive aid is required for task completion, the goal is to improve function to the point where the aid will not be needed. The device should be modified or discontinued as active motion and activity tolerance increase, and these changes should be presented to the patient as signs of progress.

Patients may be reluctant to perform tasks related to the cause of their burns, such as preparing meals if their injury was caused by a kitchen fire. It is crucial that these fears be identified and addressed. Intervention activities should include education in safety precautions and performance of the fear-provoking tasks with therapist supervision. Safety precautions should be discussed before the intervention session so they can be practiced during the activity.

Prior to discharge, the patient and therapist should address any significant permanent impairment that will interfere with resumption of previous or modified life roles. The need for wheelchairs, custom prosthetic devices, household modifications, adaptive driving equipment, computerized home technology assistive devices, or other durable medical equipment should be addressed and all items ordered so they will be available for later use during the outpatient rehabilitation phase.

Long-Term Rehabilitation Phase: Predischarge Planning

The long-term rehabilitation phase of burn recovery is greatly influenced by the patient's previous performance patterns. Extended hospitalization and postdischarge daily outpatient treatment schedules can prevent a patient from resuming familiar roles as family member, student, or provider. It is important in this phase that patients recognize their progress and begin to assume previous roles on at least a part-time basis in preparation for discharge.

Burn patients and their family members must be educated about anticipated home care activities before discharge from the hospital. Education—throughout hospitalization—about what can be expected after discharge can aid in this process. Before discharge, the patient and caregivers should have opportunities to practice dressing changes, skin care, and application of compression garments and splints. Written instructions should be provided, reviewed and practiced regarding

- Wound and skin care;
- Use of medications and moisturizers;
- Positioning recommendations;

- Home exercise programs (including both therapeutic and recreational activities);
- Care of splints and self-help devices;
- Compression garments and scar conformers;
- Sun protection, use of sunblock lotion, or SPF clothing; and
- Need for environmental modifications (as appropriate in home, school, work, and social settings).

The patient and family members should demonstrate a thorough understanding of and independence in the practice and content of the home program before discharge. A list of contacts and phone numbers should be provided in case questions or concerns arise before the first outpatient appointment. Occupational therapists attend weekly multidisciplinary team rounds where patients' discharge preparedness is discussed and responsibilities for family training are delineated.

Long-Term Rehabilitation Phase: Intervention

During the outpatient rehabilitation phase of recovery, burn patients may go through countless physical and emotional changes despite continuous and comprehensive patient education. Once home, patients begin to experience both the functional and social consequences of a serious burn injury. Changes in self-image, work roles, and social relationships all have a direct effect on motivation and compliance with therapy recommendations. Although patients may eat and dress independently at discharge, they may return to the clinic unable to raise a spoon to their mouth. Providing adaptive equipment should not be the first response to this problem and may not resolve the issue, because many factors can contribute to such a change in activity performance. Identifying the underlying cause behind a lost ability is the first step toward developing an appropriate intervention response. Although scar contracture is the most common cause, other physical and emotional factors can also contribute to performance problems. Many survivors, whether experiencing psychopathology, posttraumatic growth, or adaptive psychosocial rehabilitation, are in need of assistance (Fauerbach, Pruzinsky, & Saxe, 2007) that may reach beyond the apparent burn wound.

Before discharge from the hospital, a patient's strength and endurance may be adequate for independence in daily living. Once home, differences between the hospital and home environments may be so great that fatigue may set in before noon. This feeling of fatigue may be caused by the lack of emotional as well as physical energy. The normal reaction is to rest instead of participating in home activities and outpatient therapy. The patient may lose his or her momentum and, as a result, strength remains poor or decreases; scars tighten, causing decreased flexibility; and the patient becomes increasingly dependent on others. For this reason, outpatient visits initially should be scheduled to begin shortly after discharge with frequent follow-up visits so that patients can receive the physical and emotional support they often need to get them through this difficult adjustment period.

Outpatient treatment activities are similar to those used during inpatient rehabilitation, but their intensity and frequency increase. They should include a daily exercise program that emphasizes massage, skin conditioning, and stretching, followed by strengthening activities. Although all these activities should be done frequently throughout the day, scar massage and stretching can improve a patient's participation in all activities especially if done prior to the therapeutic activities.

Compression therapy continues, with the therapist closely monitoring the compression garments for proper fit, signs of deterioration, the need for underlying conformers or inserts, and overall effectiveness as evidenced by a decrease in vascular symptoms. Although many therapists use pressure garments and conformers to minimize scar height and maintain pliability, continuous activity is necessary to oppose the contractile forces of the scar. There are times when a scar contracture is so strong that prevention of further loss of motion may seem to be the only goal. Without addressing the scar first, there will be a loss in functional movement and independence in activities. A scar band may become unstable and tend to break down repeatedly, opening new wounds. Stretching these contractures with static progressive splinting, in a position of gentle tension, often allows the open wound to heal while slowly gaining ROM. However, scars that chronically break down will eventually require surgical intervention to restore active mobility and skin durability.

Because scar control and remodeling are easier during the early stages of wound maturation, limitations in self-care ability can be resolved if appropriate treatments are implemented promptly and the patient participates actively. In addition to other outpatient treatment activities, performing basic self-care is an effective, practical, and meaningful way to increase strength, endurance, flexibility, and coordination.

In some cases, burn depth, extent, and involvement of underlying structures are so severe that long-term adaptations are necessary for the patient to perform tasks independently. The adaptations should be simple and designed to use all available active ROM. As scars mature and soften, performance skills should gradually improve if ROM has been maintained. Tendon and joint adhesions can also eventually resolve if patients use all their available motion and continue with stretching exercises. It is important not to introduce adaptation early in the treatment without first applying compensatory techniques and adaptive equipment. A burn patient's scar contractures are relative to the amount of accommodation that is provided to the pattern of the scar.

Once scars mature, they no longer require positioning, splinting, or exercise but still require lifelong precautions. For example, the skin helps regulate body temperature through perspiration. The loss of sweat and oil glands in larger areas of deep burns and grafted areas can result in higher risk of heat stroke in spite of the body's attempt to compensate by increased perspiration from unburned areas. The patient is at risk of dehydration and will need increased fluid intake when in warm environments. There is also a need to protect all burn, graft, and donor sites from all sun exposure with hats, sun protective or SPF clothing, and sunblock lotion. Unprotected depigmented scars will sunburn rapidly, and all scars less than a year old are at risk for uneven hyperpigmentation resulting in undesirable cosmetic results. Therefore, it is recommended that the burn patient use an oil-free, PABA-free, UVA/UVB sunscreen lotion with a SPF rating of 50 or higher. Full-length pants, long-sleeved shirts, and hats are also recommended when outside to protect the scars from both reflected and direct sun exposure.

Depending on their personalities and coping skills, many burn patients with permanent physical limitations develop their own adaptive methods to accomplish specific tasks. These individuals may consider extensive adaptations to be an encumbrance or an embarrassment. If they have to use adaptive equipment, it tends to be small enough to fit in a pocket or purse, such as a button aid. This positive change of perspective usually occurs during the outpatient rehabilitation phase and is a sign that the patient is accepting permanent changes in his or her life context and is developing new performance patterns.

Early in the outpatient rehabilitation phase, patients may have little interest in daily activities because of the emotional effect of the injury. Depression and anxiety are common during recovery and are often manifested in noncompliance or apathy, both of which slow progress toward functional and emotional independence. During this adjustment period, burn patients may receive comfort and encouragement by talking with other burn survivors or by attending a burn support group. Burn centers often have family and patient retreats for coping and support services and are connected to national organizations such as the Phoenix Society for Burn Survivors (see www.phoenix-society.org). Talking with a more experienced burn survivor facilitates understanding by offering a personal perspective and physical evidence that things will get easier and better with time and continued effort.

During the long-term rehabilitation phase, therapy should include opportunities to practice work and leisure skills that incorporate past skills and current interests related to employment, home management, education, and play. Depending on the patient's length of hospital stay, some of these activities may have been initiated during the inpatient rehabilitation phase. Starting on the first outpatient visit to therapy and continuing until discharge, the start of each therapy session begins with the patient and therapist reviewing current ADL difficulties and addressing possible adaptations to work or home schedules, physical environments, and independent home programs. Practicing specific tasks improves the patient's performance of the task itself and also the underlying performance components. Activities that support current leisure and social interests should be incorporated into intervention sessions so that a balance of work and play are fostered as IADLs are resumed.

During outpatient intervention sessions, IADL skills are practiced including vocational tasks, use of public or private transportation, home management and maintenance tasks, and use of communication and computer devices. When possible, the patient's personal home and work-related equipment, (e.g., home cleaning materials, hand tools, work station materials, cell phone, laptop computer, motor vehicle) should be brought to therapy sessions so the therapist can assist with the analysis of task technique and suggest any needed adaptations.

Often only simple temporary adaptations are required, such as knob adaptations for a washing machine, computer software modifications, or a padded steering wheel and large gearshift knob for a patient with stiff or fused finger joints. A patient with minimal elbow movement because of heterotopic ossification may need to continue using long-handled devices to perform independent self-feeding, dressing, and personal grooming tasks until surgical intervention is possible. With more severe functional loss, such as with limb amputations or permanent neurological deficits, prostheses and costly custom modifications may be necessary, such as foot-powered driving controls, bathroom safety equipment, home entry ramps, or computerized home environment control systems. When the need for such equipment is anticipated, the social worker or case manager should be notified long before discharge from the hospital.

Leisure interests and social roles should not be neglected during the rehabilitation phases. If a previous leisure activity has been discarded because of permanent functional loss, it should be promptly replaced with a new social or recreational activity. This may involve learning new skills (e.g., using public transportation for the first time, learning strategies for facing the public after a disfiguring burn). Leisure activities should be incorporated into therapy routines as early as possible, for both their physical and emotional therapeutic value.

If permanent disability precludes resumption of previous work roles, leisure roles take on more importance, and past interests should be encouraged. An uncomfortable motion is often better tolerated when performed during a leisure activity or play activity (Melchert-McKearnan, Deitz, Engel, & White, 2000), and movement tasks can be made more tolerable by incorporating them into such activities. However, the therapist should be careful not to suppress the patient's interest by turning the leisure task into an "exercise."

During the long-term rehabilitation phase, the patient's need for ongoing therapy should diminish. As he or she returns to part-time work or attends school, occupational recovery will be promoted Therefore, outpatient therapy appointments gradually should be reduced in frequency. When the patient achieves the skills needed to live independently at home and can return to school or work full-time, then he or she should be discharged from ongoing outpatient therapy. However, because full burn scar maturation may not occur until 12 or more months after injury, a patient may still be wearing pressure garments or night splints even after resuming a preinjury routine. Pressure garments and splints need to be checked for excessive wear and possible modification at least every 2–3 months, possibly during the patient return visits to the burn outpatient clinic. On these occasions, the patient should be re-evaluated to monitor the status of maturing scars, performance skills, and psychosocial adjustment.

Psychosocial adjustment continues during the outpatient phase of burn recovery as the patient examines personal interests and values. The patient may grieve over lost roles and abilities and accept the permanent changes resulting from the burn. These losses often include not only vocational and leisure skills but also past social roles and body image. These psychological issues will need to be addressed throughout the rehabilitation process through coordinated efforts by professionals on the burn care team.

Facial Scars

In addition to limiting jaw and neck ROM, distortions in facial structures caused by contracting scars and hypertrophy can produce severe disfigurement, including altered nasal contours, ectropion or everted eyelids that expose the conjunctivas, everted lips, contracted oral commissures, and missing features such as the nose and ears. Eye contractures can adversely affect sight and cause corneal dryness with excessive tearing and nasal drainage. Mouth contractures, or microstomia, can cause problems with talking, eating, and excessive salivation and can interfere with oral hygiene.

Any of these conditions can have a devastating effect on the patient's ability to function in society and are difficult to correct later. For this reason, early and frequent facial exercises are critical to reduce the potential for tight facial skin. Elastic facemasks and rigid, plastic molded masks may be used and combined with thin, flexible conformers to flatten and shape developing facial and head scars and maintain normal feature contours. The garments are custom made and should be checked and possibly replaced every 6–8 weeks to ensure correct compression. They are usually worn with underlying silicone gel, elastomer, or thermoplastic inserts to distribute the pressure over and around facial contours and with an overlying chin strap to maintain neck contours.

Various facial reconstructive procedures can improve both mobility and appearance. When facial distortion caused by scarring is extensive, scar excision and autografting, and laser treatment for less severe burns, can usually improve appearance once wound maturation is complete. When the wounds are mature, the patient may be referred to a cosmetologist trained in corrective makeup blending for the face or other body areas. Burn survivor networks often recommend products. Although the appearance of facial scars may be improved with surgical reconstruction and the use of special camouflaging makeup, the patient will eventually have to realize that he or she will never look the same as before the injury. With the support of others, he or she can learn to accept a new body image.

Neuromuscular and Heterotopic Ossification Complications

Heterotopic ossification is an abnormal calcification process occurring in and around damaged joints, most often in the elbow or shoulder, that can severely limit joint movement and interfere with the ability to perform everyday tasks. The best intervention is to preserve as much range of motion as possible through nonaggressive active–assistive ROM, frequent active ROM, and splinting. Adapted devices may also be indicated for performing everyday activities.

Peripheral neuropathy is a common complication of severe burn injury in patients who are older, critically ill, have an electrical injury, or have a history of alcohol abuse (Kowalske, Holavanahalli, & Helm, 2001). Polyneuropathy is most common among patients with burns greater than 15% full thickness, are older than 40 years of age, and who stay in the ICU for more than 20 days. Patients with electrical burns may have a direct electrical injury to the nerve or may develop neuropathy from postinjury edema. Patients with a history of alcohol abuse may have a mild underlying abnormality of nerve function that would predispose them to postburn neuropathies. Peripheral nerve damage can be caused by infections, neurotoxicities, and metabolic abnormalities and are evident as a symmetrical distal weakness that slowly improves over time. Localized nerve stretch and compression injuries can occur because of improper or prolonged positioning in bed or on the operating room table. Prolonged tourniquet use or extreme edema combined with tight dressings can also contribute to neuropathy and should be avoided. Diligent proper positioning can prevent most of these injuries. This includes avoiding prolonged elbow immobilization, positioning the lower extremities in neutral rotation and knee extension (to prevent the frog leg position), and avoiding prone positioning with arms overhead.

When neuropathies persist and do not spontaneously resolve, it is important that strength and sensory recovery be reevaluated periodically throughout rehabilitation. The patient should be taught sensory reeducation techniques to promote sensory recovery. ADL-related safety precautions also should be practiced to avoid further injury that could result from residual weakness or decreased protective sensation.

Pediatric Considerations

Pediatric burn patients represent a unique set of challenges because extensive rehabilitation requires commitment of families and resources at high intensity for years after a severe burn. A child's functional, developmental, and emotional well-being are challenged during a burn injury. Occupational therapists often have a dual role as the child's direct, hands-on therapist and the family's instructor and counselor, especially when the family has suffered loss of home or loved one. The family also may be dealing with guilt or anger about the cause of the child's burn.

Occupational therapists working with pediatric patients must develop rapport with caregivers and family. Children are often anxious, crying, and creating stress throughout the environment. Caregivers and family must understand the treatment course, the basics of the physiological response of wound healing, and the commitment required to care for the child at home. Without their understanding, commitment, and dedicated participation, children who suffer severe burns often have a poor prognosis. Contractures from hypertrophic scars are preventable and can be managed through prescribed treatment—but mismanagement or neglect of tightening scars crossing joints leads to disability, dysfunction, and need for continued hospitalizations and tissue releases. The importance of engaging families in the care of burn patients cannot be overemphasized. Families and caregivers often become the primary therapists for their children when they are discharged from burn centers. Home treatment prescribed by occupational therapists often requires hours of daily stretching of scar tissue, scar massage, application of splints and compression garments, changing of dressings, grading of activities, and returning children to schools and communities. Whereas etiology, depth of burn, and the number of surgeries are medical predictors of outcome; family education, demographics, problem solving, and planning are strong psychosocial predictors of the pediatric patient's functional outcomes 6 months' post-burn injury (Tyack & Ziviani, 2003).

Small children tend to heal and scar differently from older children and adults. Children less than 5 years of age have a higher potential for hypertrophic scarring of both burn and donor sites because of prolonged scar maturation. Smaller muscles, hypermobile joints, and inability to cooperate put them at higher risk for contractures than adults. Contractures and the binding properties of tight scar may also inhibit normal growth in smaller children, especially in the hands and feet. Therefore, the surgical team may intervene earlier with surgical releases and reconstruction for children than they would for an adult with a similar scar.

Children are more likely to experience emotional regression, especially during the acute phase. The physical and social restrictions resulting from contractures and disfigurement can interfere with meeting developmental milestones. For this reason, it is helpful to obtain information from parents and family members regarding developmental milestones met by children before the burn, so that if regression occurs, appropriate interventions can be initiated while the patient is still in the hospital.

For school-age children, a school re-entry program should be initiated before discharge. This foreknowledge helps ease the resumption of the student role for the child. It also can help improve acceptance by other children who may not otherwise understand the cause of the disfigurement and the need for splints, adapted equipment, and scar compression garments. Summer camps for burned children, often cosponsored by local firefighter organizations, also help children adjust by placing them in settings where they can socialize with peers who also have been burned.

Geriatric Considerations

Elderly patients may not form hypertrophic scars as readily as younger patients, but their scars may stay fragile longer and may heal more slowly. Degenerative joint disease, osteoporosis, cardiopulmonary complications, diabetes, deconditioning, and other pre-existing conditions in the elderly person may further complicate rehabilitation. Care must be taken during active–assistive or passive ROM exercises not to overstretch joints that may have been restricted by age-related joint disease even before the burn injury. Burns to elderly persons often result from engaging in unsafe ADL or IADL practices related to slower cognitive and motor reflexes and skin sensitivity. Elderly people, who may have been failing at independent living being burned, are often placed in nursing care or require extensive family support at discharge. As the demographics in the United States move toward an aging population, elderly people will present a unique challenge to burn centers, including medical management, public health burn prevention programs, and ongoing community support.

Sexuality

Sexual activity is an occupational performance area that should be addressed during the inpatient rehabilitation phase of recovery well before discharge. Following a serious burn, multiple factors can interfere with sexual activity, including decreased mobility due to scar contractures or limited joint ROM, decreased physical strength and poor endurance, loss of sensation, hypersensitivity or pain, fragile skin and skin inflexibility, or erectile dysfunction due to scarring. Pain, poor body image, depression, performance anxiety, and lack of information are also serious deterrents to resumption of sexual activity.

The therapist should obtain a history from the patient regarding his or her basic understanding of sexual practices and related issues, including birth control, safe sex practices, personal hygiene, social and cultural influences, and personal preferences regarding sex-related issues. An activity analysis is needed to assess the patient's positioning and educational needs. Information regarding sexual performance should be provided on several occasions along with copies of or recommendations for information about sexual performance. The occupational therapist can offer solutions for specific anticipated problems related to physical disability, such as the need for positional adaptations, lubrication, skin care, hygiene, or use of adapted aids. Only a sexual counselor or professional with advanced training in sexual counseling should provide in-depth sexual therapy (Burton, 2001).

Community Mobility

If a burn patient has a permanent functional impairment that prevents driving a standard vehicle, he or she will need to consider options available for personal transportation in the community. The local public transportation department may offer ample services for persons with physical impairments. Use of these services should be investigated as an economic alternative prior to ordering costly personal transportation adaptations.

Should personal vehicle adaptation be preferred, the occupational therapist must consider the patient's physical and cognitive capabilities for driving and transferring in and out of the vehicle, the types of adaptations that will be needed, the extent of driver education needed for safe driving, and prescribed medications that may affect safe operation of a vehicle. This assessment should be performed by a professional with special training and experience in determining what kind of vehicle or equipment is necessary and appropriate for an individual. Efforts should be made to prescribe the least amount of modification necessary so that the patient can make maximum use of his or her capabilities. A prescription is then written for the modifications or vehicle needed. The prescription is also helpful to insurance or state agencies that may assist in funding the purchase.

The cost of vehicle modifications varies widely depending upon the type of adaptive equipment needed. The patient may take advantage of services and organizations that provide funding for adaptive vehicles and equipment. These include insurance companies, state rehabilitation service agencies, and local service organizations. The U.S. Department of Veterans Affairs provides grants and reimbursement for adaptive equipment for service-related disabilities.

Case Study 13.1. Zowie

Zowie is a 9-month-old child who was caught in a trailer fire when a pot of grease erupted in flames on the stove while her grandmother was home. Zowie's grandmother rescued three children from the fire, but Zowie sustained burns to both upper extremities. She was initially taken to an outside hospital and then transferred to the burn center for intensive treatment.

Occupational therapy was consulted upon admission to the burn center. Zowie was evaluated within 24 hours, and the acute rehabilitation phase was initiated. Occupational therapy noted eschar to both her palms and forearms up to mid-humeral upper extremities. The depth of the burn on the dorsal aspect of her hand and fingers was partial thickness. Her palm, forearm, and mid-upper extremity were full thickness in nature. Zowie's mother was interviewed to assess her developmental status and premorbid behavior. Antideformity hand splints were fabricated and applied within 24 hours, positioning her in a neutral position at the proximal interphalangeal joints with metacarpal phalangeal joints flexed 70–90 degrees. Her wrists were placed in 20 degrees of extension with wrist splints. Both of her upper extremities received ultrasound dopplers to evaluate the perfusion to her hand and were placed on pillows and towels above her heart level to reduce edema.

By the 5th day in the burn center the medical decision to proceed with surgery for the deep burns was made by the attending surgeon. Surgery included excision of dead tissue down to subcutaneous tissue and grafting of tissue from the patient's buttock and thigh to the full-thickness burns of the upper extremities. Surgery was performed by a burn surgeon, effectively creating wound closure to prevent infection. This prepared Zowie for continued work toward normal function and development. The burn surgeon excised to the fat layer of the upper extremities and applied grafted skin to the dorsum of her hand and the upper extremities. Sheet grafts were applied with the seams of grafts avoiding the joints to prevent contractures and joint stiffness. The occupational therapist was asked to come to the operating room to review the graft placement and to apply splints on Zowie's hands and elbows to prevent graft shearing and maximize the functional position of the grafted areas. Zowie was immobilized for 5 days postoperatively for graft adherence in wet dressings.

Occupational therapy reviewed splint fit and monitored Zowie's comfort during the 5 days of immobilization to prevent discomfort related to the splints as well as to promote optimal positioning. At Day 5, Zowie's dressings were removed and the occupational therapist was asked to review the surgical outcome. The grafts appeared well adhered, while the palms remained open with red "beefy" granulation tissue noted on both hands. The surgeon decided not to graft the palms due to the complicated rehabilitation course of having a circumferentially grafted hand. The OT began the intensive course of teaching Zowie's mother, who had a background as a nursing assistant, how to dress her daughter's hand. Dressings were applied to promote the most natural movement to allow Zowie to explore her environment and demonstrate independent finger movement and gross grasp.

Once grafts were adhered and Zowie was medically stable, the burden rested with the therapy team to provide a safe and timely discharge. During the intermediate rehabilitation phase, Zowie and her parents received daily treatment and training from the occupational and physical therapy team. The goals were to have splints provided and in place and for the parents to understand and demonstrate wound care, the stretching program, and the scar maturation process. Zowie was discharged from the hospital but remained nearby in a home-like setting provided by the hospital. Zowie and her parents returned to occupational therapy daily to evaluate the healing of her open palm wounds and stretching. Having Zowie nearby allowed her parents to test their skills with home care and home therapy with the supervision of the hospital therapists. Zowie soon began demonstrating play activity, crawling, and functional use of her upper extremities.

Because Zowie and her family had lost their home in the fire, having Zowie nearby gave the family time to focus on her treatment while finding a place to live. As family members would be the primary caregivers after Zowie's discharge from therapy services, the family's having a safe home environment was important. Zowie returned to occupational therapy for follow-up care weekly, then monthly, and finally quarterly to guide her care, make adjustments to home exercise programs, and evaluate her developmental progress.

Zowie began her story at 9 months of age, and the story will continue for years to come as she remains in the long-term rehabilitation phase of her recovery. Occupational therapy worked with the care team, family, surgeons, and patient to prevent contractures and deformity while supporting Zowie's return to a home environment in which she could continue to grow and develop.

Table 13.2. Application of PEO Model: Zowie

Person	Environment	Occupation
- 9-month-old - Full thickness burns to both upper extremities - Excision and grafting of burns - Harvest sites to thighs - Normal, engaging, developing child	- Trailer burned - ICU/floor status - Hospital housing - Family financial hardships with loss of home and expenses - Rural living	- Meeting developmental milestones - Eating/IADLs - Crawling/mobility - Daughter/social participation - Play

Note. ADLs = activities of daily living; ICU = intensive care unit; PEO = person–environment–occupation.

Case Study 13.2. Rebecca

Rebecca is a 24-year-old woman who sustained 54% TBSA burns after being ignited when lighting a cigarette beside a gas grill. Rebecca panicked and jumped out of her second-story apartment and then lost consciousness. She was transported to a local hospital and then transferred to a Level I burn center for further management of her burns and traumatic injuries. This incident occurred 5 days before Christmas.

Rebecca had superficial burns to her face, deep partial-thickness burns to her chest, and full-thickness burns (25% TBSA) to both arms and legs. Due to the significant nature of the burns to her left leg and arm, fasciotomies had to be done within the first hours of admittance to the burn center to preserve her extremities. Rebecca also was given a tracheotomy and placed on a ventilator due to the possibility of inhalation injury. She was placed in a Miami-J collar to protect her cervical spine after sustaining a high fall. Little information was known about Rebecca's previous medical history and life roles, as no family or friends were present at the burn center. She was nonresponsive due to intubation and heavy sedation.

Rebecca's family was contacted, and the goal was set to return Rebecca successfully to independence as a young adult. The occupational therapists at the burn center completed an evaluation of her burn wounds and other injuries within the first 24 hours of admittance to determine her immediate needs for positioning and splinting and to develop therapeutic goals with the burn team. She was promptly placed in bilateral antideformity hand splints to provide optimal positioning of her hands while she was in an acute and critical phase of rehabilitation.

Despite Rebecca's nonresponsiveness, the OTs and OTAs treated her every day with passive ROM stretches to bilateral upper extremities, positioning her extremities to decrease edema and educating the family about the burn rehabilitation process. Throughout her hospital admission, she endured several operative grafting procedures: split-thickness autografts to her left hand, left upper extremity, right upper extremity, and bilateral lower extremities. Occupational therapy staff assisted with all procedures by fabricating and placing Rebecca in appropriate splints for immobilization to promote optimal healing to the skin grafts.

As Rebecca became alert and coherent, her therapy was complicated by poor pain tolerance. It was important for the OT, nurses, and her family to encourage her to engage in her rehabilitation. Frustration of the family became apparent as Rebecca was slow to recover and her endurance and participation were minimal. Day by day, Rebecca regained strength and cognitive understanding of the importance of her continued integration and active participation in her physical and occupational therapy in order to regain independence.

When Rebecca was discharged, it was important for her to continue her rehabilitation on a daily basis with the OTs within the burn center clinic. She began to have significant hypertrophic scarring to her bilateral upper extremities. These were limiting her active ROM and independence in ADLs. She also required ongoing psychiatric assistance to develop a more positive self-image and address posttraumatic stress disorder symptoms. She was weaned from daily occupational therapy in order to provide her the opportunity to be as independent as possible with her home exercise program, wound care, scar management, ADLs, and IADLs. Rebecca continued to seek out new life roles with ongoing support of the burn center staff and volunteers.

Table 13.3. Model of Human Occupation: Rebecca

Volition	Habituation	Performance Capacity
Personal causation: decreased by sedation in acute inpatient	Changes in daily routines: hospital schedule/medication/therapy	Physical limitations
Decreased personal motivations caused by disbelief in ability	Decreased independence in ADLs	Decreased ROM, active and passive
Values: decreased feeling of living worthiness and belonging	Lack of social engagement	Surgery intervention, splinting needs
Loss of quality of life due to self-image	Physical environment altered from familiar environment/home	Decreased engagement in occupations
Interests: poor motivation to become socially involved	Saw self as worker (waitress) or friend; now as "patient"	Scar bands
Decreased aesthetic arousal		
Previous life roles temporarily diminished		

Note. ADLs = activities of daily living; ROM = range of motion.

Case Study 13.3. John

John sustained a 60% total body surface area burn on May 31, the result of a diesel steam engine explosion while he was at work. At the time of his burn he was 55 years of age. His burns were to his hands, both upper extremities, both lower extremities, head, neck, and anterior and posterior trunk, and he sustained a positive inhalation injury. Because of the inhalation injury and the large percentage of burns, John was intubated on a ventilator and pharmacologically sedated. The burns to his lower extremities were full-thickness and required fasciotomies, while the burns to his hands and upper extremities were full-thickness and required escharotomies.

Occupational therapy evaluated the patient the day following his admission. Because of the deep depth of the hand burns, the OT fabricated and fitted bilateral antideformity hand splints to the patient on his first full day in the burn center. The splints held the patient's hands in an intrinsic plus position to prevent deformity over the course of his rehabilitation. While the patient was sedated, the splints were worn at all times except during his bath and daily therapy. Therapy for John's hands included removing his positional hand splints and passively ranging all joints of his hands, including his wrists, followed by reapplication of the splints. Two days after his admission, John had autografting to his lower extremities, and the OT fabricated and molded bilateral knee extension splints afterward. The splints remained in place for 5 days. During this period, John returned to the operating room to have his hands autografted. Antideformity splints were reapplied to his hands for 5 consecutive days. When his hands were out of the OR splints, the OT would passively range the joints in his hands and wrists.

John was intubated and sedated during the first 2 ½ months of his hospitalization. During this period, occupational therapy interventions focused on positioning, splinting, and passive ROM to prevent burn scar contractures that could ultimately lead to lack of function. John was treated at bedside 6 days each week for 45 minutes to 1 hour. A member of his immediate family was present daily in the burn center to provide support and daily interaction. The OT kept the family informed about the purpose of therapy and incorporated them into his therapy program as much as possible.

When John was weaned from the ventilator and started to participate actively in his therapy, the focus was active ROM exercises and stretching exercises to prevent burn scar contracture. Positional splinting continued at night for his hands. In conjunction with physical therapy, John would ambulate to the occupational therapy clinic and participate in his daily exercise program. The OT continued to passively range his hands to attempt to achieve end range of each joint, because active scarring tightness prevented full active ROM. His facial scars were very active during this time; he had limited facial movement and tightness in the commissures of his mouth. The OT fabricated a dynamic mouth-stretching splint for prolonged stretching to prevent further tightening. Stretching exercises for his elbows were incorporated as well, because tightness was beginning to develop there, again the result of scar contracture.

Case Study 13.3. John *(cont.)*

After 5½ months in the burn center, John had progressed to the point that he could ambulate to occupational therapy without the assistance of the PT, and his wounds were almost completely closed. However, his active ROM in bilateral hands and upper extremities was limited because of active burn scarring, keeping him from completing his ADLs. He was able to feed himself with a built-up handle fork and setup assistance but was unable to dress himself, complete simple hygiene activities, or toilet independently.

It was decided with the burn team to discharge John to a local extended-stay hotel setting and have him return daily for outpatient occupational therapy to focus on hand therapy. He left for the hotel with his wife and one of his daughters in November and returned for therapy in the burn center daily. Over the next 5 weeks, dynamic MP flexion splints, dynamic wrist extension splints, and dynamic PIP flexion splints were made for use in his therapy program. He wore them at least three times daily for 15 minutes each session. When not using the splints, he would exercise to passively and actively stretch joints of his hands.

The OT fitted John with compression garments to his hands and upper extremities in late December to prevent vascular symptoms. As his mobility improved with intensive therapy, it was decided that he could return to his home the day before Christmas. Occupational therapy continued in the form of outpatient therapy at a local facility after John returned home.

A year after his accident, John had not returned to work. He was, however, totally independent in his self-care and beginning to drive. He continued with outpatient therapy to work on improving strength and endurance.

The OT in the burn center continues to follow this patient 3 years later, to provide therapy following his reconstructive procedures. He has undergone several reconstructive procedures to improve active ROM, including z-plasties, tenotomy of lateral bands, carpal tunnel release, little finger arthrodesis, nerve decompressions, and commissure releases.

Table 13.4. Biomechanical Model: John

Joint Range of Motion	Strength	Endurance
Previous baseline measurements	Previous baseline measurements	Age
Goniometer	Dynonometer	Prolonged ICU status
Escharotomies vs. fasciotomies	Continuous rehabilitation, BTE	Multiple surgeries over the course of many years
Progressive varieties of splints	Engaging in therapeutic activity	Proper nutrition and energy conservation

Note. BTE = Baltimore Therapeutic Equipment Work Simulator; ICU = intensive care unit.

Summary

Burn survivors require intensive services to regain independence and manage their physical changes. Occupational therapy's broad scope of practice and holistic frame of reference are uniquely suited to address the expansive trauma undergone by burn survivors. Occupational therapy's focus should be to create therapeutic goals and relationships with patients and families to provide an avenue toward independence. Addressing not only the physical dysfunction but also the spiritual and emotional limitations created by the burn injury—and understanding how these affect patients' self-image and motivation—is critical for optimal healing. Burn survivors often discover who they really are—not an image, not a role, but a strong and persistent person, fueled by a thirst to engage with the environment and live a meaningful and purposeful life. Both occupational therapists and burn survivors often are both changed through this unique engagement.

Study Questions

1. In the initial and acute stage of a burn, how should the patient's extremities be positioned?
2. What is an example of a limitation or obstacle a patient with hand burns may have in each area of the *Occupational Therapy Practice Framework* (AOTA, 2008a) (e.g., self-care)?
3. When does an occupational therapist begin therapeutic ROM with a patient?
4. How long does it take for a scar to mature, and what can patients do to manage their scars?
5. In what splint position should the burned hand be placed to prevent contracture?
6. How frequently should ROM exercises be done?

Acknowledgments

Writing and editing this chapter required a team effort, just as in burn care. We would like to recognize Beth Bale, OTA, for all her hard work and photography captions; Candice Woliver, OTR, for her research and background work on identifying references; and Sandra Utley Reeves, OTR, for her work in earlier editions of this chapter.

References

Addy, L. (2006). *Occupational therapy evidence in practice for physical rehabilitation*. Oxford, England: Wiley-Blackwell.

American Burn Association. (2007). *ABA/ACS Verification Review Committee*. Retrieved July 15, 2009, from http://www.ameriburn.org/verification_about.php

American College of Surgeons. (2006). Optimal care of the injured patient. In *Guidelines for the operation of burn centers* (Chapter 14). Chicago: Author.

American Occupational Therapy Association (2008a). Occupational therapy practice framework: Domain and process (2nd ed.). *American Journal of Occupational Therapy, 62,* 625–683.

American Occupational Therapy Association. (2008b). Physical agent modalities: A position paper. *American Journal of Occupational Therapy, 62,* 691–693.

Baum, C. M., & Christiansen, C. H. (1997). Person–environment–occupational performance: A conceptual model for practice. In C. Christiansen & C. Baum (Eds.), *Occupational therapy: Enabling function and well-being* (pp. 48–69). Thorofare, NJ: Slack.

Breines, E. B. (2001). Therapeutic occupations and modalities. In L. W. Pedretti & M. B. Early (Eds.), *Occupational therapy: Practice skills for physical dysfunction* (pp. 503–525). St. Louis, MO: Mosby.

Burton, G. U. (2001). Sexuality and sexual dysfunction. In L. W. Pedretti & M. B. Early (Eds.), *Occupational therapy: Practice skills for physical dysfunction* (pp. 212–225). St. Louis, MO: Mosby.

Dewey, W. S., Hedman, T. L., Chapman, T. T., Wolf, S. E., & Holcomb, J. B. (2007). The reliability and concurrent validity of the figure-of-eight method of measuring hand edema in patients with burns. *Journal of Burn Care and Rehabilitation Research, 28,* 157–162.

Edgar, D. (2009). Burn rehabilitation starts at time of injury: An Australian perspective. [Letter]. *Journal of Burn Care and Rehabilitation Research, 30*(2), 367.

Engrav, L., Garner, W., & Tredget, E. (2007). Hypertrophic scar, wound contraction, and hyper-hypopigmentation. *Journal of Burn Care and Rehabilitation Research, 28*(4), 593–595.

Fauerbach, J., Pruzinsky, T., & Saxe, G. (2007). Psychological health and function after burn injury: Setting research priorities. *Journal of Burn Care and Rehabilitation Research, 28*(4), 587–592.

Feldman, M., Evans, J., & O, S. J. (2008). Early management of the burned pediatric hand. *Journal of Craniofacial Surgery, 19*(4), 942–950.

Helm, P., Herndon, D., & deLateur, B. (2007). Restoration of function. *Journal of Burn Care and Rehabilitation Research, 28*(4), 611–614.

Herndon, D. (2007). *Total burn care* (3rd ed.). London: W. B. Saunders.

Kielhofner, G. (1995). *A model of human occupation: Theory and application* (2nd ed.). Baltimore: Williams & Wilkins.

Kowalske, K., Greenhalgh, D., & Ward, S. (2007). Hand burns. *Journal of Burn Care and Rehabilitation Research, 28*(4), 607–610.

Kowalske, K., Holavanahalli, R., & Helm, P. (2001). Neuropathy after burn injury. *Journal of Burn Care and Rehabilitation Research, 22,* 353–357.

Law, M., Cooper, B., Strong, S., Stewart, D., Rigby, P., & Letts, L. (1996). The Person–Environment–Occupation Model: A transactive approach to occupational performance. *Canadian Journal of Occupational Therapy, 63,* 9–23.

Lund, C., & Browder, N. (1944). The estimation of area of burns. *Surgical Gynecology and Obstetrics, 79,* 352–355.

Melchert-McKearnan, K., Deitz, J., Engel, J. M., & White, O. (2000). Children with burn injuries: Purposeful activity versus rote exercise. *American Journal of Occupational Therapy, 54,* 381–390.

Morien, A., Garrison, D., & Keeney Smith, N. (2008). Range of motion improves after massage in children with burns: A pilot study. *Journal of Bodywork and Movement Therapies, 12,* 67–71.

Okhovatian, F., & Zoubine, N. (2006) A comparison between two burn rehabilitation protocols. *Burns, 33*(4), 429–434.

Reeves, S. U. (2001). Burns and burn rehabilitation. In L. W. Pedretti & M. B. Early (Eds.), *Occupational therapy: Practice skills for physical dysfunction* (pp. 898–923). St. Louis, MO: Mosby.

Richard, R., Baryza, M. J., Carr, J. A., Dewey, W. S., Dougherty, M. E., Forbes-Duchart, L., et al. (2009). Burn rehabilitation and research: Proceedings of a consensus summit. *Journal of Burn Care and Rehabilitation Research, 30*(4), 543–573.

Richard, R. L., Hedman, T. L., Quick, C. D., Barillo, D. J., Cancio, L. C., Renz, E. M., et al. (2008). A clarion to recommit and reaffirm burn rehabilitation. *Journal of Burn Care and Rehabilitation Research, 29*(3), 425–432.

Richard, R., Stanley, M. (1994). *Burn care and rehabilitation: Principles and practice*. Philadelphia: F. A. Davis.

Richard, R., & Ward, S. (2005). Splinting strategies and controversies. *Journal of Burn Care and Rehabilitation Research, 26*(5), 392–398.

Schneider, J., Hoavanahalli, R., Helm, P., O'Oneil, C., Goldstein, R., & Kowalske, K. (2008). Contractures in burn injury part II: Investigating joints of the hand. *Journal of Burn Care and Rehabilitation Research, 29*(4), 606–613.

Tyack, Z. F., & Ziviani, J. (2003). What influences the functional outcome of children at 6 months postburn? *Burns, 29*(5), 433–444.

Whitehead, C., & Serghiou, M. (2009). A 12-year comparison of common therapeutic interventions in the burn unit. *Journal of Burn Care and Rehabilitation Research, 30*(2), 281–287.

Chapter 14

Everyday Living for Individuals With Cognitive Deficits After Alzheimer's Dementia and Traumatic Brain Injury

BEATRIZ C. ABREU, PHD, OTR, FAOTA, AND SYBIL M. YANCY, MOT, OTR

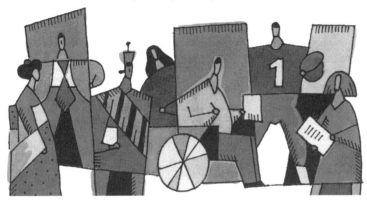

KEY WORDS

Alzheimer's dementia (AD)

Alzheimer's dementia stages

brain cortex lobes

cognitive rehabilitation

frontal lobe

Glasgow Coma Scale (GSC)

Mini-Mental Status Examination (MMSE)

occipital lobes

parietal lobes

Post-Traumatic Amnesia Scale (PTA)

stages of Alzheimer's dementia

temporal lobe

traumatic brain injury (TBI)

traumatic brain injury stages

HIGHLIGHTS

- Cognitive rehabilitation approaches are interventions that therapists use to design remediation and compensation programs for persons with Alzheimer's dementia (AD) and traumatic brain injury (TBI).

- The nature and location of a brain injury have an effect on the client's behavior and therefore can influence the evaluation and intervention process.

- Executive function behaviors are higher cortical processes that include problem solving, self-awareness, self-monitoring, self-regulation, and response inhibition.

- Executive dysfunction AD and TBI may be associated with decreased instrumental activities of daily living, such as bathing, money management, community integration, and social skills.

- Quantitative and qualitative data are collected during the evaluation process to understand clients' stories and are an important part of clinical reasoning.

- Persons with AD and TBI at a severe phase may not achieve functional improvement, and functional outcomes may not be appropriate. Appropriate critical outcomes for these clients are physical, mental, and spiritual.

- Rehabilitation is a collaborative effort requiring the coordinated efforts of the entire rehabilitation team, the client, and the family group.

OBJECTIVES

After reading this material, readers will be able to

- Define Alzheimer's dementia (AD) and traumatic brain injury (TBI),

- Describe the physiological basis for cognitive disabilities in AD and TBI,

- Describe the stages of cognitive decline in AD and stages of recovery in TBI,

- Outline evaluation strategies for persons with AD and TBI,

- Describe the challenges to occupational performance experienced by individuals with AD and TBI, and

- Describe adaptive strategies equipment or environmental modifications useful for optimal performance of everyday activities.

The purposes of this chapter are to describe the challenges to occupational performance experienced by individuals with cognitive disabilities because of Alzheimer's dementia (AD) and traumatic brain injury (TBI); to illustrate evaluation strategies; and to describe adaptive strategies, equipment, or environmental modifications useful for optimal performance of everyday activities for people with AD or TBI.

Alzheimer's Dementia and Traumatic Brain Injury

Dementia includes a group of disorders characterized by memory and other cognitive deficits. There are many causes for dementia, including AD, cerebral vascular disease, head trauma, and HIV/AIDS, among others. Dementia of all types has been classified according to the area of damage. Classifications include cortical damage, including Alzheimer's and Picks disease; subcortical damage secondary to Huntington's and Parkinson's

disease; and mixed type, such as multi-infarct dementia. Readers should refer to the *Diagnostic and Statistical Manual of Mental Disorders* for further classification of dementia (*DSM–IV–TR*; American Psychiatric Association, 2000).

AD is a progressive and irreversible neurological disease that frequently leads to dementia and is characterized by a slow, steady cognitive and functional decline (Davis, Hoppes, & Chesbro, 2005; Papp, Walsh, & Snyder, 2009; Sikkes, de Lange-de Klerk, Pijnenburg, Scheltens, & Uitdehaag, 2009). In many countries, the prevalence of AD is about 1.5% at age 65, doubling every 4 years after age 65. In the United States, there are approximately 5.3 million people with AD (Alzheimer's Association, 2009).

TBI, on the other hand, is a nonprogressive and remediable neurological condition, although some practitioners' challenge this idea and conceptualize TBI as the beginning of a disease process. They believe that TBI, at any stage of recovery, is a dynamic but chronic condition process (Masel, 2009). TBI is usually caused by a blow to the head, either from an external object or due to internal forces caused by high-speed acceleration or deceleration. In the United States, there are over 1.5 million occurrences of TBI each year, with 51% of the injuries caused by motor vehicle accidents (Centers for Disease Control and Prevention, 2009). Many of these accidents are alcohol related. Falls, assaults, and sports injuries (Brain Injury Association of America, 1998) account for the remaining 49%. Older adults are most likely to sustain TBI because of a fall. Young adults are most likely to sustain TBI in an accident (Breed et al., 2008). More than two-thirds of TBI cases are individuals under the age of 30. Young males between the ages of 14 and 24 have the highest rate of injury. TBI is considered the signature injury of the Iraq and Afghanistan wars, due to both combat- and noncombat-related activities (Han et al., 2009).

Cognitive deficits caused by AD and TBI influence the individual's everyday living, leading to an increased need for occupational therapy services in both institutional and home settings (see Box 14.1). In addition, cognitive impairments play a critical role in all types of learning, affecting health and participation across populations of all ages, diagnoses, and practice areas. Occupational therapists and occupational therapy assistants need to understand more fully the effect of such cognitive impairments on daily living activities in order to provide effective evaluation and intervention strategies. Both conditions cause great health care costs and burdens of care.

The relationship between cognition and everyday living for patients with cognitive deficits is complex, dynamic, and difficult to comprehend. Although there are no simple answers when dealing with AD and TBI, we will present a practical approach for evaluation and intervention. One general—and perhaps obvious—principle that may be applied to the relationship between cognition and daily living skills is that the more severe the cognitive deficit, the more dependent the individual will be. There is extensive information about cognition and cognitive impairments in both the cognitive psychology and neuropsychology literature; an in-depth review of this knowledge is beyond the scope of this chapter.

Evidenced-Based Practice for People With Alzheimer's Dementia and Traumatic Brain Injury

Evidence-based practice (EBP) is the formal gathering and synthesis of information from research findings by using systematic research review in order to determine best clinical practice (Abreu & Chang, 2011). EBP methods are one way to create and sustain a competent environment in the workplace. EBP describes a critical process—to search; evaluate; reject or accept; and finally, integrate evaluation and intervention result findings into clinical decision making or practice reasoning. EBP enables practitioners to upgrade their knowledge; improve their understanding of research methods; and promotes the development, refinement, and testing of

occupational therapy evaluations and interventions (Johnston & Case-Smith, 2009).

The EBP literature on brain injury supports the significant role and contribution of occupational therapists in providing evaluation and intervention guidelines for awareness of deficits after such injury (Hart, Seignourel, & Sherer, 2009; O'Keefe, Dockree, Moloney, Carton, & Robertson, 2007). We will discuss some of these contributions later in this chapter.

Although EBP values quantitative evidence, other research methodologies also provide valuable knowledge about AD and TBI. Qualitative research integrates the meaning and perceptions of persons affected by these two conditions. Therapists need to combine both qualitative and quantitative findings into their practice, but they must also remember that evidence in health care is provisional, lacking, emergent, and incomplete.

At this stage, there is some evidence to validate the use of occupational therapy interventions for AD or TBI, but further research is needed in order to generalize the evidence to practice.

Challenges to Everyday Living in Individuals With Alzheimer's Dementia and Traumatic Brain Injury

When cognitive changes first appear because of AD and TBI, individuals and family groups may not fully realize the scope and devastating effect that these conditions will have on their entire social support system and their community integration.

Box 14.1. The Brain and Behavior: Current Understandings

The field of cognitive neuropsychology focuses on the functional consequences of disease and injury to the brain. Theories are rapidly evolving, but there is agreement that

- The brain has highly specialized areas of function for memory, reasoning, sensation, motor control, and emotion; thus, injuries exhibit unique characteristics depending on the areas of the brain affected.
- Multiple sensory pathways can be used to process information, so a lesion in one area can influence one function but not another.
- Human behavior is influenced not only by cognition but also by emotional (affective) and

motivational states. These are influenced by environmental changes.
- Although tremendous advances are being made in neuroimaging, the complexity of the brain and the lack of valid predictive models do not yet permit reliable and precise mapping of functional cognition.
- Executive dysfunction after brain damage may be associated with decreased instrumental activities of daily living such as bathing, money management, community integration, and social skills.
- Brain functions extend beyond learning and memory and are necessary for producing the cortisol response to psychosocial stress.

The behavioral changes caused by such deficits extend far beyond the individual who has incurred the disability. Family groups, including immediate family members, friends, allied health professionals, and others, become caregivers and will spend a tremendous amount of time assisting cognitively impaired individuals to manage their activities of daily living (ADLs). Any one of these caregivers can frequently become overworked and stressed when faced with new roles and responsibilities, including helping the clients with severe AD and TBI to communicate their symptoms, especially pain (Gitlin, Winter, Dennis, & Hauck, 2007). Factors such as the relationship between caretaker and client; the client's cognitive, behavioral, and psychological abilities; and the caregiver's gender may affect the burden of care (Campbell et al., 2008). The emotional state of the caretakers is often adversely affected; they become candidates for counseling and guidance themselves (Ulstein, Sandvik, Wyller, & Engdal, 2007).

Occupational therapists and occupational therapy assistants, as part of a multidisciplinary health care team, may be able to use purposeful activity and ordinary occupation to promote health and achieve functional outcomes with clients, family groups, and health care staff by using retraining and compensatory strategies. For example, to address the problem of elderly people with wandering dementia and brain injury as it continues to grow, some practitioners are advocating microchips that track a person's location in order to enhance safety and decrease the burden of care (Harada et al., 2008).

Two of the most common problems after AD and TBI are memory impairments and the lack of awareness of deficits (Abreu et al., 2001; Hart et al., 2009; Ownsworth, Turpin, Andrew, & Fleming, 2008; Toglia & Kirk, 2000). People with AD and TBI show awareness deficits specifically after frontal lobe damage (Salmon et al., 2008). Lack of awareness is associated with poor rehabilitation compliance and functional outcomes. Awareness of deficits is the discrepancy between client and caretaker's ratings on client's performance. Frequently, persons after moderate and severe TBI rate themselves at a higher level of functioning than do their relatives and therapists (Abreu et al., 2001; Hart et al., 2009). Awareness of deficits appears to improve with time and with occupational therapy interventions (Goverover, Johnston, Toglia, & DeLuca, 2007).

AD and TBI are two acquired, persistent conditions that affect multiple areas of cognitive function. The illness trajectories followed by AD and TBI

are quite different. In AD, clients show deterioration in thinking, behavior, and occupational performance over time. In TBI, clients show recovery, followed by a plateau in thinking, behavior, and functional ability over time.

Rehabilitation for both AD and TBI can incorporate occupational therapy intervention approaches, including remediation, utilization of adaptive techniques or equipment, and environmental modifications. The primary focus for AD is on adaptive strategies and environmental modification. Strategies include both restoring lost skills and adaptation of the task or the environment. For example, memory deficit strategies may involve external cues in the environment to trigger an individual's recall, and the restoration approach may utilize paper-and-pencil tasks to retrain individuals in math and money management.

Behavior Changes Associated With Brain Damage

The nervous system and the brain control all functional behavior. The *nervous system* is an organized group of nerve and other non-neural cells that receive, integrate, and transmit information. After AD and TBI, the brain is significantly damaged. Four major structures of the brain that are commonly affected by AD and TBI are the frontal, parietal, temporal, and occipital lobes (see Figure 14.1). A brief identification, by brain lobe, of the performance component impairments that are present in these conditions follows.

Frontal Lobes

The *frontal lobes* are located in the most forward section of the brain, one on each side of the midline. Damage to the frontal lobes causes both cognitive and motor dysfunction. These lobes are associated with *executive functions*—a term used to describe the higher mental processes. Executive function behaviors include planning, choosing, and initiating goal-directed behaviors; self-awareness, self-monitoring, and self-regulating behaviors by self-detecting and correcting errors in performance; cognitive flexibility and problem solving by generating multiple response alternatives; and response inhibition by persisting in the face of distractions.

Research has shown that executive dysfunction following AD and TBI may be associated with decreased instrumental activities of daily living (IADLs) such as bathing, money management, community integration, and social skills (Reid-Arndt, Nehl, & Hinkebein, 2007). The ability to use social

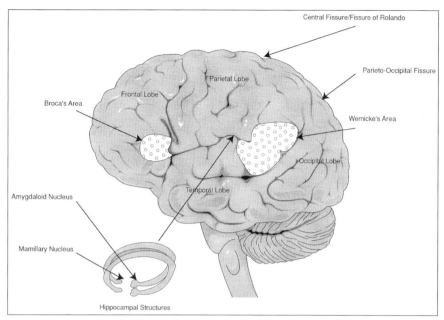

Figure 14.1. The lateral view of the brain showing the locations of the structures affected by AD and TBI.

skills flexibly, according to rules, is also an executive function behavior (Godfrey & Shum, 2000).

Broca's aphasia may also occur with damage to the lower portion of the lobe, resulting in the inability to speak or understand spoken or written language. In addition, certain pathological motor responses such as grasp reflex and groping responses with the hands may occur, which present a challenge for hand use in occupational performance. Individuals with injury to the frontal lobes may experience deficits in how to position the hand for grasping familiar or unfamiliar objects, or may overshoot or undershoot when reaching for objects.

Parietal Lobes

The *parietal lobes* are located between the frontal and the occipital lobes. They process somato-sensory information, visual–motor information in regard to the guidance of hand movement and manipulation of objects, and spatial cognition. Damage in the parietal lobes may produce impairments in arithmetic (*dyscalculia*), writing (*agraphia*), reading (*dyslexia*), and drawing because of difficulty in recognizing objects, abstract letters, and numbers.

Parietal lobe dysfunction may also produce motor planning and sequencing problems such as apraxia. Functionally, damage to the parietal lobes may result in a decreased ability to discriminate between right and left and to neglect objects and body parts contralateral to the brain lesion, resulting

in ADL problems in tasks such as dressing or grooming. Common occupational performance challenges associated with this condition are getting lost, bumping into walls, and hitting affected extremities. In general, clients may be unsafe and require supervision from family and caretakers.

Temporal Lobes

The *temporal lobes* are located below the frontal and parietal lobes. They play a role in processing auditory input, visual object recognition, emotion, spatial navigation, spatial and object memory, and long-term storage of sensory input. Damage to the temporal lobes can result in decreased visual (nonverbal) and auditory memory and impairment of emotional memories. This is especially true when there is damage to the hippocampus (spatial navigation and memory) or the amygdala (emotion), both of which are located within the temporal lobes and can lead to *anterograde amnesia* (loss of memory for all events after the trauma).

There is an area in the posterior portion of the left frontal lobe, the *Wernicke's area*, which affects speech and language. Damage to this area can result in *Wernicke's aphasia,* or loss of comprehension of the spoken and often the written word, and is considered a form of extreme "word deafness." Other symptoms include music perception deficits in the right lobe and loss of external timing. The occupational performance effect is disorganization of everyday living and inability to understand instructions and forgetfulness during ADLs, IADLs, work, play, and leisure. Although clients can speak, many of their utterances are disorganized, illogical, and without content.

Occipital Lobes

The *occipital lobes* are located behind the parietal and temporal lobes, beneath the occipital bone in the back of the skull. Damage to the occipital lobes may cause a variety of deficits in the perception of color, form, and movement. They have multiple connections with other lobes, such as dorsal routes to the parietal visual lobe areas and ventral routes to the temporal visual lobe areas. The occipital interconnections with the parietal lobe function in various aspects of object recognition (form) and motion (such as the automatic postural adjustments of preshaping of the hand for grasping objects).The occipital interconnections with the temporal lobe also take part in object recognition (form and color) and identifying objects in the visual world.

Occipital lobe damage may lead to multiple impairments such as the inability to read *(alexia)*; object agnosias; or recognition problems with objects, faces, numbers, and words. Visual–spatial disorientation *(topographical disorientation)* can also be present. Blindness and visual field cuts can occur from damage at different levels of the visual system. The occupational performance challenges associated with this area of impairment are reduced safety in ADLs; IADL, and work, play, and leisure activities such as reading, math calculations, writing, and driving.

Specific Changes in Cognition and Daily Living After Alzheimer's Dementia

Alzheimer's dementia is a progressive, degenerative disease of uncertain causes that manifests itself in damage to the brain. Rombouts and colleagues (2003) and Silverman and colleagues (2003) are among the researchers who have proposed a multitude of causes for AD, including abnormal proteins and neurochemical, immunological, toxic, viral, and genetic causes.

AD is named after Dr. Alois Alzheimer, who first described the disease in 1907. The brains of persons with AD typically show pathology of the cytoskeleton of neurons in the cerebral cortex, a structure crucial for cognitive function. Microscopic analysis of the brain postmortem in these persons shows dead neurons, with changes in the neuron nucleus and cytoplasm that eventually disappear with the advance of the disease. A chemical transformation of the neuron related to abnormal secretion of brain protein (tau and amyloid protein) leads to a formation of a tangled bundle of fibrils that emerges in the site where neurons were located. These fibril tangles are called "tombstones" of neurons (Bear, Connors, & Paradiso, 2001).

AD is the fourth leading cause of death in persons over 65 years of age, and incidence increases in individuals over 85. The disease is marked by a loss of cognitive abilities that is not considered part of the normal aging process. Some of the symptoms of AD include apathy, lack of awareness of any cognitive deficits, memory deficits, decreased initiation, decreased processing speed, face and name recognition deficits, and decreased verbal fluency (Breed et al., 2008; Turró-Garriga et al., 2009).

Stages of Cognitive Changes in Alzheimer's Dementia

The stages used to categorize issues in cognition and daily living management associated with AD are *mild*, *moderate*, and *severe* (Reisberg, 1984; Reisberg, Ferris, De Leon, & Crook, 1982). The stages used to describe and predict the behaviors expected to emerge during the course of the disease are not rigidly defined but can guide occupational therapy interventions. Mini-Mental Status Examination (MMSE) scores are frequently used to classify the severity of cognitive impairment (Folstein, Folstein, & McHugh, 1975); the scale ranges from 0 to 30 points, with scores above 27 considered *normal*; 20 to 26 indicating *mild Alzheimer's*; 10 to 19 indicating *moderate Alzheimer's*; and below 10 indicating *severe Alzheimer's*.

On average, people with AD who do not receive treatment lose 2–4 MMSE points each year, painting a grim picture of dementia. Practitioners may develop a clearer understanding of the complexities involved in treating AD when they better understand the social issues associated with the disease. These include the social stigma attached to dementia; a diagnostic process that is frequently based on subjective factors; the dehumanizing treatment some clients with AD are subject to once a diagnosis is made; and that some disruptive behaviors observed in clients are (incorrectly) viewed as normal reactions to increased anxiety (Herskovits, 1995; Ronch, 1996). Because of such social phenomena associated with AD, occupational therapists and occupational therapy assistants should seek to understand the factors that contribute to effective caregiving and strive to promote the preservation of personal identity and compassion.

First Stage of Alzheimer's Disease: Mild

The first stage begins with the appearance of symptoms that include forgetfulness, repetition of questions, and difficulty in using words. Forgetfulness includes the inability to recall information after brief (short-term memory) or extended (long-term memory) periods of time. An example of forgetfulness would be the inability to remember names and to recall recent events, conversations, or object placements. (Please note that age- or stress-related forgetfulness does not indicate the presence of AD and does not, like AD, interfere with daily living.)

During the first stage of AD, most clients encounter difficulties with the initiation, speed, amount, and quality of performance of ADLs and begin to require assistance and supervision. They become forgetful, which begins to affect their performance at their job. Clients get confused about travel directions and begin to miss appointments. Judgment and problem-solving skills are impaired, and they exhibit money management problems. As the clients become more passive and more forgetful, family members notice personality and behavioral changes such as episodes of irritability and sleep disturbances. This stage may last from 2 to 4 years, during which time clients usually reside at home.

Second Stage of Alzheimer's Disease: Moderate

During the second stage, which may last from 2 to 10 years, the symptoms worsen, and the necessity for supervision and assistance by caregivers increases. Symptoms include difficulty with short- and long-term memory, leading to *confabulation*— clients invent stories to fill in the blanks of memory loss. In addition, clients encounter difficulty recognizing family and friends as well as remembering their visits. The difficulty in finding their words is increased, and they may be unable to dress and bathe independently. Supervision for mobility and travel is required, and clients exhibit a decreased ability to read, write, and perform mathematical calculations. Changes in body weight occur, and the client becomes restless, suspicious, and tends to sleep often. At this stage, most individuals are unable to maintain jobs. The caregivers must offer moderate but constant supervision in order for the individual to perform daily activities in a safe fashion.

Third Stage of Alzheimer's Dementia: Severe

In the final stage of AD, there is a global decline of all daily functions and a complete loss of judgment. In this stage, clients are unable to judge right from wrong and are dependent on 24-hour supervision and maximal assistance. This severe stage may last from 1 to 3 years. Clients have little capacity for self-care; become incontinent; and require help eating, dressing, bathing, and toileting. They sleep more frequently and for longer periods of time. They may groan and scream and become disoriented. Clients are unable to recognize family, friends, and even themselves. Some suffer a marked weight loss. Many family groups are forced to place their loved ones in nursing homes or long-term care institutions where they can receive the most effective care and intervention.

Clients with dementia who have lost their self-identity and self-care management skills still maintain the capacity for love, affection, satisfaction, joy, pain, fear, and anxiety. Therefore, practitioners need to devise management and coping strategies that will enable the clients and their family groups to gain some relief.

Specific Changes in Cognition and Daily Living After Traumatic Brain Injury

Stages of Recovery After Traumatic Brain Injury

The immediate or primary brain injuries following head trauma are classified as either a closed or a penetrating head injury. A *closed head injury* is one with no penetration of the brain by a foreign object. A *penetrating head injury* involves just such a violation. These injuries can be localized or diffuse. *Localized injuries* are specific to certain areas of the brain; *diffuse injuries* have a more generalized affect, and many structures are involved.

TBI is a complex diagnosis; for this chapter, three stages of cognitive function will be used to describe the recovery of abilities, as well as the progression and leveling off of thinking and behavior. In TBI, the trajectory of recovery generally depicts an upward progression as opposed to the regression shown in AD. TBI clients may advance from the severe to the moderate to the mild stage. Some symptoms may diminish over time but others may persist.

Two of the most common scales used to characterize particular aspects of recovery after TBI are the Glasgow Coma Scale (GCS) and the Post-Traumatic Amnesia (PTA) measures (Giacino, Kezmarsky, DeLuca, & Cicerone, 1991; Teasdale & Jennett, 1974). The GCS is based on the duration of prolonged unconsciousness or deep sleep, while the PTA is based on the duration of memory loss of the period preceding the injury. The memory loss is also called *retrograde amnesia*. These scales can be used to categorize and predict the functional outcome for the clients.

The GCS consists of a 15-point scale used to rate eye opening and motor and verbal responses. The PTA is a measurement obtained by estimating the duration of the memory loss from the moment of trauma to the time of evaluation, at which point clients are able to demonstrate the ability to communicate about memory. The GCS and PTA are used to classify brain injury severity. In general, lower scores on the GCS and a greater PTA duration indicate a more severe injury.

There are three severity classifications of TBI. *Mild impairment* includes those clients who may not have been rendered unconscious, who achieved GCS scores of 13–15, and who had a memory loss after trauma of from 5 minutes to 1 hour as measured by the PTA. *Moderate impairment* refers to clients who endured a period of unconsciousness, achieved a GCS score of 9–12, and PTA duration of less than 24 hours. *Severe impairment* includes clients who sustained coma, with GCS scores below 8 and PTA duration of more than 24 hours.

The three TBI severity classifications are also used to predict functional outcomes. Many people can live functional and productive lives after severe brain injury. The reader is cautioned not to confuse the severity classifications of TBI using GCS and PTA with the stages of recovery described in the following section. These three stages describe distinct periods and behaviors during TBI recovery. They are dynamic and may result in motor and or cognitive disabilities that range from severe to mild.

First Recovery Stage: Severe

Damage from TBI varies depending on the nature of the blow or forces applied to the head and brain. Many TBI clients incur severe damage and begin their recovery in this first stage. Some clients may have survived only thanks to advances in medical technology. As a result, their family groups must confront the ethical challenge of prolonged life in a coma or vegetative state. Although many of these groups hope for functional improvement, some clients will remain totally dependent. There are three levels within the first stage of recovery: (1) coma, (2) persistent vegetative state, (3) reactive level.

During *coma*, individuals are bedridden and lack meaningful interaction with people and the environment. These clients have a sleep-and-wake rhythm pattern and may be able to move reflexively showing grasping, chewing, sucking, and postural reflexes. During this period, clients are totally dependent in self-care management.

From coma, clients may move to a *persistent vegetative level* where they are able to control respiration, blood pressure, digestive, and excretory functions but are still totally dependent on others for self-care management.

After the *vegetative state*, the clients may progress to the final level of the first stage, where they become more responsive and begin to interact with the environment. The range of physical and cognitive skills for individual clients in this stage may vary greatly. The same is the case for the rate of recovery of physical and cognitive: They do not necessarily proceed at the same time or the same pace. Clients may exhibit the physical capabilities to perform self-care but are unable to do so because of low arousal, severe impairment in awareness of disability, poor judgment, and limited problem-solving skills. Regardless of their apparent physical recovery, clients may be confused and agitated and are unable to take care of themselves in a safe fashion. They may need help bathing, dressing, eating, and going to the toilet, and they may require assistance with mobility. They may be able to talk, yet have communication problems because they are disoriented in time, person, and place.

Late recovery after 12 months in coma, although rare, has been reported in the literature, supporting that even after more than a year, there is a possibility of improvement in motor and cognitive functions up to a moderate disability (Sancisi et al., 2009). Cranioplasty and long-term rehabilitation programs using eye-blinking responses and microswitch-based technology have also been used, supporting claims that clients in vegetative states can learn (Lancioni et al., 2009). Many other clients come out of their coma after days or months and continue to make progress and advance to the second stage of recovery.

Second Recovery Stage: Moderate

In the second stage of recovery, clients may increase their cognitive and physical capabilities and require less assistance and supervision. As in the first stage, the recovery of cognitive and physical capabilities may occur at different rates. Some clients may show moderate cognitive improvement but minimal physical or motor recovery of the upper and or lower extremities. In the second stage, clients are more purposeful and interact more appropriately with the environment and may be able to follow instructions but may demonstrate difficulty with detecting, processing, and responding to stimuli. Their behaviors are characterized varioiusly as distractible, impulsive, slow, hyperactive or hypoactive, and repetitive *(perseveration)*.

They may have difficulty with short- and long-term memory, including recall and recognition of names, faces, objects, and locations. Clients may also be unable to remember family and friends, when they ate, when or if they took a shower, and if they had traveled. They may have problems reading, writing, and doing simple math. Many may be able to perform cash transactions independently but require supervision in budgeting and banking.

Clients in this stage often exhibit emotional changes that affect their relationships with others. They may become irritable, short-tempered, and disinhibited, leading to cursing and sexually inappropriate behavior. In general, TBI clients are likely to express emotional distress after injury and have sleep disturbances. They may have both verbal and nonverbal speech and language problems that take the form of responses inappropriate to the situation and are irrelevant, incoherent, or demonstrate misunderstanding of the intentions of others. Some clients have trouble with intonation and gesture. Their speech may not have the inflection necessary to communicate meaning, making them sound robotic.

During this stage, caregivers must provide constant supervision in order to provide a safe environment for self-care. Clients may not regain their former employment status but may be able to perform other productive activities. Some individuals progress to the third stage of recovery, but others remain fixed at this level for the rest of their lives.

Third Recovery Stage: Mild

The third stage of recovery includes those clients who have successfully completed Stage 2 and those individuals with a mild closed head injury. Clients who sustain mild TBI may not experience coma or, if they have post-traumatic memory loss, it is of brief duration.

Two examples of people at risk for mild TBI due to head concussions are athletes who participate in high-contact sports (Meehan & Bachur, 2009) and military personnel following combat (Schneiderman, Braver, & Kaney, 2008). More than 70% and up to 90% of all traumatic head injury is considered mild TBI (Shores et al., 2008). Some studies have suggested that cognitive deficits after mild TBI dissipate 1–3 months postinjury. Other have shown that even people who were only briefly stunned, or knocked unconscious by a blast or blow, may experience chronic symptoms for years postinjury (Belanger, Uomoto, & Vanderploeg, 2009; Kennedy et al., 2007; Ruff, Ruff, & Wang, 2008). Symptoms include posttraumatic stress disorder symptoms (PTSD), headaches, and executive function problems. Executive functions are complex and interacting cognitive functions that govern and regulate all purposeful behaviors, including planning and organization; decision making and sequencing; self-monitoring and self-initiating; and sustaining actions and others (Gordon, Cantor, Ashman, & Brown, 2006; Zgaljardic, Mattis, & Charness, in press). Executive dysfunction leads to a variety of difficulties in IADLs such as financial management, writing letters, calculating, driving, planning the week, and using public transportation. It represents one of the most significant barriers to social skills flexibility and community integration.

In addition, sleep disturbances are frequently present after TBI. This may pose multiple problems; clients may tend to be drowsy during the day, which may lead to decreased participation and performance during therapy. Drowsiness also makes it more difficult to maintain attention to daily task demands. Nighttime drowsiness may lead to increased falls and behavioral disturbances (Makley et al., 2008).

In the third stage, IADLs are usually the primary areas of concern, such as poor social skills and difficulty functioning independently in the community. The Community Mobility Assessment was developed to assess adolescents with acquired brain injury to determine if they are safe and capable of going out alone in the community (Brewer, Geisler, Moody, & Wright, 1998). TBI can also affect satisfaction in other areas of life such as leisure or sexual enjoyment.

In a study assessing satisfaction-of-life of patients with severe TBI, Quintard et al. (2002) found that 36% were dissatisfied with their leisure activity, and 32% were dissatisfied with their sexual life. Compared with individuals without disability, individuals with TBI report more frequent physiological difficulties influencing their energy for sex, sex drive, and ability to initiate sexual activities, as well as physical difficulties influencing body positioning, body movement and sensation (Hibbard, Gordon, Flanagan, Haddad, & Labinski, 2000). Psychosocial disability in individuals with TBI may result in a lack of involvement in leisure activities

(Hall et al., 1994). The occupational therapist should be alert to these issues and be prepared to help clients or refer them to others for appropriate counseling or intervention.

The three stages provide general guidelines that may help practitioners describe and predict the behaviors that emerge during recovery. They are not homogeneous across or within cognitive, motor, or functional areas. For example, recovery rates for short- and long-term memory may not be the same for any given client. In addition, clients may not achieve the same level of proficiency in feeding and bathing. These stages provide a general guideline of the potential progression of recovery for TBI clients. As practitioners consider the persistent nature of symptoms and their impact on the client's self-image and support system, this section might help them better appreciate the psychological and social consequences of TBI on clients and their families.

Evaluation of Cognition Performance Components and Occupational Performance

One objective of occupational therapy evaluations is to gather information that can guide intervention, whether it is remedial or adaptive. Many centers use both standardized and nonstandardized evaluations of cognitive and motor disabilities, functional performance, and participation after TBI and AD (Hartman-Maeir, Katz, & Baum, 2009; Lange, Spagnolo, & Fowler, 2009; Temple et al., 2009; Turner, Fricke, & Darzins, 2009; Unsworth, 2008).

Practitioners use a variety of evaluation methods, including direct observation of performance, specific questioning, formal questionnaires, and family groups' or other caretakers' information. Regardless of the evaluation measures used, practitioners must describe and document how the client responds to cues and repetition during the evaluation process. A client's behavioral changes in response to cues and repetition can predict functional outcomes and benefits expected from rehabilitation. Cues and prompts that were beneficial during evaluation of performance components, function, and participation are also used in the development of intervention strategies.

General Evaluation Strategies

The use of standardized and nonstandardized measurements for the evaluation of cognition and ADLs is common in the rehabilitation process (see Box 14.2). Measurement strategies are used to describe, classify, and assign numbers to behaviors in order to establish a baseline for intervention, to monitor changes, and to provide information useful for discharge planning. The authors use two perspectives, a bottom-up and a top-down (Abreu, 1981, 1998; Abreu & Peloquin, 2005).

The *bottom-up perspective* is used to measure specific impairment within performance components, such as cognition. The *top-down perspective* is used to measure and describe occupational performance, participation, community integration, and well-being. Successful rehabilitation results from using a confluent, free-flowing application of both perspectives.

Confluence denotes a fluid movement back and forth between perspectives (Peloquin, 1996). This results in simultaneous attention being given to both performance components and everyday living occupations and habits. This evaluation model balances an understanding of the specific nature of impairments with an understanding of people as occupational beings. It rejects the commonplace assumption that practitioners must choose between holism and reductionism, instead promoting the use of both perspectives (Abreu, 1998). No causality or directional relationship is implied or necessary in order for this model to be effective (Wood, Abreu, Duval, & Gerber, 1994).

During evaluation, practitioners must analyze the processing strategies used by clients during task performance. In addition, they must examine the conditions that can affect the performance positively or negatively, including the use of cues and test repetition (Abreu & Toglia, 1987; Toglia, 1991). The authors advocate using a process-oriented approach to probe clients and analyze their ability to change with practice and benefit from instructions and cues.

Identifying Cognitive Performance Necessary for Everyday Living

Cognitive evaluation strategies are dynamic, using test repetition, external cueing, and environment modifications, such as strategically placed reminder signs. Therapists using these strategies can measure the client's cognitive deficits and can determine the conditions that improve or cause deterioration in performance (Abreu & Toglia, 1987). Standardized measures use scores to indicate how well the client performed relative to norms. In contrast, nonstandardized measures do not incorporate norms. Tables 14.1 and 14.2 show examples of measures used for both AD and TBI. Therapists should select various standardized and nonstandardized measurement tools to survey at least four different performance components.

Box 14.2. The Assessment Process

Standardized and nonstandardized measurements for the evaluation of cognition and ADLs are commonly used to describe, classify, and assign numbers to behaviors in order to establish a baseline for intervention, to monitor changes, and to provide information useful for discharge planning.

- Successful rehabilitation results are reported using a confluent, free-flowing application of both a bottom-up perspective used to measure specific impairment within performance components such as cognition and a top-down perspective used to measure functional performance, participation, community integration, and well-being.
- A process-oriented evaluation approach is recommended to probe clients and analyze their ability to change with practice and benefit from instructions and cues.
- Cues and repetitions are used to determine the most efficient methods of instruction and training.
- Four performance components evaluations are as follows: (1) cognitive function; (2) awareness, including error detection and error correction; (3) movement and postural control; and (4) body alignment in action or at rest.
- The Functional Independence Measure (FIM™) is widely used to measure functional status of basic daily living skills after TBI and AD.
- IADLs in AD and TBI evaluations should include bathing, meal planning, handling finances, and shopping.
- Qualitative measures and strategies are required in order to keep a humanistic orientation with therapists acting as observers, recorders, and collaborators.

Table 14.1. Alzheimer's Dementia Evaluations

Test	Purpose	Reference
Alzheimer Home Assessment	To evaluate the home environment's legibility and stability to ensure safety	Painter, J. (1996). Home environment considerations for people with Alzheimer's disease. *Occupational Therapy in Healthcare, 10,* 45–63.
Cleveland Scale of Daily Living (CSADL)	To measure physical skills, IADLs, communication skills, and social behaviors	Patterson, M. B., Mack, J. L., Neundorfer, M. M., Martin, R. J., Smyth, K. A., & Whitehouse, P. J. (1992). Assessment of functional ability in Alzheimer's disease: A review and a preliminary report on the Cleveland Scale of Activities of Daily Living. *Alzheimer's Disease and Associated Disorders, 6,* 145–163.
Clifton Assessment Procedures for the Elderly (CAPE)	To measure physical disability, apathy, communication, and social disturbances	Pattie, A. H., & Gilleard, C. J. (1979). *Clifton assessment procedures for the elderly (CAPE).* Sevenoaks, Kent, UK: Hodder & Stoughton.
Clinical Dementia Rating (CDR)	To measure and follow the natural history (i.e., irrespective of intervention) of senile dementia of the Alzheimer's type	Morris, J. C. (1993). The clinical dementia rating (CDR): Current version and scoring rules. *Neurology, 43*(11), 2,412–2,414.
Echelle Comportement et Adaption (ECA)	To measure physical independence, social integration, occupation, orientation, mobility, and language	Ritchie, K., & Ledesert, B. (1991).The measurement of incapacity in the severely demented elderly: The validation of a behavioural assessment scale. *International Journal of Geriatric Psychiatry, 6,* 217–226.
Global Deterioration Scale (GDS)	To assess the clinically identifiable and ratable stages of primary degenerative dementia and age-associated memory impairment	Reisberg, B., Ferris, S. H., De Leon, M. J., & Crook, T. (1982). The Global Deterioration Scale for assessment of primary degenerative dementia. *American Journal of Psychiatry, 139,* 1136–1139.
Kitchen Task Assessment (KTA)	A functional measure that records the level of cognitive support required by a person with AD	Baum, C., & Edwards, D. F. (1993). Cognitive performance in senile dementia of Alzheimer's type: The Kitchen Task Assessment. *American Journal of Occupational Therapy, 47,* 431–436.

(Continued)

Table 14.1. Alzheimer's Dementia Evaluations *(cont.)*

Test	Purpose	Reference
London Psychogeriatic Rating Scale (LPRS)	To measure mental disorganization, confusion, physical disability, socially irritating behavior, and disengagement	Hersch, E. L., Kral, V. A., & Palmer, R. B. (1978). Clinical value of the London psychogeriatric rating scale. *Journal of American Geriatrics Society, 26,* 348–354.
Structured Assessment of Independent Living Skills (SAILS)	To measure language, orientation, money-related skills, IADLs, and social interaction	Mahurin, R. K., De Bettignes, B. H., & Pirozzolo, F. J. (1991). Structured Assessment of Independent Living Skills: Preliminary report of a performance measure of functional abilities in dementia. *Journal of Gerontology: Psychological Sciences, 46,* 48–66.
Direct Assessment of Functional Abilities (DAFA)	Designed as a direct performance measure of IADL status for patients with dementia	Karagiozis, H., Gray, S., Sacco, J., Shapiro, M., & Kawas, C. (1998). The Direct Assessment of Functional Abilities (DAFA): A comparison to an indirect measure of instrumental activities of daily living. *The Gerontologist, 38,* 113–121.
Direct Assessment of Functional Status	Direct assessment of functional status	Loewenstein, D., et al. (1989). A new scale for the assessment of functional status in Alzheimer's disease and related disorders. *Journal of Gerontology: Psychological Sciences, 44,* 114–112.
Mini-Mental Status Examination (MMSE)	Short, simple, qualitative measure of cognitive performance	Folstein, M. F., Folstein, S. E., & McHugh, P. R. (1975). Mini-Mental State: A practical method for grading the cognitive-state of patients for the clinician. *Journal of Psychiatric Research, 12,* 189–198.
Blessed Dementia Rating Scale	To quantify the degree of intellectual and personality deterioration in people with dementia, based on their ability to deal with the practical tasks of everyday life as well as on simple psychological tests	Blessed, G., Tomlinson, B. E., & Roth, M. (1968). The association between quantitative measures of dementia and of senile change in the cerebral grey matter of elderly subjects. *British Journal of Psychiatry, 114,* 797–811.

Note. AD = Alzheimer's disease; IADLs = instrumental activities of daily living.

Table 14.2. Traumatic Brain Injury Evaluations

Test	Purpose	Reference
Coma/Near Coma Scale (CNC)	To monitor increased responsiveness to stimulation, indicating the severity of sensory, perceptual, and primitive response deficits at the coma level	Rappaport, M., Doughtery, A. M., & Kelting D. L. (1992). Evaluation of coma and vegetative states. *Archives of Physical Medicine and Coma Rehabilitation, 73,* 628–634.
Recovery Scale (CRS)	To monitor increased responsiveness to stimulation, indicating the severity of sensory, perceptual, and primitive response deficits at the coma level	Giacino, J. T., Kezmarsky, M. A., DeLuca, J., & Cicerone, K. D. (1991). Monitoring rate of recovery to predict outcome in minimally responsive patients. *Archives of Physical Medicine and Rehabilitation, 72,* 897–900.
Sensory Stimulation Assessment Measure (SSAM)	To monitor increased responsiveness to stimulation, indicating the severity of sensory, perceptual, and primitive response deficits at the coma level	Rader, M. A., Alston, J. B., & Ellis, D. W. (1989). Sensory stimulation of severely brain-injured patients. *Brain Injury, 3,* 141–147.
Western Neuro Sensory Stimulation Profile (WNSSP)	To monitor increased responsiveness to stimulation, indicating the severity of sensory, perceptual, and primitive response deficits at the coma level	Ansell, B. J., & Keenan, J. E. (1989). The Western Neuro Sensory Stimulation Profile: A tool for assessing slow-to-recover head injury patients. *Archives of Physical Medicine and Rehabilitation, 70,* 104–108.
Awareness Questionnaire	To measure cognitive, behavioral/affective, and motor/sensory factors	Sherer, M., Bergloff, P., Boake, C., High, W., Jr., & Levin, E. (1998). The Awareness Questionnaire: Factor structure and internal consistency. *Brain Injury, 12,* 63–68.
Self-Awareness Deficits Interview	To evaluate self-awareness using qualitative methods	Fleming, J. M., Strong, J., & Ashton, R. (1996). Self-awareness of deficits in adults with traumatic brain injury: How best to measure? *Brain Injury, 10,* 1–15.

(Continued)

Table 14.2. Traumatic Brain Injury Evaluations *(cont.)*

Test	Purpose	Reference
Community Integration Questionnaire (CQI)	To measure handicap in homelike setting, social network, and integration into productive activities	Willer B., Ottenbacher, K. J., & Coad, M. L. (1994). The Community Integration Questionnaire: A comparative examination. *Archives of Physical Medicine and Rehabilitation, 73*, 103–111.
Functional Independence Measure (FIM)	To measure disability using average daily minutes of assistance from another person	Corrigan, J., Smith-Knapp, K., & Granger, C. V. (1997). Validity of the Functional Independence Measure for persons with traumatic brain injury. *Archives of Physical Medicine and Rehabilitation, 78*, 828–834.
Head Injury Symptom Checklist	To measure impairment in mild TBI	McLean, A., Dikmen, S., Temkin, N., Wyler, A. R., & Gale, J. I. (1984). Psychosocial functioning at one month after injury. *Neurosurgery, 14*, 393–399.
Medical Outcome Study SF–36	To measure physical health and role limitations	Ware, J. E. (1993). *SF–36 health survey manual and interpretation guide.* Boston: Health Institute, New England Medical Center.
		Clark, F., Azen, S., Zemke, R., Jackson, J., Carlson, M., Mandel, D., et al. (1997). Occupational therapy for independent-living older adults: A randomized controlled trial. *JAMA, 278*(16), 1321–1326.
Assessment of Motor and Process Skills (AMPS)	To evaluate household task performance	Darragh, A. R., Sample, P. L., & Fisher, A. G. (1998). Environment effect of functional task performance in adults with acquired brain injuries: Use of the Assessment of Motor and Process Skills. *Archives of Physical Medicine and Rehabilitation, 79*, 418–423.
		Cooke, K. Z., Fisher, A. G., Mayberry, W., & Oakley, F. (2000). Differences in activities of daily living process skills of persons with and without Alzheimer's disease. *Occupational Therapy Journal of Research, 20*, 87–105.
Autobiographical Memory Interview (AMI)	To assess autobiographical memory (the capacity to recall facts and incidents from one's own life) in order to help understand the nature of any memory deficit, to assist in intervention, to individualize subsequent management, and to facilitate research investigating anterograde vs. retrograde amnesia	Published by Thames Valley Test Company, Suffolk, England (1990). Distributed in North America by National Rehabilitation Services, 117 North Elm Street, P.O. Box 1247, Gaylord, MI 49735; tel: 517-732-3866; fax: 517-732-6164
Contextual Memory Test (CMT)	To assess awareness of memory capacity, use of strategy, and recall in adults with memory dysfunction; can be used as a screen to determine the need for further evaluation or to indicate how responsive the individual is to memory cues, thereby indicating need for compensatory or remedial treatment	Published by Therapy Skill Builders (1993), a division of The Psychological Corporation, 555 Academic Court, San Antonio, TX 78204-2498; tel: 800-228-0752; fax: 800-232-1223

Note. TBI = traumatic brain injury.

The first component is *cognitive function,* or the manner in which clients gather information from the environment. This includes attention, memory, and problem solving. Therapists may use a cancellation test, which assesses both speed and accuracy, to evaluate attention. Memory can be tested with a simple recall schema for auditory and visual memory. Simple mathematics problems may be used for problem solving.

The second component is *awareness of disability,* which may be tested via an interview process.

Therapists may ask if clients are aware of any problems, determine whether they recognize errors, and see if they predict that they are going to have problems in the future.

The third component includes *movement and postural control* and is tested when practitioners observe individuals performing arts, crafts, or other activities. Finally, the fourth component includes the *client's body alignment,* observed while the body is in action and at rest. Advanced technology in pressure mapping allows clinicians to objectively and directly measure postural adjustment of trunk and extremities while the client is seated on a wheelchair, standing, in motion, and also while weight-bearing with the hands (Abreu, Jones, & Opacich, 2007; Abreu et al., 2007; Reistetter, Abreu, Bear-Lehman, & Ottenbacher, in press). The evaluation of both cognitive and motor components is essential because motor performance is a reflection of cognitive process.

Evaluating Everyday Living Skills

The Functional Independence Measure (FIM™) is widely used to measure the functional status of basic daily living skills after TBI and AD. IADLs in AD and TBI evaluations may involve meal planning, handling finances, and shopping (these are frequently self-reported or informant-based questionnaires or both) and performance-based assessments (Sikkes et al., 2009).

However, other quantitative and qualitative measures and strategies are required in order to maintain a humanistic orientation that has therapists actively observing, recording, and collaborating. Therapists use narrative and performance analysis to explain and predict behavior based on four client characteristics: (1) lifestyle status, (2) life stage, (3) health status, and (4) level of disadvantage. Therapists interview clients and family groups, asking questions about each area.

- Questions on lifestyle focus on communication, work, and day-to-day operations, including personal characteristics and the use of economic resources. A sample question is "How would you describe your lifestyle before your accident?"
- A life-stage status sample question is "How would you describe the physical, emotional, and spiritual characteristics of your life today?" Relevant factors include age, marital status, accomplishments, and losses. Another question is "What was your latest accomplishment?"
- Therapists survey the client's health status, including premorbid conditions and changes in behavior or condition following the accident or illness. "How was your health before the illness?"

Notice that these questions require receptive- and expressive-language skills. The therapist may need to simplify and shorten the questions for people with speech, language, and cognitive impairments.

For a determination of the level of disadvantage experienced by the client, therapists investigate the degree of personal and social restrictions. Examples might be a client's inability to attend movies, shop, cook, or provide in any way for family members or others. "What support system does your community offer to people with brain injury?" Therapists evaluate the client's motivation, goals, actions, and capacity through an analysis of his or her performance of ordinary occupations and activities. Therapists use both standardized and nonstandardized measures to assess the client's ability in ADLs. The scoring of the client's performance is based on his or her level of independence—independent, mild, moderate, or maximum assistance.

Persons with AD and TBI appear to retain procedural memory of "knowing how" to do particular activities better than declarative memory of "knowing what" to do for particular activities (Cooke, Fisher, Mayberry, & Oakley, 2000). These differences are used for evaluation and intervention directed toward increasing functional independence. However, it is unclear how cognitive components relate and affect ADL and IADL performance (Nygard, Amberla, Bernspång, Almkvist, & Winblad, 1998). Therefore, we need to continue to evaluate and study their relationship.

Adaptive Strategies, Equipment, and Environmental Modifications for Everyday Living

Intervention alternatives for persons with cognitive deficits are varied and complex. The goals are to maintain, restore, and improve everyday living; to promote health; and to modify through compensation, adaptation (Moyers, 1999), and prevention. The use of cueing and the repetition of tasks continue as a basic theme in intervention strategies, whether the intervention is for remediation or compensation. Cues and repetition are used to determine the most efficient methods of instruction and training.

Following neurological decline, clients may have difficulty changing the way they perform their ADLs, and IADLs (Miller & Butin, 2000; Reistetter, Chang, & Abreu, 2009), including meal planning and preparation. These are universal, personal, cultural, and social activities in which one engages regularly. Persons with AD or TBI can have deficits in language comprehension, organization, judgment, memory, attention, problem solving, planning, awareness of deficits, sensation, vision, reaction time, and time management. These may pose hazards in the kitchen environment (Zhang et al., 2003).

Therapists provide advice on adapting kitchen environments and equipment for maximum safety and success. Occupational therapists teach clients, caretakers, and family groups cognitive strategies emphasizing simplification, planning, organization, and categorization. Some strategies used to increase safety are checklists to ensure tasks are completed in an orderly fashion; memory books; marking through steps already performed; adaptive equipment to compensate for physical limitations; enlarged directions for the visually impaired; auditory timers; simplified directions; and reduced and simplified stimuli, such as doing one task at a time rather than multitasking.

General Intervention Strategies

Presented below are four dynamically interrelated intervention strategies for individuals both with AD and TBI. They are (1) drugs and medications, (2) cognitive rehabilitation, (3) human connection, and (4) caregiver education (see Box 14.3).

Drugs and Medications

Frequently, drugs and medications can reduce AD and TBI symptoms of cognitive and motor dysfunction. Pharmacological interventions after TBI include a variety of medications, including methylphenidate, donepezil, and bromocriptine for the treatment of cognitive disturbances, beta-blockers for controlling aggressiveness, and progesterone as a neuroprotective drug. Botulinum toxin type A injections for spasticity reduction are also frequently used with good supportive evidence at the impairment level, such as increased range of motion and and muscle tone, but many studies do not follow up for generalization in functional performance. (Further discussion of this complex topic is beyond the scope of this chapter.)

Cognitive Rehabilitation

Cognitive rehabilitation approaches are interventions that remediate or compensate for cognitive deficits. Therapists use these approaches to design programs for AD and TBI (Katz, 1998). The foundation for cognitive learning strategies is cognitive psychology. Cognitive learning strategies include teaching clients to process, structure, and modify information that is not directly observable, such as awareness and memory. Therapists facilitate clients' efficiency with specific ADL tasks, situations, and rules of behavior. For example, clients are encouraged to use imagery, conscious awareness, and self-monitoring techniques such as using checklists, slowing down before rechecking answers, and self-talk. The assumption when using cognitive learning strategies is that the client's motivation in everyday living activities lies in their desire to master competency and enjoy independence. The clients' conscious awareness and self-monitoring abilities determine the selection of cognitive strategies.

The foundation for behavioral learning strategies is behavior modification. Therapists use these techniques to teach clients to modify their observable behaviors, such as ADLs (Giles & Clark-Wilson, 1993; Jacobs, 1993). Therapists facilitate appropriate social behaviors when decreasing behaviors such as

---

Box 14.3. The Intervention Process

Four dynamically interrelated intervention strategies for both individuals with AD and TBI are as follows: (1) drugs and medications, (2) cognitive rehabilitation, (3) human connection, and (4) caregiver education.

- Drugs and medications can reduce AD and TBI symptoms of cognitive and motor dysfunction.
- Cognitive rehabilitation can use behavioral learning strategies through behavior modification techniques to modify specified behaviors, such as incontinence, biting, hitting, and screaming, by using reward and punishment.
- Cognitive rehabilitation can use cognitive learning strategies through practices such as conscious awareness, and self-monitoring techniques such as using checklists, slowing down, and self-talking.
- Human connection strategies can use emphatic communication, caring touch, and the reconstruction of rituals and habits (e.g., the morning routine, television viewing, outings).
- Caretaker education in how to deal with the responsibilities of caregiving and the effects of cognitive deficit can reduce the burden of care and increase quality of life of family groups.
- The three intervention phases—preparation, performance, and review—are used to establish emotional and social connections and goals, to teach compensation and functional performance, to bring closure at the end of each session, and to document and adjust goals and timetables.

incontinence, biting, hitting, screaming, and crying are present. They identify possible functional relationships of cause and effect, such as reward and punishment, to shape specified behaviors. The assumption is that clients are motivated to perform self-care by their positive or negative environmental reinforcements. Behavioral learning strategies require a very rigorous program involving the entire health care team. Most practitioners use a combination of cognitive and behavioral learning strategies.

Human Connection

The foundations for human connection strategies include universal principles of wellness, social science, and occupational science. Human connection helps us regain or preserve a person's meaningful and emotional experiences (Wilcock, 1998; Zemke & Clark, 1996). Examples of human connection strategies are empathic communication; caring touch; and the reconstruction of rituals and habits such as the morning routine, television viewing, and outings (Clark, 1993; Crepeau, 1995; Peloquin, 1995; Zemke, 1995).

All clients have the need for social interconnections; they help them maintain a sense of well-being regardless of their cognitive deficits (Abreu, 1998; Hasselkus, 1998; Herskovits, 1995). Therapists must try to understand their client's experience of disability, the trajectory of their illness, their loss of well-being, and their disruption of self. They need to use human connection strategies for everyday living skills management because these emotional experiences are essential to the achievement of a holistic intervention.

Caregiver Education

Caregiver education strategies include identifying and describing the client's needs and characteristics to the caregiver group. These help prepare families and friends for their new roles. Although there are numerous reports on family-focused intervention, there are limited guidelines for these strategies. Therapists must use sociological principles to develop an approach to caregiving and consider cultural differences. Haley and colleagues have shown that African-American caregivers often report less depression than White family groups when assisting AD clients (Haley et al., 1996). Other studies suggest that Hispanic caregivers have strong family relationships, values, and norms that shape their caregiving roles (Cox & Monk, 1993).

For AD, therapists must advise family groups how to deal with puzzlement, fear of genetic linkages, and the responsibilities of caregiving for an individual with substantial cognitive deficit. They must also inform caregivers of the need for respite services and support groups. In the later stages of dementia, caregivers must be prepared to deal with nursing care decisions, guardianship, and informed consent.

For TBI, therapists must advise family groups about confusion, awareness of disability, and other effects of cognitive impairment. They should also inform clients and family groups of community resources and support groups. In cases involving chronic and severe impairment, placement, guardianship, and informed consent should be addressed.

Intervention Phases

Most intervention involves three phases: (1) preparation, (2) performance, and (3) review. To be effective, each phase requires collaboration among practitioners, clients, and family groups.

Preparation Phase

In the first phase, therapists work with clients and family groups to establish emotional and social connections and to have the clients express their goals. There are three parts to the preparation phase. First, the therapists, clients, and family groups *establish a trusting and relaxed rapport* through conversation, stress reduction, and meditation techniques. Next, therapists help clients become aware of and focus their attention on the *goals and projected outcomes* of intervention. Therapists may use instruction and cueing with multiple senses to increase the awareness of intervention (e.g., use of visual and auditory instructions). Finally, therapists and clients *develop strategies* to maximize the client's ability to organize and process information during preparation for self-care and other ADLs. The instructional information used may have to be divided into component parts to make it more understandable.

Performance Phase

In the performance phase, the goal is to improve or compensate for the clients' memory and learning ability and increase their satisfaction with their progress. This involves the use of practice, feedback, and environmental modification, based on the clients' evaluation and goals. Therapists, clients, tasks, exercise, and occupations all contribute to the environmental change or contextual modification during intervention.

Practice consists of clients' planned repetition of actions and behaviors at a predetermined frequency for a predetermined duration. An example would be for clients to repeat the action of putting on a sweater 3 times in a half-hour 3 times a week. Therapists and caregivers use feedback to provide helpful responses to clients during practice, adjusting their feedback depending on the client's performance. The frequency varies depending on the clients' cognitive and physical recovery level, as indicated by performance tests. Clients may be independent (100%) or require mild (90%), moderate (50%), or maximum assistance (25%). If the initial evaluation performance score is less than 50%, therapists will use constant feedback; however, if the score is above the 50%, the therapist will use less.

Environmental modifications are used simultaneously with feedback and include adaptation by clients, therapists, and family groups to their surroundings and changing the objects within them. There are two types of environments. A *congruent environment* is one that is simple and familiar, requiring minimal cognitive-processing demands. Making soup at home with no time constraints is an example of a congruent and stable environment. A *contextual interference environment* is a more complex surrounding that requires maximal processing demands. An example would be the client making full-course meals in an unfamiliar kitchen with a time limit. Contextual interference makes the immediate intervention goal more difficult to achieve but, if used properly, can strengthen the learning pattern. Clients whose performance requires mild assistance benefit by training in distracting, variable environments with contextual interferences. On the other hand, clients requiring moderate and maximum assistance benefit by training in nondistracting, stable, predictable environments.

Review Phase

At the end of each intervention session, therapists bring closure by re-evaluating and documenting client progress, comparing current to prior performance. Based on this constant reevaluation, therapists, clients, and family groups readjust goals and timetables. It is important to note that chronic clients who are maximally dependent in ADLs, such as self-care, may not achieve significant functional progress. With these clients, the focus must be on humanistic connection and well-being. Examples of strategies used in each phase are given in Table 14.3 and Table 14.4, which list examples of intervention strategies for AD and TBI.

Measuring Intervention Outcomes

Outcome measurement is an attempt to quantify the quality of therapeutic services in terms of effectiveness or achievement of goals, efficiency or optimal rate of progress, and value or cost containment. Both standardized and nonstandardized measures quantify rehabilitation results. AD and TBI clients in the severe phase may not achieve functional improvement. Therefore, functional outcomes are not always appropriate. A critical outcome for these clients is physical, mental, and spiritual wellness. Other tools at the community and participation level may be appropriate. Please refer to the evaluation tables.

Summary

Management of AD and TBI is a collaborative effort requiring the coordinated efforts of the entire rehabilitation team, the client, and the family group. This collaboration allows constant monitoring of daily living skills and consistency in approaches to patients, particularly those with cultural differences. While both AD and TBI can profoundly affect cognition, the trajectories of the conditions are quite different. AD results in progressive cognitive decline, requiring greater assistance as the client becomes more dependent on others for care. TBI, in contrast, is often characterized by the client's ability to relearn skills or adaptive approaches that enable increased independence in performing the activities necessary for daily living. In each condition, when cognitive impairment is moderate or severe, careful attention must be given to the use of cues and prompts to support the client's performance of daily activities.

Because of the demands of care, the burden placed on family caregivers can be significant. Therapy personnel can educate family members about appropriate techniques for client assistance at home and offer strategies to prevent burnout. Because health is more than the absence of illness; effective intervention plans involve strategies to foster community integration, which provides an opportunity for clients and family groups to develop healthy lifestyles (Wilcock, 1998).

Effective intervention plans enable clients to perform meaningful occupations that foster connections with others and provide as much autonomy and self-determination as possible. Given the challenges of daily living management for individuals with cognitive deficits after AD and TBI, achieving these aims remains both an art and a science.

Table 14.3. Intervention Phases for Alzheimer's Dementia and Traumatic Brain Injury

Preparation Phase	Identify the most effective means for interacting with the client and influencing performance by identifying and assessing various *regulators*—the relevant characteristics in the environment that can help individuals direct and organize their response to action, derived from language, people, circumstances, and conditions that surround an individual.

Language regulators: Nature of instructions that are most effective for the client:
- *Verbal instructions:* Language used, level, volume, speed, inflections, concreteness, complexity, general cues, specific cues, give-away cues, hierarchy.
- *Written instructions:* Language used, level, speed of presentation, size, concreteness, complexity general cues, specific cues, give-away cues.
- *Gestural instructions:* Language used, speed, concreteness, general cues, specific cues, give-away cues.
- *Pictorial instructions:* Line drawings, black-and-white pictures, color pictures, two-dimensional, three-dimensional.
- *Tactile/kinesthetic instructions:* Amount of hand guidance, tactile proprioceptive pressure used, speed of movement, general cues, specific cues, give-away cues.

Sociocultural regulators: Client's value judgment on the meaningfulness of the skill.

Physical regulators: Physical attributes that control actions of that skill, such as temporal and spatial attributes (location and target speed).

Identify the most effective environment for interacting with the client and influencing performance (identify and assess the environmental affordances and barriers).
- *Physical appearances:* Physical affordances and attributes that may or may not control action. They can conceal or make goal of the skill more salient, such as color, texture, size.
- *Practice location:* Real-life or simulated environments (e.g., client's room, gym, kitchen, bathroom, shops).
- *Practice frequency and intensity:* Amount of repetition of specific skill and time of analysis dedicated to the practice of each skill in one training session.
- *Nature of feedback:* Verbal, nonverbal, general, specific, give-away, or face-saving hierarchy.
- *Feedback frequency and intensity:* Constant, immediate, delayed, infrequent, (i.e., 100% feedback = every trial; 50% = 5 times out of every trial).

Performance Phase

List the client's goals by common denominator.

Analyze underlying skills for each goal.

Analyze pretreatment, concurrent, and post-treatment practice strategies.

Bottom up (micro) sample goals, The client is—
- Able to orient eyes, head, and neck 100% of the time during a variety of postures in 1 week.
- Able to realign and adjust to self-initiated postural control during dressing tasks 75% of the time in 2 weeks.
- Able to realign and adjust to externally initiated postural control during dressing tasks 75% of the time in 3 weeks.
- Able to increase body response during self-care from 12 seconds to 7 seconds in 1 week.

Top down (macro) sample goals, The client is—
- Able to perform favorite occupation safely in 3 weeks, while standing.
- Able to perform more than one activity, task, or role safely in 2 weeks.
- Able to engage in favorite social recreation (i.e., dancing) in 2 weeks.

General Rules
- Instruct learners on the importance of practice as it relates to posture (i.e., home, institution, community safety).
- Involve family members during the practice. They can help validate the client's responses.
- During the initial trial, allow the client to respond without modification. Then adapt the modification strategies during the next trials.
- Notice, discover, and recognize gross and subtle changes in visual, auditory, vestibular, and proprioceptive stimuli.

Review Phase
- Performance is tested after an interval long enough to have practice effects dissipated.
- Determine the performance effect of random, variable, and blocked practice.
- Question client/family about their satisfaction or dissatisfaction with the results of the treatment session.
- Adjust or expand goals in an interdisciplinary context.

Table 14.4. Treatment Strategies for Alzheimer's Dementia and Traumatic Brain Injury in Performance Areas

Targeted Action	Retraining for Mild Cognitive Impairment	Compensation for Moderate Cognitive Impairment	Total Caregiving for Severe Cognitive Impairment
PERSONAL HYGIENE			
Unable to brush hair	• Clients are taught to simplify and organize task in parts: right side, left side, front. • Therapists' cues match clients' most beneficial sensory modality (auditory, visual, tactile, kinesthetic). • Clients are taught to say steps aloud before and during task.	• Clients are given checklist with steps and sequences. • Clients are taught one-handed techniques. • Therapists appropriately modify brushes: larger or smaller, heavier or lighter, bright colors. • Therapists appropriately modify location of brush: constant, fixed position to match any perceptual or cognitive loss. • Therapists appropriately modify mirror location and size.	• Use caregiver assistance for part or whole task.
Unable to perform oral hygiene	• Clients are taught to use toothbrush and floss in parts: front teeth first, followed by left, right, and back teeth.	• Clients are provided battery-operated toothbrushes, taught one-handed flossing.	• Use caregiver assistance for part or whole task.
Unable to bathe and shower	• Clients are taught to simplify and organize task in steps: temperature control—cold water before hot; regulation; clean critical body areas.	• Clients are given checklist with steps and sequences. • Clients are given bathtub and shower seats, adapter shower handles, soaps on a rope, rubber mats, and handrails.	• Use caregiver assistance for part or whole task.
DRESSING			
Unable to perform upper dressing	• Clients are taught to arrange garments in specific order and dress in specific sequence. • Clients are taught to say steps aloud before and during task.	• Clients are given checklist with correct steps and sequences. • Clients are given pictures/photos of correct steps as cues. • Clients are taught one-handed techniques. • Therapists appropriately modify clothing: larger sizes; hook-and-loop fasteners, snaps, button aids, zipper aids.	• Use caregiver assistance for part or whole task.
Unable to perform lower dressing Unable to put shoes on feet Unable to put on prosthetic devices	• Clients are taught to arrange garments in specific order and dress in specific sequence. In addition postural control training in bed, sitting on a chair, or standing. • Clients are taught to say steps aloud before and during task.	• Clients are given checklist with correct steps and sequences. • Clients are given pictures/photos of correct steps as cues. • Clients are taught one-handed techniques. • Therapists appropriately modify clothing: elastic pants, hook-and-loop fasteners, button aids, zipper aids, long-handled shoehorns, shoe aids, stocking aids.	• Use caregiver assistance for part or whole task.

(Continued)

Table 14.4. Treatment Strategies for Alzheimer's Dementia and Traumatic Brain Injury in Performance Areas *(cont.)*

Targeted Action	Retraining for Mild Cognitive Impairment	Compensation for Moderate Cognitive Impairment	Total Caregiving for Severe Cognitive Impairment
EATING			
Unable to indicate food needs	• Clients are taught to remember specific time schedule.	• Clients are taught to set alarm clocks to remember schedules. • Clients are taught to use memory notebook or visual aids to point out needs to others.	• Use caregiver assistance for part or whole task.
Unable to get/set up food	• Clients are taught mobility techniques to get food within reach. • Clients are taught to organize and arrange utensils within visual field and easy reach (low placement).	• Clients are taught appropriate techniques to use: one-handed technique, switch handedness, or using two hands in a specific way. • Therapists set up food location to help client.	• Use caregiver assistance for part or whole task.
Unable to select and/or use utensils	• Clients are taught to organize and arrange utensils within visual field and easy reach before starting to eat. • Clients are taught to look all over place setting before starting to eat to locate utensil location.	• Therapists set up utensil location to help clients. • Therapists arrange kitchen drawers with utensil facing open end of drawer and handles pointing toward rear. • Therapists appropriately modify utensils: large or small handles, heavier or lighter, colorful; one-handed knives provided.	• Use caregiver assistance for part or whole task.
Unable to eat/drink food	• Clients are taught oral–motor retraining. • Clients are taught swallowing retraining. • Clients are taught to take small bites and drink fluids to encourage swallowing (refer to neurodevelopmental motor techniques).	• Therapists appropriately modify consistencies: thicker liquid, using straws. • Therapists appropriately modify drinking cups: larger, smaller, heavier, lighter, colorful, and personalized with picture or name. • Therapists appropriately modify use of napkins as bibs. Modify for motor un-coordination: scoop dish, plate guard, skid mat.	• Use caregiver assistance for part or whole task.
IADLs			
Unable to perform community mobility	• Clients are taught to increase self-awareness, goal setting, planning, and self-monitoring.	• Clients are provided with the opportunity to use a variety of maps to remember geographic locations. • Clients progress through repeated rehearsals and shadowing experiences on specific routes before providing opportunities for independent mobility trips.	• Use caregiver assistance for part or whole task. • For clients with dementia, compensatory strategies need to provide environmental cues to enhance successful orientation and way-finding. These include adequate seating in wheelchairs, lighting, smooth terrain, clear and redundant signage, and environmental cues for access or nonaccess.

Table 14.4. Treatment Strategies for Alzheimer's Dementia and Traumatic Brain Injury in Performance Areas *(cont.)*

Targeted Action	Retraining for Mild Cognitive Impairment	Compensation for Moderate Cognitive Impairment	Total Caregiving for Severe Cognitive Impairment
IADLs			
Unable to perform money management	• Clients are cued to use self-monitoring techniques such as step-by-step instruction guidelines, using calculators, and practicing in mock situations.	• Clients may reduce their bank and checking account transactions or get assistance from a caregiver. • Clients are taught math skills for cash transactions.	• Compensation for loss of memory or spatial understanding (i.e., way around the building). • Destination orientation. • Use caregiver assistance for part or whole task.
PLAY AND LEISURE			
Unable to choose, perform, and engage in intrinsically motivating and pleasurable activities. (Play is an attitude. It is not so much what activity or occupation you perform as a fun-seeking activity, it is how you do it.)	• Clients are provided with opportunities to participate in occupations, games, and hobbies that are playful and fun. • Structure and unstructured play and leisure activities are promoted. • Spontaneity, humor, improvisation, and creativity fostered. • Spontaneous and organized play opportunities are provided, including competitive and non-competitive, intellectual and physical games and sports.	• Clients are provided with opportunities to participate in occupations, games, and hobbies that are playful and fun. • Structure and unstructured play and leisure activities are promoted. • Spontaneity, humor, improvisation, and creativity fostered. • Spontaneous and organized play opportunities are provided, including competitive and non-competitive, intellectual and physical games and sports.	• Opportunities for hobbies and enjoyable occupation are provided with caregiver assistance. • Spontaneity, humor, improvisation, and creativity fostered. • Spontaneous and organized play opportunities are provided, including competitive and noncompetitive, intellectual and physical games and sports.
WORK AND PRODUCTIVE ACTIVITY			
Client cannot perform productive activities (Work and play are culturally biased performance areas. For some people, the same activity may be perceived as work; for others, it is play and leisure.)	• Assist client in identifying incentives for return to work (e.g., job protection, financial benefits). • Provide opportunities to explore work accommodations such as adaptations of hours, job redesign, and change of workplace. • Office-based supported employment (advisement or coaching). • Agency-based supported employment (community training consultations, job sharing, contractual arrangements). • Natural supported employment (supported employment, employer or supervisor training as mentor, co-worker assistance).	• Provide opportunities to modify clients' disorganized behaviors to foster a sense of productivity, job skills, and vocational training. • Office-based supported employment with cues, structure, and supervision (advisement or coaching). • Agency-based supported employment with cues, structure, and supervision (community training consultations, job sharing, contractual arrangements). • Natural supported employment with cues, structure, and supervision (supported employment, employer or supervisor training as mentor, coworker assistance).	• Provide opportunities to increase work samples (e.g., sitting tolerance, standing tolerance, dexterity, and understanding instructions). • Provide simulated work in the facility or home to model ability to accept supervision, get along with coworker, sustain productivity for long hours, and tolerate frustration.

(Continued)

Table 14.4. Treatment Strategies for Alzheimer's Dementia and Traumatic Brain Injury in Performance Areas *(cont.)*

Targeted Action	Retraining for Mild Cognitive Impairment	Compensation for Moderate Cognitive Impairment	Total Caregiving for Severe Cognitive Impairment
WORK AND PRODUCTIVE ACTIVITY			
Client cannot perform housework, caregiving, volunteer work, or part-time work	• Clients are provided with opportunities for housework such as making the bed, cleaning own house/room, clearing and setting table, completing yard work, and using garbage disposal. • Clients are provided with opportunities for caregiving to persons, children, pets, and plants as needed. • Clients are provided to do volunteer work in community (e.g., church, synagogue, mosques, and other places of worship; nursing homes; political parties; community organizations). • Clients are provided to do part-time jobs such as washing windows, yard work, washing clothes, washing car, babysitting, and pet setting.	• Clients are provided with opportunities for housework with cues and supervision, such as making the bed, cleaning own house/room, clearing and setting table, completing yard work, and using garbage disposal.	• Clients perform parts of these activities.

Note. IADLs = instrumental activities of daily living.

Study Questions

1. What are some common impairments affecting everyday living in individuals with TBI or AD?
2. How much evidence is currently available for occupational therapy treatment of both populations?
3. What are the similarities and differences in the stages of recovery in TBI and AD?
4. What factors interact to impact community mobility in individuals with TBI?
5. Which IADL typically demonstrates the earliest decline in individuals with AD?

Acknowledgments

The Moody Foundation, Grant 2005-24, supported this work. We also gratefully acknowledge Renee Pearcy, CPS/CAP, for her research assistance.

References

Abreu, B. C. (Ed.). (1981). *Physical disabilities manual.* New York: Raven Press.

Abreu, B. C. (1998). The quadraphonic approach: Holistic rehabilitation for brain injury. In N. Katz (Ed.), *Cognition and occupation in rehabilitation: Cognitive models for intervention in occupational therapy* (pp. 51–97). Rockville, MD: American Occupational Therapy Association.

Abreu, B. C., & Chang, P.-F. J. (2011). Evidence-based practice. In K. Jacobs & G. L. McCormack (Ed.), *The Occupational therapy manager* (5th ed., pp. 331–347). Bethesda, MD: AOTA Press.

Abreu, B. C., Heyn, P., Reistetter, T. A., Patterson, R. M., Buford, W. L., Jr., Masel, B., et al. (2007). Postural control comparisons of able-bodied horseback riders and riders with brain injury. In B. Engel & J. MacKinnon (Eds.), *Enhancing human occupation through hippotherapy: A guide for occupational therapy* (pp. 92–99). Bethesda, MD: AOTA Press.

Abreu, B. C., Jones, J. S., & Opacich, K. (2007). Hippotherapy and evidence-based practice. In B. Engel & J. MacKinnon (Eds.), *Enhancing human occupation through hippotherapy: A guide for occupational therapy* (pp. 70–75). Bethesda, MD: AOTA Press.

Abreu, B. C., & Peloquin, S. M. (2005). The Quadraphonic Approach: A holistic rehabilitation model for brain injury. In N. Katz (Ed.), *Cognition and occupation across the life span: Models for intervention in occupational therapy* (2nd ed., pp. 73–109). Bethesda, MD: AOTA Press.

Abreu, B. C., Seale, G. S., Scheibel, R. S., Huddleston, N., Zhang, L., & Ottenbacher, K. J. (2001). Levels of self-awareness after acute brain injury: How patients' and rehabilitation specialists' perceptions compare. *Archives of Physical Medicine and Rehabilitation, 82*(1), 49–56.

Abreu, B. C., & Toglia, J. P. (1987). Cognitive rehabilitation: A model for occupational therapy. *American Journal of Occupational Therapy, 41*, 439–448.

Alzheimer's Association. (2009). Alzheimer's disease facts and figures. *Alzheimer's and Dementia, 5*(3), 1–74.

American Psychiatric Association. (2000). *Diagnostic and statistical manual of mental disorders* (4th ed., text rev.). Washington, DC: Author.

Ansell, B. J., & Keenan, J. E. (1989). The Western Neuro Sensory Stimulation Profile: A tool for assessing slow-to-recover head injury patients. *Archives of Physical Medicine and Rehabilitation, 70*, 104–108.

Baum, C., & Edwards, D. F. (1993). Cognitive performance in senile dementia of Alzheimer's type: The Kitchen Task Assessment. *American Journal of Occupational Therapy, 47*, 431–436.

Bear, M. F., Connors, B. W., & Paradiso, M. A. (2001). *Neuroscience: Exploring the brain* (2nd ed.). Baltimore: Lippincott Williams & Wilkins.

Belanger, H. G., Uomoto, J. M., & Vanderploeg, R. D. (2009). The Veterans Health Administration system of care for mild traumatic brain injury: Costs, benefits, and controversies. *Journal of Head Trauma Rehabilitation, 24*(1), 4–13.

Blessed, G., Tomlinson, B. E., & Roth, M. (1968). The association between quantitative measures of dementia and of senile change in the cerebral grey matter of elderly subjects. *British Journal of Psychiatry, 114*, 797–811.

Brain Injury Association of America. (1998). *Facts about traumatic brain injury*. Retrieved December 5, 2006, from http://www.biausa.org/elements/aboutbi/factsheets/factsaboutbi_2008.pdf

Breed, S., Sacks, A., Ashman, T. A., Gordon, W. A., Dahlman, K., & Spielman, L. (2008). Cognitive functioning among individuals with traumatic brain injury, Alzheimer's disease, and no cognitive impairments. *Journal of Head Trauma Rehabilitation, 23*(3), 149–157.

Brewer, K., Geisler, T., Moody, K., & Wright, V. (1998). A community mobility assessment for adolescents with an acquired brain injury. *Physiotherapy Canada 50*(2), 118–122.

Campbell, P., Wright, J., Oyebode, J., Job, D., Crome, P., Bentham, P., et al. (2008). Determinants of burden in those who care for someone with dementia. *International Journal of Geriatric Psychiatry, 23*(10), 1078–1085.

Centers for Disease Control and Prevention. (2009). *Traumatic brain injury in the United States: Emergency department visits, hospitalizations and deaths*. Retrieved April 7, 2009, from www.cdc.gov/ncipe/pub-res/tbi_in_ us_04/tbi_ed.htm

Clark, F. (1993). Occupation embedded in a real life: Interweaving occupational science and occupational therapy (1993 Eleanor Clarke Slagle Lecture). *American Journal of Occupational Therapy, 47*(12), 1067–1078.

Clark, F., Azen, S., Zemke, R., Jackson, J., Carlson, M., Mandel, D., et al. (1997). Occupational therapy for independent-living older adults: A randomized controlled trial. *JAMA, 278*(16), 1321–1326.

Cooke, K. Z., Fisher, A. G., Mayberry, W., & Oakley, F. (2000). Differences in activities of daily living process skills of persons with and without Alzheimer's disease. *Occupational Therapy Journal of Research, 20*(2), 87–105.

Corrigan, J., Smith-Knapp, K., & Granger, C. V. (1997). Validity of the Functional Independence Measure for persons with traumatic brain injury. *Archives of Physical Medicine and Rehabilitation, 78*, 828–834.

Cox, C., & Monk, A. (1993). Hispanic culture and family care of Alzheimer's patients. *Health and Social Work, 18*(2), 92–100.

Crepeau, E. B. (1995). The practice of the future: Putting occupation back into therapy In C. B. Royeen (Ed.), *AOTA self-study series: Rituals*. Rockville, MD: American Occupational Therapy Association.

Darragh, A. R., Sample, P. L., & Fisher, A. G. (1998). Environment effect of functional task performance in adults with acquired brain injuries: Use of the Assessment of Motor and Process Skills. *Archives of Physical Medicine and Rehabilitation, 79*, 418–423.

Davis, L. A., Hoppes, S., & Chesbro, S. B. (2005). Cognitive–communicative and independent living skills assessment in individuals with dementia: A pilot study of environmental impact. *Topics in Geriatric Rehabilitation, 21*(2), 136–143.

Fleming, J. M., Strong, J., & Ashton, R. (1996). Self-awareness of deficits in adults with traumatic brain injury: How best to measure? *Brain Injury, 10*, 1–15.

Folstein, M. F., Folstein, S. E., & McHugh, P. R. (1975). Mini-Mental State: A practical method for grading the cognitive-state of patients for the clinician. *Journal of Psychiatric Research, 12*, 189–198.

Giacino, J. T., Kezmarsky, M. A., DeLuca, J., & Cicerone, K. D. (1991). Monitoring rate of recovery to predict outcome in minimally responsive patients. *Archives of Physical Medicine and Rehabilitation, 72*, 897–900.

Giles, G. M., & Clark-Wilson, J. (1993). *Brain injury rehabilitation: A neurofunctional approach*. San Diego: Singular.

Gitlin, L. N., Winter, L., Dennis, M. P., & Hauck, W. W. (2007). A non-pharmacological intervention to manage behavioral and psychological symptoms of dementia and reduce caregiver distress: Design and methods of Project ACT. *Clinical Interventions in Aging, 2*(4), 695–703.

Godfrey, H. P. D., & Shum, D. (2000). Executive functioning and the application of social skills following traumatic brain injury. *Aphasiology, 14*(4), 433–444.

Gordon, W. A., Cantor, J., Ashman, T., & Brown, M. (2006). Treatment of post-bi executive dysfunction: Application of theory to clinical practice. *Journal of Head Trauma Rehabilitation, 21*(2), 156–167.

Goverover, Y., Johnston, M. V., Toglia, J., & DeLuca, J. (2007). Treatment to improve self-awareness in persons with acquired brain injury. *Brain Injury, 21*(9), 913–923.

Haley, W. E., Roth, D. L., Coleton, M. I., Ford, G. R., West, C. A. C., Collins, R. P., et al. (1996). Appraisal, coping, and social support as mediators of well-being in Black and White family caregivers of patients with Alzheimer's disease. *Journal of Consulting and Clinical Psychology, 64*, 121–129.

Hall, K. M., Karzmark, P., Stevens, M., Englander, J., O'Hare, P., & Wright, J. (1994). Family stressors in traumatic brain injury: A two-year follow-up.

Archives of Physical Medicine and Rehabilitation, 75(8), 876–884.

Han, S. D., Suzuki, H., Drake, A. I., Jak, A. J., Houston, W. S., & Bondi, M. W. (2009). Clinical, cognitive, and genetic predictors of change in job status following traumatic brain injury in a military population. *Journal of Head Trauma Rehabilitation, 24*(1), 57–64.

Harada, T., Ishizaki, F., Nitta, Y., Nitta, K., Shimohara, A., Tsukue, I., et al. (2008). Microchips will decrease the burden on the family of elderly people with wandering dementia. *International Medical Journal, 15*(1), 25–27.

Hart, T., Seignourel, P. J., & Sherer, M. (2009). A longitudinal study of awareness of deficit after moderate to severe traumatic brain injury. *Neuropsychological Rehabilitation, 19*(2), 161–176.

Hartman-Maeir, A., Katz, N., & Baum, C. M. (2009). Cognitive Functional Evaluation (CFE) process for individuals with suspected cognitive disabilities. *Occupational Therapy in Health Care, 23*(1), 1–23.

Hasselkus, B. R. (1998). Occupation and well-being in dementia: The experience of day-care staff *American Journal of Occupational Therapy, 52*(4), 423–434.

Hersch, E. L., Kral, V. A., & Palmer, R. B. (1978). Clinical value of the London psychogeriatric rating scale. *Journal of American Geriatrics Society, 26*, 348–354.

Herskovits, E. (1995). Struggling over subjectivity: Debates about "self" and Alzheimer's disease. *Medical Anthropology Quarterly, 9*, 146–164.

Hibbard, M. R., Gordon, W. A., Flanagan, S., Haddad, L., & Labinski, E. (2000). Sexual dysfunction after traumatic brain injury. *Neurorehabilitation, 15*(2), 107–120.

Jacobs, H. E. (1993). *Behavior analysis guidelines and brain injury rehabilitation: People, principles, and programs.* Gaithersburg, MD: Aspen.

Johnston, M. V., & Case-Smith, J. (2009). Development and testing of interventions in occupational therapy: Toward a new generation of research in occupational therapy. *OTJR: Occupation, Participation and Health, 29*(1), 4–13.

Karagiozis, H., Gray, S., Sacco, J., Shapiro, M., & Kawas, C. (1998). The Direct Assessment of (Functional Abilities (DAFA): A comparison to an indirect measure of instrumental activitiues of daily living. *The Gerontologist, 38*, 113–121.

Katz, N. (1998). *Cognition and occupation in rehabilitation: Cognitive models in occupational therapy.* Bethesda, MD: American Occupational Therapy Association.

Kennedy, J. E., Jaffee, M. S., Leskin, G. A., Stokes, J. W., Leal, F. O., & Fitzpatrick, P. J. (2007). Posttraumatic stress disorder and posttraumatic stress disorder-like symptoms and mild traumatic brain injury. *Journal of Rehabilitation Research and Development, 44*(7), 895–920.

Lancioni, G. E., Singh, N. N., O'Reilly, M. F., Sigafoos, J., de Tommaso, M., Megna, G., et al. (2009). A learning assessment procedure to re-evaluate three persons with a diagnosis of post-coma vegetative state and pervasive motor impairment. *Brain Injury, 23*(2), 154–162.

Lange, B., Spagnolo, K., & Fowler, B. (2009). Using the Assessment of Motor and Process Skills to measure functional change in adults with severe traumatic brain injury: A pilot study. *Australian Occupational Therapy Journal, 56*(2), 89–96.

Loewenstein, D., et al. (1989). A new scale for the assessment of functional status in Alzheimer's disease and related disorders. *Journal of Gerontology: Psychological Sciences, 44*, 114–112.

Mahurin, R. K., De Bettignes, B. H., & Pirozzolo, F. J. (1991). Structured Assessment of Independent Living Skills: Preliminary report of a performance measure of functional abilities in dementia. *Journal of Gerontology: Psychological Sciences, 46*, 48–66.

Makley, M. J., English, J. B., Drubach, D. A., Kruez, A. J., Celnik, P. A., & Tarwater, P. M. (2008). Prevalence of sleep disturbance in closed head injury patients in a rehabilitation unit. *Neurorehabilitation and Neural Repair, 22*(4), 341–347.

Masel, B. (2009). *Conceptualizing brain injury as a chronic disease.* Vienna, VA: Brain Injury Association of America.

McLean, A., Dikmen, S., Temkin, N., Wyler, A. R., & Gale, J. I. (1984). Psychosocial functioning at one month after injury. *Neurosurgery, 14*, 393–399.

Meehan, W. P. III, & Bachur, R. G. (2009). Sport-related concussion. *Pediatrics, 123*(1), 114–123.

Miller, P. A., & Butin, D. (2000). The role of occupational therapy in dementia—C.O.P.E. (Caregiver Options for Practical Experiences). *International Journal of Geriatric Psychiatry, 15*(1), 86–89.

Morris, J. C. (1993). The clinical dementia rating (CDR): Current version and scoring rules. *Neurology, 43*(11), 2412–2414.

Moyers, P. A. (1999). The guide to occupational therapy practice. *American Journal of Occupational Therapy, 53*, 247–322.

Nygard, L., Amberla, K., Bernspång, B., Almkvist, O., & Winblad, B. (1998). The relationship between cognition and daily activities in cases of mild Alzheimer's disease. *Scandinavian Journal of Occupational Therapy, 5*(4), 160–166.

O'Keefe, F., Dockree, P., Moloney, P., Carton, S., & Robertson, I. H. (2007). Awareness of deficits in traumatic brain injury: A multidimensional approach to assessing metacognitive knowledge and online-awareness. *Journal of the International Neuropsychological Society, 13*, 38–49.

Ownsworth, T. L., Turpin, M., Andrew, B., & Fleming, J. (2008). Participant perspectives on an individualized self-awareness intervention following stroke: A qualitative case study. *Neuropsychological Rehabilitation, 18*(5/6), 692–712.

Painter, J. (1996). Home environment considerations for people with Alzheimer's disease. *Occupational Therapy in Healthcare, 10*, 45–63.

Papp, K. V., Walsh, S. J., & Snyder, P. J. (2009). Immediate and delayed effects of cognitive interventions in healthy elderly: A review of current literature and future directions. *Alzheimer's and Dementia, 5*, 50–60.

Patterson, M. B., Mack, J. L., Neundorfer, M. M., Martin, R. J., Smyth, K. A., & Whitehouse, P. J. (1992). Assessment of functional ability in Alzheimer's disease: A review and a preliminary report on the

Cleveland Scale of Activities of Daily Living. *Alzheimer's Disease and Associated Disorders, 6,* 145–163.

Pattie, A. H., & Gilleard, C. J. (1979). *Clifton assessment procedures for the elderly (CAPE).* Sevenoaks, Kent, UK: Hodder & Stoughton.

Peloquin, S. M. (1995). The fullness of empathy: Reflections and illustrations. *American Journal of Occupational Therapy, 49*(1), 24–31.

Peloquin, S. M. (1996). Using the arts to enhance confluent learning. *American Journal of Occupational Therapy, 50*(2), 148–151.

Quintard, B., Croze, P., Mazaux, J. M., Rouxel, L., Joseph, P. A., Richer, E., et al. (2002). Life satisfaction and psychosocial outcome in severe traumatic brain injuries in Aquitaine. *Annales de Readaptation et de Medecine Physique, 45*(8), 456–465.

Rader, M. A., Alston, J. B., & Ellis, D. W. (1989). Sensory stimulation of severely brain-injured patients. *Brain Injury, 3,* 141–147.

Rappaport, M., Doughterty, A. M., & Kelting D. L. (1992). Evaluation of coma and vegetative states. *Archives of Physical Medicine and Coma Rehabilitation, 73,* 628–634.

Reid-Arndt, S. A., Nehl, C., & Hinkebein, J. (2007). The Frontal Systems Behaviour Scale (FrSBe) as a predictor of community integration following a traumatic brain injury. *Brain Injury, 21*(13–14), 1361–1369.

Reisberg, B. (1984). Stages of cognitive decline. *American Journal of Nursing, 84*(2), 225–228.

Reisberg, B., Ferris, S. H., De Leon, M. J., & Crook, T. (1982). The Global Deterioration Scale for assessment of primary degenerative dementia. *American Journal of Psychiatry, 139,* 1136–1139.

Reistetter, T., Abreu, B. C., Bear-Lehman, J., & Ottenbacher, K. J. (in press). Unilateral and bilateral upper extremity weight-bearing effect on upper extremity impairment and functional performance after brain injury. *Occupational Therapy International.*

Reistetter, T., Chang, P.-F. J., & Abreu, B. C. (2009). Showering habits: Time, steps, and products used after brain injury. *American Journal of Occupational Therapy, 63,* 641–645.

Ritchie, K., & Ledesert, B. (1991).The measurement of incapacity in the severely demented elderly: The validation of a behavioural assessment scale. *International Journal of Geriatric Psychiatry, 6,* 217–226.

Rombouts, S. A. R. B., van Swieten, J. C., Pijnenburg, Y. A. L., Goekoop, R., Barkhof, F., & Scheltens, P. (2003). Loss of frontal fMRI activation in early frontotemporal dementia compared to early AD. *Neurology, 60,* 1904–1908.

Ronch, J. L. (1996). Assessment of quality of life: Preservation of the self. *International Psychogeriatrics, 8,* 267–275.

Ruff, R. L., Ruff, S. S., & Wang, X.-F. (2008). Headaches among Operation Iraqi Freedom/Operation Eduring Freedom veterans with mild traumatic brain injury associated with exposures to explosions. *Journal of Rehabilitation Research and Development, 45*(7), 941–952.

Salmon, E., Perani, D., Collette, F., Feyers, D., Kalbe, E., Holthoff, V., et al. (2008). A comparison of unawareness in frontotemporal dementia and Alzheimer's disease. *Journal of Neurology, Neurosurgery, and Psychiatry, 79*(2), 176–179.

Sancisi, E., Battistini, A., Di Stefano, C., Simoncini, L., Simoncini, L., Montagna, P., et al. (2009). Late recovery from post-traumatic vegetative state. *Brain Injury, 23*(2), 163–166.

Schneiderman, A. I., Braver, E. R., & Kang, H. K. (2008). Understanding sequelae of injury mechanisms and mild traumatic brain injury incurred during the conflicts in Iraq and Afghanistan: Persistent postconcussuive symptoms and posttraumatic stress disorder. *American Journal of Epidemiology, 167*(12), 1446–1452.

Sherer, M., Bergloff, P., Boake, C., High, W., Jr., & Levin, E. (1998). The Awareness Questionnaire: Factor structure and internal consistency. *Brain Injury, 12,* 63–68.

Shores, E. A., Lammel, A., Hullick, C., Sheedy, J., Flynn, M., Levick, W., et al. (2008). The diagnostic accuracy of the Revised Westmead PTA Scale as an adjunct to the Glasgow Coma Scale in the early identification of cognitive impairment in patients with mild traumatic brain injury. *Journal of Neurology, Neurosurgery, and Psychiatry, 79*(10), 1100–1106.

Sikkes, S. A. M., de Lange-de Klerk, E. S. M., Pijnenburg, Y. A. L., Scheltens, P., & Uitdehaag, B. M. J. (2009). A systematic review of Instrumental Activities of Daily Living Scales in dementia: Room for improvement. *Journal of Neurology, Neurosurgery, and Psychiatry, 80,* 7–12.

Silverman, J. M., Smith, C. J., Marin, D. B., Mohs, R. C., & Propper, C. B. (2003). Familial patterns of risk in very late-onset Alzheimer disease. *Archives of General Psychiatry, 601,* 90–197.

Teasdale, G., & Jennett, B. (1974). Assessment of coma and impaired consciousness. A practical scale. *Lancet, 2,* 81–84.

Temple, R. O., Zgaljardic, D. J., Abreu, B. C., Seale, G. S., Ostir, G. V., & Ottenbacher, K. J. (2009). Ecological validity of the neurophysical assessment battery screening module in post-acute brain injury rehabilitation. *Brain Injury, 23*(1), 45–50.

Toglia, J. P. (1991). Generalization of treatment: A multicontext approach to cognitive perceptual impairments in adults with brain injury. *American Journal of Occupational Therapy, 45*(6), 505–516.

Toglia, J., & Kirk, U. (2000). Understanding awareness deficits following brain injury. *NeuroRehabilitation, 15,* 57–70.

Turner, C., Fricke, J., & Darzins, P. (2009). Interrater reliability of the Personal Care Participation Assessment and Resource Tool (PC–PART) in a rehabilitation setting. *Australian Occupational Therapy Journal, 56*(2), 132–139.

Turró-Garriga, O., López-Pousa, S., Vilalta-Franch, J., Turón-Estrada, A., Pericot-Nierga, I., Lozano-Gallego, M., et al. (2009). Estudio longitudianl de la apatiá en pacientes con enfermedad de Alzheimer. *Revista De Neurologia, 48*(1), 7–13.

Ulstein, I. D., Sandvik, L., Wyller, T. B., & Engdal, K. (2007). A one-year randomized controlled psychosocial intervention study among family carers of dementia patients: Effects on patients and carers. *Dementia and Geriatric Cognitive Disorders, 24*(6), 469–475.

Unsworth, C. A. (2008). Using the Australian Therapy Outcome Measures for Occupational Therapy (AusTOMs–OT) to measure outcomes for clients following stroke. *Topics in Stroke Rehabilitation, 15*(4), 351–364.

Ware, J. E. (1993). *SF–36 health survey manual and interpretation guide.* Boston: Health Institute, New England Medical Center.

Wilcock, A. A. (1998). *An occupational perspective of health.* Thorofare, NJ: Slack.

Willer B., Ottenbacher, K. J., & Coad, M. L. (1994). The Community Integration Questionnaire: A comparative examination. *Archives of Physical Medicine and Rehabilitation, 73,* 103–111.

Wood, W., Abreu, B., Duval, M., & Gerber, D. (1994). Occupational performance and the function approach. In C. B. Royeen (Ed.), *AOTA self-study series: Cognitive rehabilitation.* Bethesda, MD: American Occupational Therapy Association.

Zemke, R. (1995). Habits. In C. B. Royeen (Ed.), *AOTA self-study series: The practice of the future: Putting occupation back into therapy.* Rockville, MD: American Occupational Therapy Association.

Zemke, R., & Clark, F. (Eds.). (1996). *Occupational science: The evolving discipline.* Philadelphia: F. A. Davis.

Zgaljardic, D. J., Mattis, P. J., & Charness, A. (in press). Executive dysfunction. In K. Kompoliti & L. Verhagen (Eds.), *Encyclopedia of movement disorders.* Oxford, England: Elsevier.

Zhang, L., Abreu, B. C., Seale, G. S., Masel, B., Christiansen, C., & Ottenbacher, K. J. (2003). A virtual reality environment for evaluation of a daily living skill in brain injury rehabilitation: Reliability and validity. *Archives of Physical Medicine and Rehabilitation, 84*(8), 1118–1124.

Chapter 15

Strategies to Enable Meaningful Everyday Living for People With Psychiatric Disabilities and Other Mental Health Needs

CAROL HAERTLEIN SELLS, PHD, OTR, FAOTA, AND
VIRGINIA C. STOFFEL, PHD, OT, FAOTA, BCMH

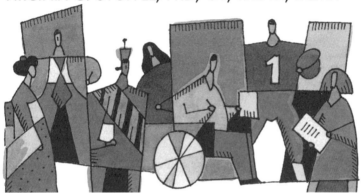

KEY WORDS

assertive community treatment

case management

Clubhouse model

community support program (CSP)

co-occurring disorders

empowerment models

marginalized populations

procovery

psychoeducational approaches

serious mental illness/psychiatric disability

HIGHLIGHTS

- Mental health care provided by occupational therapists extends beyond those with psychiatric disabilities to populations in society that have been marginalized.

- Stigma interferes with the ability of people with mental health needs to meet their occupational performance goals.

- Engagement in meaningful occupations may be the most significant indicator of a high quality of life for people with mental health needs.

- The occupational therapy process starts with an occupational profile that determines the client's priorities for services.

- There are many good assessment instruments available to help occupational therapists determine all the factors that will influence a client's ability to engage in occupations.

- The occupational role of parenting has recently received more attention for people with psychiatric disabilities.
- The role of occupational therapists with marginalized populations, including the homeless, victims of natural disasters, and war veterans, needs to expand in the future.

OBJECTIVES

After reading this material, readers will be able to

- Describe the impact of the major psychiatric disabilities on occupational performance;
- Identify the role of occupational therapy in achieving desirable outcomes for people with psychiatric disabilities;
- Identify the role of occupational therapy in meeting the occupational performance needs of special populations with mental health issues, including refugees, people living in extreme poverty, war veterans, and other potentially marginalized populations;
- Identify useful assessments for people with psychiatric disabilities;
- Identify strategies that enable enhancement of occupational performance, including the psychoeducational approach, case management, assertive community treatment, empowerment models, psychiatric rehabilitation, and building community supports; and
- Discuss research on outcomes of intervention for people with psychiatric disabilities.

The quotation on the right reflects the hopes and dreams of hundreds of people served by occupational therapists every day. The authors of this chapter are university professors. The people they work with are university students, whose aspirations are not much different from those of the hundreds of people with psychiatric disorders with whom the authors have worked over the past two decades. Just as professors strive to help students reach their goals, how can occupational therapists and occupational therapy assistants support the millions of people with psychiatric disorders and other mental health needs in their efforts to reach those same goals?

The *Occupational Therapy Practice Framework* (2nd ed., American Occupational Therapy Association [AOTA], 2008; hereinafter the *Framework*) clearly states the domain of concern for the profession to be "supporting health and participation in life through engagement in occupation" (p. 625). This reflects a focus on helping people become full participants in community life through active engagement in meaningful occupations in the contexts of their choice.

Full participation is often denied people with mental illness or other mental health needs—often associated with poverty and marginalization—by stigma. Public perception plays a role in opening and closing doors of opportunity to people who seem to "belong" or "not belong." Although an extensive discussion of occupational justice and related topics of occupational deprivation, marginalization, and rights is beyond the scope of this chapter, they will be briefly reviewed here to underscore their relevance to occupational therapy practice for all people with mental health needs.

For occupational therapists and occupational therapy assistants to have an impact on promoting full participation in community life, they must be prepared to make changes in the environment through advocacy and public policy, through participation in anti-stigma campaigns, and through public information and awareness. Kathleen Crowley (2000), in her book *The Power of Procovery in Healing Mental Illness: Just Start Anywhere*, suggests that hope and taking practical, everyday steps toward living a productive and fulfilling life—by starting anywhere—are key elements of the "procovery" process. Creating supportive environments and addressing participation restrictions go hand in hand with helping a client rebuild his or her dreams and create a life beyond mental illness. Expanding the focus of

Speaking of fantasies, I once had one: That I was one of millions of mental health clients who all lived in the communities of our choice, in our own places, with our own kitchens, our own furniture, our own bathrooms, our own food and clothing.... We shared our communities with all kinds of people...we did things together, helped each other, and laughed and cried with each other....we all had decently paying, fulfilling jobs.

Howie the Harp, 1995, p. xiii

recovery from mental illness to include the pursuit of occupational justice is a key theme in this chapter.

Role of Occupational Therapy

Occupational therapists and occupational therapy assistants can provide a wide range of services for people with psychiatric disabilities (also referred to as *consumers*). Occupational therapy services are designed to address all areas of occupation, including basic activities of daily living (ADLs), including rest and sleep, and those instrumental activities (IADLs) necessary for living in the community. But occupational therapy also addresses the categories of education, work, play, and leisure. Ultimately, then, occupational therapists focus on enabling productive and satisfying participation in a person's total round of daily activities.

Services for people with psychiatric disabilities may focus on one or more of these areas. The emphasis may be on evaluating and restoring performance patterns, modifying activity demands, or establishing the performance skills necessary to support occupational performance. The context in which the consumer participates is often overlooked, but it may be the most critical influence on successful adaptation to the demands of daily life.

Case Study 15.1 illustrates how areas of occupation, performance skills and patterns, context, and activity demands all interact to affect the quality of occupational therapy services for one consumer.

This chapter focuses on strategies used to meet the occupational needs of people with serious mental illnesses, particularly schizophrenia. It also reviews other conditions, such as mood disorders, personality disorders, substance abuse, co-occurring disorders, and condtions unique to special populations, such as refugees and war veterans. It is the authors' belief that occupational therapy intervention for people with mental health needs should focus on occupational performance and should occur in the communities where the consumers live.

Psychiatric Disorders

The most common mental health or social marginalization conditions occupational therapists see include schizophrenia, mood disorders, personality

---

Case Study 15.1. B.T.

B.T. is a 40-year-old man with a 22-year history of mental illness, specifically chronic schizophrenia and dependent personality disorder. He had his first psychotic incident during exam week of his first semester in college. Following a hospitalization of several months, he returned to the university to continue his education. For about 3 years he was able to live on his own and attend classes with the help of two roommates and his mother.

As the time approached to make an employment decision, and when his roommates graduated and moved away, B.T. experienced another psychotic episode, with severe depression. This hospitalization was for a longer period, extended by his setbacks any time a trial discharge or extended home pass occurred. The intervening years, from this point until the age of 37, consisted of several hospitalizations, group home placements, and brief periods of living with his mother. Each setting seemed only to increase his dependence and his belief that he was unable to meet his most basic self-care needs.

At age 37, B.T. was admitted to a community support program (CSP) and initially attended groups in a day treatment setting. These groups focused on learning the skills that would lead to more independence in his daily life (e.g., personal hygiene, meal preparation, grocery shopping, financial management, home management). Once he found an apartment, with the help of his occupational therapist/case manager, he began the process of doing those activities independently.

An occupational therapy assistant now meets with B.T. every other week to help him with his grocery shopping. He prepares his own meal plan and shopping list prior to the trip. B.T. is independent in most tasks but needs some encouragement and support to deal with difficult situations, such as the crowds at the grocery store or confronting the landlord about repairs.

B.T. credits the one-on-one feedback and the constant encouragement of his occupational therapist/case manager and other CSP staff with his ability to live on his own for the last 3 years. "I thought I took care of myself before, but I really didn't know how. I only knew how to get others to take care of me. With the help of my occupational therapist, I now know that I can take care of myself and my apartment. I'm even budgeting my money so I can take a trip soon!" As B.T. acquired the knowledge and skills necessary for living on his own, his self-esteem and motivation increased to the point where he was willing to engage in necessary IADLs.

Table 15.1. Primary Psychiatric Disorders Seen by Occupational Therapists and Occupational Therapy Assistants

Disorder/Condition	Symptoms	Onset and Duration	Prognosis and Treatment
Schizophrenia	2 or more of the following for 1 month: delusions, hallucinations, disorganized speech, disorganized or catatonic behavior, negative symptoms, social or occupational dysfunction below level achieved prior to onset.	Late adolescence or early adulthood onset, with an acute episode; fluctuating remissions and exacerbations throughout lifespan.	Majority has chronic disability and marginal functioning; prognosis improves with late onset. Treatment includes medications, social skills training, psychoeducational approaches, family support, and community support programs.
Mood disorder: Depressive disorder	5 or more of the following for 2 weeks: depressed mood; diminished interest in activities; weight loss or gain; insomnia or hypersomnia; psychomotor agitation or retardation; loss of energy restlessness; irritability; feelings of worthlessness, guilt, or helplessness; poor concentration; and recurrent thoughts of death.	Onset at any age between childhood to older adult, with highest incidence for ages 25–34; one or more factors—genetic, psychological, and environmental—linked to cause; duration is dependent upon the severity, with most people experiencing long periods of depression that are recurrent throughout their lifespan.	Recurrent episodes likely to occur throughout lifespan. Treatment includes psychotherapy and medications, specifically selective serotonin reuptake inhibitors (SSRIs) and monoamine oxidase inhibitors (MAOIs).
Mood disorder: Bipolar disorder	Depressive episode alternating with a distinct period of expansive, elevated, or irritable mood of 1 week duration with 3 or more of the following: grandiosity, decreased need for sleep, pressured speech, flight of ideas, distractibility, increase in goal-directed activity or psychomotor agitation, excessiveness in activities with potential negative results.	Onset can occur from childhood to adulthood with episodes of mania and depression recurring throughout one's life; most who suffer from bipolar disorder are free of symptoms between episodes (average interval of 2.5 years); a small percentage experience chronic constant symptoms.	Severity of symptoms determines seriousness of impact. Treatment includes medications (mood stabilizers, i.e., Lithium, and antidepressants) and psychotherapy including cognitive–behavioral and psychoeducational approaches and family therapy.
Personality disorders	Characterized by an enduring pattern of inner experience and behavior that deviates from expectations of culture in 2 of the following areas: cognition, affect, interpersonal functioning, and impulse control. The pattern is inflexible and pervasive, leading to significant impairment in social or occupational functioning.	Adolescent or early adulthood onset; patterns of behavior are stable and of long duration.	The course of the disorder is life-lasting, and prognosis is unpromising due to resistance to treatment. Treatment approaches include pyschodynamic therapy, cognitive therapy, dialectical behavioral therapy, social skills training, assertiveness training, and psychoeducational approaches.
Substance use disorders	Dependence characterized by maladaptive patterns causing significant impairment with 3 of the following over 12 months: increased tolerance; withdrawal symptoms; unintended excessiveness; unsuccessful efforts to control use; excessive focus on use; changes in social, occupational, or recreational function; continued use despite knowledge of problems. Abuse characterized by 1 of the following over 12 months: failure to fulfill major role obligations, recurrent use in dangerous situations, legal problems, and continued use despite knowledge of problems.	Adolescent to adulthood onset. Higher risk noted for males with less education; unmarried, separated, or divorced more than once; and younger age. Duration can be life-long, with frequent remissions and abuse of substances. Course and family/genetic patterns vary considerably among substances used.	Prognosis varies among substances used; prevalence drops with age; up to 35% do not improve or progressively deteriorate until death; up to 25% have stable remission via long-term abstinence or nonproblem drinking; up to 40% alternate between short-term abstinence and problem drinking. Treatment includes 12-step programs, medications, group and individual psychotherapy, and community interventions.

Sources: American Psychiatric Association (2000) and Hersen & Van Hasselt (2001).

disorders, and substance use disorders, which are often co-occurring (Table 15.1). A brief introduction to these diagnoses is provided below. Readers are directed to the *Diagnostic and Statistical Manual of Mental Disorders*, (*DSM–IV–TR;* American Psychiatric Association [APA], 2000) or other resources (Morrison, 2007; Sadock & Sadock, 2007) for more detailed information.

Schizophrenia is a pervasive and usually chronic disorder that is diagnosed when a person shows deterioration from a previous level of function in personal care, social relationships, or work and education. A wide range of characteristics may occur in schizophrenia, not all of which are found in everyone diagnosed with the condition.

Mood disorders include a wide range of conditions, from depressed mood secondary to bereavement to severe depressive and bipolar disorders. Impairment in areas of occupation varies considerably between conditions of depression and mania.

People with *personality disorders* have exaggerations of traits found in people without psychiatric disturbances, such as detached and limited emotional responses *(schizoid disorder),* distrust and suspiciousness *(paranoid disorder),* grandiosity and self-absorption *(narcissistic disorder),* and orderliness and perfectionism *(obsessive–compulsive disorder).* People with personality disorders typically have long-term behavioral patterns that are dysfunctional throughout life; the affected person learns little or nothing from life experiences. Only when the personality decompensates in the face of a crisis or the person seeks help for another psychiatric condition is the disorder typically diagnosed.

People who have histories of *substance use disorders* often have other psychiatric diagnoses, called *co-occurring disorders* (e.g., the person with depression who drinks to avoid feelings of hopelessness) or have a situational response to a physical condition (e.g., the person who abuses prescription drugs to cope with pain and develops a physical and psychological dependence on them). *Abuse* is defined as recurrent use that interferes with some aspect of functioning, such as fulfilling role obligations, or use that is physically hazardous, such as driving while impaired (APA, 2000). *Dependence* is more severe than abuse; it interferes with most aspects of function and includes increased tolerance for the substance, unsuccessful efforts to decrease use, and possible elicitation of withdrawal symptoms upon cessation of use (APA, 2000).

Co-occurring disorder (COD), the concurrent presence of at least one substance-related disorder and one mental disorder (Center for Substance Abuse Treatment, 2007), is accurately identified when all the diagnostic criteria for both conditions are present, as delineated by the *DSM–IV–TR* (APA, 2000). Because the mental health care delivery system often precludes identification and thus treatment of both conditions concurrently, the correct diagnosis may be overlooked.

The most recent available data from the National Survey on Drug Use and Health (Substance Abuse and Mental Health Services Administration [SAMHSA], 2007) indicates that 2.7 million people, or 1.2% of adults, had a co-occurring major depressive episode and substance use disorder. Compared to the estimated 24.3 million people (10.9% of the adult population) with serious psychological distress, defined as a "non-specific indicator of past year mental health problems, such as anxiety or mood disorders" (SAMHSA, 2008, p. 1), those with COD represent a relatively small number. But the complexities involved in the diagnosis and treatment of a person with COD require special consideration.

Dysfunction in Occupational Performance

The focus in occupational therapy treatment for people with mental health needs should be on occupational performance, regardless of the psychiatric diagnosis or precipitating events that lead to dysfunction. Occupational performance is a highly complex process that may involve aspects such as the person's performance skills and patterns, physical and social context, societal norms, and relationships with others. An ADL such as bathing is associated with knowledge of hygiene, healthy behavior, and use of the necessary supplies and equipment; with the motivation to respond to sociocultural norms of acceptable cleanliness; with routines and habits that support daily hygiene; and with the ability to recognize and respond to feedback from others regarding the practice of adequate bathing routines. It also requires sufficient motor coordination to manipulate faucets and shampoo bottles; strength, mobility, and balance to enter and exit the tub; sensitivity to temperature so as to regulate warmth of water; kinesthetic awareness to wash all body parts; and judgment and sequencing ability to organize bathing tasks.

A person with a psychiatric disorder is unlikely to bathe if he or she is indifferent to social and cultural expectations and feedback from others, lacks sufficient self-esteem to maintain his or her own health, lacks the sensory or neuromusculoskeletal abilities and skills to use equipment and supplies in a particular environment, or is unable to cognitively process the demands of bathing. Difficulty in carrying out ADLs may increase when one has impairments in executive functions, habits, routines, and interpersonal skills (e.g., seeking help), or lacks meaningful life roles.

The same parameters that influence the ability to bathe can be applied to activities across the spectrum of occupation, work, education, play, leisure, and social participation. For example, employment seeking and acquisition require knowledge of resources for job opportunities, cognitive and process functions to understand and complete job applications, information exchange and relational skills to participate in an interview, and sufficient self-knowledge to match a job opportunity with one's best interests. Participation in family life requires clear understanding of one's roles within the family; communication and interpersonal skills to convey needs, wants, and expectations; and sensitivity to and knowledge of the social context of the family.

Impairment in areas of occupation may appear as total lack of performance, partial or incomplete performance, performance that does not meet socially accepted standards, or performance that is insufficient to meet the person's needs. The consequences of performance in ADL and IADL may be particularly problematic for people with psychiatric disabilities because these tasks are essential for survival on a daily basis and include the foundational skills (acceptable personal hygiene, adequate nourishment, health management, and awareness of safety and emergency responses) needed to be successful in the occupations of work, education, leisure, and social participation.

The impairments seen in ADL and IADL among people with psychiatric disabilities and other mental health needs are the focus of this chapter. The manifestation of impairments differs with the type of psychiatric disability.

ADL Impairments

Changes in personal care and hygiene may be among the most noticeable early symptoms for people with schizophrenia and mood disorders. They typically appear as a person moves from substance abuse to a substance-dependence disorder and as symptoms exacerbate for both conditions in a co-occuring disorder. Dysfunction in ADL is not characteristic of people with personality disorders. When it is present, dysfunction represents not a deficit in performance skills but a symptom of the disorder (e.g., the exaggerated trait that character-

izes the particular disorder, such as unkempt appearance in a person with socially isolated schizoid personality).

Early in the disease process of schizophrenia, the person may cease or change personal hygiene and grooming habits. Women may adopt inappropriate and attention-seeking uses of makeup (e.g., excessive eye shadow and liner or unusual lipstick color and application). Changes in dress are common, and the person often becomes unkempt, slovenly, or dirty. Inappropriate attire is often seen, such as clothes that are too casual or dressy for the occasion or are inappropriate for the weather, especially for people with a long history of the disease. Changes in dress sometimes occur in response to hallucinations or delusional thinking as described in Case Study 15.2.

A typical secondary effect of deterioration in personal hygiene and grooming is adverse responses from other people. Family and friends may react with concern or denial, but strangers almost always will respond with avoidance, contributing to the person's delusional thought processes, social withdrawal, or other symptomatic behavior. The interaction of declining hygiene and grooming and interpersonal rejection becomes a self-perpetuating, downward cycle for people with schizophrenia. These interactive dynamics are important for occupational therapy personnel to understand, as they illustrate how context and performance interact to influence self-perception and create additional barriers to social participation.

Eating habits of people with schizophrenia may deteriorate, and they may have a total disregard for good nutrition. They may start overeating at meals, eat junk food in excess, or avoid certain foods or meals secondary to delusions or hallucinations. People with early signs of the illness (occurring in late adolescence through early adulthood) may never have developed the process skills that facilitate good self-care (e.g., temporal organization and adjustment to social norms). More often, those who have had frequent or long-term hospitalizations lose per-

---

Case Study 15.2. R.F.

R. F. is a 40-year-old man diagnosed with continuous paranoid schizophrenia who always wears a long-sleeved shirt, and often a sweater or jacket too, even in very warm weather. He feels he must do this to keep the panther tattooed on his forearm from biting him or from coming alive and attacking someone else.

formance skills (Bonder, 1995), along with motivation and interest in maintaining performance patterns of care routines, and they stop responding to external cues in the environment (e.g., time, events, temperature).

The range of ADL dysfunction in people with mood disorders is wide, from no apparent changes to the inability to get out of bed and engage in any occupational behaviors. The deficits seen in personal hygiene and grooming care are not from loss of performance skills and patterns or actual changes in mental or physical functions; rather, they are secondary symptoms of the altered mood and subsequent behavioral and thought disturbances. Because of the habitual nature of the performance of most ADLs, however, direct intervention at the level of occupational performance not only can re-establish performance patterns but also can improve self-perception and encourage the actual use of performance skills as the client engages in occupations.

Altered appetite is a fairly common change in ADLs for people with depression. This change may appear as decreased eating, which results in weight loss and potentially inadequate nutrition, or increased appetite secondary to agitation, resulting in weight gain. Personal hygiene, grooming, and dressing may be neglected as a result of depressed mood, loss of interest, impaired concentration, and lethargy.

In contrast, people in the manic episode of a bipolar disorder may change their dress or appearance as they act on increased goal-directed activities in the areas of work or social or sexual activities (e.g., a woman who starts engaging in sexual indiscretions wears provocative clothing, or a man who makes a sudden job switch or changes his social circle grows a beard and long hair). Changes in patterns of sleep and rest also are characteristic of a manic episode.

The ADL dysfunctions seen among people who have personality disorders involve enduring deviations from their cultural expectations and are consistent with the particular type of disorder. For example, a woman with narcissistic personality disorder may use excessive makeup and dress seductively as part of attention-seeking behavior (Bonder, 1995). The impulsivity of a person with borderline personality disorder may lead to abandonment of hygiene and eating routines as value systems fluctuate and relationships waiver.

People with substance use disorders may exhibit ADL impairment as loss of interest in eating or lack of attention to personal hygiene, grooming, and other daily self-care as the need for the substance supersedes all other occupations. Central nervous system changes are most apparent during intoxication but may persist; if abuse continues, the changes may cause impairment in performance skills, which in turn will lead to deficits in all areas of occupation. When this is coupled with any of the above conditions in a COD, the potential for deterioration of performance skills and patterns is greatly increased.

IADL Impairments

Because IADLs are "activities to support daily life within the home and community that often require more complex interactions" (AOTA, 2008, p. 631), they put considerably more demands on underlying performance skills, particularly process skills, communication and interaction skills, and performance patterns necessary for satisfactory function. Again, the manifestations of dysfunction will vary depending on the psychiatric disorder that is present.

For people with schizophrenia, especially of a more severe and enduring nature, IADLs that are particularly problematic include financial management, health management and maintenance, home establishment and management, meal preparation and cleanup, and safety procedures and emergency responses. Daily medication management is often difficult and usually has to be supervised by someone else. Reminders of appointments for medication checkups or physical health assessments also may be needed. Because of impairments in communication and interaction skills, shopping and community mobility may suffer.

The tendency toward social isolation also interferes with functional communication and, consequently, getting need fulfillment at several levels. For example, even though he or she experiences hunger, someone with schizophrenia living in a group home environment may not seek information from others regarding the time of the next meal. This lack of initiative may cause him or her to miss the call or reminder for that meal. Instead of eating a meal, the person typically will find his or her way to the vending machine and fill up on junk food. Consequently, nutritional needs go unmet.

When a person experiences a depressive disorder, IADL impairments will be most apparent in activities requiring processing and communication and interaction skills. Managing daily medications may be impaired because of lowered concentration. Appearance of clothes may suffer due to disinterest and disorganization. Care of others, financial management, meal planning and preparation, home establishment and management, and shopping—all of which require considerable energy, initiation, and organization—will become difficult, if not impossible, for the person with depression. Functional communication may be impaired as the depressed mood, loss of interest, and behavioral manifestations elicit negative reactions and avoidance responses from others. The impulsivity and excessiveness seen in a manic episode will interfere with the person's ability to attend to the complexities inherent in completing many IADLs. Inability to carry out individual and interpersonal tasks may ultimately result in the complete upheaval of daily life for someone with bipolar disorder who is experiencing either mania or depression.

As people with substance use disorders focus on obtaining substances, they may experience a loss of motivation and eventual loss of the performance patterns and skills necessary for IADLs such as care of others, financial management, meal planning and preparation, home management, and shopping. The disruption they eventually experience in home life will likely alter the entire spectrum of their daily life activities and carry over into other areas of occupational performance. For the individual with COD, the challenges posed by their mental illness to successfully engaging in critical IADLs are complicated by the focus on securing and using substances.

One occupational role area that may be overlooked for a person with a psychiatric disability is that of parenting. Given that women with mental illness have children at the same rate as other women, but with high separation and divorce rates that leave them caring for their children with little support (Ackerson, 2003), there is a need to consider parenting as an important IADL. The safety and welfare of children with parents who live with serious mental illness underscore the importance of building parenting skills and needed supports and services to assist families in remaining intact (Bybee, Mowbray, Oyserman, & Lewandowski, 2003).

Rest and Sleep

Disturbances of sleep and rest, including insomnia, daytime sleepiness, and fatigue, are common and legitimate complaints among people with psychiatric disabilities, especially those with anxiety-related disorder (Sateia, 2009). Disorders of sleep are often a side-effect of the medications used to treat symptoms of a wide range of psychiatric disorders (APA, 2000; Ferentinos et al., 2009). The *Framework* includes "rest and sleep" as an identified area of occupation within the domain of occupational therapy assessment and intervention for the first time. It is described as the "activities related to obtaining restorative rest and sleep that supports healthy active engagement in other areas of occupation" (AOTA, 2008, p. 632), with an emphasis on the establishment of routines, creation of a physical environment, and use of techniques that induce rest and sleep. Although there is extensive research in the psychiatry, neuropsychiatry, quality-of-life, and related literature on characteristics and treatment of sleep and rest disturbance, the area has not been addressed to any extent within the occupational therapy literature. A study on time use among people receiving services from an Assertive Community Treatment Association program found that the clients spent almost 9 hours in sleep, which is considered more than necessary for a balance of time-use patterns associated with health and well-being (Krupa, McLean, Estabrook, Bonham, & Baksh, 2003). Green (2008) notes that sleep is addressed sporadically in the occupational therapy literature. He suggests that, given the amount of time one spends in sleep, as well as the number of conditions that affect sleep that are addressed by occupational therapists, a closer examination of issues related to rest and sleep is warranted. This seems especially true for occupational therapists who work with people with psychiatric disabilities.

Education

Defined as "activities needed for learning and participating in the [learning] environment" (AOTA, 2008, p. 632), the occupational area of *education* presents unique challenges for people with psychiatric disabilities. The onset of several of the adult psychiatric disabilities occurs in late adolescence and early adulthood, often disrupting educational plans and endeavors. Some of the impairments in performance skills and patterns associated with the various disorders are likely to preclude the kind of planning and goal-directed activity necessary for success in educational occupations. For example, the disorganized thought processes and delusional ideation associated with schizophrenia may prevent use of the communication and interaction skills necessary to plan an academic course of study or participate in a classroom environment. The current literature examines the impact of one program (Gutman et al., 2007) on the educational pursuits and activities of people with psychiatric disabilities (reviewed below).

Mood disorders are characterized by disruptions in performance patterns, particularly maintenance of routines, which makes it difficult to comply with the schedule and routine of being a student. Among people with the psychiatric disabilities reviewed in this chapter, however, educational achievements are typically highest among those with mood disorders (Tse, 2002).

The impairments in performance skills, particularly cognitive, emotional regulation, and communication and social skills (AOTA, 2008) that are characteristic of many personality disorders will likely interfere with making realistic educational plans and following through on them. Such impairments also prevent people with personality disorders from accurately judging the social norms and role expectations of a student and functioning in an educational setting.

Alcohol abuse among college students often interrupts the educational plans of young adults; for a subset of that population who are especially at high risk, alcohol abuse may lead to lifelong problems with substances (Larimer & Cronce, 2002). Once the habit of substance abuse is established, it dominates daily life and overrides the performance skills and patterns needed for engagement in education occupations (Moyers & Stoffel, 2001). When this is coupled with the onset of a psychiatric disability that can occur in young adulthood and results in a COD, it is extremely challenging to regain a focus on educational goals and plans.

The presence of a psychiatric disability does not preclude a person from high levels of educational achievement, as evidenced by such accomplished people as Abraham Lincoln, Virginia Woolf and Ernest Hemingway, Beethoven and Schumann, and John Nash (NAMI, n.d.).

Work

The importance of work to people with schizophrenia, specifically paid employment rather than volunteer activities or day treatment, cannot be overemphasized. Eklund, Hansson, and Alhqvist, (2004) found that the satisfaction with daily occupations of persons with schizophrenia who were competitively employed was significantly greater than that of those involved in volunteer and other community-based activities. The values placed on paid employment and the worker role (i.e., financial, productivity, meaning) in Western society are held by all segments of the population, including those with serious psychiatric disabilities.

Entering or re-entering the workforce is thus a highly desired, yet often unattainable, goal for people with psychiatric disabilities (Nagle, Cook, & Polatajko, 2002). It has been reported that people with a major psychiatric disability generally do not work and thus experience a sense of uselessness and diminished meaning in life (Lloyd & Samra, 2000).

A growing body of occupational therapy literature addresses work and employment issues for people with all types of disabilities, including the psychiatric disabilities reviewed here—particularly people with the serious mental illness of schizophrenia (Chan, Tsang, & Li, 2009; Eklund et al., 2004; Liu, Hollis, Warren, & Williamson, 2007; Oka et al., 2004).

The onset of schizophrenia in late adolescence or young adulthood may disrupt early work opportunities and vocational development. If one of the most consistent predictors of vocational function for people with mental illnesses is their employment history (Lloyd & Samra, 2000; Tsang, Ng, & Chiu, 2002; Gioia & Brekke, 2003), the person with schizophrenia may be particularly disadvantaged in never having the opportunity to develop the employment-seeking and acquisition skills or vocational performance patterns that are critical to success. A study of 20 young men and women with schizophrenia in the United States (Gioia & Brekke, 2003) found that they had greater vocational success when requesting "job accommodations" to respond to unexpected symptoms (through the Americans with Disabilities Act of 1990), such as status quo job assignments and flexible job hours, rather than climbing the employment ladder. The difficulty in communication and interaction skills seen in people with schizophrenia, and identified as a major problem in successful employment (Tsang et al., 2002), may make requesting those accommodations difficult. *Integrated, supported employment*, an approach developed by Tsang (Chan et al., 2009) and described as "individual job placement with support and the additional necessary element of social skills training," was shown to be effective in a case study of a 41-year-old woman with a severe mental illness (Chan et al., 2009).

The involvement of a suitable support system—a family member, case manager, or supported employment counselor—may be necessary for even that first step toward returning to employment. Possibly one of the most socially debilitating effects of schizophrenia—the side effects of foot tapping or pin-rolling finger motions that appear when symptoms are managed with medications (Bonder, 1995)—may bring embarrassing attention from others and entirely preclude entering and sustaining employment in the competitive job market.

People with mood disorders may have higher educational levels than those with other psychiatric disabilities; consequently, they are more likely to have vocational histories and job performance skills. Practice guidelines from New Zealand for people with bipolar disorder emphasize quick job placement (Tse, 2002) and the "place-then-train" supported employment model over the "train-then-place" approach that emphasizes protected employment options and typically, low-skill jobs. Because job histories may not match educational achievement in people with bipolar disorder, the emphases in occupational therapy should be on maintaining a sense of hope; increased self-awareness; and good fit among the client, the job, the support system, and the wider context (Tse & Walsh, 2001; Tse & Yeats, 2002).

Personality and substance use disorders present patterns of behaviors that are not conducive to success in employment, although the patterns may be disruptive at different points in the person's life. Because personality disorders endure over a lifetime, they will affect early employment experiences and may lead to situations of unemployment or underemployment similar to those with other psychiatric disabilities. Substance use disorders in the stage of abuse may not initially cause problems in the occupational area of work. As dependence develops, job performance skills will be compromised, and role fulfillment in employment situations will become impaired. Substance use, coupled with a mental illness in the form of a COD, may lead to substance abuse when job frustrations and disappointments occur, making treatment of the mental illness more challenging and often overlooked as substances abuse leads to dependence.

More attention has been paid to the employment of people with psychiatric disabilities in the past several years, both outside of and within occupational therapy. Swedish authors have described a strategy to address the problem of workforce reentry for people with psychiatric disabilities (Gahnstrom-Strandqvist, Liukko, & Tham, 2003). The "social working cooperative" provides a setting for psychiatric rehabilitation that incorporates real work activities and opportunities for social connection. Such cooperatives are based on principles of democracy, responsibility, permissiveness, and community—"living–learning situations." Researchers in Japan retrospectively evaluated the long-term impact of a vocational rehabilitation program that combined occupational therapy and supported employment on duration of hospitalizations, time spent living in the community, and social adjustment for 52 participants with schizophrenia discharged from a psychiatric hospital (Oka et al., 2004). They concluded that the program was more effective when participants had the continued involvement of the clinical team and the support of

their families. Another study suggests that even though barriers to job seeking may be removed through supported employment programs, effort is still required by individuals to prepare oneself for work and to make ongoing effort to secure jobs (Liu et al., 2007).

The most current thinking in the area of employment for people with psychiatric disabilities suggests that successful employment requires effort by the individual, ongoing and sustained involvement of service providers, and community and family supports. Finally, concepts such as *return to work, work hardening, work outcomes,* and *work disability* have not been developed for people with psychiatric disabilities as extensively as for those with physical impairments. It has been suggested that work capacity evaluation and subsequent work preparation and work-hardening programs be made available to people with psychiatric disabilities, given the employment issues seen with this population (Tsang et al., 2002).

Play and Leisure

Although games and leisure activities typically are used as treatment modalities for people with psychiatric disorders, the literature gives little attention to them. Yet, "leisure is considered to be an important part of life for every individual. This is even more so for people with limited employment prospects and life options" (Lloyd, King, Lampe, & McDougall, 2001, p. 107).

Many types of play and leisure participation require motor, process, and communication and interaction skills that become impaired with many psychiatric disabilities. For example, as a result of the side-effects of medications mentioned earlier, a person with schizophrenia may be unable to engage in games requiring mobility and coordination skills. Someone in the manic phase of a bipolar disorder may have unrealistic expectations of his or her ability to succeed in competitive games. People with personality disorders may pursue play and leisure activities that minimize interaction with others, such as computer games, or collecting items, which can be done individually, and noncompetitive sports activities. When in the abuse stage, substance use typically is the focus of leisure participation; it replaces other leisure and play participation as abuse becomes dependence.

Unemployment or underemployment also affect play and leisure participation because they result in reduced financial resources. The time of onset of several psychiatric disabilities, as well, may prevent the development of many of the play and leisure interests pursued by adults. Still, people in a mental health rehabilitation program reported that their leisure participation was a source of intellectual stimulation, enjoyable relationships with others, and relaxation at a higher level than that reported by a population without diagnosed mental illness (Lloyd et al., 2001). For people with a COD, leisure participation is complicated by the need to replace old activities associated with "using" and to change social contacts (Hodgson, Lloyd, & Schmid, 2001). Leisure participation is important for the recovery process and to prevent relapse (Hodgson & Lloyd, 2002).

Social Participation

Social participation, the "organized patterns of behavior that are characteristic and expected of an individual of a given position within a social system" (AOTA, 2008, p. 633), is typically a challenge for people with psychiatric disabilities. Social participation can occur at the level of the community, of the family, or with peers. It has probably been most successfully operationalized for people with severe mental illnesses in the well-known Fountain House, or clubhouse, model of community-based mental health services (described later in this chapter). This model asserts that all roles and functions of an organization or social system are carried out by the clubhouse members with the support of a small staff, thus enabling social participation at the community level.

Social participation in the family has received more attention in the past decade as organizations that support people with severe mental illness have recognized the challenges faced by clients in their roles as parents. Ackerson (2003) notes that the child welfare system focuses on parental fitness and attempts to identify when parental rights ought to be terminated. On the other hand, Ackerson further notes that providision of specialized supports and services to parents with psychiatric disabilities is often overlooked by mental health professionals. Miller (2008) found that parents living with serious mental illness found great joy in their children and that the meaningfulness of parenting provided motivation to take care of themselves and more actively engage in mental health services.

Occupational Therapy Evaluation

The first consideration in evaluating a person with a psychiatric disability is deciding just what to assess: occupational performance, performance skills and patterns, the context or contexts in which occupa-

tional performance will occur, activity demands, or client factors. The *Framework* suggests that the first step in an occupational evaluation is the creation of an occupational profile that identifies the person's occupational history and experiences; gains an awareness of the typical patterns of daily living; and determines his or her interests, values, and needs with regard to current and future occupational goals. Guidelines for completion of the occupational profile are provided in the *Framework* (AOTA, 2008); the process to conduct formal and informal interviews is described by Page (2008).

Other tools that can be used to create the occupational profile include the Occupational Performance History Interview (OPHI–II; Kielhofner et al., 2004) and the Occupational Circumstances Assessment Interview and Rating Scale (OCAIRS; Forsyth et al., 2005), which are both based on the Model of Human Occupation and available from the Model of Human Occupation (MOHO) Clearinghouse at http://www.moho.uic.edu/. These instruments are suggested because they are well developed, theory based, administered in uniform manner, and psychometrically sound.

Once the client-identified priorities are established, specific evaluations can be selected to provide a clearer picture of his or her occupational performance in selected contexts. Naturalistic observation of actual performance in the areas of occupation in which the person is currently engaged using tools such as the Occupational Therapy Task Observation Scale (OTTOS; Margolis, Harrison, Robinson, & Jayaram, 1996), the Comprehensive Occupational Therapy Evaluation (COTE; Brayman, 2008) or the Observed Tasks of Daily Living–Revised (OTDL–R; Goverover & Josman, 2004), combined with a structured interview, such as the Canadian Occupational Performance Measure (COPM; Law et al., 1998), can help identify areas of performance or environments needing further evaluation and highlight client factors and performance skills. The COPM is one of the most widely studied assessments in occupational therapy, for its use both in guiding intervention and in measuring outcomes (Baptiste, 2008; Carswell et al., 2004; McColl et al., 2005). It has been used successfully in mental health practice (Chesworth, Duffy, Hodnett, & Knight, 2002; Pan, Chung, & Hsin-Hwei, 2003; Warren, 2002).

Evaluation of the client and his or her chosen environments is consistent with the psychiatric rehabilitation assessment process as described by Mac-Donald-Wilson, Nemec, Anthony, and Cohen (2001), who suggested that the skills and resources present and needed by the person to achieve his or her rehabilitation goal should be the focus of such an evaluation. Useful assessment instruments should be "clear, brief, environmentally specific, and skills and/or resources-oriented" (p. 430). Assessment instruments for the cultural, physical, social, and other aspects of context and environments (AOTA, 2008) have not been developed specifically for populations with psychiatric disorders, with the exception of some quality-of-life measures discussed below.

A review of measures of environmental factors by Rigby, Cooper, Letts, Stewart, and Strong (2005) identified potential instruments that assist the occupational therapist to better evaluate the person–environment interaction that supports or limits occupational performance. This reference provides detailed information about the purpose, clinical utility, standardization, psychometrics, and resources for each instrument. Some potentially useful tools for people with psychiatric disorders cited by Rigby et al. include the Home Environment, Multidimensional Scale of Perceived Social Support (MSPSS), Life Stressors and Social Resources Inventory–Adult Form (LISRES–A), the Work Environment Impact Scale, and the Work Environment Scale (WES; Rigby et al., 2005).

The underlying client factors and performance skills affecting occupational performance may include impaired attention, memory, or thought; altered body awareness and self-concept; and lack of knowledge and judgment. These factors often can be analyzed simultaneously with occupational performance. Evaluation should begin at the level of performance; client factors, contexts, and performance skills and patterns can be considered as necessary. This perspective allows the therapist to assist someone with psychiatric disabilities to focus on what is "necessary and fulfilling" (Bonder, 1993, p. 214) to be able to engage in meaningful occupations, not on whether he or she is depressed or isolated. It may be helpful at some level of evaluation and intervention to identify the relationship between the person's social isolation and depression, but it is probably more meaningful to assist in developing financial management and communication skills so that the person can afford to eat one meal a day at the local coffee shop and in doing so be part of an important social context and experience social participation.

Chapter 3 outlines several instruments that assess occupational performance, many of which can be used with clients with psychiatric disorders. Many assessments for use in mental health practice have been developed in the past three decades, including observational tools, self-report checklists and questionnaires, interviews, and mixed-method assessments (Hemphill-Pearson, 2008; Law, Baum, & Dunn, 2005). It is highly recommended that occupational therapists and occupational therapy assistants take advantage of and use the multitude of tools available and continue to contribute to their development.

Several home assessment instruments have been developed to specifically measure underlying mental functions of people with psychiatric disorders, including the Allen Cognitive Level Screen–5 (Allen et al., 2008), the Executive Functions Performance Test (EFPT; Baum et al., 2008), the Routine Task Inventory–Expanded (RTI–E; Katz, 2006) and the Lowenstein Occupational Therapy Cognitive Assessment–Second Edition (Su, Chen, Tsai, Tsai, & Su, 2007). Occupational therapists and occupational therapy assistants should evaluate the validity, reliability, administration procedures, clinical utility, and other supporting information for any instrument before using it in an intervention setting.

Other dimensions of participation that might influence occupational performance for people with psychiatric disabilities include life roles, use of time, and perceived quality of life. The assessment texts by Hemphill-Pearson (2008) and Law et al. (2005) are excellent resources for assessments that address the performance patterns of roles and time use. Dimensions of perceived quality of life have been discussed in the psychiatric rehabilitation literature for the past 30 years and in the occupational therapy literature for the past decade (Aubin, Hachey, & Mercier, 1999; Bejerholm & Eklund, 2007; Boyer, Hachey, & Mercier, 2000; Chan, Krupa, Lawson, & Eastabrook, 2005; Laliberte-Rudman, Yu, Scott, & Pajouhandeh, 2000). The Quality of Life Measure for Persons With Schizophrenia (QOLM–S; Laliberte-Rudman, Hoffman, Scott, & Renwick, 2004) is an assessment developed from qualitative data on people with schizophrenia and incorporates concepts of occupational performance. It is a promising tool that will enhance occupational therapy services for this population. The Satisfaction With Life Scale (Test, Greenberg, Long, Brekke, & Senn Burke, 2005) is an 18-item self-report tool reflecting subjective satisfaction with life for persons with serious mental illness in four areas: (1) living situation, (2) social relationships, (3) employment/work, and (4) self and present life. The domain scores might aid in goal setting and measuring outcomes associated with life satisfaction and mental health recovery.

Adaptive Strategies for Occupational Performance

Helping clients with psychiatric disabilities develop strategies to manage ADLs, IADLs, work, education, and the other areas of occupation can take many forms, including psychoeducational (PE) approaches, case management, assertive community treatment (ACT), psychiatric rehabilitation, empowerment models, and community supports. Most of the programs found in the occupational therapy literature use an academic or educational model to address ADLs and IADLs for people with psychiatric disabilities (Eaton, 2002; Fike, 1990; Friedlob, Janis, & Deets-Aron, 1986; Neistadt & Cohn, 1990; Remien & Christopher, 1996; Ziv, 2000). Psychoeducational models are found within and outside of the occupational therapy literature and often are described in connection with the strategies mentioned earlier.

Psychoeducation Models

The notion that one can use educational approaches to change occupational performance in ADLs and IADLs and to change the habits and routines of clients is grounded in the belief that therapy is learning. This concept is not new; references to teaching and learning in therapy have appeared in the occupational therapy literature since the 1960s (Box 15.1). Applying principles of psychoeducation, The Bridge Program was developed by the occupational therapy faculty at Richard Stockton College to help people with psychiatric disabilities succeed in higher education (Gutman et al., 2007). Sixteen participants successfully completed the program; one month later, 75% continued in educational coursework. Quantitative and qualitative measures indicated improvement in the academic and social skills needed to pursue higher education.

Behavioral Approaches

Behavioral approaches consist of cause–effect associations, shaping, reinforcement, behavior modification, habituation, and sensitization. They are most effective for people with psychiatric disabilities who also have the following characteristics:

- Their cognitive abilities are impaired by psychoses (e.g., acute schizophrenia, severe depression).
- They have normal attention span and memory abilities (e.g., personality disorders).
- They are in situations in which the environment is unchanging and responses require little or no judgment in determining what to do (e.g., people living in group homes).

Cognitive Approaches

Cognitive approaches focus on teaching how learning occurs; on transferring learning; and on role playing, rehearsal, imagery, and memory enhancement techniques. They are best used in the following circumstances:

- The client must learn to do situational problem solving (e.g., select appropriate clothing for weather conditions).
- The client has deficits in attention span, memory, or other cognitive abilities (e.g., a person with central nervous system damage, such as someone with a long history of substance use).
- The skills being learned need to be generalized or transferred to other situations (e.g., using acceptable eating behaviors in a restaurant).

Case Study 15.3 demonstrates how behavioral and cognitive approaches may be combined with client-centered practices that emphasize goals im-

---

Box 15.1. Strategies and Characteristics of Psychoeducational Approach

Specific strategies common to PE programs include

1. Verbal, written, visual, and experiential learning in various areas of daily living, including technology-based learning.
2. Community outings to relate learning to real-life experiences and apply the new skills to the real environment.
3. Role-playing, rehearsal, and education games.

Characteristics suggested for a consumer's successful involvement in a PE program are

1. Person is able to learn.
2. Enrollment in the program is voluntary.
3. Participants in the program are students and instructors, not patients/clients and staff.
4. Students set their own goals for learning.
5. Involvement in the program is time-limited (imparts a sense of urgency to acquire skills or knowledge).
6. There is some financial cost to students.

Sources: Bakker & Armstrong, 1976; Lillie & Armstrong, 1982.

Case Study 15.3. T.R.

The format of a men's wellness group for those receiving case management services in the mental health center is open-ended and addresses the needs of clients as determined by group members on a day-to-day basis. All male participants in the program attend the group, the focus of which varies depending on whose issues are being dealt with on a given day. Group members assume a supportive peer role and give feedback to each other about how to accomplish the goals each participant has set for himself. For some, the goal may be to eat more healthy foods: The members then share ideas on planning and cooking nutritious meals; on how to shop in a grocery store, food pantry, or farmers' market; or provide help on how to read labels on prepared food for nutritional content.

T.R. initially remained a quiet, background participant in most of the group sessions. Some staff and members had difficulty approaching him because of his body odor and disheveled appearance. When T.R. spoke, it was about his goal of finding a girlfriend and developing a relationship. His peers were able to share with T.R. the effect that his hygiene had on others and how that might keep people from approaching and getting to know him. The group used role-playing and rehearsal (i.e., cognitive techniques) to help him improve his personal hygiene and to learn how to use the machines at the laundromat. A group shopping trip helped him begin to overcome his anxiety about being in crowds and having a store clerk approach him. After a few weeks of attending the group, T.R. arrived one day in clean clothes and with a more pleasing odor. One of the group members shared an extra bottle of aftershave a present (i.e., reinforcement, a behavioral technique).

---

portant to the client when helping him or her adopt socially acceptable standards of personal hygiene.

When implementing the PE approach, it is important to take the "mystique" out of learning; that is, it is important to tell learners that behavior patterns are learned, that everyone goes through essentially the same learning process, and that behavior can be acquired or changed. As Lamb (1976) stated when describing PE model for people with long-term psychiatric disorders, it is crucial to help consumers "realize that the basic skills of everyday living are learned skills" (p. 877). The key to success is consumer involvement in establishing the goals for learning, in establishing curriculum, and in taking some responsibility for its implementation. The occupational therapist must "take some responsibility" as well, by helping clients to establish goals, whether they be learning to use a washer and dryer, reading a recipe, or completing a job application. Ng and Tsang (2002) described the importance of setting realistic goals for a population of 25 psychiatric inpatients: Upon completion of a program for setting goals called the Goal Attainment Program, 92% of participants wanted to leave the hospital, and 72% aspired to competitive employment.

Another key factor is conducting the program away from the site of mental health treatment, if possible. By doing so, the consumer can acquire "a new identity, that of student, and feels he can participate in activities outside of mental health centers just like other people in the community. That, plus the information imparted to him in the course,

helps the student move beyond the mental health system" (Lamb, 1976, p. 877).

The adoption of PE strategies into occupational therapy services for people with psychiatric disabilities is also described by Crist (1986) in a program for community living skills; in Jacobs, Selby, and Madsen's (1996) description of supporting college students with serious mental illness; in Neistadt and Marques' (1984) program for independent living skills training; in O'Sullivan, Gilbert, and Ward's (2006) description of a healthy living program; in a food skills program developed by Porter, Capra, and Watson (2000); and in Weissenberg and Giladi's (1989) program for adolescents to acquire habits and skills. For the most part, these programs emphasize complex IADLs, work, and education tasks needed to function in community settings.

Case Management

Case management has been described as a "service which assists clients in negotiating for services that they both need and want" (Cohen & Nemec, 1988, p. 27). Descriptions of case management also may emphasize coordination and allocation of services with limited resources, as is more common with European-based models (Ziguras, Stuart, & Jackson, 2002).

An extensive body of literature describes case management approaches and strategies to assist people with psychiatric disabilities. Recent literature describes variations of earlier case management concepts to include strengths-based case management

(Brun & Rapp, 2001), intensive case management (Kuno, Rothbard, & Sands, 1999), and the continuous treatment team model (Johnsen, Samberg, Caslyn, Blasinsky, Landow, & Goldman, 1999). One study reported that consumers involved in intensive case management over a 2-year period had fewer emergency visits and increased social networks and that families had experienced a reduced burden of care (Aberg-Wistedt, Cressell, Lidberg, Liljenberg, & Osby, 1995).

Although there are variations in case management practices, nearly all have the following characteristics: establishing a close relationship with the consumer; working with the consumer in his or her own environment; assessing skills and training in areas such as self-care, symptom management, and money management; linking consumers to preferred service providers; and advocating for service improvement (Cohen, Nemec, Farkas, & Forbess, 1988). Services may be provided by teams or individuals.

Hodge and Giesler (1997) have developed case management practice guidelines and identified three levels of intensity for case managers, based on the needs of the client. Levels I and II case management involve having the case manager teach independent living skills in the client's natural environment; Level III services are directed primarily toward finding the community resources matched to the client's needs.

Occupational therapists and occupational therapy assistants are well suited to serve as case managers for people with psychiatric disabilities. The occupations of ADLs, IADLs, education, work, and play or leisure are the centerpiece of the occupational therapist's knowledge base. In addition, the therapist's knowledge of activity analysis, therapeutic use of self, the importance of meaningful occupation, and the interdisciplinary team approach provide a solid foundation for the case manager role.

Assertive Community Treatment

The ACT program was developed by Leonard Stein, Mary Ann Test, and Arnold Marx in the early 1970s at Mendota Mental Health Institute in Madison, Wisconsin (Stein & Santos, 1998). This comprehensive, multidisciplinary program offers full-support case management services in the community with staff whose expertise informs group decision making. By working with the community and families in a collaborative process, the model ACT program has had powerful outcomes that demonstrate success in community living and working (summarized in Stein and Santos, 1998). ACT programs have been reviewed and studied extensively in the United States (Becker, Meisler, Stormer, & Brondino, 1999; McGrew, Pescosolido, & Wright, 2003; McGrew, Wilson, & Bond, 2002); in Canada (Dewa et al., 2003; Krupa et al., 2003; Neale & Rosenheck, 2000; Prince & Prince, 2002; Schaedle, McGrew, Bond, & Epstein, 2002); and in Europe (Falk & Allebeck, 2002; Ford et al., 2001; Gournay, 1999). The approach is generally accepted as having "shaped the delivery of mental health care over the past 25 years" (Dixon, 2000, p. 759).

Occupational therapy can offer an ACT team concrete expertise in ADL and IADL assessment and training. The typical ACT assessment includes an ADL and IADL assessment that covers food and nutrition skills, maintenance and housekeeping skills, personal hygiene and grooming skills, mobility skills, recreation and leisure skills, social skills, communication skills, interpersonal relationships, money management and banking skills, time management, problem-solving and decision-making skills, and safety skills (Stein & Santos, 1998). Occupational therapists are skilled in assessing the client's capacity for independent living as well as the context needed to support his or her optimal function. Pitts (2001); Auerbach (2002); and Krupa, Radloff-Gabriel, Whippey, and Kirsh (2002) all wrote about the contributions of occupational therapy to ACT programs and agree that the focus on occupations and enhancing community adjustment and quality of life are consistent with desired occupational therapy intervention outcomes for people with psychiatric disabilities.

Personal Assistance in Community Existence

Empowerment models for people with psychiatric disabilities, sometimes referred to as *consumer/survivor models*, give consumers considerable control over services; in fact, consumers may actually provide services (Ahern & Fisher, 1999; Chinman, Rosenheck, Lam, & Davidson, 2000; Liberman & Kopelowicz, 2002; Spaniol & Koehler, 1994). The Personal Assistance in Community Existence (PACE) philosophy is based on five elements of recovery: (1) relationships, (2) beliefs, (3) self-identify, (4) community, and (5) skills (Ahern & Fisher, 2001). Laurie Ahern, a successful journalist, and Daniel Fisher, a biochemist and psychiatrist, are survivors of mental illness and nationally known writers and speakers on recovery for people who have been labeled with a mental illness. Their PACE philosophy emphasizes the reality that people do fully recover from even the most serious mental illnesses and must do so at their own pace. In addition, people must

- Believe they will recover,
- Have someone who believes in them and also believes they will recover,
- Have economic support and a social identity,
- Have a positive sense of self,
- Be a part of a "collective voice" for security and identity, and
- Acquire self-management and self-help skills.

Other premises of consumer-driven models include the belief that mental illness is caused by severe emotional distress and loss of social roles, rather than a permanent brain disorder, and that the most important relationships are with peers and those who provide encouragement and support, not with mental health professionals. These approaches and beliefs are consistent with interventions and beliefs about serious mental illness in nonindustrial societies (Gureje, Olley, Olusola, & Kola, 2006) and in the Vermont Longitudinal Study and the Soteria Project (discussed in the outcomes section below).

Psychiatric Rehabilitation

The literature on psychiatric rehabilitation has become rich with principles and outcomes supporting people with psychiatric disabilities living full lives in their communities of choice. The emphasis on rehabilitation over treatment focuses on improved functioning and life satisfaction; present and needed skills and supports; teaching skills; and coordinating and modifying resources—all instead of focusing on "cure," symptomology, and medications (Anthony, Cohen, Farkas, & Gagne, 2002).

Occupational therapy practitioners are one of several types of professionals who contribute to the rehabilitation process. Tse and Walsh (2001) reflected on the importance of hope in vocational recovery for people with bipolar affective disorder. Brown (2001) suggested that self-awareness of sensory processing may help people with mental illness find environments that facilitate optimum occupational functioning.

The basic principles of psychiatric rehabilitation include a focus on improving capabilities and competencies; enhancing the consumer's environmental supports; eclectically using various techniques; improving vocational, residential, and educational outcomes; instilling hope; and actively involving the client in the rehabilitation process (Anthony et al., 2002). Wisconsin's Blue Ribbon Commission on Mental Health (1997) applied these principles to its reorganization of the state mental health program and has advocated shifting the paradigm of care from treatment to rehabilitation to recovery. In this vision of recovery, the client attains a productive and fulfilling life regardless of mental illness. Occupational therapists and occupational therapy assistants can help the client build meaningful life roles leading to full, active participation in his or her community of choice.

Clubhouse Models

Consistent with a psychiatric rehabilitation model is the clubhouse model of psychosocial rehabilitation, often referred to as the Fountain House Model. The model is based on the New York City institution of the same name, established in 1948, where people with serious mental illness joined together to support one another as they adjusted to community living and helped one another find jobs (Fountain House, n.d.). The International Center for Clubhouse Development (ICCD) lists in its 2008 International Directory (available at http://www.iccd.org /search_form.php) clubhouse programs in 29 countries and at more than 210 sites in the United States. The ICCD has established standards and sponsors training and accreditation programs. Clubhouse staff and members work side-by-side and operate as generalists to meet the needs and interests of the members (Dougherty, 1994).

Given the good fit between the domain of occupational therapy (i.e., "supporting health and participation in life through engagement in occupation," [AOTA, 2008, p. 626]), and the following description from the ICCD Web site, occupational therapy practitioners are well suited to contribute to clubhouse programs (Stoffel, 2007):

> A Clubhouse is a place where people who have had mental illness come to rebuild their lives. The participants are called members, not patients and the focus is on their strengths not their illness. Work in the clubhouse, whether it is clerical, data input, meal preparation, or reaching out to their fellow members, provides the core healing process. Every opportunity provided is the result of the efforts of the members and small staff, who work side by side, in a unique partnership. One of the most important steps members take toward greater independence is transitional employment, where they work in the community at real jobs. Members also receive help in securing housing, advancing their education, obtaining good psychiatric and medical care and maintaining

government benefits. Membership is for life so members have all the time they need to secure their new life in the community. (ICCD, n.d.)

Occupational therapists and occupational therapy assistants are employed at a number of clubhouses throughout the United States and worldwide (see Box 15.2).

Community Supports

The integration of people with psychiatric disabilities into the community is a challenge to all people with an interest in community mental health, including consumers, family members, mental health professionals, policy makers, housing professionals, and employers. Paul Carling (1975) and his colleagues at the Center for Community Change have identified several principles that underlie successful integration. Almost 30 years ago, they called for a radical shift in thinking about needs of people with psychiatric disabilities and how they are served. Note that these principles are particularly consistent with those of a client-centered approach in occupational therapy as described by Law (1998). The principles proposed by Carling (1975) and supported by Bonder (1995) may be summarized as follows:

- All people, regardless of any differences, belong in a community.
- People with differences can be integrated into typical neighborhoods, work situations, and community social situations.
- Support is necessary for all people and their families (not just those who are "different") and should be offered in regular places in the community.
- Relationships between people with and without labels are crucial; each group has much to teach the other.
- Service users and their families should be involved in the design, operation, and monitoring of all services and should have the power to hold services providers accountable.
- Success in housing, work, and social relationships is primarily a function of whether a person has the skills and supports that are relevant to that environment or relationship.
- People's needs and relationships change over time; services and supports should be available at various levels of support for as long as a person needs them.

Box 15.2. Fairweather Model

Another community based model for mental health, the Fairweather Model, provides a unique peer-supported environment upholding major principles of rehabilitation and recovery. The original Fairweather model included the development of "lodges," wherein individuals with serious and persistent mental illness lived and worked together in a peer-supported environment (Fairweather, 1964; Fairweather & Fergus, 1988). The program sought to empower consumers to take an active role in society relatively autonomous from staff supervision and to combat the stigma of mental illness.

Today, lodges are typically community-based homes that house 4–8 persons in an interdependent community culture. Residents live together and share daily household IADL responsibilities. Compensated work is a primary aspect of the Fairweather model, as is the emphasis on mutual decision making and meaningful engagement in daily activity. Lodges are often supervised by a coordinator who serves to assure the healthy daily functioning of the lodge community. Basic tenets of the lodge include (1) members have a stake in the system, (2) they are given much autonomy, (3) their role is voluntary, (4) the system offers opportunities for advancement, and (5) individuals are expected to fulfill the roles of society (Onaga, 1994).

Despite its emergence in the 1960s and the existence of over 100 Fairweather lodges in the United States, the model has only recently again been highlighted in research-based literature (e.g., Haertl, 2005, 2007; Haertl & Minato, 2006). Research supports the lodge model's effectiveness in promoting a family-like culture, reducing hospitalization rates, increasing quality of life, decreasing total cost to the community, and increasing the number of hours worked and rate of pay. The national Fairweather organization, The Coalition for Community Living, has developed Fidelity Standards outlining criteria to evaluate programs (Trepp & Onaga, 2004). These standards emphasize principles consistent with supportive environments. For more information on the Fairweather model, see the National Coalition for Community Living (http://theccl.org/).

Information in this section provided by Kristine Haertl, PhD, OTR/L.

Issues that must be addressed in communities for full participation of people with psychiatric disabilities include access to and support in housing, employment, education, health and dental care, and resocialization. Occupational therapists and occupational therapy assistants are well suited to address those needs for mental health consumers. They must position themselves in community agencies, work to establish informal networks for clients, and empower consumers to help themselves.

Intervention Outcomes for People With Psychiatric Disabilities

Occupational therapy outcomes for people with psychiatric disabilities should focus on enhanced occupational performance and role competence; improved adaptation in response to occupational challenge; health and wellness; participation in desired occupations; prevention of occupational deprivation; satisfactory quality of life; the ability to advocate for oneself; and occupational justice (AOTA, 2008).

It has long been known that in nonindustrial nations (e.g., Sri Lanka, Nigeria, India), treatment outcomes for people with serious mental illnesses, particularly schizophrenia, are superior to those in industrial nations (e.g., Denmark, the United Kingdom, the United States; Waxler, 1979). The Vermont Longitudinal Study and the Soteria Project (Mosher, 1999) found results in the United States similar to those in nonindustrial nations for people with schizophrenia (Harding, Brooks, Ashikaga, Strauss, & Breier, 1987; DeSisto, Harding, McCormick, Ashikaga, & Brooks, 1995).

The common features of successful intervention approaches are an emphasis on psychotropic medications; limited inpatient hospitalization (if any); and quick return to the community, which may be the family, the village or town or, in the case of Soteria House, a supportive, protective residential environment. The approach allows the client to resume his or her usual work, IADLs, and social occupations and routines as soon as possible. The research makes a compelling case for the resumption of meaningful occupations and occupational roles as soon as possible for anyone diagnosed with a serious mental illness or experiencing a relapse of symptoms.

Several authors have described positive relationships between engagement in occupation, recovery from mental illness, and the desired outcomes of occupational therapy interventions, as noted earlier. A study in Montreal confirmed that "perceived competence in daily tasks and rest, and pleasure in work and rest activities are positively correlated with subjective quality of life" (Aubin et al., 1999, p. 53). Another Canadian study found that activities that bring enjoyment to people with serious mental illness also were associated with excitement, a sense of accomplishment, relaxation, social connectedness, and interest, demonstrating a relationship between health and wellness and engagement in occupations (Emerson, Cook, Polatajko, & Segal, 1998).

Likewise, in Sweden it was found that characteristics of meaningful occupations were closely related to support for "living a life approaching normality, and . . . creating a natural arena of social interaction . . . and a sense of well-being" (Hvalsoe & Josephsson, 2003, p. 61). Kelly, McKenna, Parahoo, and Dusoir (2001) studied people with serious mental illness in Northern Ireland and also found a positive correlation between involvement in activities and self-reported quality of life. People with serious mental illness in England reported that the opportunity to engage in occupation at a workshop and a drop-in center was empowering and gave them a sense of purpose and a reason to stay healthy (Mee & Sumison, 2001). Another randomized, controlled study of people with serious mental illness in England found that participation in occupational therapy in the community resulted in significant improvement in relationships, independence, and recreation (Cook, Chambers, & Coleman, 2009).

The study of the influence of occupation and its meaning on desired occupational therapy outcomes for people with severe psychiatric disabilities is in its infancy and is currently most active outside the United States. Eklund and colleagues are contributing to this knowledge with their thoughtful descriptive research on temperament, character, self-esteem, psychopathology, social networks, locus of control, engagement in work, and other characteristics and their relationship to occupational performance (Bejerholm & Eklund, 2007; Eklund, 2006, 2007; Eklund & Bejerholm, 2007). The research to date offers encouraging and compelling evidence that engagement in occupations greatly benefits people whose lives have been disrupted by mental illness.

Occupational Performance Needs of Special Populations With Mental Health Issues

In the past decade, occupational therapists have begun to pay closer attention to groups of people who are unable to participate in chosen areas of occupation, often because of extreme poverty, relocation, and other conditions outside of their control (Kronenberg, Algado, & Pollard, 2005). Although the profession has advocated for people with disabilities throughout its history, the focus on occupational needs of populations and communities outside of traditional health delivery systems provides new perspective on the direction that occupational therapy may take in the future.

The initial impetus for the current work occurred outside of the United States; however, the situations that arose during the aftermath of Hurricane Katrina gave face to the fact that even in one of the richest countries in the world, at any given point in time, people may not have access to meeting their most basic ADLs, rest, and sleep needs, much less participate in meaningful occupations such as work and education. Several writers in occupational therapy (Christiansen & Townsend, 2010; Kronenberg et al., 2005; Kronenberg & Pollard, 2006; Townsend, 2003; Whitford, 2000; Wilcock, 1999; Wilcock & Townsend, 2000) have contributed greatly to our understanding of concepts of social justice, occupational justice, occupational deprivation, occupational marginalization, and related concepts (Braveman & Bass-Haugen, 2009).

Closely related to social and occupational justice are concerns about the prevalence of health inequities that exist for populations, especially related to ethnic and racial status (Bass-Haugen, 2009). An extensive review of the literature on these important topics is well beyond the scope of this chapter. However, a brief description of the mental health issues of two marginalized populations, their occupational functioning and performance needs, and potential adaptive strategies are provided. Our hope is that they will stimulate readers to consider occupational therapy as a valuable and important in meeting these populations' mental health needs, and that these populations be considered within the broader category of those who can benefit.

The first example considers refugees from war-torn countries in Asia and Africa who relocate to the United States, often under the umbrella of religious organizations and often into midsized urban areas in northern climates with historically homogeneous, primarily White populations. Over approximately 20 years, starting in the late 1970s, over 100,000 Hmong refugees, most from Thailand, resettled in the United States. Many of the original transplants were veterans who had fought alongside the United States in the Vietnam War; their children and grandchildren now comprise the vast number of Hmong in the United States. Wisconsin

has the third highest number of Hmong citizens among the states (Rogers, 2006).

Historical and personal experience in working with these refugees suggests that the transition from lives as farmers in an agrarian-dominated society to life in urban America was filled with confusion, missteps, and alienation (Ingersoll, 2004). The profession of occupational therapy was not actively involved in the resettlement of the Hmong (to our knowledge), and the only publication that appeared regarding the role of occupational therapy focused on the consideration of culture when assessing Hmong children with development disabilities in the schools (Meyers, 1992).

Since that time the Hmong refugees and their descendents have become successful members of American society, with high rates of academic achievement, business and home ownership, and service as elected officials. Hmong immigrants and their families now enjoy full integration into their communities (Ingersoll, 2004). But consider the potential challenges with areas of occupation, occupational performance, and mental health issues they faced upon arriving in the United States. One man recounted that as a newly arrived teenager he moved into a hotel with his family for a short time. The family did not know how to turn the shower on and off, drain the tub, or work the thermostat (Ingersoll, 2004). In a resettlement context, challenges for parents in being unable to secure basic needs for their children can create anxiety, grief, anger, and depression. It can be something as seemingly simple as how to locate, travel to, and then complete shopping tasks for food, clothing, and other sustenance needs. Imagine coming from a refugee camp and then having to purchase food items at a warehouse grocery store, or navigating through a mall to find shoes for your children. The authors of chapters in the *Occupational Therapy Without Borders: Learning From the Spirit of Survivors* (Kronenberg et al., 2005), address these issues for populations in communities around the world. The same concerns can be assumed for displaced populations in the United States.

Another example of a potentially marginalized population that might not typically be considered are the young war veterans returning to families, communities, places of employment, and educational institutions following service in Afghanistan and Iraq. A study of 30 of these young veterans found that they experience occupational performance challenges across the areas of IADLs, sleep, education, and social participation in families (Plach, 2009). In addition, when screened for a number of potential mental health problems, 77% screened positive for potential depression, 53% for problem drinking, 40% for a possible mild traumatic brain injury, and 23% for posttraumatic stress disorder.

They recount adjustment issues to the areas of occupation that are most important to them, such as completing their education and spending quality time with their families, and a paucity of services addressing their unique mental health needs, especially if they live far away from veterans' affairs services. Without sufficient support and opportunity to resolve the occupational performance issues they face, this population of young veterans has the potential to become marginalized in society, as occurred with so many of the veterans from the Vietnam War.

Opportunities for occupational therapists to engage with young veterans and provide assistance may come at institutions of higher education, especially those housing occupational therapy education programs, where they could conduct problem-solving groups to help student veterans meet role demands, provide relaxation training to cope with stressors, and support recreational efforts that minimize use of alcohol.

Occupational therapists also may see young veterans in orthopedic and hand clinics or in places of employment where they serve as ergonomic consultants and offer additional services to address mental health needs that may not be considered elsewhere. Again, offering psychoeducational groups that address the concerns of this population in areas such as sleep, hygiene, pain management, and alcohol abuse may be outside of the traditional occupational therapy role in these settings but may go a long way toward aiding the transition of young veterans who do not receive services elsewhere.

In conclusion, the roles of occupational therapists in serving the mental health needs of real and potentially marginalized populations in the United States received little attention in the occupational therapy literature until the last decade. As a result, the opportunity to expand occupational therapy's "borders" of service to ensure that all people have the chance to pursue occupational goals now seems more achievable.

Summary

In this chapter, the role of occupational therapy personnel in providing services to individuals with psychiatric disabilities was reviewed. The most prevalent disorders requiring adaptive living strategies, including schizophrenia, mood disorders, personality disorders, and substance abuse disorders were described. The behavioral patterns associated with each condition were described from the standpoint of their interference with the occupational performance (particularly ADLs and IADLs) and life roles necessary for employment and for living in the community. Adaptive strategies for enabling individuals with psychiatric disabilities to manage life tasks and roles were described, including psychoeducational models, behavioral approaches, and cognitive approaches. Various case management approaches were described, including ACT, PACE, and Clubhouse models. Throughout the chapter, it was emphasized that successful programs for psychiatric rehabilitation in the community require an integrated, multidisciplinary approach, support systems for clients and their families, well-developed relationships among staff and indivduals requiring care, and opportunities for developing skills.

Study Questions

1. What are the symptoms, onset, duration, prognosis, and treatment of the major psychiatric disabilities?
2. What are the similarities and differences in impairment in occupational performance among people with different types of psychiatric disabilities?
3. What are the desired outcomes of occupational therapy for people with psychiatric disabilities, and what is the role of occupation in achieving them?
4. What are the differences between the PACT and PACE approaches to recovery for people with psychiatric disabilities?
5. How does an occupational therapist's professional preparation match the kinds of programs and focus that a Clubhouse program offers?
6. What are the principles for integrating people with psychiatric disabilities within the community?

References

Aberg-Wistedt, A., Cressell, T., Lidberg, Y., Liljenberg, B., & Osbey, U. (1995). Two-year outcome of team-based intensive case management for patients with schizophrenia. *Psychiatric Services, 46,* 1263–1266.

Ackerson, B. J. (2003). Parents with serious and persistent mental illness: Issues in assessment and services. *Social Work, 48,* 187–194.

Ahern, L., & Fisher, D. (1999). *Personal assistance in community existence: Recovery at your own PACE.* Electronic version. Lawrence, MA: National Empowerment Center. Retrieved November 23, 2009, from www.power2u.org

Ahern, L., & Fisher, D. (2001). An alternative to PACT: Recovery at your own PACE. *Mental Health Special Interest Quarterly, 24,* 3–4.

Allen, C. K., Austin, S. L., David, S. K., Earhart, C. A., McCraith, D. B., & Riska-Williams, L. (2008). *Manual for the Allen Cognitive Level Screen–5 (ACLS–5) and Large Allen Cognitive Level Screen–5 (LACLS–5).* Camarillo, CA: ACLS and LACLS Committee. Available at www.ssww.com

American Occupational Therapy Association. (2008). Occupational therapy practice framework: Domain and process (2nd ed.). *American Journal of Occupational Therapy, 62,* 625–683.

American Psychiatric Association. (2000). *Diagnostic and statistical manual of mental disorders* (4th ed., text rev.). Washington, DC: Author.

Americans with Disabilities Act of 1990, Pub. Law 101–336, 104 Stat. 327.

Anthony, W. A., Cohen, M. R., Farkas, M. D., & Gagne, C. (2002). *Psychiatric rehabilitation* (2nd ed.). Boston: Boston University, Center for Psychiatric Rehabilitation.

Aubin, G., Hachey, R., & Mercier, C. (1999). Meaning of daily activities and subjective quality of life in people with severe mental illness. *Scandinavian Journal of Occupational Therapy, 6,* 53–62.

Auerbach, E. (2002). An occupational therapist in an assertive community treatment program. *Mental Health Special Interest Section Quarterly, 25(1),* 1–2.

Bakker, C. B., & Armstrong, H. E. (1976). The adult development program: An educational approach to the delivery of mental health services. *Hospital and Community Psychiatry, 27,* 330–334.

Baptiste, S. (2008). Client-centered assessment. The Canadian Occupational Performance Measure. In B. J. Hemphill-Pearson (Ed.), *Assessments in occupational therapy mental health: An integrative approach* (2nd ed., pp. 34–47). Thorofare, NJ: Slack.

Bass-Haugen, J. D. (2009). Health disparities: Examination of evidence relevant for occupational therapy. *American Journal of Occupational Therapy, 63,* 24–34.

Baum, C. M., Connor, L. T., Morrison, T., Hahn, M., Dromerick, A. W., & Edwards, D. F. (2008). Reliability, validity, and clinical utility of the Executive Function Performance Test: A measure of executive function in a sample of people with stroke. *American Journal of Occupational Therapy, 62,* 446–455.

Becker, R. E., Meisler, N., Stormer, G., & Brondino, M. J. (1999). Employment outcomes for clients with severe mental illness in a PACT model replication. *Psychiatric Services, 50,* 104–106.

Bejerholm, U., & Eklund, M. (2007). Occupational engagement in persons with schizophrenia: Relationships to self-rated variables, psychopathology, and quality of life. *American Journal of Occupational Therapy, 61,* 21–32.

Bonder, B. (1993). Issues in assessment of psychosocial components of function. *American Journal of Occupational Therapy, 47,* 211–216.

Bonder, B. (1995). *Psychopathology and function* (2nd ed.). Thorofare, NJ: Slack.

Boyer, G., Hachey, R., & Mercier, C. (2000). Perceptions of occupation performance and subjective quality

of life in persons with severe mental illness. *Occupational Therapy in Mental Health, 15(2),* 1–15.

Braveman, B., & Bass-Haugen, J. D. (2009). Social justice and health disparities: An evolving discourse in occupational therapy research and intervention. *American Journal of Occupational Therapy, 63,* 7–12.

Brayman, S. (2008). The Comprehensive Occupational Therapy Evaluation. In B. J. Hemphill-Pearson (Ed.), *Assessments in occupational therapy mental health: An integrative approach* (2nd ed., pp. 113–124). Thorofare, NJ: Slack.

Brown, C. (2001). What is the best environment for me: A sensory processing perspective. *Occupational Therapy in Mental Health, 17(3/4),* 115–126.

Brun, C., & Rapp, R. C. (2001). Strengths-based case management: Individuals' perspectives on strengths and the case manager relationship. *Social Work, 46,* 278–288.

Bybee, D., Mowbray, C. T., Oyserman, D., & Lewandowski, L. (2003). Variability in community functioning of mothers with serious mental illness. *Journal of Behavioral Health Services and Research, 30,* 269–289.

Carling, P. J. (1975). *Return to community: Building support systems for people with psychiatric disabilities.* New York: Guilford.

Carswell, A., McColl, M. A., Baptiste, S., Law, M., Polatajko, H., & Pollock, N. (2004). The Canadian Occupational Performance Measure: A research and clinical literature review. *Canadian Journal of Occupational Therapy, 71,* 210–222.

Center for Substance Abuse Treatment. (2007). *Definitions and terms relating to co-occurring disorders* (COCE Overview Paper 1, DHHS Publication No. SMA 07-4163). Rockville, MD: Substance Abuse and Mental Health Services Administration & Center for Mental Health Services.

Chan, A. S. M., Tsang, H. W. H., & Li, S. M. Y. (2009). Case report of integrated supported employment for a person with a severe mental illness. *American Journal of Occupational Therapy, 63,* 238–244.

Chan, P. S., Krupa, T., Lawson, J. S., & Eastabrook, S. (2005). An outcome in need of clarity: Building a predictive model of subjective quality of life for persons with severe mental illness living in the community. *American Journal of Occupational Therapy, 59,* 181–190.

Chesworth, C., Duffy, R., Hodnett, J., & Knight, A. (2002). Measuring clinical effectiveness in mental health: Is the Canadian Occupational Performance an appropriate measure? *British Journal of Occupational Therapy, 65,* 30–34.

Chinman, M. J., Rosenheck, R., Lam, J. A., & Davidson, L. (2000). Comparing consumer and nonconsumer case management services for homeless persons with serious mental illness. *Journal of Nervous and Mental Disease, 188,* 446–453.

Christiansen, C. H., & Townsend, E. A. (Eds.). (2010). *Introduction to occupation: The art and science of living* (2nd ed.). Upper Saddle River, NJ: Prentice-Hall.

Cohen, M., & Nemec, P. (1988). Trainer orientation. In M. Cohen, P. Nemec, & M. Farkas (Eds.), *Case management training technology.* Boston: Boston University, Center for Psychiatric Rehabilitation.

Cohen, M., Nemec, P., Farkas, M., & Forbess, R. (1988). Training module: Introduction. In M. Cohen, P. Nemec, & M. Farkas (Eds.), *Case management training technology.* Boston: Boston University, Center for Psychiatric Rehabilitation.

Cook, S., Chambers, E., & Coleman, J. H. (2009). Occupational therapy for people with psychotic conditions in community settings: A pilot randomized controlled trial. *Clinical Rehabilitation, 23,* 40–52.

Crist, P. H. (1986). Community living skills: A psychoeducational community-based program. *Occupational Therapy in Mental Health, 6(2),* 51–64.

Crowley, K. (2000). *The power of procovery in healing mental illness: Just start anywhere.* Los Angeles: Kennedy Carlisle.

DeSisto, M. J., Harding, C. M., McCormick, R. V., Ashikiga, T., & Brooks, G. W. (1995). The Maine and Vermont three-decade studies of serious mental illness I: Matched comparison of cross-sectional outcomes. *British Journal of Psychiatry, 167,* 331–342.

Dewa, C. S., Horgan, S., McIntyre, D., Robinson, G., Krupa, T., & Estabrook, S. (2003). Direct and indirect time inputs and assertive community treatment. *Community Mental Health Journal, 39,* 17–32.

Dixon, L. (2000). Assertive community treatment: Twenty-five years of gold. *Psychiatric Services, 51,* 759–765.

Dougherty, S. J. (1994). The generalist role in Clubhouse organization. *Psychosocial Rehabilitation Journal, 18,* 94–95.

Eaton, P. (2002). Psychoeducation in acute mental health settings: Is there a role for occupational therapists? *British Journal of Occupational Therapy, 65,* 321–326.

Eklund, M. (2006). Occupational factors and characteristics of the social network in people with persistent mental illness. *American Journal of Occupational Therapy, 60,* 587–594.

Eklund, M. (2007). Perceived control: How is it related to daily occupation in patients with mental illness living in the community? *American Journal of Occupational Therapy, 61,* 535–542.

Eklund, M., & Bejerholm, U. (2007). Temperament, character, and self-esteem in relation to occupational performance in individuals with schizophrenia. *OTJR: Occupation, Participation and Health, 27,* 52–58.

Eklund, M., Hansson, L., & Alhqvist, C. (2004). The importance of work as compared to other forms of daily occupations for well-being and functioning among persons with long-term mental illness. *Community Mental Health Journal, 40,* 465–477.

Emerson, H. A., Cook, J., Polatajko, H., & Segal, R. (1998). Enjoyment experiences as described by persons with schizophrenia: A qualitative study. *Canadian Journal of Occupational Therapy, 65,* 183–192.

Fairweather, G. W. (Ed.). (1964). *Social psychology in treating mental illness: An experimental approach.* New York: Wiley.

Fairweather, G. W., & Fergus, E. O. (1988). *The Lodge Society: A look at community tenure as a measure of cost savings.* East Lansing: Michigan State University.

Falk, K., & Allebeck, P. (2002). Implementing assertive community care for patients with schizophrenia. *Scandinavian Journal of Caring Sciences, 16,* 280–286.

Ferentinos, P., Kontaxakis, V., Havaki-Kontaxaki, B., Paparrigopoulos, T., Dikeow, D., Ktonas, P., et al. (2009). Sleep disturbances in relation to fatigue in major depression. *Journal of Psychosomatic Research, 66,* 37–42.

Fike, M. L. (1990). Considerations and techniques in the treatment of multiple personality disorder. *American Journal of Occupational Therapy, 44,* 984–990.

Ford, R., Barnes, A., Davies, R., Chalmers, C., Hardy, P., & Muijen, M. (2001). Maintaining contact with people with severe mental illness: 5-year follow-up of assertive outreach. *Social Psychiatry Psychiatric Epidemiology, 36,* 444–447.

Forsyth, K., Deshpande, S., Kielhofner, G., Henriksson, C., Haglund, L., Olson, L., et al. (2005). *The Occupational Circumstances Assessment Interview and Rating Scale (OCAIRS), Version 4.0.* Chicago: Model of Human Occupation Clearinghouse, Department of Occupational Therapy, College of Applied Health Sciences, University of Illinois at Chicago. http://www.moho.uic.edu/

Friedlob, S. A., Janis, G. A., & Deets-Aron, C. (1986). A hospital-connected halfway house program for individuals with long-term neuropsychiatric disabilities. *American Journal of Occupational Therapy, 40,* 271–277.

Gahnstrom-Strandqvist, K., Liukko, A., & Tham, K. (2003). The meaning of the working cooperative for persons with long-term mental illness: A phenomenological study. *American Journal of Occupational Therapy, 57,* 262–271.

Gioia, D., & Brekke, J. S. (2003). Use of the Americans with Disabilities Act by young adults with schizophrenia. *Psychiatric Services, 54,* 302–304.

Gournay, K. (1999). Assertive community treatment—Why isn't it working? *Journal of Mental Health, 8,* 427–429.

Green, A. (2008). Sleep, occupation, and the passage of time. *British Journal of Occupational Therapy, 71,* 339–347.

Goverover, Y., & Josman, N. (2004). Everyday problem solving among four groups of individuals with cognitive impairments: Examination of the discriminant validity of the Observed Tasks of Daily Living–Revised. *OTJR: Occupation, Participation and Health, 24,* 103–112.

Gureje, O, Olley, B. O., Olusola, E. O., & Kola, L. (2006). Do beliefs about causality influence attitudes toward mental illness? *World Psychiatry 5(2),* 104–107.

Gutman, S. A., Schindler, V. P., Furphy, K. A., Klein, K., Lisak, J. M., & Durham, D. P. (2007). The effectiveness of a supported education program for adults with psychiatric disabilities: The Bridge Program. *Occupational Therapy in Mental Health, 23(1),* 21–38.

Haertl, K. L. (2005). Factors influencing success in a Fairweather Model mental health program. *Psychiatric Rehabilitation Journal, 28,* 370–377.

Haertl, K. L., (2007). The Fairweather Mental Health Housing Model—A peer-supported environment: Implications for psychiatric rehabilitation. *American Psychiatric Rehabilitation Journal, 3,* 149–162.

Haertl, K., & Minato, M. (2006). Daily occupations of persons with mental illness: Themes from Japan and America. *Occupational Therapy in Mental Health, 22,* 19–32.

Harding, C. M., Brooks, G. W., Ashikaga, T., Strauss, J. S., & Breier, A. (1987). The Vermont Longitudinal Study of persons with severe mental illness, I: Methodology, study sample, and overall status 32 years later. *American Journal of Psychiatry, 144,* 718–726.

Hemphill-Pearson, B. J. (Ed.). (2008). *Assessments in occupational therapy mental health: An integrative approach* (2nd ed.). Thorofare, NJ: Slack.

Hersen, M., & Van Hasselt, V. (2001). *Advanced abnormal psychology* (2nd ed.). New York: Kluwer Academic/Plenum.

Hodge, M., & Giesler, L. (1997). *Case management practice guidelines for adults with severe and persistent mental illness.* Ocean Ridge, FL: National Association of Case Management.

Hodgson, S., & Lloyd, C. (2002). Leisure as a relapse prevention strategy. *British Journal of Therapy and Rehabilitation, 9,* 86–91.

Hodgson, S., Lloyd, C., & Schmid, T. (2001). The leisure participation of clients with a dual diagnosis. *British Journal of Occupational Therapy, 64,* 487–492.

Howie the Harp. (1995). Preface. In P. J. Carling, *Return to community: Building support systems for people with psychiatric disabilities* (pp. xiii–xvii). New York: Guilford.

Hvalsoe, B., & Josephsson, S. (2003). Characteristics of meaningful occupations from the perspectives of mentally ill people. *Scandinavian Journal of Occupational Therapy, 10,* 61–71.

Ingersoll, B. (2004, May 18). *For Hmong, a new home.* Retrieved August 31, 2009, from http://www.madison.com/wisconsinstatejournal/local/74542.php

International Center for Clubhouse Development. (n.d.). *How ICCD Clubhouses can help.* Available online at http://www.iccd.org

Jacobs, B. L., Selby, S., & Madsen, M. K. (1996). Supporting academic success: A model for supported education in a university environment. *Occupational Therapy in Health Care, 10*(2), 3–13.

Johnsen, M., Samberg, L., Caslyn, R., Blasinsky, M., Landow, W., & Goldman, H. (1999). Case management models for persons who are homeless and mentally ill: The ACCESS demonstration project. *Community Mental Health Journal, 35,* 325–346.

Katz, N. (2006). *Routine Task Inventory–Expanded: Manual 2006* [Prepared and elaborated on the basis of Allen, C. K. (1989 unpublished)]. Retrieved May 12, 2009, from http://www.allen-cognitive-network.org/index.php/allen-model/assessments/48-routine-task-inventory-expanded-rti-e

Kelly, S., McKenna, H., Parahoo, K., & Dusoir, A. (2001). The relationship between involvement in activities and quality of life for people with severe and enduring mental illness. *Journal of Psychiatric and Mental Health Nursing, 8,* 139–146.

Kielhofner, G., Mallinson, T., Crawford, C., Nowak, M., Rigby, M., Henry, A., et al. (2004). *The Occupational Performance History Interview–II, Version 2.1.* Chicago: Model of Human Occupation Clearinghouse, Department of Occupational Therapy, College of Applied Health Sciences, University of Illinois at Chicago. http://www.moho.uic.edu/

Kronenberg, F., Algado, S. S., & Pollard, N. (2005). *Occupational therapy without borders: Learning from the spirit of survivors.* Edinburgh, Scotland: Elsevier.

Kronenberg, F., & Pollard, N. (2006). Political dimensions of occupation and the roles of occupational therapy. *American Journal of Occupational Therapy, 60,* 615–625.

Krupa, T., Radloff-Gabriel, D., Whippey, E., & Kirsch, B. (2002). Reflections on occupational therapy and assertive community treatment. *Canadian Journal of Occupational Therapy, 69,* 153–157.

Krupa, T., McLean, H., Estabrook, S., Bonham, A., & Baksh, L. (2003). Daily time use as a measure of community adjustment for persons served by assertive community treatment teams. *American Journal of Occupational Therapy, 57,* 558–565.

Kuno, E., Rothbard, A. B., & Sands, R. G. (1999). Service components of case management which reduce inpatient care use for persons with serious mental illness. *Community Mental Health Journal, 35,* 153–167.

Laliberte-Rudman, D., Hoffman, L., Scott, E., & Rensick, R. (2004). Quality of life for individuals with schizophrenia: Validating an assessment that addresses client concerns and occupational issues. *OTJR: Occupation, Participation and Health, 24,* 13–21.

Laliberte-Rudman, D., Yu, B., Scott, E., & Pajouhandeh, P. (2000). Exploration of the perspectives of persons with schizophrenia regarding quality of life. *American Journal of Occupational Therapy, 54,* 137–147.

Lamb, H. R. (1976). An educational model for teaching skills to long-term patients. *Hospital and Community Psychiatry, 27,* 875–877.

Larimer, M. E., & Cronce, J. M. (2002). Identification, prevention, and treatment: A review of individual-focused strategies to reduce problematic alcohol consumption by college students. *Journal of Studies on Alcohol, Supplement No. 14,* 148–163.

Law, M. (Ed.). (1998). *Client-centered occupational therapy.* Thorofare, NJ: Slack.

Law, M., Baptiste, S., Carswell, A., McColl, A., Polatajko, H., & Pollack, N. (1998). *Canadian Occupational Performance Measure* (3rd ed.). Ottawa, Ontario: CAOT Publications ACE.

Law, M., Baum, C., & Dunn, W. (2005). *Measuring occupational performance: Supporting best practice in occupational therapy* (2nd ed.). Thorofare, NJ: Slack.

Liberman, R. P., & Kopelowicz, A. (2002). Teaching persons with severe mental disabilities to be their own case managers. *Psychiatric Services, 53,* 1377–1379.

Lillie, M. D., & Armstrong, H. E. (1982). Contributions to the development of psychoeducational approaches to mental health service. *American Journal of Occupational Therapy, 36,* 438–443.

Liu, K. W. D., Hollis, V., Warren, S., & Williamson, D. L. (2007). Supported-employment program processes and outcomes: Experiences of people with schizophrenia. *American Journal of Occupational Therapy, 61,* 543–554.

Lloyd, C., & Samra, P. (2000). OT and work-related programmes for people with a mental illness. *British Journal of Therapy and Rehabilitation, 7,* 254–261.

Lloyd, C., King, R., Lampe, J., & McDougall, S. (2001). The leisure satisfaction of people with psychiatric disabilities. *Psychiatric Rehabilitation Journal, 25,* 107–113.

MacDonald-Wilson, K. L., Nemec, P. B., Anthony, W. A., & Cohen, M. R. (2001). Assessment in psychiatric rehabilitation. In B. F. Bolton (Ed.), *Handbook of measurement and evaluation in rehabilitation* (3rd ed.; 423–448). Gaithersburg, MD: Aspen.

Margolis, R. L., Harrison, S. A., Robinson, H. J., & Jayaram, G. (1996). Occupational Therapy Task Observation Scale (OTTOS)©: A rapid method for rating task group function of psychiatric patients. *American Journal of Occupational Therapy, 50,* 380–385.

McColl, M. A., Law, M., Baptiste, S., Pollock, N., Carswell, A., & Polatajko, H. J. (2005). Targeted applications of the Canadian Occupational Performance Measure. *Canadian Journal of Occupational Therapy, 72,* 298–300.

McGrew, J. H., Pescosolido, B., & Wright, E. (2003). Case managers' perspectives on critical ingredients of assertive community treatment and on its implementation. *Psychiatric Services, 54,* 370–376.

McGrew, J. H., Wilson, R. G., & Bond, G. R. (2002). An exploratory study of what clients like least about assertive community treatment. *Psychiatric Services, 53,* 761–763.

Mee, J., & Sumison, T. (2001). Mental health clients confirm the motivating power of occupation. *British Journal of Occupational Therapy, 64,* 121–128.

Meyers, C. (1992). Hmong children and their families: Consideration of cultural influences in assessment. *American Journal of Occupational Therapy, 46,* 737–744.

Miller, H. (2008). *Using Photovoice to explore the experiences of parenting while living with a mental illness.* Unpublished master's thesis, University of Wisconsin–Milwaukee.

Mosher, L. (1999). Soteria and other alternatives to acute psychiatric hospitalization: A personal and professional review. *Journal of Nervous and Mental Disease, 187,* 142–149.

Morrison, J. (2007). *Diagnosis made easier: Principles and techniques for mental health clinicians.* New York: Guilford.

Moyers, P. A., & Stoffel, V. C. (2001). Community-based approaches for substance use disorders. In M. Scaffa (Ed.), *Occupational therapy in community-based practice settings* (pp. 318–342). Philadelphia: F. A. Davis.

Nagle, S., Cook, J. V., & Polatajko, H. J. (2002). I'm doing as much as I can: Occupational choices of persons with severe and persistent mental illness. *Journal of Occupational Science, 9,* 72–81.

NAMI (nd.). *People with mental illness enrich our lives.* Retrieved November 24, 2003, from http://www.nami.org/Content/ContentGroups/Helpline1/People_with_Mental_Illness_Enrich_Our_Lives.htm

Neale, M. S., & Rosenheck, R. A. (2000). Therapeutic limit setting in an assertive community treatment program. *Psychiatric Services, 51,* 499–505.

Neistadt, M. E., & Cohn, E. S. (1990). *An independent living skills model for Level I fieldwork.* Bethesda, MD: American Occupational Therapy Association.

Neistadt, M. E., & Marques, K. (1984). An independent living skills training program. *American Journal of Occupational Therapy, 38,* 671–676.

Ng, B. F. L., & Tsang, H. W. H. (2002). A program to assist people with severe mental illness in formulating realistic life goals. *Journal of Rehabilitation, 68*(4), 59–66.

Oka, M., Otsuka, K., Yokoyama, N., Mintz, J., Hoshino, K., Niwa, S., et al. (2004). An evaluation of a hybrid occupational therapy and supported employment program in Japan for persons with schizophrenia. *American Journal of Occupational Therapy, 58,* 466–475.

Onaga, E. E. (1994). The Fairweather Lodge as a psychosocial program in the 1990s. In L. Spaniol, M. Brown, L. Blankertz, D. Burnham, J. Dincin, K. Furlong-Norman, et al. (Eds.), *An introduction to psychiatric rehabilitation* (pp. 206–214.). Columbia, MD: International Association of Psychosocial Rehabilitation Professionals.

O'Sullivan, J., Gilbert, J., & Ward, W. (2006). Addressing the health and lifestyle issues of people with a mental illness: The health living programme. *Australasian Psychiatry, 14,* 150–155.

Page, M. S. (2008). Interviewing in occupational therapy. In B. J. Hemphill-Pearson (Ed.), *Assessments in occupational therapy mental health: An integrative approach* (2nd ed., pp. 15–33). Thorofare, NJ: Slack.

Pan, A. W., Chung, L., & Hsin-Hwei, G. (2003). Reliability and validity of the Canadian Occupational Performance Measure for clients with psychiatric disorders in Taiwan. *Occupational Therapy International, 10,* 269–277.

Pitts, D. (2001). Assertive community treatment: A brief introduction. *Mental Health Special Interest Section Quarterly, 24*(4), 1–2.

Plach, H. L. (2009). *Assessing the needs of young veterans across the occupational performance areas of self-care, leisure, and productivity.* Unpublished master's thesis, University of Wisconsin–Milwaukee.

Porter, J., Capra, S., & Watson, G. (2000). An individualized food-skills progamme: Development, implementation and evaluation. *Australian Occupational Therapy Journal, 47,* 51–61.

Prince, P. N., & Prince, C. R. (2002). Perceived stigma and community integration among clients of assertive community treatment. *Psychiatric Rehabilitation Journal, 25,* 323–331.

Remien, R. H., & Christopher, F. (1996). A family psychoeducation model for long–term rehabilitation. *Physical and Occupational Therapy in Geriatrics, 14*(2), 45–59.

Rigby, P., Cooper, B., Letts, L., Stewart, D., & Strong, S. (2005). Measuring environmental factors. In M. Law, C. Baum, & W. Dunn (Eds.), *Measuring occupational performance: Supporting best practice in occupational therapy* (2nd ed.). Thorofare, NJ: Slack.

Rogers, M. G. (2006). *Hmong resettlement*. Retrieved August 31, 2009, from http://www.legis.state.wi.us/LRB/pubs/ttp/ttp-06-2004.html

Sadock, B. J., & Sadock, V. A. (2007). *Kaplan and Sadock's synopsis of psychiatry: Behavioral sciences/clinical psychiatry* (10th ed.). Baltimore: Lippincott Williams & Wilkins.

Sateia, M. J. (2009). Update on sleep and psychiatric disorders. *Chest, 135,* 1370–1379.

Schaedle, R., McGrew, J. H., Bond, G. R., & Epstein, I. (2002). A comparison of experts' perspective on assertive community treatment and intensive case management. *Psychiatric Services, 53,* 207–210.

Spaniol, L., & Koehler, M. (1994). *The experience of recovery*. Boston: Boston University, Center for Psychiatric Rehabilitation, Sargent College of Allied Health Professions.

Stein, L. I., & Santos, A. B. (1998). *Assertive community treatment of persons with severe mental illness*. New York: W. W. Norton.

Stoffel, V. C. (2007). Perception of the Clubhouse experience and its impact on mental health recovery (Doctoral dissertation, Cardinal Stritch University, Milwaukee, Wisconsin). Available from *ProQuest Digital Dissertations Database* (Publication No. AAT 3279196).

Su, C., Chen, W., Tsai, P., Tsai, C., & Su, W. (2007). Psychometric properties of the Lowenstein Occupational Therapy Cognitive Assessment–Second Edition in Taiwanese persons with schizophrenia. *American Journal of Occupational Therapy, 61,* 108–118.

Substance Abuse and Mental Health Services Administration, Office of Applied Studies. (2007). *The NSDUH report: Co-occurring major depressive episode (MDE) and alcohol use disorder among adults.* Rockville, MD: Author.

Substance Abuse and Mental Health Services Administration, Office of Applied Studies. (2008). *The NSDUH report: Serious psychological distress and receipt of mental health services.* Rockville, MD: Author.

Test, M. A., Greenberg, J. S., Long, J. D., Brekke, J. S., & Senn Burke, S. (2005). Construct validity of a measure of subjective satisfaction with life of adults with serious mental illness. *Psychiatric Services, 56,* 292–300.

Townsend, E. (2003). Reflections on power and justice in enabling occupation. *Canadian Journal of Occupational Therapy, 70,* 74–87.

Trepp, J., & Onaga, E. (2004). *Fairweather Lodge fidelity: Principles, practices, outcomes, and satisfaction.* East Lansing, MI: Coalition for Community Living.

Tsang, H. W. H., Ng, B. F. L., & Chiu, F. P. F. (2002). Job profiles of people with severe mental illness: Implications for rehabilitation. *International Journal of Rehabilitation Research, 25,* 189–196.

Tse, S. (2002). Practice guidelines: Therapeutic interventions aimed at assisting people with bipolar affective disorder achieve their vocational goals. *Work, 19,* 167–179.

Tse, S. S., & Walsh, A. E. S. (2001). How does work work for people with bipolar affective disorder? *Occupational Therapy International, 8,* 210–225.

Tse, S., & Yeats, M. (2002). What helps people with bipolar affective disorder succeed in employment: A grounded theory approach. *Work, 19,* 47–62.

Warren, A. (2002). An evaluation of the Canadian Model of Occupational Performance and the Canadian Occupational Performance Measure in mental health practice. *British Journal of Occupational Therapy, 65,* 515–521.

Waxler, N. E. (1979). Is outcome for schizophrenia better in nonindustrial societies? The case of Sri Lanka. *Journal of Nervous and Mental Disease, 167,* 144–158.

Weissenberg, R., & Giladi, N. (1989). Home economics day: A program for disturbed adolescents to promote acquisition of habits and skills. *Occupational Therapy in Mental Health, 9,* 89–103.

Whitford, G. (2000). Occupational deprivation: Global challenge in the new millennium. *British Journal of Occupational Therapy, 63,* 200–204.

Wilcock, A. A. (1999). *An occupational perspective on health.* Thorofare, NJ: Slack.

Wilcock, A. A., & Townsend, E. (2000). Occupational terminology interactive dialogue. *Journal of Occupational Science, 7,* 84–86.

Wisconsin Blue Ribbon Commission on Mental Health. (1997). *The Blue Ribbon Commission on Mental Health: Final report.* Madison, WI: Office of the Governor.

Ziguras, S. J., Stuart, G. W., & Jackson, A. C. (2002). Assessing the evidence on case management. *British Journal of Psychiatry, 181,* 17–21.

Ziv, N. (2000). Application of the psychoeducational therapy approach in an occupational therapy group for women with depression. *Israel Journal of Occupational Therapy, 9,* E64.

Chapter 16

Living With Vision Loss

DON GOLEMBIEWSKI, MA, CVRT, AND JANE CHARLTON, MSED

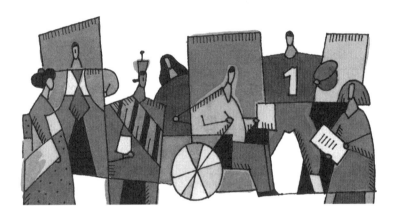

KEY WORDS

Braille

cataracts

central vision loss (CVL)

diabetic retinopathy

eccentric viewing

glaucoma

global positioning satellite (GPS)

legal blindness

macular degeneration (AMD)

no light perception (NLP)

peripheral vision loss (PVL)

photophobia

self-protection techniques

severe visual impairment

sighted guide technique

Snellen chart

HIGHLIGHTS

- The rate of severe visual impairments increases as people age.
- Macular degeneration is the leading cause of severe visual impairment in North America.
- Occupational performance will vary greatly depending on the type of diagnosis and related vision loss whether central, peripheral, or general.
- All vision loss is not the same.
- Occupational performance can be improved dramatically with environmental adaptations such as increased lighting, controlled glare, and enhanced color contrast.
- The use of a sighted guide is the safest way for a person with a severe visual impairment to travel.
- Tactual labels and enlarged print improve IADL functioning.
- Adjustment to severe vision loss is as unique as each person experiencing it.

- Technological advances such as computer access and GPS systems for mobility are improving the occupational functioning of people with severe visual impairments.

OBJECTIVES

After reading this material, readers will be able to

- Describe the challenges to occupational performance (everyday living) experienced by individuals with each of the major age-related eye conditions;
- Describe the functional visual impact of each of the major age-related eye conditions;
- Define the terms used to classify the levels of vision loss;
- Describe the phases of adjustment to a severe loss of vision;
- List the factors that improve the potential for increased independence in occupational performance;
- Describe adaptive strategies, equipment, and environmental modifications for optimal performance in daily activities for people with vision loss;
- Describe the impact that lighting, texture, and color contrast have on occupational performance of people with severe visual impairments;
- List the benefits of early service intervention for people with a severe vision loss;
- Describe the protections of the Americans with Disabilities Act for people with vision loss; and
- Describe the use and benefits of using a GPS system.

This chapter describes the visual impairments, short of total blindness, most commonly associated with aging. It details strategies that allow individuals with these conditions to function with confidence and independence. Many of the strategies, tools, and approaches also apply to younger people and those who are congenitally blind—a relatively small percentage of the population having difficulty seeing (Kirchner & Schmeidler, 1997).

A severe vision loss will negatively affect virtually all activities of daily living (ADLs) of people living with low vision (Carroll, 1961; Mayo Clinic, 2009). This functional impact will be different for each person and will vary in an intensity that may not be in proportion to the severity of the loss. Thus, the information presented in this chapter only touches on the full range of adaptive strategies and aids available to this highly diverse population. The chapter focuses on modifying the environment for activity limitations in the crucial performance areas of communication, mobility, ADLs, leisure, and work.

Definitions of Visual Acuity

Visual acuity levels neither dictate nor necessarily limit one's ability to function; they may be used to explain performance problems. Eye care providers (i.e., ophthalmologists, optometrists) report visual acuity levels using the following designations (Corn & Koenig, 1996):

- *No light perception (NLP)* means total blindness. People with NLP are totally blind and must use a variety of compensatory sensory skills to function. Hearing, the only other long-distance sense, must be used for mobility and to gather critical information about the environment. A person with NLP should be encouraged to learn Braille, a tactual means of reading and writing, and the use of assistive technology (AT) for compensatory purposes.
- *Light perception (LP)* is the ability to perceive light only. LP can be useful in determining whether household appliances or lights are on, whether it is daytime, or whether window shades are open.
- *Light projection (L. Proj.)* is the ability not only to see light but also to determine the direction of the source. L. Proj can be essential in aiding mobility and in spatial orientation.
- *Hand movement (HM)* designates the ability to see movement or gross forms, such as a doctor's hand moving in front of the patient. HM ability is useful in orientation and safe travel and in observing other environmental activity. HM is an unreliable predictor of function but is a recordable level of vision when an eye chart is not distinguishable.
- *Counts fingers (CF)* or *finger counting (FC)*, often used in conjunction with "at 2 feet" or another distance, also is an unreliable and seldom used designation of vision. This designation is neither truly objective nor exact, but it

occasionally may be seen in medical reports. People with CF may be able to see a coffee cup on their desk or read newspaper headlines.

- *Snellen notation* is the tested level of vision that coincides with each line of progressively smaller print letters a patient is able to read on a Snellen chart. The use of the Snellen eye chart with the familiar large capital "E" or "O" on the top line is the standard tool for the measurement of distance acuity. Depending on the chart, the top line with large type may measure vision of 20/400 or 20/200. As each line of type decreases in size, the acuity level increases. The bottom line on most charts represents vision of 20/15.

Legal Blindness and Severe Visual Impairment

Clinical *legal blindness* is defined as having vision of 20/200 or less (using the Snellen eye chart measurement) in the better eye with best spectacle-corrected visual acuity (BSCVA) or having a visual field that encompasses (or *Subtends)* an angle of 20 degrees or less.

The first part of this definition states how clearly one can see (i.e., "acuity"). The second part states how much area of the potential visual field one sees. Vision of 20/200 means the person *sees* at 20 feet what someone with 20/20 (i.e., "normal" or "perfect") vision sees at 200 feet. The "normal" visual field with both eyes (i.e., binocular vision) will approach 180 degrees (Jose, 1983).

The National Center for Health Statistics defines *severe visual impairment* as a self- or proxy-reported inability to read standard newsprint. The loss of vision may be due to a loss of visual acuity, loss of visual field, or a decrease in range of motion of the head or eyes (Centers for Disease Control and Prevention [CDC], 2009). Lighthouse International (2009) defines vision impairment while using corrective lenses as

- Some trouble seeing or rating vision as poor or very poor,
- Inability to recognize someone familiar across the room,
- Inability to read regular newspaper print, or
- Blindness in one or both eyes.

Prevalence of Severe Visual Impairment and Blindness

Age-related vision loss is the second most prevalent disability among older adults (Lighthouse International, 2009).

Based on data from the 2004 National Health Interview Survey, among people ages 18 or older, approximately 19 million (8.8%) report having trouble seeing, even when wearing glasses or contact lenses (Lighthouse International, 2009). Among the 9.3 million people between ages 45–64 years, 15% report some form of visual impairment. Among people ages 65 or older, an estimated 21% (7.3 million) report some form of vision impairment. At ages 75 or older, 4.3 million people (26%) report visual impairments.

People with serious eye conditions cannot routinely expect their vision to remain stable. For people, vision will likely change very gradually over time. For some, vision may fluctuate on a daily or even hourly basis. Ophthalmologic reports will have specific measurements of components of vision but often do not tell the entire story of how those components affect a person's ability to function visually.

Impaired Visual Acuity

Whereas total blindness is a condition readily comprehended, people often misunderstand visual acuity in people who are severely visually impaired (Tuttle & Tuttle, 2004). Just as everyone has different physical abilities, each person with low vision can be expected to have a unique ability to see. Approximately 80%–85% of all people who are legally blind have some level of useful vision (Flax, Golembiewski, & McCaulley, 1993). Therefore, most people have the ability to see something, such as large print, the shapes of houses or furniture, trees or people, the action on television, or simply light and dark, and they are able to use their sight for purposeful activities. To complicate matters however, many people with severe vision loss have visual abilities that fluctuate and cannot be predicted. Physical or mental fatigue, poor lighting, glare, motivation, and other factors impact the ability to see. This uncertainty and variability can make service delivery challenging.

Each major eye condition causes a somewhat typical vision loss. However, age at onset of condition, duration of condition, other eye conditions, other health concerns, personal motivation, and environmental factors can all affect how well and how much each person sees, and how they are able to use or process what they see. Regardless of the condition, however, a person with any severe visual impairment may experience feelings of isolation, depression, inadequacy, and self-doubt.

Common Eye Conditions

Macular degeneration, glaucoma, diabetic retinopathy, and cataracts are the leading causes of age-related vision loss in the United States (CDC, 2009). Each condition is described in the following sections.

Macular Degeneration

Macular degeneration, or *age-related macular degeneration (AMD),* is a condition that affects central visual acuity, primarily in those over the age of 50. The vision loss may begin bilaterally, or in one eye and later, the other. Major concerns of clients with AMD include an inability to read small print, drive a car, see their grandchildren's faces, set their thermostat or stove dials, or see themselves in a mirror (Lighthouse International, 2009).

Many people with AMD find that using optical aids such as magnifiers, telescopes, video magnifiers, or closed circuit TVs (CCTVs) lets them read and function at a much more satisfactory level. *Eccentric viewing* exercises and techniques may also help people with AMD use the viable area of their visual field (Flax et al., 1993). Eccentric viewing is a way to locate and use the area of best visual function on the retina. As one turns one's eyes, the *central scotoma,* or blind spot, moves with the visual field. To make best use of the remaining useful portion of the visual field, the person must not look directly at the object of concern but rather toward the best area of the peripheral field.

People with AMD or other conditions affecting central vision must learn to use side or peripheral vision in a different way. The technique is to visualize an area that can be seen as though it were the face of a large clock showing only the 12, 3, 6, and 9, then imagine a central spot or target in the middle of the clock face. To use eccentric vision, a person must follow 5 steps to discover the location of the area of best remaining vision:

1. Sit comfortably about 10 feet from a familiar static object (e.g., a picture on the wall, the refrigerator, a bookcase).
2. Use only the better eye (cover the other eye).
3. Look directly at the center of the target object. If done properly, the target should seem to disappear or appear blurrier because it is being lined up with the central blind spot.
4. Look slightly above the target, or at "12 o'clock." If the target becomes clearer or easier to see, practice the exercise several times.
5. Continue looking from the center of the target to each of the other clock times. The target will appear and disappear, but when the best acuity spot is located, always look to that "time" for best vision.

Even if one position works, complete the exercise to find any other areas of useful vision.

It is important to remember that, to see the target most clearly, you must not look directly at it. Remember also that eccentric viewing techniques will not restore vision but will help to get the most use out of remaining vision.

Diabetic Retinopathy

Diabetic retinopathy is a condition that affects the retinas of some diabetic individuals (Figure 16.1). The *retina,* or innermost layer of the eye, receives images transmitted through the cornea and contains the rods and cones, which are sensory receptors. Diabetes may cause hemorrhages or blood vessel changes that affect the retina and thus interfere with vision. The entire visual field may become involved, causing severe functional limitations often characterized by episodes of highly fluctuating vision.

It is common for a person with diabetic retinopathy to say they feel as if they have cobwebs or lint on their eyes, and they want to keep brushing it off. Others say that everything they see has a reddish tint. They may experience poor vision early in the day, with improvement through the morning followed by a mid-afternoon decline and another improvement late in the day. This fluctuation may be caused by blood sugar levels, the settling of vitreous debris, or the level of natural light.

People with diabetic retinopathy may need to adjust the timing of certain tasks, especially in the morning. Filling insulin syringes in advance, for example, or reading fine print may be better accomplished the night before or late morning.

A person with a recent hemorrhage may require stronger magnification, better color contrast, larger print, or the continual use of optical filters to reduce associated glare. A simple, low-cost adaptation to improve color contrast in reading material is to place a yellow-colored acetate sheet over the printed page.

The severity and location of the diabetic hemorrhage or scar tissue may require stronger magnification, computer speech output, audible books, increased task lighting, or personal assistance to accomplish tasks.

Glaucoma

Glaucoma is another leading cause of blindness in the United States. Glaucoma damage is the result of a build up of pressure within the eye that damages the optic nerve. This increased pressure causes a decrease of vision in the peripheral field (commonly known as "tunnel vision").

As the term suggests, people with tunnel vision cannot see things on either side without turning

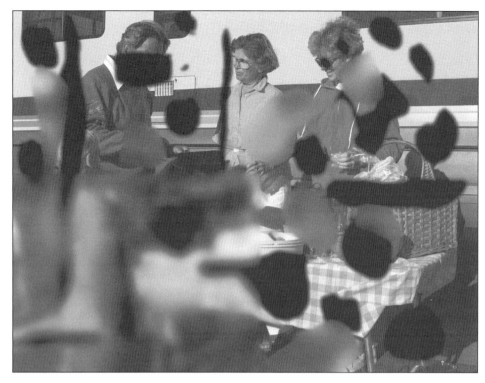

Figure 16.1. Vision of a person with diabetic retinopathy.

their head. An individual with glaucoma may have 20/20 vision in the central part of the visual field—which may be only 10 degrees in size. People with glaucoma may find their reading ability relatively unchanged. Their ability to use their peripheral vision, however, on stairs, icy sidewalks, or in dim lighting, is greatly diminished.

Cataracts

Cataracts, another common condition affecting the older population, are opacity or cloudiness of the normally clear lens inside the eye. The lens is responsible for properly focusing light onto the retina. Cataracts are caused by aging, disease, trauma, or other factors; people often liken the effect to "looking through a dirty windshield or a gauze curtain" (Lighthouse International, 2009).

A person with cataracts will find increasing problems with glare from oncoming vehicle headlights at night and with adjusting to outside light after exiting a dark building, at the beach, or after a fresh snowfall on a sunny day. People who have cataracts often function well with optical aids. Some use broad-brimmed hats and a variety of optical filter sunglasses for everything from sitting on the beach to washing dishes in front of a window to department store shopping under artificial lights.

The medical treatment for cataracts is surgery, most often with the implantation of an artificial lens.

Presbyopia

Presbyopia is a reduction in accommodative ability that occurs with age (Mayo Clinic, 2009). *Accommodation* refers to the ability of the eyes to adjust or focus. Presbyopia, commonly beginning between the ages of 42 and 45, is characterized by the inability to focus on near objects such as fine print in a book. Presbyopia is a normal consequence of aging and is not cause for alarm. It does cause functional complications, especially when combined with serious eye conditions.

Occupational Performance Consequences of Eye Conditions

For rehabilitation providers, the occupational performance consequences of eye conditions are of most concern. In the following sections, visual impairments resulting from central, peripheral, and overall or general vision loss are described. Case studies illustrate how selected individuals experienced these conditions and how they adapted to their visual impairment.

Central Vision Loss

Central vision is often referred to as *identification* or *fine detail* vision, as it is what people use to determine what they see (Case Studies 16.1 and 16.2,

Case Study 16.1. Central Vision Loss (AMD)

R.L. is 83 years of age with a confirmed diagnosis of AMD. He was unable to see newspaper headlines and contended that he could not see well enough to do certain household chores. His wife was concerned about his vision and how it was limiting him. One day, she lost a sewing needle in a shag carpet and was unable to locate it. R.L., however, was able to see it—leaving his wife very confused about his vision. Why couldn't he see well enough to help her but could find a very small item for which she had searched at length? After the functional limitations of AMD were explained to her, she understood his inability to see fine detail while maintaining his ability to see peripherally.

Because doing dishes is a tactual job, the occupational therapist helped R.L. and his wife work out a compromise. He would do more housework, and she would be responsible for more of the visual tasks such as balancing the checkbook.

Case Study 16.2. Central Vision Loss (AMD)

M.M. has AMD and misses seeing photographs of her grandchildren. She generally sees the shapes of people sitting in front of her, but she cannot recognize them. She can see rings on someone's finger but not whether they are wearing glasses or makeup.

One concern is that friends do not understand the impact of AMD. She can walk to the nearby grocery store and independently do her shopping with the assistance of a small lighted magnifier, but she does not see well enough to acknowledge friendly waves from across the street. In her neighborhood, this snub is considered serious. The occupational therapist encouraged M.M. to inform her friends of her inability to recognize people from a distance and to carry a white cane for identification purposes. She routinely offers friends a copy of a brochure on AMD she picked up from her ophthalmologist's office.

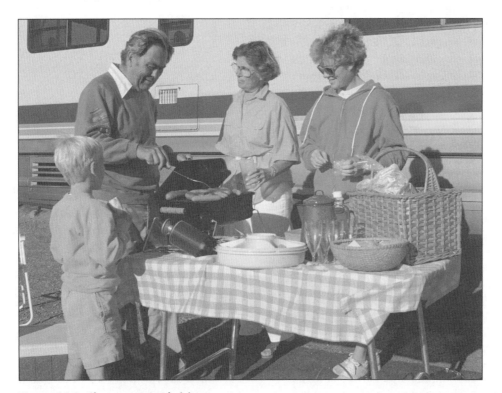

Figure 16.2. Clear or normal vision.

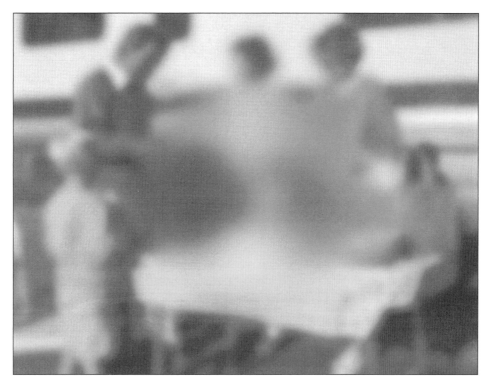

Figure 16.3. Vision of a person with central vision loss.

Figures 16.2 and 16.3). *Central vision loss (CVL)* will therefore cause an individual to lose central or fine detailed vision. Color discrimination ability, located centrally on the retina, will also be severely affected. A simple analogy is to consider the normal circular visual field as a donut complete with donut hole. Individuals with CVL will see the donut but not the hole.

Without the benefit of fine detail vision, the person will see better using eccentric or peripheral vision (see above). It is not unusual for a person with CVL to be unable to read newspaper headlines from inches away but able to see a fly in the corner of the ceiling or a bit of paper on the floor. Moreover, people with CVL often will complain of not being able to see photographs or recognize faces from across the table but may be able to see whether that person's shoes are shined.

Peripheral Vision Loss

People with *peripheral vision loss (PVL)* have a narrow visual field (Case Study 16.3, Figure 16.4). If an object is not immediately in the center field of vision, it will not be seen. *Peripheral vision* is sometimes referred to as the *orientation vision,* because it tells people where they are in relation to objects in the

Case Study 16.3. Peripheral Vision Loss (Glaucoma)

P.T. has advanced glaucoma. He lives alone in a very small home in a rural area. He has a strong network of natural supports on which he relies. His visual field is less than 10 degrees in his left eye, and he has no light perception in the right. His acuity is unknown. He is able to read some print quite slowly, usually one letter at a time, when extremely bright task lighting is available. He has given up trying to walk alone outside except in very bright sunlight, for which he uses sunglasses.

P.T. experienced his vision loss at least in part because he refused to follow his medication regimen. He explained that his uncle had glaucoma and lost all vision over a 10-year span despite taking drops to relieve the pressure. Because he refused to take the proper medication, he permanently lost his vision to glaucoma much faster.

Because optical aids were no longer an option, P.T. relied on talking books and volunteer readers; tactual markings for his appliances, medications, and household items; and a white cane for his walks.

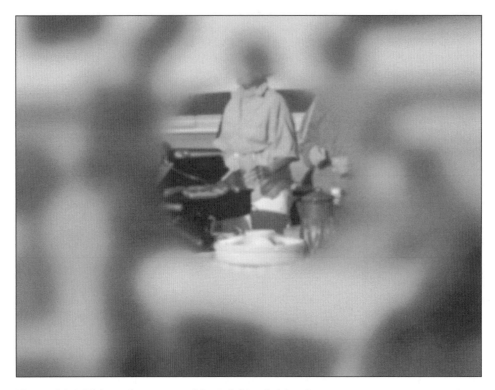

Figure 16.4. Vision of a person with peripheral vision loss.

environment. It is also the area of best vision in low-light environments.

People with PVL must continually scan their environment to view, in series, what people with a normal field see instantly. Often, low-lying objects such as coffee tables, steps, rugs, or uneven pavement cause serious difficulties.

PVL will limit activities where peripheral (side) vision is necessary and limit independent mobility,

especially in low-light situations. Many people with PVL function best when adequate task lighting, a color-contrasting background, and centrally presented objectives are available.

General Vision Loss

Someone with *general vision loss* may experience a loss of vision in part or all of the field of vision (Case Study 16.4, Figure 16.5). Cataracts or diabetic retinopathy may be the cause of the loss. Any portion of the visual field may be affected, and visual acuity will be variable.

Adjustment to Blindness or Low Vision

Blindness shares much with other disabling conditions in the stages of the adjustment process. Seven phases of adjusting to life with blindness have been identified (Tuttle & Tuttle, 2004):

1. Trauma,
2. Shock and denial,
3. Mourning and withdrawal,
4. Succumbing and depression,
5. Reassessment and reaffirmation,

Case Study 16.4. General Vision Loss

B.A. has diabetes and greatly fluctuating vision. Her vision in the morning is cloudy, and everything appears dark. Turning on bright lights helps, but she sometimes needs to control the indoor glare by wearing optical filter sunglasses. When she reads, she tries to look around or past her numerous hemorrhages and retinal scars that seem to move about. By mid-morning, her vision seems to clear so she tries to do her reading then with her back to the brightest window. Later her vision may become cloudy for a time before getting relatively clear again during the evening hours.

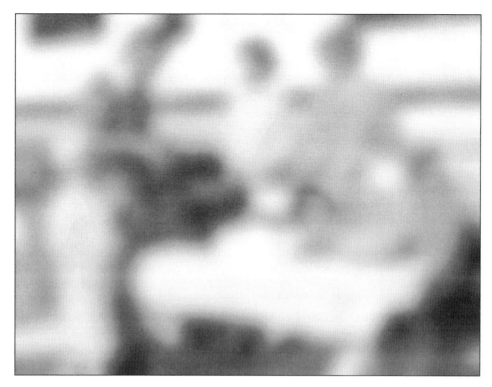

Figure 16.5. Vision of a person with general vision loss.

6. Coping and mobilization, and
7. Self-acceptance and self-esteem.

Each individual will feel the effects of blindness or low vision differently. For example, someone who has been highly active, or has relied on driving, or has been an outdoor enthusiast may have difficulty with a perceived need to adopt a more sedentary lifestyle. Conversely, an avid reader who develops AMD may feel much more loss than someone who has never enjoyed reading.

Social factors are an important part of adjusting. Because blindness limits the ease of mobility, such as driving across town or walking to the corner coffee shop, people who have lost vision may not have the same freedom of movement that they did previously. To avoid feelings of isolation, social contacts should be continued and new ones explored. This can be difficult to achieve, however, as making and maintaining social contacts often requires transportation. A source of transportation is also required to complete activities such as grocery shopping and attending appointments. Thus, it is imperative that the vision-impaired person know the affordable transportation options available to him or her (e.g., senior citizen vans, taxi services, volunteer drivers).

Evaluation of Occupational Performance

Because of the individualized nature of visual abilities, evaluation is necessary to help target service needs. This section describes two assessment tools. The first, Assessment for Vision Rehabilitation Therapy Services (Golembiewski, 2009), is verbally administered to screen potential recipients of vision rehabilitation services. It is designed for ease of use by professionals and nonprofessionals alike.

Each of the functional areas is queried in three steps. Can you accomplish the task? If not, is it due to a vision loss? And do you want assistance with the visually restricting task? Although there are limitations with assessments that are not performance-based, this tool is meant as a simple means of identifying those who are truly appropriate for vision rehabilitation services. It is intended as a basis for formulating a plan of service (see Appendix 16.A).

The second assessment instrument is meant to be administered either in the client's home or in an institutional facility. This assessment, which is not standardized, identifies the need for adaptive aids and techniques that can be recommended by an individual qualified to provide rehabilitation services for people with blindness or low vision. The need

Table 16.1. Functional Assessment of People Who Are Blind or Visually Impaired

Category	Performance Items
Vision	Near vision Intermediate vision Distance vision Current optical aid use Illumination Absorptive lenses Clinical low-vision exam
Orientation and mobility	Sighted guide Self-protective techniques Doorways Indoor travel Room familiarization Outdoor travel Automobiles Searching techniques Cane Orientation and movement specialist
Communications	Braille Script writing Typing and keyboarding Using the telephone Using a tape recorder Telling time Library service
Personal management	Grooming and hygiene Clothing care and identification Money handling Table etiquette Diabetic concerns Medication management Knowledge of eye disease Acceptance of eye condition
Home management	Cleaning Laundry Household organization Minor repairs and tool use Safety
Food preparation	Safety Labeling Reading and saving recipes Shopping Timing Pouring and measuring Cutting, peeling, slicing, and spreading food Using appliances Addressing dietary and nutritional concerns
Leisure activities	Social and support groups Crafts and hobbies Table games Sewing Sports
Community resources	Aging network

Case Study 16.5. Severe Vision Loss

K.T. was despondent over his severe vision loss. The biggest effect on him was a self-imposed withdrawal from his "coffee club" group of fellow retirees at a nearby café. All were long-time friends who shared similar life experiences, sports allegiances, and sense of community connections. After K.T.'s vision declined, he felt the others were now being overly protective and treating him like a blind person, not as "good, old K.T." For example, one friend apologized profusely after asking if everyone had seen the recent football game. A painful silence that followed made everyone feel uncomfortable. K.T. didn't feel they understood him at all, so he gave up his coffee group.

Eventually, he heard of a support group for people with vision loss that met every month at the local senior center. Everyone was welcome, although most attendees were over 70. No dues were collected, and the aging office provided transportation. After a few meetings that included discussions of dealing with the sighted world and living as a blind person, K.T. began to accept his vision loss and was able to better understand how he was misinterpreting his friends' comments. He then resumed meeting with his coffee buddies and was able to Monday-morning quarterback as he always had. He even told a joke about a dog guide for the blind, which easily and permanently broke the ice.

Case Study 16.6. Advanced Glaucoma

M.L., 18 years old, has Down syndrome and advanced glaucoma. His visual acuity report is unreliable because of communication limitations and his questionable responses to standard tests. When M.L. showed a seemingly drastic and sudden functional decrease, the special education teacher contacted the vision rehabilitation specialist for a consultation. Review of the the classroom environment revealed that M.L.'s desk had been turned so he faced a large bank of windows looking out on an open area covered with snow. Turning the desk toward the light not only didn't help, it caused severe problems with glare and photophobia. After rotating the desk so that M.L.'s back was to the windows, he was able to resume visual tasks as before.

and color-contrast changes in the environment, orientation and mobility, communication, household organization, food preparation, and personal management (see Case Studies 16.5 and 16.6).

Environmental Lighting and Contrast

Proper lighting is critical to enabling someone with vision loss to best use his or her residual vision (Jose, 1983). Too much, too little, or poorly directed light will hinder the ability to perform ADLs (Tuttle & Tuttle, 2004). Improving household lighting is perhaps the least expensive but most beneficial of all adaptations that a person with visual impairments can make.

Any work area should be illuminated by a general light source, with focused task lighting added as needed. The light source must be kept below eye level or be positioned behind or to the side of the individual. Halogen stand lamps, gooseneck, or other types of flexible and portable lighting are an ideal source of extremely bright task lighting. Lampshades should be used to help eliminate glare and to direct light to the targeted work area. Environmental light can be more useful if the work area is adjusted so the light streams from the back or side of the task area. Rotating the task area or work surface from facing toward a window to a position facing away from a bright light source can often increase functional vision. Adjusting window shades or blinds will also minimize glare.

Many people use flashlights with ultra-bright krypton or halogen bulbs for portable task lighting. These are useful for setting thermostats or stove and laundry dials and for seeing in dark areas of closets, drawers, or hallways.

areas identified will form the basis for the individualized plan for services developed for the client. Items included in this performance-based assessment are listed in Table 16.1.

Intervention for People With Vision Loss

Intervention options for people with vision loss can be organized according to the standard categories outlined in Chapter 4: *remediation* (teaching and training), *compensation* (changing the task or environment), *disability prevention* (encouraging performance of tasks that prevent health problems and encouraging safe task methods), and *health promotion* (encouraging engagement in meaningful, balanced, and healthy occupations and environmental interactions).

This chapter focuses on compensatory strategies that permit accomplishing activities of daily living (ADLs), including environmental modifications and specific procedures and techniques for accomplishing tasks using other sensory cues. The following sections describe compensatory strategies for lighting

Case Study 16.7. Photophobia

C.D. had a combination of eye conditions and severe photophobia. She had trouble in bright outdoor conditions, on overcast days, and even indoors. After a few trials with optical filters, she realized that her three situations each required different levels of light transmission and tints for her to be most comfortable. A high light transmission (40%) amber lens allowed her to use her vision best indoors for some reading, a medium level (10%) gray was best for overcast days, and a dark green low transmission (2%) was necessary on bright days. The best environment for her to read print was in natural light, so she positioned her reading desk by the brightest window available. Because the light was also irritating, however, she used the amber lenses for reading.

The need for or tolerance of certain light levels is highly individual and needs to be assessed by trials with various light levels. These can establish the optimum visual environment that will improve performance and prevent fatigue.

Photophobia

Photophobia is discomfort caused by abnormally increased sensitivity to bright sunlight or reflected light from water, snow, or even highly polished floors (Duffy, 2002; see also Case Study 16.7). Some people with extreme photophobia experience discomfort even indoors and especially from natural light on overcast days.

If glare is a problem, sunglasses with absorptive lenses or optical filters that block infrared and ultraviolet light may be helpful. Sunglasses that control glare and absorb irritating light are available in different colors, shades, and percentages of light transmission. Many people with photophobia or unstable conditions need different lenses for indoor and outdoor conditions.

Color Contrast

To enhance visual abilities for accomplishing ADLs, one should widely incorporate the practical use of color contrast into all environmental features. The use of light dishware that stands out clearly against dark, solid-color tables or tablecloths is recommended. Two cutting boards should be available: a light-colored one for dark foods and a dark one for light foods. Contrasting or brightly colored items should be strategically placed to help locate furniture such as coffee tables and the backs or arms of chairs. Colored tape strips can be added to countertop edges, doorsills, and steps to improve contrast. High-contrast electrical outlet switchplate covers and cabinet handles can make them easier to find. Contrasting or bright fluorescent tape added to tool handles will make them easier to locate on dark work surfaces.

Because some people have a decreased ability to distinguish color, especially in low-light conditions, high contrast is especially important for environmental landmarks. A simple cafeteria tray may be used not only to keep craft supplies from rolling away but also to increase color contrast. If possible, have a dark and a light tray available to contrast with the predominant color of the supplies. If only dark trays are available, consider applying white or light contact paper or electrical tape to one side to provide better contrast.

In most instances, solid colors are best for background surfaces. Floral or festive patterns or other busy backgrounds for tablecloths or other work surfaces act as camouflage (Figure 16.6). Avoid boldly

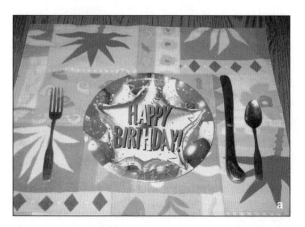 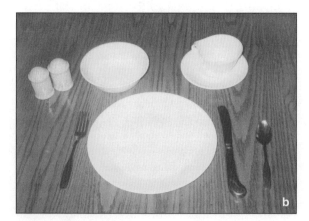

Figure 16.6. Avoid busy backgrounds, and use solid colors to enhance contrast.

patterned wallpaper or tabletop work surfaces. Electrical outlets, eating utensils, and tools are difficult to locate on these types of backgrounds.

Orientation and Mobility

Orientation is a term for knowing where one is, where one is going, and how one is going to get there; *mobility* is the means of getting there (see Case Studies 16.8 and 16.9). The most comfortable, widely used, safe, and efficient way to assist people who are blind or have low vision in traveling is use of a *sighted guide*. Certified orientation and mobility specialists are professionals trained in providing travel instruction to people who are blind. State and private agencies for the blind can provide information on obtaining their services.

For outdoor or more advanced independent travel, clients may require instruction in the use of telescopic aids, a white cane, electronic mobility devices, or a dog guide. State agencies for the blind and private agencies can provide information on white cane safety laws and the regulations governing legal use of a cane.

Sighted Guide Technique

This technique has the blind person holding the guide's arm just above the elbow, walking a half-step behind and to the side of the guide. In this position, someone who is blind or has low vision can

> **Case Study 16.9. Visual Field Cut**
>
> A stroke caused **S.L.** to have a visual field cut and left her confused about her location, even while in her own home. She was concerned about determining her location and the direction she must travel. A cuckoo clock with its audible tick-tock provides the orientation to her current location and to the direction to the other rooms in her home.

safely follow the guide's body movements as the two walk (Figures 16.7 and 16.8).

The guide and the person to be guided first make contact with their arms. The guide verbally offers assistance; the person needing assistance will move his or her hand up above the guide's elbow, keeping the thumb on the outside of the guide's arm. The four fingers should be on the medial side of the guide's arm and should maintain a firm and comfortable grip. The opposite shoulders of the traveling partners should be one behind the other (Hill & Ponder, 1976).

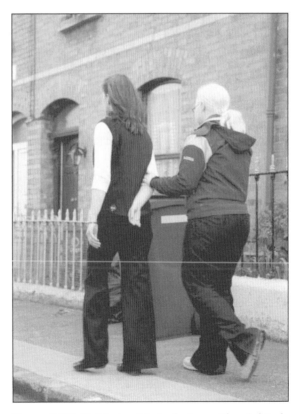

Figure 16.7. Sighted guide technique. The sighted guide moves her arm behind her back to negotiate a narrow pathway.
Photo credit: National Council for the Blind of Ireland. Used with permission.

> **Case Study 16.8. Glaucoma**
>
> **M.T.** is a widower living alone on the farm he has called home for more than 40 years. Despite his vision impairment, he thoroughly enjoys going to his workshop in one of his outbuildings. Glaucoma has reduced his visual field to a small tunnel, and his remaining vision does not work well in low-light conditions. M.T. placed a wind chime near his back doorway and strung a thin rope on posts from his house to the outbuilding. The rope gives him the guidance he needs, and the wind chime, given the right breeze, helps him locate the back door when he is elsewhere on his property. M.T. also uses a radio at his back door to provide an audible directional beacon toward which to walk. In his barn, M.T. must negotiate around a few low beams. He strategically placed lengths of bailing twine about three feet in front of all low obstructions. These soft warning signs alert him and have saved more than a few bumps on the head.

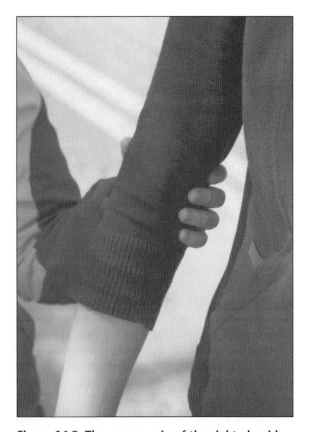

Figure 16.8. The proper grip of the sighted guide technique.
Photo credit: National Council for the Blind of Ireland. Used with permission.

The question of which side is best for the process is based on a number of factors, most notably personal preferences. Strength, hand dominance, the need for a support cane, hearing loss, the need to carry a package or purse, and other factors affect this decision. Most experienced travelers find they are able to travel equally well on either side of a sighted guide. Also, with experience, most sighted guide partnerships require less verbal input about the travel environment. Travel companions can safely carry on conversations just as others friends do.

Sighted guide techniques are adapted for specific situations, as follows:

- *Room familiarization.* Room familiarization begins at the primary entrance to a room. The blind person should be guided around the perimeter of the room. The guide should emphasize locating all permanent or semipermanent landmarks, such as light switches and electric outlets, windows, furniture, closet doors, and hanging plants.
- *Narrow spaces.* To negotiate narrow spaces, the guide moves the guiding arm to the

middle of his or her back as a sign for the blind person to walk directly behind the guide, with arm extended for increased distance from the guide. This keeps the blind person from walking on the heels of the guide and enables single-file travel through narrow or congested areas.
- *Curbs and stairs.* At each change of elevation, whether at a curb or a flight of stairs, the sighted guide should pause and describe the change. It is generally safer for the guide to keep his or her weight forward when ascending and backward when descending.
- *Seating.* The guide should lead the blind person to the chair so that his or her body comes in contact with the chair. The guide then places the blind person's hand on the back of the chair to provide a reference point.
- *Doorways.* After describing the direction in which the door opens (toward or away) and on which side it is hinged, the sighted guide always should go through doorways first. Revolving doors may cause problems for some slow-walking travelers; in those cases, the guide should use a different door, or the blind person should practice using revolving doors with the guide during less busy times.
- *Automobiles.* The guide should describe the direction in which the vehicle is pointing. After the passenger door is opened, the guide places one of the blind person's hands on the roof and the other on the top edge of the open door.

It is neither safe nor efficient to attempt to guide a blind person by pushing from behind. In this position, the guide will not readily see uneven pavement, patches of ice, water, or otherwise slippery surfaces. Moreover, sudden noises or safety concerns may cause a clumsy resistance to the guide's efforts. Finally, no one is in front of the blind person to act as a buffer or stabilizer should a stumble occur or an immediate stop become necessary.

Self-Protection

Self-protection techniques are necessary even in a familiar home environment. One technique involves holding one hand (usually the nondominant one) at shoulder height, palm out, with the hand just below eye level (Figure 16.9). The dominant hand is held diagonally across the body, palm inward, in front of the opposite upper thigh. This positioning in front of the face and across the torso will provide safe coverage from open cupboards, closet doors, and narrow poles.

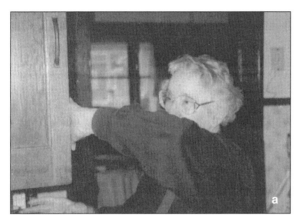
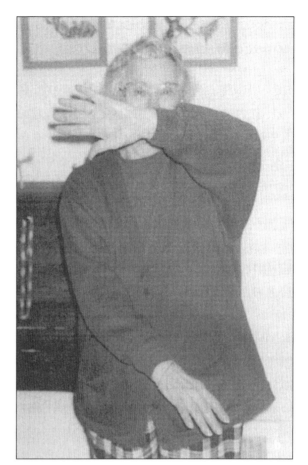

Figure 16.9. Two examples of self-protection techniques.

Trailing and Squaring Off

Trailing is a popular mobility technique that is used indoors. To trail a wall, the arm closest to the wall is extended out in front of the body; the back or side of that hand brushes along the wall as the individual moves forward. Trailing helps to maintain a straight line of travel and helps to locate doorways and other landmarks along the way. In the kitchen or bathroom, trailing can be done along a countertop. Trailing can also be done while traveling with a long white mobility cane. In this situation, the cane can be held diagonally across the body, with the tip of the cane remaining in contact with the wall/floor interface.

Squaring off is done by putting one's back, heels, and head against a flat surface. By starting to travel this way, the individual is off to a straight start, and heading in the desired direction.

Ascending and Descending Stairs

Blind or visually impaired persons will understand the importance of allowing their canes to touch each step when ascending stairs so they can easily determine when they are at the top. When descending, the cane must be kept in a stationary position, extended in front of the traveler, just slightly higher than the edge of the step. This positioning allows the cane tip to reach the floor before the traveler's feet when coming to the end of a flight of stairs.

Indoor Cane Techniques

There are a variety of cane techniques, such as diagonal technique, constant contact, and two-point, that should be explored as a part of mobility training.

Outdoor Travel Techniques

For outdoor or more advanced independent travel, formal instruction from a trained orientation and mobility professional is required. In addition to orientation and sensory development training, this instruction may include work with dog guides, telescopic aids, electronic mobility devices, and a variety of cane techniques. It may specifically involve sidewalk travel, crossing intersections, analyzing traffic patterns, and using public transportation. Instruction typically will take place in the individual's neighborhood, community, place of employment, at an adjustment training center, or at a combination of several of these locales.

Using a Global Positioning System for Travel

Certainly one of the most significant innovations in technology for travelers who are blind or visually impaired is the development of a global positioning system (GPS) device with speech output. GPS is a navigation system that uses approximately 25 satellites to accurately determine any location on earth.

In addition to a receiver, an accessible GPS for those with vision loss requires visual impairment navigation software. This software can either be loaded onto a portable personal digital assistant (PDA) with voice output, where a receiver would be a separate device, or the software may be incorporated with a receiver into a single unit. Using GPS and assistive technology gives blind and visually impaired travelers unprecedented independence. Before GPS was available, the only way these travelers could obtain information about what was around them was to ask someone with sight.

Accessible GPS can provide information on almost every aspect of travel. It can provide directions for either a walking route or directions to help a driver navigate, it can search for points of interest by key words, and it can identify locations within 30 feet. For example, an accessible GPS can provide a list of Italian restaurants within a specific distance range, giving address and directions to the choice selected. In addition, individuals can program future destinations into the GPS from their homes so that they can prepare for and review a route before actually traveling. While on a route, the accessible GPS provides vital information such as street names; cardinal directions; when, where, and which way to make turns; and the distance needed to travel before reaching intersections, points of interest, and the final destination.

While accessible GPS offers exciting opportunities, it does not lessen the need for orientation and mobility training and does not take the place of either a cane or a dog guide. The traveler must use logic and common sense and combine his or her own knowledge, such as the use of landmarks and environmental clues, with the information the GPS provides. Users should have strong basic orientation and mobility skills and must remember accessible GPS is a tool that enhances, not grants, the ability to travel independently.

Communication

Oral Communication

As with other types of disabilities, such as hearing loss, people with blindness and vision loss are sometimes treated inappropriately by individuals who do not understand their conditions. The following guidelines provide useful suggestions for polite, respectful, and appropriate interactions with people who have vision loss.

- When offering assistance, speak in a normal tone of voice unless you know of a hearing loss. Speak directly to the blind person, not the sighted guide, if one is present.
- Always introduce yourself by name; voice recognition is not always reliable, especially in a crowded or noisy environment.
- Inform the blind person when leaving. No one wants to appear foolish by starting to talk to someone who is no longer there.
- Use words like "look" and "see" as you do in everyday conversations; attempts to use substitutes are usually awkward and may make everyone less comfortable.
- When helping a blind person with dining, use the "face of the clock" method of orientation to describe the location of food (e.g., the peas are at two o'clock, the meat is at six, and the french fries are at ten; see Figure 16.10). The same method can be used for locating utensils, condiments and other items. Make sure you're visualizing the clock from the blind person's perspective, not your own.
- Be specific when giving directions. Use right and left, behind or in front.
- Avoid gestures, pointing and nonspecific terms such as "over there" and "that way." Rather than saying "It is right there," say,

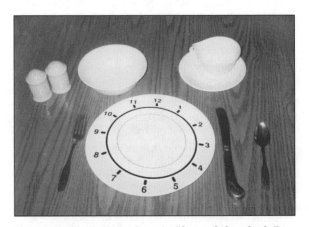

Figure 16.10. Orientation via "face of the clock."

"The blue candy dish is in front of you and to the right" or "It is at 2 o'clock."

- Never move furniture without informing the blind person who is familiar with a particular arrangement.

Written Communication

Whenever possible, print size should be large, using clear block letters, and be black on either white or yellow, or vice versa. Avoid ornate, serif, and condensed typefaces. Most colored or patterned paper should also be avoided. Some people find that yellow paper offers better contrast for reading print; an alternate approach is to use a sheet of yellow acetate or a report cover over black print on white paper.

Announcements and other notices should be posted in large print on bulletin boards in public places. One strategy used in senior centers is to post all headlines in very large type, thereby allowing people with low vision to see the subject of the posting and read the document with optical aids or to request further assistance when indicated.

The most basic handwriting task is that of signing one's name. For some, it can be the single most important aspect of increasing their sense of well-being and confidence. Everyone should be encouraged to sign his or her own name. Darkening the signature line with a bold pen can provide enough guidance for some people with low vision to sign their name.

Writing Guides and Templates

A signature guide may be as simple as a credit card–sized piece of thin cardboard or plastic, usually black, with a rectangular window cut out (see Figure 16.11 and Case Study 16.10). Other guides may be metal, and some have an elastic band allowing the writer to easily make the tails of letters below the line. The guide is placed over the signature space, creating a structurally rigid barrier or frame. With practice

Figure 16.11. Black plastic signature guide.

and encouragement, people can sign their name. Suggest using natural motions or use "auto pilot"— often the faster one signs his or her name after a lengthy nonwriting period, the better it looks.

Other important concerns with cursive writing include inability to stay on the line and writing on a slant, not crossing Ts or dotting Is and being uncertain of the need to correct mistakes. For people with relatively good vision, the first option is to use lined paper, which is available in various sizes of line width and boldness. This paper makes it easier to stay on the line. Some people use different paper of different line sizes for different purposes. Narrow-lined paper is suitable for writing personal letters that do not necessarily need to be reread. Very wide-lined paper is more useful for writing that will be later referenced, such as an address book, a recipe, or a shopping list.

A black script-writing template of plastic or cardboard may be even more helpful for people with less vision. These templates force the writing to conform to the space available and assure parallel lines. Paper clips hold the writing paper firmly. Using the various widths of bold-line pens makes it easier to see where the writing starts and stops.

Case Study 16.10. AMD

L.B. moved from her small town in South Carolina to northern Wisconsin to die. She came to live with her daughter because of an inoperable condition that caused her physician to predict only a 2-month life expectancy.

When seen by the local rehabilitation teacher from the state, she agreed to enroll in the talking book program to help pass the time. A signature was required to receive services, but L.B. was unable to sign her name for a few years because of AMD.

She was shown a black plastic signature template and assigned a practice regimen. With time and encouragement, she progressed to writing letters to her relatives and friends in South Carolina. After more practice, she was able to write telephone messages for her daughter's home-based business. This allowed better customer service, saved the cost of call forwarding to an answering service, and boosted her self-confidence as well. Because of her charming personality and wonderful South Carolina accent, she was a true asset to the business—and obviously lived longer than the predicted 2 months.

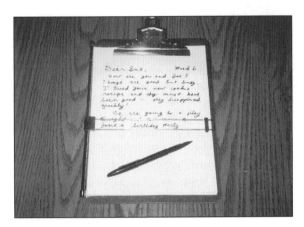

Figure 16.12. MARKS script-writing guide.

A MARKS writing guide is a clipboard-type device that holds writing paper in place and uses a line-sized frame that is moved down the page (Figure 16.12). As the writer reaches the end of each line, he or she moves the frame down to the next line. Writing paper that is embossed with raised lines is another useful aid. Envelopes can be addressed using a MARKS-type guide or envelope templates with windows cut out for each line of the address.

Braille

Braille is a system of reading and writing using a configuration of six raised dots in a rectangular pattern resembling a muffin pan (Ashcroft & Henderson, 1963; see also Figure 16.13). Louis Braille, a blind Frenchman, developed the system for his own use. Prior to the development of Braille, other systems of tactual reading were tried, but not until Braille was developed did blind people have the ability to become truly literate by writing in addition to reading raised symbols.

Braille may be used not just for reading and writing text; it may also be used for labeling items such as medicines, canned goods, or playing cards. Braille may be written with a Perkins Brailler, which looks somewhat like an antique typewriter, or with

1	2	3	4	5	6	7	8	9	0
a	b	c	d	e	f	g	h	i	j
k	l	m	n	o	p	q	r	s	t
u	v	x	y	z		w			

Figure 16.13. The Braille alphabet.

a portable slate and stylus. Computer-embossed Braille is becoming more readily available.

Electronic Communications and Other Helpful Devices

Telephones

There are many ways to adapt a telephone so that visually impaired people can use it independently. These include using large print, bold print, and raised numbers, which allows easier location of the buttons. Many phones have volume controls for people with hearing loss. Voice recognition telephones are available for people who have physical limitations in addition to vision loss. Cellular telephones have recently become accessible to people with visual impairments. Several cellular telephone models are now available with speech output, large-print buttons, and touch displays.

Many styles of large-print telephones are available. Speed dial buttons may be tactually or visually marked for easy location. It is possible to adapt older rotary telephones by installing large-print dial overlays or tactual markers; large-print push-button adapters may be applied to standard push-button telephones.

Standard push-button telephones can be dialed using three fingers that cover each row of numbers. The index finger pushes the one, the middle finger pushes the two, and the ring finger pushes the three. To reach the second row of four through six, the user simply moves the three fingers down one row, and so forth.

Most telephone companies offer exemptions from directory assistance charges for assistance calls made by people who are blind or visually impaired. Each company may have different regulations and eligibility policies, which should always be checked to avoid unpleasant surprises.

In 1996, the U.S. Congress amended the Telecommunications Act (Section 255) to ensure that telephone services and telephones, both traditional and wireless, are accessible to people with disabilities. The Federal Communications Commission (FCC) oversees communication law, including the Section 255 disability provisions in the Telecommunications Act.

How to Get an Accessible Telephone (American Foundation for the Blind, n.d.) contains step-by-step instructions about shopping for a phone and for filing complaints with the FCC. It is available in standard-print, large-print, or Braille formats from the American Foundation for the Blind, Information Center, 11 Penn Plaza, Suite 300, New York, NY 10001;

800-232-5463; afbinfo@afb.net; http://www.afb.org/section255.asp.

Tape Recorders

Cassette tape recording is another option for the storage and retrieval of information. People can mail taped letters to friends using special cassette mailers that qualify for "Free Matter for the Blind" mailing privileges. A letter is recorded, placed in a special mailer, and put in a mailbox. Most of these mailers have double "from" and "to" labels. The "from" and "to" addresses are reversed on each side, and are designed for repeated round trip use. Other mailers contain a reversible postcard-like label that is placed in a clear window.

Access to printed material is becoming easier as more devices that convert text to speech are developed. Small portable devices, for example, such as digital talking book players, allow people who are blind or visually impaired to download books from a variety of sources, including the National Library Service and the Bookshare program.

Digital Voice Recording

Small digital voice recorders are available as convenient and portable note-taking devices. Several companies manufacture portable Braille notetakers with speech output that not only act as PDAs but also can create and store documents, surf the Web, send and receive emails, and play music.

Volunteer Reader Services

Perhaps the single most frequently used means of reading is to secure the services of a sighted volunteer or paid reader. Volunteers may be coordinated through religious organizations, aging units, government offices, and private agencies.

Computers

Job Access With Speech (JAWS) and Zoom Text are two types of AT software for computer access by people with low vision. JAWS enables voice output, and Zoom Text enlarges text on computer monitors.

Personal Digital Assistants and Braille Notetakers

PDAs are now available for blind and low vision users as well. BrailleNote from Pulse Data International and Braille Lite Millennium from Freedom Scientific are the two most common accessible PDAs. Both have a refreshable Braille display and voice output in a portable package.

Both can send and receive Windows-style e-mail accounts by using Microsoft's Outlook or Qualcomm's Eudora.®

Basic and Instrumental Activities of Daily Living

Grooming and Hygiene

Techniques for shaving can be discussed and practiced, initially using a razor without the blade or with an electric shaver. Using an electric shaver relies simply on touch. If someone had been familiar with shaving and is comfortable with a specific type of shaver, that should be the type with which to practice. Magnifying mirrors, some with lights, help with makeup and shaving.

Many people simply dispense toothpaste onto a finger or directly into their mouths if they are the only one using that particular tube of toothpaste.

Medication Identification

Wrapping rubber bands around the bottles may easily identify similar prescription bottles (Figure 16.14). Large-print index cards can also be used to identify medications. A 7-day pillbox can help manage medication use.

Household Organization

Organization is especially important for people with vision loss. Every household item should have its place and be in it when not in use. Cleaning supplies or toxic substances in similarly shaped containers must be labeled in large print or by tactual means. The standard array of commercially available organizational aids, including assorted bins, pocket folders,

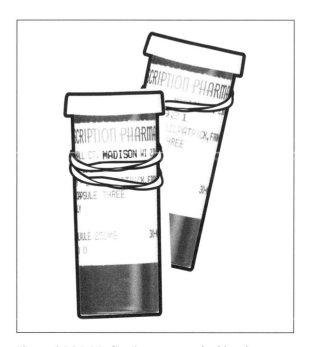

Figure 16.14. Medications are marked by the number of rubber bands.

files, and large-print or tactual labels can all be used to put and keep household items in their place. Textures, smells, colors, shapes, sizes, sounds, and other properties of objects can all be incorporated into a discussion of organization techniques.

Marking and Labeling

People with vision loss have a wide variety of marking and labeling aids available. Textures, bright colors, high-contrast markings, and various shapes can be used to mark and distinguish like-shaped items, dial settings, controls, clothing, tools, and other items. Following is a sampling of available aids.

- Hi-Marks is a bright orange, glue-like material that comes in a tube. Dots, bumps, letters, and lines can be drawn providing both a visual and tactual mark. Stoves, thermostats, microwave ovens, laundry equipment, radios, and virtually any dial on any appliance can be easily marked. Spot-N-Line is a similar tactual marking aid available in black or white. Both materials are durable and inexpensive but may be difficult for a blind or severely visually impaired person to independently apply as precisely as needed.
- Bump Dots in black or white are soft foam dots with sticky backing used for marking various items.
- Beads may also be glued in place as tactual landmarks. Bright nail polish may be used for marking dials.
- Bold felt-tip pens are ideal for labeling purposes. For reusable labels, index cards may be marked in bold letters and attached to canned goods by rubber bands (Figure 16.15). After use, the index cards can be placed in an envelope—becoming the next shopping list.

Simplicity is usually the best approach to marking appliance dials. One or two temperatures are all that may be needed to mark an oven. If 325 degrees is the most common oven temperature, with practice, 350 degrees may be reliably estimated from the known 325-degree mark. Many manufacturers will supply tactually marked dials or overlays for their products.

Clothing may be identified in several ways:

- Braille tags may be sewn into clothing in a nonvisual spot away from the skin.
- Some people use different sizes of buttons in different locations to distinguish between similar items.
- One way to keep socks in pairs is to use plastic disks with star-shaped cutouts in different

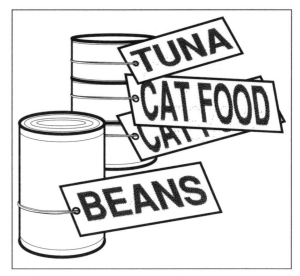

Figure 16.15. Large-print labels for food identification.

shapes in which the socks are always kept when not being worn. They can remain attached through washing and drying and are stored that way. When the socks are being worn, the disks are kept in a spot where they are easy to locate. Simply attach to the socks as they are put into the laundry hamper. The shapes allow easy identification. Others use different sizes of safety pins to distinguish colors.

- Some people organize closets into sections of "go together" clothes or group outfits together on the same hanger. Using the "simpler is better" approach, clothing details such as textures, buttons, or other distinguishing features can suffice for many people.

Money Management

Coin identification is taught by tactually exploring the rim or edges of coins with a thumbnail (Figure 16.16). Pennies and nickels, the two least valuable coins, have smooth edges; dimes and quarters have a milled or ridged edge. The size differences between smooth and ridged coins make correct identification simple.

Coin purses with separate channels for each denomination of coin are helpful in organizing change. Any type of small container—cannisters for (predigital) 35mm film or prescription bottles in various sizes—can be used to keep coins separated (Flax et al., 1993).

Paper money can be organized by folding the different denominations in various ways (Figure 16.17). One dollar bills may be left unfolded, the fives may be folded in half so they are almost a square, the tens

450

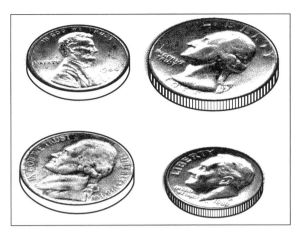

Figure 16.16. The edges of coins make identification easier.

might be folded in half the lengthwise, and a twenty can be folded like a ten and then folded over a second time. Another common way to handle paper money is to put the different denominations in different compartments of a wallet or purse. Still another method to simplify the identification of bills is to

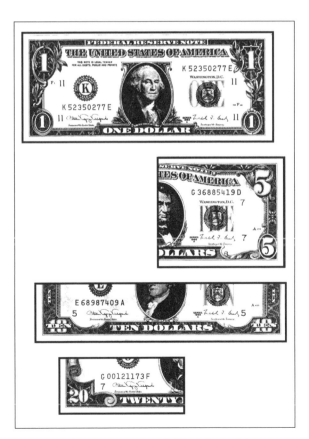

Figure 16.17. Paper money folded for quick identification.

limit the paper money to just ones and fives and keep them in separate compartments or pockets.

Using checks for purchases or paying bills is often the only option. A number of approaches can be effective, including the use of large-print checks, raised line checks, or one of the many available plastic or metal check templates. Contact the bank for information on the availability of accessible checks. Some people use bold line markers to highlight the lines on personal checks. Large-print check registers can make financial recording easier for people with low vision.

Black plastic check templates have window cutouts to match the information fields. The Keitzer Check Guide is made of thicker plastic that makes a thicker border to restrict the writing.

Credit and debit cards are convenient way to make purchases. The card can also function as a signature guide, as it underlines the signature line on the receipt. Have the clerk place the card under the signature space to make signing easy.

Systematic Searching Patterns

People with vision loss find it useful to search for dropped objects in an organized or patterned way. For example, after listening for the sound of the object hitting the floor, turn to face that location, and then search for it in that direction. Either a circular pattern, with gradually increasing concentric circles radiating outward or an up-over-and-back, grid-like pattern may be tried. In all regards, a methodical pattern will ensure complete coverage and be less frustrating.

Telling Time

Large-print, Braille, and talking watches are all available from specialized suppliers (Figure 16.18). Some people adapt existing equipment by tactual or large-print means.

Meal Planning and Shopping

Food preparation includes numerous and varied activities and skills that must be mastered in sequence, including

- Menu development;
- Shopping;
- Reading recipes;
- Distinguishing among ingredients that seem similar;
- Peeling, chopping, slicing, and dicing;
- Accurately pouring and measuring;
- Setting oven and stovetop temperatures;
- Timing; and
- Safely handling hot utensils.

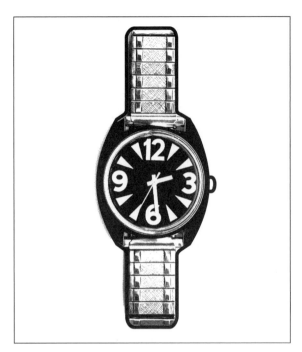

Figure 16.18. Large-print watch.

Reading large-print, Braille, or cassette-recorded cookbooks can help develop menu items. Recipes may be put in large print, Braille, or on cassette tape; cookbooks are available in the same formats.

Shopping is easier when a list of items to be included in a weekly menu is planned in advance. Index card labels for canned goods can be used in addition to a standard shopping list. Shopping assistance can usually be secured from store personnel or optical aids can be employed. Many communities offer online grocery shopping and delivery.

Canned goods are identified by shapes, label designs, and often by their sound when shaken. Some people use large-print labels on index cards with a hole punched in a corner attached to the can by a rubber band. Some mark the cabinet and place all like items behind that label. Small bins may be used to contain just one item, mushroom soup, for instance.

Spice containers, while appearing similar, may often be identified by smell, large print, or tactual labels.

Light-colored squares of flexible magnetic sheet can be written on with bold, permanent pens in large print or written in Braille. These can be affixed and easily reused. Some people with low vision can recognize certain brands of products by their familiar red and white stripes, for instance, but cannot read the print label. As noted, the labels can then be recycled into a "shopping list" envelope after the item is used.

Food Preparation

People who are blind or have low vision may find the following techniques helpful in preparing food:

- Dual-colored cutting boards (dark on one side and light on the other)—or two different cutting boards—can provide color contrast. Cutting boards with a funnel-shaped end enable easier transfer and placement of chopped foods.
- Kitchens must have sufficient task lighting or under-the-counter lights.
- Knives with adjustable slicing-width guides make it easier to create uniform slices of meats, breads, vegetables, and other foods.
- Liquid-level indicators emit an audible signal when the desired amount of liquid has been poured. Pouring and measuring can be practiced using cold water over a sink.
- Pouring colored liquids into a clear glass can be made easier if the glass is held against a contrasting background color (e.g., a dark wall or backsplash for pouring milk or a white background for pouring dark liquids).
- White coffee cups provide better contrast for pouring black coffee.
- By hooking an index finger over the edge or lip of a glass, one can determine when the level of the liquid reaches that point. Clients can practice over a sink or cafeteria tray to build confidence.
- Individual measuring cups or scoops are recommended and can be marked tactually or in large print. Large-print designations are available on some measuring spoons. Others may

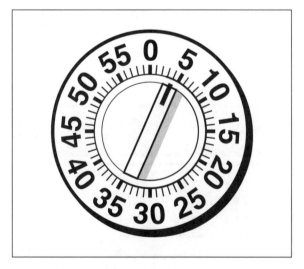

Figure 16.19. Large-print timer.

be marked with permanent bold-line pens or by filing grooves into the handles.

- Many types of large-print, audible, and Braille timers are available (Figure 16.19). Some may be marked with additional tactual or large-print embellishments to ensure ease of use.
- Safety around hot areas is always a concern for people with visual impairments. Large oven mitts protect arms when removing hot dishware from ovens.
- Every kitchen should have an operable fire extinguisher in a handy location.

Leisure Participation

Table Games

Playing cards are available in various large-print sizes, with raised line print, and in both standard and jumbo-dot Braille (Case Study 16.11). Cribbage boards with raised borders around the pegging holes allow easy counting of points. Checkerboards with indented squares, round red and square black checkers make the game accessible for totally blind players.

Braille dice are produced with raised dots on indented sides and large print dice are simply made larger. Large-print and Braille bingo cards wll allow people to play these games. Other board games are available from the catalog suppliers listed at the end of this chapter. Many people also tactually mark in Braille (or other means) selected pieces of their favorite board games.

Case Study 16.11. Low Vision

S.S. always had a close relationship with her granddaughter and enjoyed playing cards with her. Low vision, however, severely affected her ability to continue card playing. After she purchased a deck of large-print cards, she was able to continue regular card games with her granddaughter. Her vision was often good enough for her to identify the cards in good light, but she did not want to slow down a heated game with her granddaughter when the light changed. A rehabilitation teacher from the state agency for the blind helped S.S. develop proficiency at writing Braille using a slate and stylus. S.S. put the 15 Braille symbols needed for playing cards on a deck of large-print cards so that as she lost more vision, she was able to continue playing using Braille symbols.

Crafts and Hobbies

Using wire-loop needle threaders is an almost automatic way to thread sewing needles. The threader is first put into the eye of a needle using sense of touch. (As it is difficult to put the limp thread through this loop, the user should first wrap it around a toothpick.) This rigid arrangement can easily be put through the loop. After that, it is quite simple to withdraw the wire loop pulling the thread through the eye of the needle. The wire-loop needle threader may also be used to put hooks onto fishing line.

Chimney-like needle threaders also work quite well. The user places the eye of the needle down into the chimney, places the thread adjacent to the chimney, moves the slide or button that pushes a wire rod through the tower picking up the thread, and push it through the eye.

Spread-eye needles are flexible needles that have a long eye that runs nearly the entire length of the needle. Self-threading needles have a notch just above the eye. To thread this type of needle, the user places the sharp end in a bar of soap or a cork, locates the notch in the top, places the thread in the notch, and firmly pops it into the eye.

Reading

The many branches of The Library for the Blind and Physically Handicapped provide talking books on records, cassettes, or in Braille. Accessible reading materials are mailed to individuals and are returned postage-free. Applications and eligibility criteria are available from local libraries or the state or a private agency for the blind (Figure 16.20).

Social and Community Participation

Local peer support groups for visually impaired people (VIPs) are available in many communities. Local information and referral agencies or state services for the blind or private agencies can arrange connections with appropriate groups. The Lighthouse National Center on Aging and Vision is a leader in information on peer support groups (see Appendix 16.A for more information).

Community programs and resources play an important role in the service plan for people with severe vision loss. Federally mandated services under the Older Americans Act of 1965 include transportation, nutrition (both home-delivered and in group settings), and benefits counseling, available to all individuals over the age of 60. These and other in-home support services are administered through the local aging unit or area agency on aging.

Senior centers often provide a rich array of services for older people, including exercise therapy, craft classes, computer users groups, reading clubs, travel opportunities, a nutrition program, and recreation as well as peer support groups.

"Touch me" exhibits in museums, "scent walks" in botanical gardens, and audio-guided historical tours are available in many locations.

There are organizations of blind athletes who compete in sports including golf, soccer, weightlifting, goalball, beep baseball, diving, bowling, downhill and cross country skiing, windsurfing, and more. The American Foundation for the Blind offers more information at www.afb.org or by calling 1-800-232-5463.

The American Foundation for the Blind, the Lighthouse National Center for Vision and Aging, consumer groups, and special interest groups in support of specific eye conditions can provide a wealth of information and referral to local services.

Work

Some 61% of working-age adults (ages 16–64 years) classified as blind or having serious visual impair-

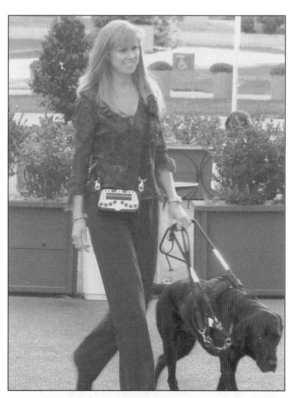

Figure 16.20. GPS technology enables persons with visual impairments to navigate to geographic locations using specially designed audio or Braille interfaces. Photo credit: Sendero Group. Used with permission.

ment are not in the labor force (U.S. Bureau of Labor Statistics [BLS], 2010). Only 22% of the 2.1 million working-age adults in this category were employed. This proportion is significantly lower than the estimated 83.8% of persons in this age group without any kind of disability who were employed (BLS, 2010).

The Americans with Disabilities Act of 1990 prohibits discrimination and ensures equal opportunity for persons with disabilities in employment, state and local government services, public accommodations, commercial facilities, and transportation. The U.S. Department of Justice provides free ADA materials. Printed materials may be ordered by calling 1-800-514-0301 (Voice) or 1-800-514-0383 (TDD). Automated service is available 24-hours a day for recorded information and to order publications.

Summary

Acquired visual deficits can be caused by health conditions such as diabetes and stroke, normal aging, and injuries to the eye. These deficits affect vision generally or can produce limitations affecting central or peripheral vision, with different functional consequences. Assessing the functional needs of individuals with low vision requires a thorough consideration of the individual's living environment and lifestyle. Many adaptive devices and techniques can be used to help people adapt to the functional challenges of vision loss.

Study Questions

1. What is the definition of legal blindness?
2. What is the definition of severe visual impairment?
3. What is the impact of each?
4. How do each of the 4 major age-related eye conditions differ in their impact on functional vision?
5. Which eye condition will have a greater impact in low light situations?
6. Describe adaptive strategies for cooking and housework for individuals with vision loss.
7. What are the most practical ways to control light and glare?
8. When and why should a person with low vision be referred to a self-help group?
9. What is the position and responsibility for a sighted guide?
10. What are the benefits and limitations of using a GPS system for mobility?
11. What protections for persons with visual impairment are afforded by the ADA?

References

American Foundation for the Blind. (n.d.) *How to get an accessible telephone*. New York: Author.

Americans With Disabilities Act of 1990, Pub. L. 101–336, 42 U.S.C. ß 12101.

Ashcroft, S. C., & Henderson, F. (1963). *Programmed instruction in Braille*. Pittsburgh: Stanwix House.

Carroll, T. J. (1961). *Blindness: What it is, what it does, and how to live with it*. Boston: Little, Brown.

Centers for Disease Control and Prevention, National Center for Health Statistics. (2009). *Vision impairment*. Atlanta: Author.

Corn, A. L., & Koenig, A. J. (1996). *Foundations of low vision: Clinical and functional perspectives*. New York: AFB Press.

Duffy, M. A. (2002). *Making life more livable*. New York: AFB Press.

Flax, M., Golembiewski, D., & McCaulley, B. (1993). *Coping with low vision*. San Diego, CA: Singular.

Golembiewski, D. (2009). *Assessment for vision rehabilitation therapy services*. Winnetka, IL: Hadley School for the Blind. (Unpublished).

Hill, E., & Ponder, P. (1976). *Orientation and mobility techniques: A guide for the practitioner*. New York: AFB Press.

Jose, R. T. (Ed.). (1983). *Understanding low vision*. New York: AFB Press.

Kirchner, C., & Schmeidler, E. (1997). Prevalence and employment of people in the United States who are blind or visually impaired. *Journal of Visual Impairment and Blindness, 91*(5), 508–511.

Lighthouse International. (2009). *Current research studies*. Retrieved March 22, 2010, from http://www.lighthouse.org/research/current-research-studies/

Mayo Clinic Health Information. (2009). *Mayo Clinic on vision and eye health: Practical answers on glaucoma, cataracts, macular degeneration, and other conditions*. Rochester, MN: Mayo Clinic on Vision and Eye Health.

Older Americans Act of 1965, Pub. Law 89–73, 79 Stat 218.

Telecommunications Act of 1996, Pub. Law 104–104, 110 Stat. 56.

Tuttle, D., & Tuttle, N. (2004). *Self-esteem and adjusting with blindness: The process of responding to life's demands* (3rd ed.). Springfield, IL: Charles C Thomas.

U.S. Bureau of Labor Statistics. (2010). *Employment status of the civilian population by sex, age, and disability status, not seasonally adjusted*. Retrieved July 2, 2010, from http://www.bls.gov/news.release/empsit.t06.htm

Appendix 16.A.

ASSESSMENT FOR VISION REHABILITATION THERAPY SERVICES

Name _____   Phone _____

Address _____   Birth Date _____

City _____   Zip _____

Are you able to read your mail, your recipes, or the newspaper?

Yes __ No __ > If "No" due to vision loss, check if help is needed. ____

Are you able to identify and properly take your medications?

Yes __ No __ > If "No" due to vision loss, check if help is needed. ____

Are you able to accurately tell time by reading your watch or wall clock?

Yes __ No __ > If "No" due to vision loss, check if help is needed. ____

Can you tell a nickel from a quarter and a $1 from a $10?

Yes __ No __ > If "No" due to vision loss, check if help is needed. ____

Can you set the correct temperature on a thermostat or oven?

Yes __ No __ > If "No" due to vision loss, check if help is needed. ____

Do any magnifiers you use for your reading work well enough?

Yes __ No __ > If "No" due to vision loss, check if help is needed. ____

Are you able to write letters, a grocery list, or sign your name?

Yes __ No __ > If "No" due to vision loss, check if help is needed. ____

Can you handle your own household cleaning if you wish?

Yes __ No __ > If "No" due to vision loss, check if help is needed. ____

Are you able to identify friends from across the room or table?

Yes __ No __ > If "No" due to vision loss, check if help is needed. ____

Are you able to follow the action or see characters on TV?

Yes __ No __ > If "No" due to vision loss, check if help is needed. ____

Are you able to identify traffic signals from across the street?

Yes __ No __ > If "No" due to vision loss, check if help is needed. ____

What are your favorite leisure activities? Can you still do them?

Yes __ No __ > If "No" due to vision loss, check if help is needed. ____

Can you shop for groceries and prepare your own meals if you wish?

Yes __ No __ > If "No" due to vision loss, check if help is needed. ____

When did you last go to your eye doctor for a checkup? _____

When did you last have your eyeglasses prescription changed? _____

Do your eyeglasses work well enough to read, watch TV, or see in the distance?

No ____ Yes____

Has anyone from an agency for the visually impaired or blind been out to see you?

No ____ Yes ____ When ____ Who _____

Do you want someone to contact you to help you with any of the above?

Yes ____ Not Yet____

REFERRAL SOURCE _____   DATE _____

PHONE _____

COMMENTS: _____
_____

Source: Hadley School for the Blind, Winnetka, IL. Used with permission.

Chapter 17

Sexuality and People With Chronic Disabilities

BERNADETTE HATTJAR, DrOT, MEd, OTR/L

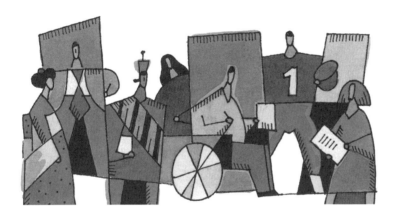

KEY WORDS

chronic disability

intimacy

sensuality

sexual activity

sexual orientation

sexual rights

sexuality

HIGHLIGHTS

- The role of occupational therapy in enabling participation in meaningful sexual activity by clients with activity limitations emphasizes client education and adaptive strategies.

- Sexual activity should be regarded as an important and necessary aspect of self-care, meeting important needs for intimacy and self-expression.

- Current generations and Baby Boomers have changing attitudes and expectations about sexuality.

- Professionals often neglect the topic of sexuality because of misinformation, discomfort, lack of knowledge, or assumptions.

- Occupational therapists can offer specific and useful recommendations for adaptive approaches to different chronic conditions that enable satisfying participation in sexual activity by their clients.

OBJECTIVES

After reading this material, readers will be able to

- Differentiate among intimacy, sexuality, and sensuality;

- Recognize occupational therapy's roles and responsibilities in addressing sexual activity with clients;

- Identify methods to introduce elements of sexuality, sensuality, and intimacy into evaluation and client-centered care for clients with chronic disabilities;

- Articulate adaptive strategies or suggestions for intimacy and sexuality for clients with chronic disabilities;

- Discuss sexuality, sensuality, and intimacy with clients at their personal comfort level; and

- Recognize the effect of chronic disability on sexual activity, roles, and occupational performance.

Sexual activity is a normal part of daily living. The *Occupational Therapy Practice Framework: Domain and Process* (American Occupational Therapy Association, 2008; hereinafter the *Framework*) identifies *sexual activity* as an activity of daily living, as "engaging in activities that result in sexual satisfaction" (p. 631).

Sexual activity is the way in which people express and share the sexual, sensual, and flirtatious part of themselves with another individual (Young, 2004). Sexual activity comprises not only the act of sexual intercourse but also the constructs of sexuality, sensuality, and intimacy.

Sexuality is a composite of many layers, including self-image, intimacy patterns, elements people find attractive or appealing in others, and mate or partner selection (Harwood & O'Conner, 1994). Adult sexuality is an essential component of our identity and self-image (Freda, 1998, p. 364; Neistadt, 1986).

Sensuality was defined as "tenderness" by Pope John Paul II (Sri, 2007) and is more literally defined as the capacity for enjoying the pleasures of the senses (Encarta, 2009). *Intimacy* is described as "a close, personal relationship" and "detailed knowledge resulting from a close or long association" (Encarta, 2009). Additionally, "intimacy" is sometimes used as a euphemism for the act of having sex (e.g., "being intimate with" another person). Intimacy can also relate to trust, consistency, and dependability in a relationship with another individual.

These components of sexual activity make us human and sexual beings. They are inherent in our persona, just as are the habitual and commonplace activities of daily living (ADLs)—dressing, bathing, toileting, and grooming. The major departure between the common ADLs and sexual activity is that occupational therapists regularly address the usual ADLs but do not regularly address sexual activity; sexual activity does not receive the same weight or level of attention as other ADLs. Sexual activity may not be a comfortable topic to discuss with clients and may be interpreted as unacceptable or unimportant (Couldrick, 1998).

Many who have explored and researched the subject of sexual activity over the past 30 years seem to agree that this area is important to address in the context of holistic treatment, but as noted, it is frequently overlooked, neglected, or misunderstood in how it is discussed or handled with clients (Kingsberg, 2006; Klein & Merritt, 2006; Sakellariou & Algado, 2006).

Demographic Connection Between Chronic Disability and Sexuality

The population in the United States is aging due to the "bulge" of the Baby Boomer generation (those born between 1946 and 1964) and the following generation, "Generation X" (those born between 1964 and the mid-1980s). Chronic diseases such as arthritis, cardiac and cardiopulmonary disease, diabetes, stroke, neurological diseases, and psychosocial dysfunction tend to increase proportionately with the aging process. A *chronic disease or disability* is defined as a disease that is slow in its progression and long in its continuance (Booth, Gordon, Carlson, & Hamilton, 2000). With the aging of the population, occupational therapists will be serving more clients with chronic conditions and age-related illnesses (Kazan, 1990; McInnes, 2003).

By 2030, it is estimated that approximately 20% of the population will be older than age 65 years, and an additional 35% of the population will be older than age 50 (McNamara, 2009). These generations are noted for embracing change and are expected to age in new, unconventional ways. Sexual activity is an inherent component of their life; as they age, they will likely continue to embrace sexual activity as a contributing factor to their well-being. Addressing sexuality with aging clients is an

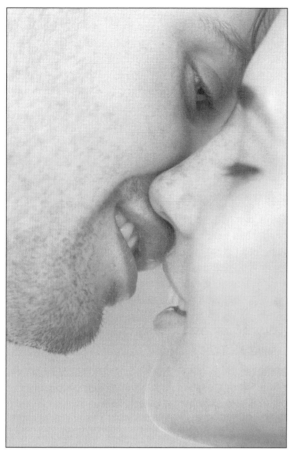

Figure 17.1. The expression of sexuality is a natural part of daily living for everyone, regardless of age or disability status.
Photo used under license from 123rf.com.

important part of holistic and client-centered care for occupational therapists.

How Important Is Sexual Activity?

Sexual images abound in the media and inundate the everyday lives of people in Western culture. Television shows, movies, music, and the Internet bombard us with explicit or implicit sexual messages daily. Individuals with chronic disabilities experience all the same messages (Young, 2004).

The perceived importance of sexual activity is highly individual. Some people place a very high value on this aspect of a relationship or lifestyle, while others place sexual activity in the "back seat," preferring companionship and friendship. However, neither age nor disability changes the basic sexual nature of the individual (Freda & Rubinsky, 1991). In other words, everybody needs somebody, but the definition of "needing" is subjective and personal.

The importance of sexuality and sexual activity to perceived well-being, quality of life, and physical health has been demonstrated in many studies (McCabe, 1997; Ventegodt, 1998). These indicated that sexual activity may reduce the risk of heart disease in men (Davey Smith, Frankel, & Yarnell, 1997) and may increase life satisfaction in the elderly population (Spector & Fremeth, 1996). Elderly clients, chronically ill clients, breast cancer clients (Harwood & O'Conner, 1994; Derogatis, 1986), and women with multiple sclerosis cited sexuality and sexual activity as being a central and primary concern in their lives. Sexual activity may promote increased life satisfaction in the chronic population. McInnes (2003) reported that sex and sexual activity can become a source of "comfort, pleasure and intimacy, and an affirmation of gender when other gender roles have been stripped away" by the chronic disease process. Other studies have shown that satisfactory adjustment to disability, illness, or injury is also accompanied by greater satisfaction with and participation in sexual activity (Bianchi, 1997; Kreuter, Sullivan, & Siosteen, 1996).

Problems with sexual activity may be of primary or secondary concern for a client, but either way, the problem is generally not addressed by occupational therapy or by health care professionals. While illness, injury, or disability may challenge "the usual way we think about sexuality" (Spica, 1989, p. 56), intervention plans that fail to consider this aspect of everyday living are incomplete. Through knowledge, the provision of information, and practical problem solving, occupational therapists can provide an important service to their clients. Addressing problems with sexual activity must be viewed as an important aspect of any client-centered, holistic assessment or intervention by occupational therapists. This personal and private area may be "the missing ADL" (Linder, 2007).

Barriers to Meeting the Sexual Information Needs of Clients

There are several obstacles that can interfere with providing effective intervention for clients regarding sexual activity and sexual function. The obstacles may arise from the occupational therapist's own attitudes and from boundaries that may be established by the client. These major obstacles are

- Insufficient knowledge of how to approach the topic of sexuality with a client and the perception (real or unfounded) of client discomfort with the topic;

Box 17.1. Sex Therapy and Counseling

Occupational therapists are not trained sex therapists or counselors. Sex therapists and sex counselors receive advanced training is all aspects of sexuality, including function and dysfunction; intervention methods; techniques for helping individuals enjoy a satisfying sex life in spite of problems, issues, or disabilities; and appropriate methods for attaining satisfaction.

- Lack of educational preparation about sexuality, a topic not fully addressed in occupational therapy education, as well as discomfort with the topic from both the client's and the occupational therapist's perspectives; and
- An assumption that another health care provider is or will be addressing this subject.

Linder (2007) and Patrica (2006) questioned how occupational therapists can effectively deal with intimate aspects of self-care, including activities like dressing, bathing, and toileting, yet neglected sexual activity in their interventions. Couldrick (1998) questioned whether the occupational therapy profession places the same level of acceptance and importance on sexual activity as it does with the more typical ADLs. A 2005 pilot study (McLaughlin & Cregan, 2005) on how sexuality and sexual activity were being addressed by health care professionals who worked with chronic population found that although clients asked health care professionals for advice on sexuality issues, the professionals did not feel that they were adequately trained to provide answers, interventions, or counseling.

People tend to be uncomfortable talking about sexuality. This becomes an additional barrier in addressing sexual concerns of clients. Occupational therapists and other health care professionals are more likely to address *technical* than *personal* issues related to sexuality with clients (McCabe, 2002), as this type of intervention aligns more closely with the traditional medical model of care. A 2002 study (Haboubi & Lincoln, 2003) found that clinical and technical problems like infertility, erectile dysfunction, and ejaculatory dysfunction were routinely addressed by physicians and other members of the health care team, especially with clients who exhibited obvious physical disability. Technical issues discussed with clients also included positioning for sexual activity, use of adaptive equipment, exercise, medication, and testing procedures, but usually not the emotional, intimate, and personal issues of sexuality. Most health care professionals tend to

adopt a clinical persona that places the client in a "sick role" by aligning their clinical practice with the traditional medical model. The sick role promotes and fosters a clinical distance between the client and health care provider. Within the medical model, other issues including sexual activity may not be considered important to address.

Clients also inadvertently face barriers to broaching the topic of sexuality or sexual activity with health care providers. These barriers are usually related to age, culture, affect, orientation, or gender.

Age

There are generational differences in comfort levels of discussing sexuality with others. In the case of a younger therapist and an older client, for example, it may be difficult to appropriately and professionally address sexual activity. Culture has changed

---

Box 17.2. The Sick Role vs. Client Empowerment

Talcott Parsons is considered the "father of the sick role" (1950s). Parsons identified four norms identified with the sick role, including

1. The individual is not responsible for their illness.
2. Normal obligations become excusable for the individual.
3. Illness is undesirable.
4. The ill should seek professional help. (as cited in Hughes, 1994)

The sick role is assumed until the client is reintegrated or disease- or illness-free, according to Parsons. The sick role may be passive, where the health care service provider takes control, or it may be a shared decision-making role (Stiggelbout & Kiebert, 1997), where the provider and client work cooperatively, thereby promoting client empowerment.

In today's health care arena, client empowerment has become more important as resources are more limited, client stays are shorter, and power is shifting from the traditional medical model to a more equitable therapist–client relationship (Smith-Gabai, 2007). LaRue and Huebner (2001) expand upon the totality of Parsons's concept by stating that it is comprised of "the physical, emotional, and sexual self." If the health care professional empowers the client, sexual activity, sexuality, and all other personal and important issues are more likely to be discussed.

---

such that the younger generation can speak more freely about sexual activity, but this may not be true for someone who is older. Occupational therapists must be aware of and sensitive to these differences as they work with clients.

Culture

In some cultures, discussing sexual activity with a nonfamily individual is considered taboo. Sexual activity, in many cultures, is simply not discussed. The opposite may also be true in cultures that consider sexual activity a normal and natural aspect of life that is freely discussed. The therapist must seek information about other cultures and potential cultural barriers in order to adequately meet the needs and expectations of the client in regard to sexual activity.

Affect

In the presence of psychological problems, the subject of sex or sexual activity may become a focal point or be totally avoided. After enduring a chronic disability or illness, a client may be fearful of resuming

his or her sexual life for fear of further injury, exacerbation of symptoms, or even death. On the other hand, some clients want to immediately resume sexual activity in spite of their condition. The therapist must secure information about the clients' physical and psychological status in order to provide informed and appropriate information.

Orientation

Sexual orientation involves a person's feelings and sense of identity. Sexual orientation is usually categorized as *heterosexual*, attraction to individuals of the opposite sex, or *homosexual*, attraction to individuals of the same sex, or *bisexual*, attraction to individuals of either sex.

Sexual orientation may or may not be apparent in how a person looks or acts (WebMD, 2009) and in no way is reflective of if they are a "good" or "bad" person. It is important for the therapist to be nonjudgmental and to use the self in a therapeutic manner in the case of client sexual orientation differences or similarities. If client or therapist

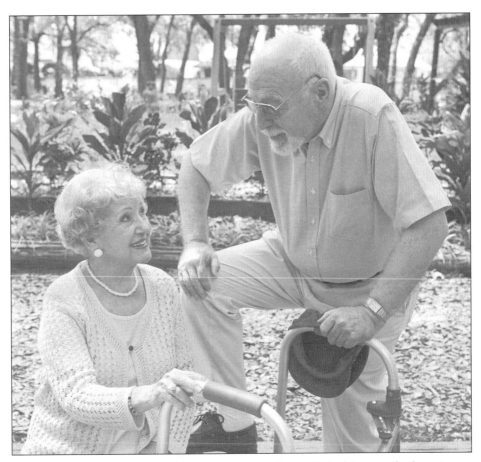

Figure 17.2. One common and incorrect assumption is that older people do not need to express their sexuality.
Photo used under license from 123rf.com.

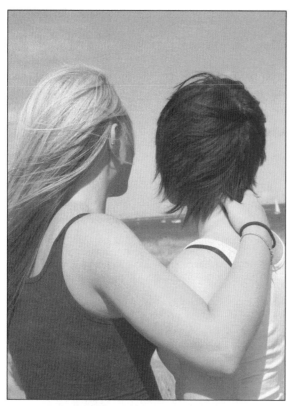

Figure 17.3. Practitioners must recognize that sexual expression takes many forms and avoid imposing their values or lifestyle preferences on their clients.
Photo used under license from 123rf.com.

discomfort is present, this may impede the therapeutic and professional process. In this case, seeking supervision or client counseling may better facilitate a positive therapeutic situation.

Gender

The client–therapist dyad is not always a same-sex composition. Having a female therapist discuss sexual activity with a male client, and vice versa, may provide stress, anxiety, or embarrassment to both parties. It is usually a good idea to provide any intervention on sexual activity with a female–female or male–male therapist–client dyad.

To appropriately address sexual activity, sex therapists have devised specific techniques for helping those with specific sexual dysfunction (Kaplan, 1974) and developed a model for determining the level of intervention needed (LoPicollo & LoPiccolo, 1978). Annon (1976) developed the PLISSIT Model, considered to be the gold standard for sexual counseling:

- *Permission.* Acknowledgment of the problem or issue without biases and without causing embarrassment.

- *Limited information.* Presentation of information within the professional's knowledge base as well as providing information about the condition that is affecting sexual performance.
- *Specific suggestions.* Positioning, use of devices to enable or enhance sexual performance, techniques, compensatory strategies, and adaptations.
- *Intensive therapy.* Specific clinical interventions that are outside the realm of occupational therapy.

The PLISSIT Model identifies levels of intervention and provides the framework for introducing and addressing sexual activity and sexuality within the confines of treatment. It can also be used to educate and train staff, clients, and caregivers (Klein & Merritt, 2006; Linder, 2007; McInnes, 2003; Weerakoon & Wong, 2003).

Functional Perspective of Sexual Activity for Occupational Therapy

Occupational therapists could provide sexual activity counseling within a rehabilitative model, rather than medical model, on the basis of their professional training and scope of practice, but this is not typically done (Kennedy, 1987). It is important to remember that occupational therapists are not sex educators or counselors and that the intent of remediation for sexual activity is framed with a functional- and meaningful-activity perspective.

Occupational therapists may deal with clients' issues surrounding sexual activity as they relate to a specific disability. Interventions geared toward helping clients return to productive and meaningful lives and to appropriate roles in their family, work, and community fall within the professional domain. In this spirit, helping clients resume an active and healthy sex life falls within the occupational therapy's scope of practice.

There are several methods occupational therapists can use to address the topic of sexual activity with a client. Using the framework established in the PLISSIT Model, information can be shared verbally or through written material within group or individual sessions. Knowing what the client is comfortable with should dictate the method in which information is disseminated. Information provided to clients should be presented at a level consistent with his or her comfort zone. It is acceptable to begin any session at a basic level and frequently ask the client if he or she understands the information and is comfortable with a continuation of the session. It is also important to know if the client is receiving the type of information expected. The therapist must be able to change approaches and delivery of information if the information is not deemed helpful or beneficial by the client.

Young (2004) provided helpful and reasonable guidelines for the therapist to consider when addressing the subject of sexual activity in a non-judgmental manner:

- The therapist should acknowledge his or her personal feelings, biases, and values and put them aside during treatment sessions.
- The therapist must have an open mind and be personally comfortable with the topic of sexual activity.
- The therapist must recognize and respect divergent viewpoints and lifestyles in relation to sexual activity.

These guidelines can provide the therapist with a useful personal system of "checks and balances" when dealing with sexual activity issues.

How Can Occupational Therapists Address Sexual Activity With Clients?

To effectively address the topic of sexual activity, components of the previously identified PLISSIT Model should be used. To gain client permission (P) to broach this subject, an interactive and client-centered assessment such as the Canadian Occupational Performance Measure (COPM; Canadian Association of Occupational Therapists, 1996) is appropriate. The COPM is client-driven regarding occupational performance activities and addresses client task performance, satisfaction, and importance. Using guided and open-ended inquiry, the therapist can ask questions about specific occupational performance and ADLs. If the client does not state the topic of sexual activity in the interview process, the therapist can ask, in general, "Are there any other areas that occupational therapy should address?" or more specifically, "Are there any personal area or activities that you would like to discuss in occupational therapy?" or very targeted, "Have you thought about more personal areas you believe are important to address? Consider things like your personal, sexual, or close relationships" (Hattjar, Parker, & Lappa, 2008). By asking these types of questions, the therapist is opening the therapeutic door for the client to address the more personal and intimate effects of his or her condition but is not prying or demanding that the topic of sexual activity be addressed.

The occupational therapist can further address sexual activity by including an "intimacy history" section in the evaluation process. Because occupational therapists are not sex therapists, the "intimacy history" should include questions that relate to the clients' occupational role, occupational function, and environmental contexts as identified in the framework of the profession, yet focally address sexual activity, sexuality, and sensuality from a psychological and individual perspective.

Box 17.3. Occupational Therapy Intimacy History

The "intimacy history" aspect of an occupational therapy evaluation should pose open-ended and nonthreatening questions to the client that relate to sexual activity. Again, the PLISSIT Model of inquiry should be adopted. Guideline questions might include the following:

1. How do you feel about your current physical status with regard to attractiveness and being desirable to your partner?
2. Are you content with your physical appearance? Is there anything you would like to change about your physical appearance?
3. Do you feel that your intimate relationship has changed since the diagnosis of your condition?
4. How much physical and/or intimate contact have you had with your partner (or others) since the diagnosis of your condition?
5. Do you detect a different type of touch or sensory input from your care provider(s) (if appropriate and the client has a care provider) as opposed to your partner? Can you identify what is different in these types of touch?
6. How do you respond to different sensations like smell, temperature, visual, auditory, and gustatory input since you were made aware of your diagnosis? Did you notice any changes in this area before receiving your diagnosis? Does this sensory input elicit memories, thoughts, and so forth?
7. Do you have concerns about resuming your intimate relationship with your partner?
8. Do you have any other concerns that you would like to address?

These questions fall well within the occupational therapy scope of practice and align with the physical, psychosocial, and sensory domain of the profession.

Knowledge Needed to Address Issues of Sexual Function and Activity Related to Disability

Prior to embarking on a discussion or intervention about sexual activity, the therapist must understand the client's disability or disease process. This is preceded by the therapist's understanding the normal sexual system in males and females, including normal anatomy, physiology, neuroanatomy, and genitalia and reproductive organs (Young, 2004). These elements along with appropriate communication skills are more likely to elicit "permission" to deal with sexual activity issues.

Masters and Johnson (1966) identified four normal sexual response stages for men and women:

1. *Excitement:* Breathing, pulse, and blood pressure begin to increase; muscle tension increases; breast and genitalia tissue begin to become engorged due to increased blood circulation; vaginal lubrication in females and penile erection in males takes place.
2. *Plateau:* Intensification of responses listed in the excitement phase occurs.
3. *Orgasm:* Men ejaculate; women experience vaginal and uterine muscle contractions; heart rate, breathing, blood pressure, and muscle tension intensify.
4. *Resolution:* All the physiologic changes return to their pre-excitement levels.

Therapists must possess a good working knowledge of professional communication skills because of the personal and intimate nature of this topic. These skills include good active listening; direct eye contact; a relaxed body position and open body language; and the ability to be compassionate, empathetic, and assertive. The therapist must sense when to probe, when to stop asking questions, when to permit the client to talk freely and openly, and when and how to terminate the channel of communication. Good communication in regard to discussions about sexual activity involves having a clear understanding of the self, the client, and the disability. Communication should transpire in a calm, quite, area that is free of distractions and interruptions.

Impact of Chronic Disease on Client Diagnosis Groups Commonly Seen in Occupational Therapy

Arthritis

Osteoarthritis and the systemic arthritis groups are characterized by pain, stiffness of joints, and fatigue. With the systemic diseases in this category, body image disturbances resulting from joint deformity may also prevail (Kazan, 1990). Pain and limited range of motion (ROM) may interfere with sexual pleasure by distracting patients from pleasurable sensations, thoughts, or fantasies (Kraaimaat, Bakker, Janssen, & Bijlsma, 1996, p. 112). Arthritis does not necessarily affect the physiological capacity for sexual arousal or fulfillment, but it may create a less spontaneous environment for potential sexual activity because of joint stiffness or the presence of pain.

Suggestions

Preplanning the time of intimate activities and sexual activity will promote physical comfort and symptom decrease. Medications can be timed so that the full effect of the analgesic will occur during sexual activity times. Joint pain and muscle relaxation can be promoted by taking warm baths or showers before sexual activity. This can be followed by gentle ROM exercises to the affected joints as a means of promoting greater and more comfortable joint movement during sexual activity.

Chronic Pulmonary Disease

Chronic pulmonary disease includes diagnoses like emphysema and bronchitis. Although this type of disease does not necessarily affect the individual's appearance or ROM, the breathing limitations that may be caused severely limit involvement in any activity, including sexual activity. Clients with pulmonary

---

Box 17.4. Strategies for Arthritis and Joint Disease

- Use joint protection techniques when deciding upon positions for sexual activity. Positions that stress the affected joints should be avoided.
- Schedule sexual activity at times when medication pain relief is at a maximum level.
- Schedule sexual activity at times when joint mobility is greatest.
- Take advantage of unaffected joints for support during sexual activity.
- A side-lying position is generally less stressful for sexual activity.
- Use pillows or bolsters to maximize comfort during sexual activity.
- Consider sensual touching, caressing, and other forms of intimacy if sexual intercourse positioning is uncomfortable. (Young, 2004)

Box 17.5. Strategies for Chronic Pulmonary Disease

- Use pillows or bolsters to improve positioning as a means of enhancing breathing ease.
- Schedule sexual activity of any kind during times where breathing is easier—usually in the afternoon or early evening.
- Utilize breathing treatments prior to sexual activity to maximize breath depth.
- Consider the use of sensual massage prior to sexual activity or intercourse.
- Promote the use of stress reduction techniques.
- Promote the use of alternative positions to decrease energy expenditure during sexual activity.

disease are activity-intolerant due to exertional dypsnea, anxiety due to frequent coughing spells (Kazan, 1990), and positional breathing changes. In the sexual activity area, for example, lying supine may decrease breathing capacity.

Suggestions

Preplanning the time of sexual activity may improve the clients breathing ability. Scheduling sexual activity at "nontraditional" times like afternoon or early evening may capture times when breathing is deeper and nourishing, whereas early morning tends to be a time when increased coughing occurs, and later in the evening, fatigue may be likely. The client should be supported in his or her use of breathing treatments to enhance breath depth prior to embarking on any sexual activity. Because pulmonary clients tend to be anxious, the use of stress reduction techniques and massage may enhance engagement in sexual activity. Suggesting alternative positions for sexual activity and incorporating energy conservation techniques can also enhance participation in.

Diabetes

The major physiological cause of dysfunction for males is *peripheral neuropathy*, more commonly referred to as the inability to achieve an erection. This has been found to be the major limiting factor in approximately 50% of males with diabetes (Kazan, 1990). Females with diabetes experience vaginal dryness, frequent fungal infections, vaginitis, and a diminished desire to engage in sexual activities. Amputation of a limb may also provide physical and psychological impediments to engagement in sexual activity because of the obvious change in the appearance of the body.

Suggestions

Because clients with diabetes commonly experience the inability to successfully engage in sexual activity, the occupational therapist can provide client education about sexual activity or sexuality issues that are present with the disease. Referral to a sex therapist or counselor can address sexual dysfunction while keeping the therapeutic relationship intact. This type of sensible referral may promote further discussion of sexual activity. With amputation, the physical and psychological effects can be dealt with effectively in a one-to-one targeted counseling arena.

Cardiac Conditions

Psychosocial and physical problems may present the cardiac client with a myriad of problems and concerns in regard to sexual activity. Anxiety, depression, and denial may psychologically affect engagement in any type of sexual activity. Pain, fatigue, and a general feeling of malaise may affect a client after cardiac episodes or cardiac surgery.

Frequently, cardiac clients are fearful of death if they engage in any type of sexual activity. It is usually prudent to wait 4–8 weeks after cardiac surgery of any type before re-engaging in sexual activity. A physician's approval should precede any discussion of and consideration of resuming sexual activity.

Box 17.6. Strategies for Diabetes

- Encourage sexual counseling because of variability of symptoms that may adversely affect sexual activity.
- Identify the use of lubrication gels or lotions to maximize comfort and to provide additional sensual stimulation for males and females.
- Encourage medication management to ensure consistent blood sugar levels during sensual or sexual activity.
- Males may want to speak to their physician regarding the use of medication for erectile dysfunction if appropriate.
- In the case of limb amputation, the residual stump, if sensate and healed, can be a source of sensual touching and assist in body positioning. Secure or safe body position should be achieved during sexual activity, as well. This may include sitting, assuming an "on top" or "on bottom" position and may represent a divergence from previously used sexual positions.

Box 17.7. Strategies for Cardiac Conditions

- Stress that sexual activity rarely results in death.
- Schedule sexual activity during times where there is energy and interest.
- If low libido or denial of sexual interest is present, encourage open communication and discussion.
- Encourage involvement in stress and anxiety reduction techniques before initiating any sexual activity.
- Secure physician approval before any initiation of sexual activity occurs. It may also be prudent to get the physician's "okay" before broaching the topic of sexual activity.
- Emphasize that the act of having sex is not the only way to demonstrate caring for the partner. Massage, sensual touching, and cuddling may set the stage for sexual activity. Time and consideration for both the client and partner are essential.

Suggestions

Because of the anxiety that may be present, aspects of sensuality may figure more prominently with this diagnosis group. Tactile and other sensory input in the form of foreplay, rest or relaxation before the initiation of sexual activity, energy conservation, and positioning suggestions may decrease client anxiety and assist in engagement in sexual activity (Calgary Health, 2008).

Spinal Cord Injury

Spinal cord injury (SCI) adaptation is the result of a gradual process that extends over a prolonged period of time. Successful sexual adjustment to this disability is influenced by the age at the time of injury, quality of social supports, physical health, gender, and severity of the injury. Losses in regard to sexual activity need to be mourned so that the remaining intact strengths can be developed. To achieve satisfying sexual adjustment, a person with a SCI will have to learn new sexual capabilities, as opposed to recapturing past abilities (Ducharme, 2000). Although sexual function varies among persons with SCI, males with cervical lesions are more likely to retain the ability to have erections, and females are more likely to retain the ability to produce vaginal lubrication. SCI clients may not experience orgasms after injury in the same manner as

prior to the injury, but many SCI clients report some feeling of pleasure or excitement, a gradual building of excitement, pleasurable muscle spasms, or skin flushing during sexual excitement (Mooney, Cole, & Chilgren, 1975).

With SCI, procreation is possible. Fertility is not permanently affected in women with a SCI. If a male with a SCI is found to have viable sperm but cannot ejaculate, he may have an electro-ejaculation medical procedure to collect sperm, followed by insemination of his partner (Freda, 1998).

Suggestions

Promoting verbalization and good communication is essential to the entire rehabilitation and community reintegration process for the SCI client. In regard to sexual activity, both the physiological and psychological components must be addressed. Sex positions and strategies should be discussed in a

---

Box 17.8. Strategies for SCI

The partner should be encouraged to touch and caress the sensate parts of the client's body. If sensation is essentially absent in a part of the body, the partner should gently describe where touching is taking place.

- The client and partner should experiment with new erogenous areas. These areas usually are located at the level of the last intact dermatome or sensate surface area of the skin (Neistadt & Freda, 1987). Good client–partner communication can facilitate the location of these areas.
- If a male SCI client is catheterized, tubing may be secured to the shaft of the penis for sexual activity. If the SCI male client knows when he has to urinate, he may experiment with taking the catheter off for short periods and engage in sexual activity at these times (Neistadt & Freda, 1987). If the SCI client is intermittently catheterized, sexual activity can be scheduled as appropriate to coincide with the catheterization schedule.
- If a female SCI client has an indwelling catheter, the catheter tube can be taped to her abdomen and the collection bag can be positioned away from her body during sexual activity (Neistadt & Freda, 1987).
- Lubricating gels or creams may be used to increase vaginal lubrication.
- Clients should be encouraged to use positions that take advantage of any movement that is present for sensual and sexual activity.

---

comfortable environment. Counseling should occur first with a counselor, followed by sessions with the counselor, client, and his or her partner. It should be stressed, in most cases, that an SCI does not necessarily mean the end of all sexual activity.

Cerebral Vascular Accident

A cerebral vascular accident (CVA) can cause a variety of physical and psychological problems, including, but not limited to, paresis; hemiparesis; hemiplegia; cognitive deficits; sensory loss or distortion; bowel and bladder problems; proprioceptive deficits; visual problems; communication disorders; feeding, eating, and swallowing deficits; and perceptual deficits. Because of the variability in the presentation of problems and deficits, libido, or sex drive, many be significantly reduced or totally absent. A decrease in ejaculatory function and peniile erection may also be present in males (Monga, Lawson, & Inglis, 1986; Zasler, 1991). CVA clients may also experience fatigue, depression, and anxiety caused by their deficits.

Because a CVA tends to affect older individuals, other health problems may be present and are exacerbated by the CVA. Additionally, the normal consequences of aging may be magnified by the CVA (Freda & Rubinsky, 1991), including decreased mobility, body changes, sensory and vision deficits, and cognitive decline.

Suggestions

The client with CVA may experience expressive or receptive aphasia, and this may create a communi-

---

Box 17.9. Strategies for CVA

- If motor loss is present, the client and partner can experiment with positions that maximize engagement, safety, and satisfaction.
- If ongoing fatigue is present, sexual activity should be scheduled at times when energy and interest are high.
- If expressive aphasia is present, the client can be educated in hand signals or use a modified communication board to ensure that feelings and needs are expressed.
- If receptive aphasia is present, the partner can utilize tactile stimulation to the skin and body parts. The partner must be aware of the client's facial gestures and vocalizations during tactile or sensory stimulation activities.
- The partner may need to be educated in alternative sexual positions if the client's motor and mobility loss are significant.

---

cation barrier in regard to communication about sexual activity. Additionally, paresis, hemiparesis, or hemiplegia and muscle tone inconsistency can create mobility and position problems for sexual activity. Because of the variability of symptoms, these issues should be addressed with the client and partner. If intervention is beyond the scope of occupational therapy practice, a referral to a sex therapist or counselor is indicated.

Sexual Rights

The Valencia Declaration on Sexual Rights places sexual activity in the mainstream of life. All individuals, whether disabled or nondisabled, male or female, young or old, and regardless of sexual orientation, have certain rights regarding sexuality and sexual activity.

The 13th World Congress on Sexology, the scientific study of sex, held in Valencia, Spain, in June 1997, identified the following sexual rights for all individuals (see http://www.cirp.org/library/ethics/valencia1997/):

- The right to freedom, which excludes all forms of sexual coercion, exploitation, and abuse, at any time and in all situations in life. The struggle against violence is a social priority. All children should be desired and loved.

- The right to autonomy, integrity, and safety of the body. This right encompasses control and enjoyment of our own bodies, free from torture, mutilation, and violence of any sort.

- The right to sexual equity and equality, which refers to freedom from all forms of discrimination, paying due respect to sexual diversity, regardless of sex, gender, age, race, social class, religion, and sexual orientation.

- The right to sexual health, including availability of all sufficient resources for development of research and the necessary knowledge of HIV/AIDS and STDs as well as the further development of resources for research, diagnosis, and treatment.

- The right to wide, objective, and factual information on human sexuality in order to allow decision making regarding sexual life.

- The right to a comprehensive sexuality education from birth and throughout the life cycle. All social institutions should be involved in this process.

- The right to associate freely, meaning the possibility to marry or not, to divorce, and to establish other types of sexual associations.

- The right to make free and responsible choices regarding reproductive life, the number and spacing of children, and the access to means of fertility regulation.

- The right to privacy, which implies the capability of making autonomous decisions about sexual life within a context of personal and social ethics. Rational and satisfactory experience of sexuality is a requirement for human development (World Congress on Sexuality, 1997).

Conclusion

Although the profession of occupational therapy purports to address the many facets of each individual to whom it provides services, it frequently does not address the most normal and natural aspect of being human: sexual activity and its components—sexuality, sensuality, and intimacy. The topic of sexual activity is frequently omitted from evaluation and interventions but can and should be introduced in a variety of ways, including client-centered evaluation and by addressing sexual activity components in evaluations and interventions.

Sexual activity is a topic that is barrier-ridden from both the client's and therapist's perspectives. Therapist comfort, knowledge seeking, and sensitivity can lower the therapeutic barriers, while clients' trust, communication, and knowledge of disease can overcome their personal barriers. Occupational therapists are in no way sex therapists or counselors but can address and remediate sexual activity problems due to their expansive knowledge base. Because sex therapists and counselors are available, a referral to these professionals is appropriate when questions, problems, or concerns are beyond our scope of practice.

All individuals have a basic human right to a sexual self regardless of disability, age, orientation, culture, or gender. To provide holistic and truly client-centered care, sexual activity—an ADL—should be given the importance it is due.

Study Questions

1. What are some specific suggestions and strategies to use in interventions with chronically disabled clients who are diagnosed with arthritis?
2. When is a referral to a sex therapist or counselor indicated in occupational therapy clinical practice? What diagnosis group or groups are most likely to warrant a referral, and why is this so?

3. What are the differences among sexual activity, sexuality, sensuality, and intimacy?
4. What is the role of occupational therapists when dealing with issues relating to sexual activity?
5. What are some professional and client barriers as they relate to addressing and intervening for sexual activity issues?
6. How can the therapeutic use of self enhance client empowerment in relation to sexual activity?
7. What model of intervention can decrease anxiety when dealing with sexual activity?
8. How can a practitioner develop open-ended questions that encourage a client to talk about sexual activity issues? Consider evaluation, evaluation components, and intervention strategies.
9. Why is it important to address sexual activity with chronic disabled clients?

References

American Occupational Therapy Association. (2008). Occupational therapy practice framework: Domain and process (2nd ed.). *American Journal of Occupational Therapy, 56,* 625–683.

Annon, J. (1976). The PLISSIT Model: A proposed conceptual scheme for the behavioral treatment of sexual problems. *Journal of Sex Education and Therapy, 2,* 1–15.

Bianchi, T. L. (1997). Aspects of sexuality after burn injury: Outcomes in men. *Journal of Burn Care and Rehabilitation, 18*(2), 183–186.

Booth, F., Gordon, S., Carlson, C., & Hamilton, X. (2000). Waging war on modern chronic diseases: Primary prevention through exercise biology. *Journal of Applied Physiology, 88,* 774–787.

Calgary Health. (2008). *Sexual and reproductive health: Sexuality and chronic illness and/or disability.* Retrieved March 24, 2008, from http://www.calgary healthregion.ca/becomm/sexual/disability.htm

Canadian Association of Occupational Therapists. (1996). *Canadian Occupational Performance Measure.* Ottawa, Ontario: CAOT Publications ACE.

Couldrick, L. (1998). Sexual issues: An area of concern for occupational therapists? *British Journal of Occupational Therapy, 61,* 493–496.

Davey-Smith, G., Frankel. S., & Yarnell, J. (1997). Sex and death: Are they related? Findings from the Caerphilly Cohort Study. *British Medical Journal, 315*(7123), 1641–1644.

Derogatis, L. (1986). The unique impact of breast and gynecological cancers in body image and sexual identity of women: A reassessment. In J. M. Varth (Ed.), *Body image, self-esteem, and sexuality in cancer patients* (2nd ed., pp. 1–14). Basel, Switzerland: Karger.

Ducharme, S. (2000). *Sexuality and spinal cord injury.* Retrieved December 4, 2009, from http://www. stanleyducharme.com/resources/sex_spinal cord_injury.htm

Encarta. (2009). *Intimacy.* Retrieved November 24, 2009, from http://www.encarta.com

Freda, M. (1998). Sexuality and disability. In M. E. Neistadt & E. Crepeau (Eds.), *Willard and Spackman's occupational therapy* (pp. 364–369). Philadelphia: Lippincott.

Freda, M., & Rubinsky, H. (1991). Sexual function in the stroke survivor. *Physical Medicine and Rehabilitation Clinics of North America, 2*(3), 643–659.

Haboubi, N., & Lincoln, N. (2003). Views of health professionals on discussing sexual issues with patients. *Disability and Rehabilitation, 25*, 291–296.

Harwood, K., & O'Conner, A. (1994). Sexuality and breast cancer. *Innovations in Oncology Nursing, 10*(2), 30–33.

Hattjar, B., Parker, J., & Lappa, C. (2008). Addressing sexuality with adult clients with chronic disabilities: Occupational therapy's role. *OT Practice, 13*(11), CE1–CE8.

Hughes, J. (1994). *Approaches to the doctor–patient relationship.* Retrieved August 3, 2007, from http://www.changesurfer.com/Hlth/DPReview.htm

Kaplan, H. (1974). *The new sex therapy.* New York: Brunner/Mazel.

Kazan, L. (1990). Chronic illness and sexuality. *American Journal of Nursing, 90*(1), 54–59.

Kennedy, G. (1987). Occupational therapists as sexual rehabilitation professionals using the rehabilitative frame of reference. *Canadian Journal of Occupational Therapy, 54*(4), 189–193.

Kingsberg, S. (2006). Taking a sexual history. *Obstetrics and Gynecology Clinics of North America, 33*, 535–547.

Klein, M., & Merritt, L. (2006). *Sexuality and disability.* Retrieved June 3, 2007, from http://www.emedicine.com/pmr/topic178.htm

Kraaimaat, F. W., Bakker, A. H., Janssen, E., & Bijlsma, J. W. J. (1996). Intrusiveness of rheumatoid arthritis on sexuality in male and female patients living with a spouse. *Arthritis Care and Research, 9*(2), 120–125.

Kreuter, M., Sullivan, M., & Siosteen, A. (1996). Sexual adjustment and its predictors after traumatic brain injury. *Brain Injury, 12*(5), 349–368.

LaRue, A., & Huebner, R. (2001). The influence of the sick role on health in rehabilitation. *Physical Disabilities Special Interest Quarterly, 24*(2), 1–4.

Linder, S. (2007). *The missing activity of daily living.* Retrieved June 3, 2007, from http://www.occupational-therapy-advanceweb.com

LoPiccolo, J., & LoPiccolo, L. (1978). *Handbook of sex therapy.* New York: Plenum.

Masters, W. H., & Johnson, V. E. (1966). *Human sexual response.* Boston: Little, Brown.

McCabe, M. P. (1997). Intimacy and quality of life among sexually dysfunctional men and women. *Journal of Sex and Marital Therapy, 23*(4), 276–290.

McCabe, M. (2002). Relationship of functioning and sexuality among people with multiple sclerosis. *Journal of Sex Research, 39*, 302–309.

McInnes, R. A. (2003). Chronic illness and sexuality. *Medical Journal of Australia, 179*, 263–266.

McLaughlin, J., & Cregan, A. (2005). Sexuality in stroke care: A neglected quality of life in stroke rehabilitation? A pilot study. *Sexuality and Disability, 23*, 213–226.

McNamara, M. (2009). *Growing old, Baby-Boomer style.* Retrieved November 26, 2009, from http://www.cbsnews.com/stories/2006/01/10/health/webmd/main1195879.shtml

Monga, T. N., Lawson, J. S., & Inglis, J. (1986). Sexual dysfunction in stroke patients. *Archives of Physical Medicine and Rehabilitation, 67*, 19–22.

Mooney, T., Cole, T., & Chilgren, R. (1975). *Sexual options for paraplegics and quadriplegics.* Boston: Little, Brown.

Neistadt, M. E. (1986). Sexuality counseling for adults with disabilities: A module for an occupational therapy curriculum. *American Journal of Occupational Therapy, 40*, 542–545.

Neistadt, M. E., & Freda, M. (1987). *Choices: A guide to sex counseling with physically disabled adults.* Malabar, FL: Robert Krieger.

Patrica, L. (2006). Addressing sexual activities in inpatient rehabilitation. *Physical Disabilities Special Interest Quarterly, 29*(4), 2–3.

Sakellariou, D., & Algado, S. S. (2006). Sexuality and occupational therapy: Exploring the link. *British Journal of Occupational Therapy, 69*, 350–356.

Smith-Gabai, H. (2007). Client empowerment. *OT Practice, 12*(13), 23–25.

Spector, I. P., & Fremeth, S. M. (1996). Sexual dysfunction after spinal cord injury. *Urology Clinics of North America, 20*, 535–542.

Spica, M. M. (1989). Sexual counseling standards for spinal cord-injured. *Journal of Neuroscience Nursing, 21*(1), 56–60.

Sri, E. (2007). *Men, women, and tenderness.* Retrieved September 4, 2007, from http://www.catholiceducation.org/articles/sexuality/se0134.htm

Stiggelbout, A., & Kiebert, G. (1997). A role for the sick role: Patient preferences regarding information and participation in clinical decision making. *Canadian Medical Journal, 157*, 383–389.

Ventegodt, S. (1998). Sex and the quality of life in Denmark. *Archives of Sexual Behaviour, 27*(3), 295–307.

Weerakoon, P., & Wong, M. (2003). *Sexuality education online for health professionals.* Retrieved June 16, 2007, from http://www.ejhs.org/volume6/Sex Ed.html

WebMD. (2009). *Sexual orientation.* Retrieved December 3, 2009, from http://www.webmdcom/sex-relationships/guide/sexual-orientation

World Congress on Sexology. (1997, June). *Valencia declaration on sexual rights.* Valencia, Spain. Retrieved December 11, 2009, from http://www2.hu-berlin.de/sexology/ECE5/was_declaration_of_sexual_righ.html

Young, M. E. (2004). *Sexuality and people with physical disabilities.* In C. Christiansen & K. M. Matuska (Eds.), *Ways of living: Adaptive strategies for special needs* (3rd ed., pp. 385–396). Bethesda, MD: AOTA Press.

Zasler, N. (1991). Sexuality in neurologic disability: An overview. *Sexuality and Disability, 9*(1), 11–27.

Chapter 18

Using Assistive Technology to Enable Better Living

DENIS ANSON, MS, OTR

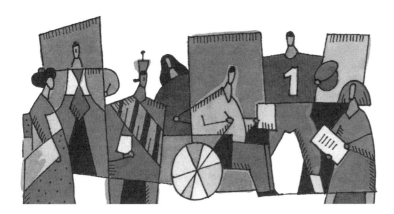

KEY WORDS

ABLEDATA

adaptive equipment

assistive technology (AT)

augmentative and alternative communication (AAC)

electronic aids to daily living (EADLs)

universal design

HIGHLIGHTS

- Assistive technology (AT) is defined by how it is used, not by what it is. Many mass-market products can be used as AT.

- The adaptive equipment that occupational therapists have used throughout the history of the occupational therapy profession are examples of AT.

- AT must be prescribed to match the skills and needs of the individual, the demands of the task, and the limitations of the environment in which it is to be used.

- The field of AT is changing rapidly. New products are introduced daily, others disappear. The Internet can be a powerful aid to the therapist in finding appropriate devices.

- Unless the client is trained in how to use the device and the training continues until using the device is natural and efficient, the intervention is likely to fail.

OBJECTIVES

After reading this material, readers will be able to

- Describe the historical role of assistive technology (AT) in occupational therapy practice;
- Provide a use-based definition of AT;
- Give examples of how AT is used by people without disabilities;
- Explain the use of AT as an avenue of intervention in occupational therapy practice;
- Describe how AT must be matched to the person, task, and environment to be effective;
- Describe the relationship of AT domains to occupational therapy outcomes; and
- Describe advantages and disadvantages of different sources of AT devices.

What Is Assistive Technology?

In Thomas Carlyle's 1833 book *Sartor Resartus*, he observes "Man is a tool-using animal. Weak in himself, and of small stature . . . without Tools, he is nothing, with Tools he is all."

Technology is commonly defined as "the practical application of knowledge for purposes" (*Merriam-Webster's Collegiate Dictionary*, 1996) or "tools." We use tools to magnify our abilities and to allow us to perform tasks that we cannot do without the tools. Without a hammer (or a rock), we cannot push a nail into wood to hold structures together. Without refrigerators, we cannot preserve perishable foods over time. Without airplanes, we cannot leap over oceans in hours. Our tools expand our abilities far beyond our intrinsic capabilities.

Assistive technology (AT) is composed of the tools that we use to allow a person with a functional limitation to perform the everyday tasks that others are able to perform without such tools. A person who is unable to walk may use a wheelchair to move from place to place. While a wheelchair does not enable "walking," it does restore mobility.

For exceptional athletes, the mobility may be well beyond the norm for those without mobility limitations. In 2009, for example, Deriba Merga, the fastest runner in the Boston Marathon, finished the race in 2 hours, 8 minutes, and 42 seconds (Boston Athletic Association, 2009a). Ernst Van Dyk, the fastest man in a wheelchair, finished more than half

an hour ahead of Merga, in just 1 hour, 33 minutes, and 29 seconds (Boston Athletic Association, 2009b). For other users, assistive devices might be used for such prosaic activities as buttoning a shirt or tying shoes.

One aspect of AT that can be confusing is that the field is not defined by the device but by the application of the device. Some assistive technologies are developed specifically for individuals with physical or sensory disabilities and are generally used only by those individuals. While it is possible for a person who can walk to use a wheelchair, wheelchairs are used almost exclusively by those who, if they can walk at all, are restricted to very short distances. Braille, the tactile alphabet of raised dots, was developed in the early 1800s as a variant of "night writing" for artillery officers. This "night writing," developed by Charles Barbier (Kimbrough, 2008), was never widely accepted, although Louis Braille's variation remains widely accepted and is, in fact, legally mandated. Braille can, with difficulty, be read by sighted people, but is very usable by a person who is blind.

Some technologies that were developed for individuals with disabilities are now widely used by those without disabilities, who may not be aware of the source of the tool. Some may not think of a curb cut as a technology, much less an assistive technology, but they were developed, and are legally required, to provide people using mobility aids with a way of crossing streets. The primary users of curb cuts, though, are not people in wheelchairs. Curb cuts are most widely used by those making deliveries to businesses; by people with wheeled luggage; and those using carts, skateboards, or carriages.

Still other technologies were developed for the convenience of able-bodied individuals but have the added benefit of enabling people with disabilities. The television remote control was developed to allow the "lazy nondisabled" to change channels without getting up from their chairs. Sound- and touch-activated light switches were developed to avoid the difficult task of flipping a toggle switch on entering or leaving a room. For the person with a disability who cannot rise from a chair, the television remote control becomes an assistive technology because it allows him or her to change channels without requiring the use of controls on the television. Similarly, when a person with mobility restrictions turns on the light by the sound of their presence in the room, the sound-activated light switch, installed for the lazy homeowner without disabilities, becomes an assistive technology.

This use-based definition of AT has significant implications for funding. When people with a disability buy an appliance, they may find that only the more expensive models have the features that make the appliance usable. A lower-cost appliance may not be usable at all or only with extreme effort. Should the insurance company be required to pay the entire cost of the appliance as an assistive technology? Should the third-party payer cover only the difference between an entry-level model and the usable one? Or should the individual with a disability be fully responsible for the cost of the appliance, as it is not marketed as an assistive technology?

AT is often discussed as being used by individuals with "disabilities." As the field has developed, however, we have discovered that many people who have significant limitations do not consider themselves to be "disabled." As people age, for example, they may find their ability to see fine detail is reduced, and their dexterity to be less than it once was. In most cases, however, people experiencing the normal changes of aging will not consider themselves to be "disabled." Because the devices developed specifically for people with acquired disability (e.g., traumatic injury or disease) can also be effectively used by those experiencing changes due to aging or developmental variation, in this chapter we will consider AT solely in terms of the enhancement of function, regardless of the source of the limitation.

Occupational Therapy Intervention and Assistive Technology

The *Occupational Therapy Practice Framework* (American Occupational Therapy Association, 2008) (hereinafter the *Framework*) makes just one reference to AT and one to universal design. This infrequency of reference may derive from the assumption that the adaptive tools used by occupational therapists are clearly assistive technologies, but it may also reflect a failure to maintain the language of occupational therapy with current terminology in related professions. While every profession has special terminology that is used to convey information between practitioners (jargon), we must ensure that the language of occupational therapy also accurately reflects our practice to those outside the profession. As will be seen, AT is pervasive throughout the practice. Each outcome area described in the *Framework* can be supported by AT.

When planning intervention for a new client, a therapist must evaluate possible avenues of intervention to maximize functional independence for that client. The possible avenues of intervention can be divided into six broad areas:

1. Reduce the impairment.
2. Compensate for the impairment.
3. Modify the activity.
4. Modify the environment.
5. Provide assistive technology.
6. Provide assistance through others.

Reduce the Impairment

Whenever possible, the rehabilitation process should restore normal functioning to the extent possible. If an individual breaks a femur, for example, there will be a period during which he or she will not be able to walk, followed by a period of weakness. Ultimately, in uncomplicated cases, full functional return is expected. In such cases, the occupational therapist might be called on to provide treatment that will provide independence during the recovery process, but major life changes and environmental adaptations will not be called for. If the client is in recovery from Guillain-Barré syndrome or a cerebrovascular accident (CVA), however, the recovery is likely to be incomplete. In spite of this, the therapist will invest intervention time and effort in reducing the impairment as much as possible. In cases of traumatic amputation, there will be no regrowth of the lost limb. However, in the process of treatment and recovery, an individual is likely to experience secondary losses such as phantom limb pain or general loss of endurance. In these cases, the effort invested in reducing impairment may address these secondary injuries, as available technologies will not regrow lost fingers or limbs.

Compensate for the Impairment

The "paucity principle" suggests that nature always does things in the way that requires the least overall effort. Normal movements are refined over time to require as little energy as possible. Following an injury or illness, however, the patterns of behavior learned over a lifetime may no longer be possible or may be less efficient.

One of the jobs of the occupational therapist is to teach the client who has sustained a disability new ways to accomplish the tasks of their daily lives with what skills and abilities remain. For a person who has experienced a CVA, such tasks often begin with one-handed dressing, including managing zippers, shoelaces, and buttons. When a person has lost his or her sight, therapists may teach orientation

Table 18.1. Occupational Therapy Outcomes and Assistive Technology

Occupational Therapy Outcome	Applications of Assistive Technology
Occupational performance	Assistive technology (adaptive devices) may be key to facilitating occupational performance. Following a CVA, a person with residual weakness may require dressing aids such as reachers, button hooks, or zipper pulls for dressing. A client with traumatic head injury may require a PDA as a cuing aid to maintain her schedule.
Adaptation	An employee with a lower-back injury may require adaptation of the workplace, including the use of power tools, adjustable workbench, or lifting aids to continue working. In a community with public transportation, lift equipped busses can allow citizens who are wheelchair-mobile to participate in community activities.
Health and wellness	An elder with low vision may need a magnifier to draw up his insulin. A woman with hearing loss may need an amplified telephone handset to communicate with her doctor's office to set up an appointment. An elderly woman with balance issues may depend on an alert pendant to call for help should she fall, allowing her to continue to live in her home of 40 years.
Participation	A former runner who lost a leg in military service uses a high-tech prosthetic to continue to complete in local races. A sailor who severed her spine in a car accident now sails and races an adapted single-hand boat. A social activist who is blind uses screen-reading technology to allow him to be a leading member of the city council.
Prevention	A talking blood pressure monitor allows a woman with diabetic retinopathy to monitor her blood pressure independently. A man with peripheral sensory loss uses a thermometer to monitor the temperature of his bathwater to avoid a repeated burn. A large-display, talking thermometer allows a mother with low vision to monitor the health of her children.
Quality of life	A young boy with multiple disabilities uses Morse code to participate in class. A nonvocal adult describes how his AAC system allowed him to become a useful member of his community. A man with a C1 level spinal lesion organizes a "Transverse Myelitis National Conference."
Role competence	A man injured on the job uses his prosthetic arm to play catch with his son. A woman with severe tremor secondary to MS uses a card holder to continue her weekly participation in the bridge club.
Self-advocacy	A large group of adults with developmental disabilities pickets the U.S. Supreme Court to oppose rule changes that would require them to live in nursing homes to continue to receive federal support. A man with an SCI is aided by his service dog in managing the hills of his coastal community. A woman who has received a communication aid 5 years after her stroke left her unable to speak initiates divorce proceedings against her abusive husband.
Occupational justice	A secretary who is blind uses a screen reader to manage appointments for her employer. A farmer uses a prosthetic limb to operate the tractors and other equipment on his farm. A woman with TBI uses a pacing-board to help moderate her speech rate, and be welcomed as a member of a panel on community revitalization.

Note. AAC = augmentative and alternative communication; CVA = cerebrovascular accident; PDA = personal digital assistant; SCI = spinal cord injury; TBI = traumatic brain injury.

and navigation using touch (the blind cane), sound (echo-location), or a service animal (seeing-eye dog). A person with chronic fatigue may be taught energy conservation strategies, including using low-force movements and building rest breaks into the schedule.

For compensatory strategies to be effective, they must be trained and practiced until the effort of using the strategy is less than that of the distorted movements resulting from the disability. Many therapists have been frustrated after having spent hours teaching adaptive dressing techniques to find that, at the 6-month checkup, the client has abandoned all such training as "too hard" or "uncomfortable." In most cases, this abandonment occurs because the compensatory techniques were not practiced to the point of mastery, and the paucity principle has driven the client back to the less demanding, but also less effective, habitual methods.

Modify the Activity

Three of the cornerstones of occupational therapy practice are activity analysis, gradation, and adaptation. When a client is no longer able to perform a meaningful activity because of a disability, the therapist may analyze the activity, identify the components of the activity that are presenting the barrier, and adapt the activity to allow it to be continued. Alternatively, the therapist may analyze a meaningful activity to find ways to use it in therapy, enhancing client motivation and effort.

When adapting or grading an activity, a key question is "What aspects of this activity can I change without it becoming a different activity?" The answer to this question may be different for different people participating in the same activity. One approach to identifying the key components of an activity is to ask the client to describe the activity in two sentences (the "two-sentence rule"). The components that the client includes in the two-sentence description are the key features of the activity for that individual and should be preserved in any grading or adaptation. All other aspects can be examined for possible changes.

For example, suppose an individual was an avid painter of landscapes prior to experiencing a stroke and would like to continue painting. Although the client has retained enough mobility to get to the areas formerly painted, managing the easel, brushes, and paints while moving over rough terrain is very frustrating. When asked to describe painting, the client speaks of mixing oils to match the colors and textures of the scene and translating the depth and colors seen onto the canvas in a way that evokes an emotional response in others. For this client, the process of mixing oils and translating vision to canvas cannot be changed, but the client might be convinced to try still-life painting in a studio.

Another client might describe the activity as finding the right view and the right light to bring the openness of the outdoors into the studio. Clearly, the needs of this client will not be met by studio work, but the client might find that scenic photography, which requires more manageable equipment, would be as enjoyable. The creative process of composing photographs matches closely that of painting, and digital manipulation (i.e., color balance, lighting) of a photograph is similar to the process of finding the right hue of paint.

In adapting an activity, the therapist must first find out which aspects of the complex activity the client enjoys and which of these remain possible and then design new activities that continue to meet the client's needs in an adapted format.

Modify the Environment

As noted in the models of AT intervention described below, an activity is performed by a person in an environment. In many cases, the nature of the environment may be a key factor in the success or failure of the individual to perform the task. For example, a person with visual deficits may find reading impossible under low light and may find walking difficult when lights reflect off the floor surface. A student with attention deficit may find it difficult to attend to a lecture when seated next to a window or when a radio is playing in the next room. Yet, the person with visual deficits may be able to read when adequate light is provided and walk without stumbling on carpet. The student with attention deficit may be able to learn quite well when seated away from competing visual and auditory distracters.

Environmental adaptation, like the other aspects of the intervention process, has been part of occupational therapy from its beginnings. Environmental adaptation has been described as being unlike the other aspects of occupational therapy practice in that the focus of attention is away from the client and on the environment in which the client will be performing activities. More accurately, effective environmental adaptation requires the therapist to examine the environment through the filter of the client's strengths and weaknesses. Because an adaptation that supports one person may hinder another, it is impossible to perform effective environmental adaptations without a detailed understanding of the client for whom the environment is being adapted. (This does not mean that universally useful environments cannot be designed, only that universally *optimal* ones cannot.)

Many aspects of environmental adaptation are relatively easy once the therapist learns to attend to the barriers. Just as an individual with limited hand function may require button hooks and adapted zipper pulls to dress independently, she may require lever door knobs to move between rooms and bar-style drawer pulls rather than knobs on kitchen cabinets. A home that has three steps to enter the front door may require that a ramp or alternative entrance be provided to allow a person in a wheelchair to continue residence. A small, push-button phone may need to be replaced with a large-button or voice-dialing phone to accommodate a person who is losing vision.

Other environmental barriers may be subtler, or relate to tasks that are performed only occasionally. A long-pile carpet with soft pad may be very comfortable to walk on but can be difficult to propel a wheelchair over. If the client does not wish to replace the carpet, it may be possible to replace the pad with a firmer, less energy-absorbing one, and retain the same carpet for improved wheeled mobility. Tasks such as replacing furnace air filters or smoke detector batteries may occur only once a year, but if these can be adapted by replacing screws with knobs or providing a track to pull detectors to a lower reach, the independence of the individual can be maintained.

Provide Assistive Technology

While the terminology is new, the concept of AT, like the other aspects of rehabilitation, has been part of occupational therapy from its earliest days. *Assistive technologies*, as defined in the Technology Related Assistance Act (Technology-Related Assistance for Individuals with Disabilties Act of 1988 as Amended in 1994, 1988), the Rehab Act (The Rehabilitation Act Amendments of 1973, as amended, 1973), and the ADA (Americans with Disabilities Act of 1990), are those technologies (both devices and services) that allow a person with a disability to perform tasks that people without disabilities are able to do without the technology. As such, all of the special tools that occupational therapists routinely provide are examples of assistive technologies. Button hooks, sock aids, and key holders allow individuals with disabilities to fasten buttons, put on socks, and turn keys, just as people without disabilities can without such tools. In modern clinical practice, the available assistive devices have grown in number and power.

As noted in the Human Interface Assessment (HIA) model (Anson, 2001), AT is provided to meet the demands of a task in a specific environment. When a therapist is considering an AT solution to enable independence, the therapist must clearly identify which aspects of the task are presenting difficulty and identify the assistive technology that provides the needed help. This is a process that is central to occupational therapy practice.

Consider an individual who has difficulty dressing and is seeing an occupational therapist. The therapist does not simply provide a buttonhook and dressing stick as the "solution" to dressing problems but instead evaluates which components of dressing

the client has difficulty with. It may be that the client has difficulty with buttons and that the buttonhook is the correct solution. But it might also be the case that the client cannot reach his feet, and a sock aid and long shoehorn are required. It might also be the case that the client is unable to reach clothes hung in the closet, and a reacher with a hanger hook is needed.

Another client may have difficulty using the telephone. If the difficulty is in hearing the speech of the caller, he or she may require an amplified handset. Or the client may have limitations in strength or endurance and finds the effort of holding the handset to be too great for extended calls. In this case, a speakerphone, handset support, or headset may provide the required assistance. The client may be unable to see the telephone keypad or lack the motor control necessary to accurately press the small buttons. In this case, a telephone with large buttons or voice dialing, or operator-assisted calling may provide the assistance needed.

In each case, the assistive technology is selected only when the specific deficit is identified. Just as there is no universal treatment plan for a person with a CVA, there is no universal assistive technology. The technology must be carefully matched to the abilities of the individual, the demands of the task to be performed, and the restrictions of the environment in which the task is to be performed.

Provide Assistance Through Others

One of the most important lessons in becoming an occupational therapist is that it is never the therapist's job to tell a client "you cannot do this task." It is the job of the therapist to determine what would be necessary for the client to do the job and the degree of success that is possible. Then the client can decide whether or not the task is worth the investment. In some cases, the answer to that question will be "No, it's not worth it."

In some cases, activities that are not worth the effort may be given up. A former rock climber, after sustaining an SCI in a fall, may decide that rock climbing is no longer worth the effort required. A long-distance runner who has lost a leg in an auto accident may find that, while running with a prosthesis is possible, he or she does not get the same feeling of freedom and lightness that made the activity enjoyable. A lumber mill worker who operated an overhead crane may discover that the adaptations necessary to allow him to continue after his stroke would cost three times his annual salary and do not constitute "reasonable accommodation" for his employer. In such cases, the individual may reasonably decide that continuing the activity is not worth the effort and spend his or her energy on other activities that remain interesting and possible.

In other cases, the need for a certain task continues, but the effort required to perform it is excessive. For example, after a high-level SCI, independent dressing might be possible but might require 3 hours to complete and exhaust the client. Yet the client must be dressed. After a head injury, a client may no longer be able to prepare meals but must still eat. With advancing dementia, a client may not be able to able to recall having taken medications, but medication management remains critical to maintaining health. In these and many other cases, assistance from another person may be required.

In cases where clients have limited amounts of physical or cognitive capacity, it may be that basic activities of daily living (ADLs) remain possible, but being independent in ADLs would take all the time and energy available to them, forcing them to abandon other enjoyable activities. In such a case, providing assistance for basic ADLs may allow clients to participate in a job, in school, or in hobbies that provide meaning to life.

Resource Allocation in Treatment

Given these six possible avenues of intervention in the case of disability, which should the therapist attempt? The singularly least helpful answer given by many expert therapists is "you do all of them." This answer is accurate, but incomplete. The therapist does all of them but does not invest equal effort in each.

In biology, the process is referred to as *dynamic allocation of resources*. At each stage of treatment, resources are adjusted to place the effort in areas that seem to offer the greatest probability of improving the overall outcome. In the early treatment sessions, the primary effort may be in restoring function and teaching adaptive strategies, with some effort to explore long-term barriers that may need to be overcome. As the therapist develops a projection of likely function at the end of treatment, more effort will be allocated to exploring environmental adaptations and assistive technologies that might be needed and planning for the acquisition and training required. The therapist will also be examining the assistance that may be available from the client's family or friends over the short term and for extended periods.

This process is based on clinical experience and can be difficult for the novice therapist to understand. To a great extent, the projection of probable intrinsic function and compensatory strategy adoption is based on the individual therapist's past experience with similar clients. Since the new therapist lacks a catalog of past clients with which to compare the new case, such projections are difficult. Similarly, the novice therapist may not have in-depth knowledge of available environmental adaptations and assistive technologies available.

For the novice therapist, then, a useful approach is to attempt to provide a functional outcome that most closely matches the "normal" or predisability level. As such, the approaches to treatment are provided in approximately the order that effort should be applied. To the extent possible, the therapist should attempt to reduce impairments. When further progress in restoring intrinsic function seems unlikely, the therapist should seek to teach compensatory strategies that will allow the client to function in his or her "typical" environment. If compensatory strategies do not allow a return to task performance, the therapist should explore ways of adapting the task (task accommodation in home and work settings). If the environment in which the task is to be performed is the source of barriers, the therapist can recommend environmental adaptations. When these efforts have resulted in the changes that are possible, but the client still faces limitations in performing a task, the novice therapist may explore assistive technologies to address the issue. When all of these accommodations do not allow the individual to perform a task independently, or when the client has decided that the effort required to perform an essential task is too great, the therapist may recommend and train a caregiver to perform the tasks.

Models of Assistive Technology Provision

Human Activity Assistive Technology

Bailey's Human Performance Model (Bailey, 1989) indicates that in order to properly model human activity, one must consider the human, the activity, and the contexts (physical, emotional, social) of the activity (Figure 18.1). Bailey's model was important for indicating that the environment of an activity can be crucial to the ability of the individual to perform successfully. Reading, for example, may be easy in a well-lit space, but the same book can be impossible to read at the back of a dark cave. Cook and Hussey (2002, 2007) extended the Bailey model to include assistive technology in their Human, Activity, Assistive Technology (HAAT) model. This model represents the person and activity as embedded within an environment or context, as does the Human Performance Model, but includes an AT component.

The HAAT model shows the interdependency of the human, the activity, and the environment with

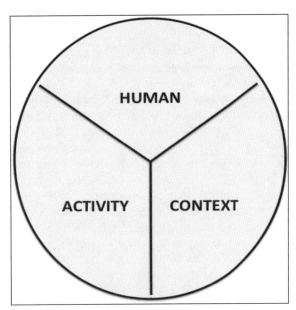

Figure 18.1. Human activity context model.

the assistive technology to provide an effective intervention (Figure 18.2). The "context" or environmental component of the HAAT model includes such aspects of the physical environment as temperature, light and sound levels, and work and floor surfaces. But it also includes such cultural aspects as the value of time, values related to belonging and independence, and social support systems. The assistive technology suggested to the client must be usable by the person, must enable performance of the activity and must be compatible with the social and physical context in which it is to be used.

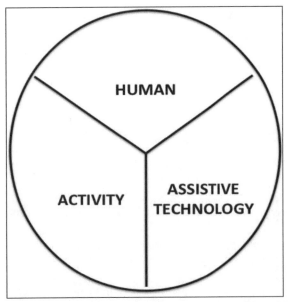

Figure 18.2. The HAAT model.

Consider the case of a young Amish boy who needed a communication aid to participate in school. The Amish do not welcome advanced technology in many aspects of their lives and generally do not have electrical power in their homes. The therapist working with this boy was able to provide a high-technology aid at school because the Amish accept technology that furthers work, and education is part of work. But the augmentative and alternative communication (AAC) device had to be charged at the school, as electrical power was not available in the home. The boy was able to use the device in his home but felt that using it to participate in social or church activities would not be acceptable. The HAAT model can help to guide the clinician in thinking through the complexities of such a situation.

Human–Environment/Technology Interface Model

The Human–Environment/Technology Interface model (Smith, 1991) more closely examines the process of human interaction with technology (Figure 18.3). In performing an activity, an individual receives information about his or her surroundings, including the state of the activity and the environment. From this information, the person determines a desired action, then acts on that desire in the form of a volitional action (the action may be movement or may be producing a mental state). The volitional action is accepted as input into the environment or technology system. The system responds to the input by changing in some way. This may be by activating a selection on a keyboard, receiving paint from a paintbrush, or signaling a need for assistance to a caregiver. This environmental response is the output of the environment or technology. If the output is perceptible to the individual, the person can respond to the changes in their environment, and the cycle begins again.

The HETI model can be particularly helpful in selecting an assistive technology. For example, a 57-year-old woman, an avid reader, was losing her vision secondary to diabetic retinopathy. Her therapist initially considered teaching the client braille, as this would allow her to access any material that is currently available in that format. However, the client, in addition to her retinopathy, was experiencing peripheral neuropathy, such that she had poor two-point discrimination in her fingers. Because of this, she was not able to discriminate the different dot patterns necessary for Braille reading. The suggested intervention failed because of an inability to perceive her environment. When the therapist suggested a talking book reader, three of the available models were rejected for having a mono-

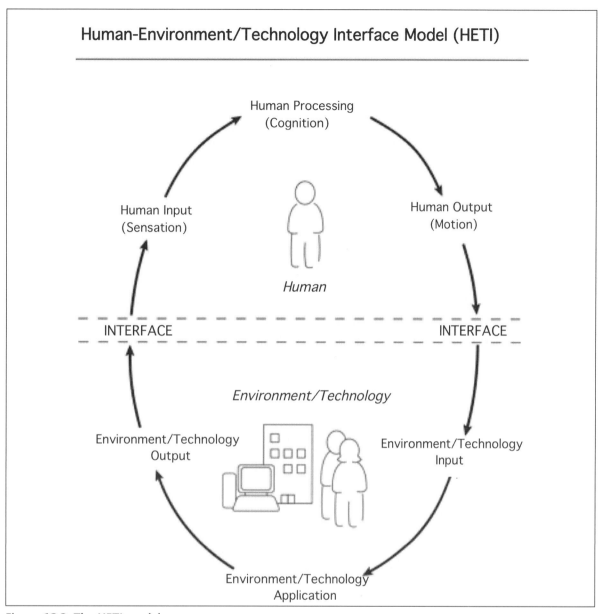

Figure 18.3. The HETI model.

tone control panel with flush controls that could not be easily discriminated. Only when a reader was found that provided easily identifiable (by sight and by touch) controls was this option accepted. The client was able to press the buttons on the device to start and stop playback and raise and lower volume, so she could read in both quiet and noisy environments. The HETI model guides the examination of the input, output, and processing components of both the person and the device.

Human Interface Assessment Model

The Human Interface Assessment (HIA) model (Anson, 2001) focuses more closely on the interface be-

tween the person and the task (Figures 18.4, 18.5, and 18.6). Any person, regardless of disability, has a range of skills and abilities. These can be represented by a stepped interface with the person's strengths extending to the right, and weaknesses extending to the left. The difference in levels of ability explains why some people are gifted artists, some are skilled at car repair, and others are effective public speakers. In some cases, the person who is gifted in one area may be significantly limited in others. The gifted public speaker may not be able to reliably change a light bulb, while the skilled auto mechanic may not be able to read functionally. When a person acquires a disability, some part of

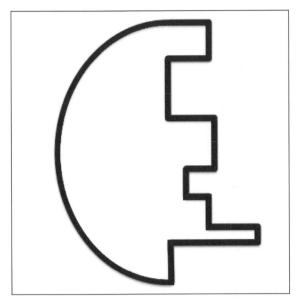

Figure 18.4. The HIA model: The human.

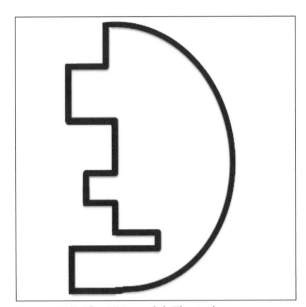

Figure 18.5. The HIA model: The task.

his or her former physical, sensory, or cognitive ability is lost. In some cases, the levels of ability will change throughout the day. As a person fatigues, the available levels of coordination and mental organization may decrease to the point that an activity that was very possible in the morning becomes extremely difficult or impossible in the evening. When evaluating a client for an AT intervention,

the clinician must develop an understanding of the strengths and limitations that the individual brings to the job.

Just as individuals have different levels of skills and abilities, tasks and environments have different levels of physical and cognitive demands. In seafood processing, the job of "picking crab bones" requires endurance for standing at a processing line

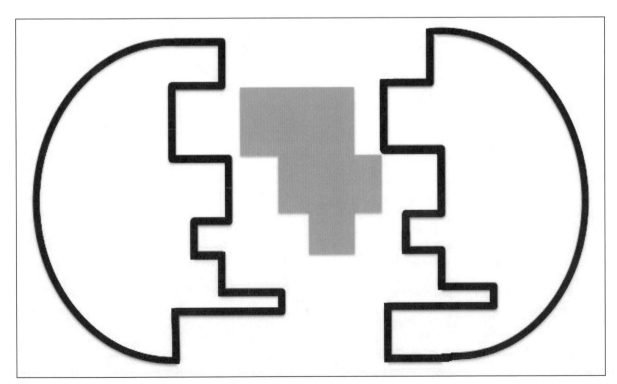

Figure 18.6. The role of assistive technology.

and vigilance to watch for "non-meat" among the crab meat moving past the worker on a conveyer belt. It also requires eye–hand coordination to pick the bones out of the moving stream of meat but does not require much strength or creativity. (Indeed, in a job like this, creativity can be a detriment.) A hod-carrier (assistant to a mason) must be able to carry bricks and mortar over rough ground and up and down ladders. An accountant requires little physical strength but must have a facility with numbers, an understanding of accountancy rules, and the ability to operate information technologies (e.g., calculators, computers). In the process of evaluating a task, the therapist must carefully evaluate the demands of the task and the environment in which it is to be performed.

In rare cases, the skills and abilities of the individual will exactly match the demands of the task and the environment. At such times, the individual will be fully engaged in the task and will be quite satisfied. In many cases, the individual will have skills that exceed the demands of the task, so that they may become bored over time and will seek new challenges.

In cases where the task does not make demands on the individual that exceed his or her skills, no AT will be required, even by an individual with functional limitations. For example, being wheelchair-mobile would be a significant barrier to a hod-carrier but would not present a barrier to an accountant, if the office were accessible. This does not mean that the person does not have functional limitations, only that the current task and environment do not impose demands that the individual cannot meet.

In many cases, the environment and the task present demands that are beyond the skills and abilities of the individual. It is the interaction between the functional limitations of the individual and the demands of the task and environment that cause disability. However, if AT is provided that extends the person's ability to meet the demands of the task, disability can be avoided.

It is important to keep in mind that, because the demands of each task are different, a person may require AT for one task and not for another. Further, the technology must match the demands of the individual tasks. An individual with functional limitations may need assistance with mobility for one task, with organization for another task, and with coordination for a third. Because technologies are designed to meet specific needs, in many cases an individual will need a variety of technologies through the day.

The HAAT, HETI, and HIA models of AT are useful tools to help the therapist organize thinking about the service delivery process. The HAAT model, the broadest of the models, reminds the therapist to examine the nature of the person, the task, the assistive technology, and the cultural and physical contexts of an AT intervention. The HETI model looks more closely at the internal and external processing of the task and reminds the clinician to examine each stage of the process for the client and the setting to ensure a match. The HIA model looks in even more detail at the abilities of the individual and the demands of the task and reminds the therapist that these abilities and demands occur at levels of function. It also describes the fit of the AT technology into the interface between the person and the task to be performed.

Domains of Assistive Technology

The National Institute on Disability and Rehabilitation Research (NIDRR) sponsors an online database of assistive technology known as ABLEDATA (2009). This resource lists over 35,000 commercial and custom-made products, of which over 22,000 are currently available. Clearly, it would not be practical to sort through all available technologies each time a device or service is needed. Some means of imposing order on the field is necessary.

One way is to divide the technologies into subgroups. There are many equally valid ways of subgrouping assistive technologies, just as there are many ways to group flowers. Flowers can be sorted by color, by climate zones, or by size, for example. Similarly, assistive technologies can be sorted by cost, by power source, or by manufacturer. For our purposes, assistive technologies will be categorized by the life activities to which they are typically applied. Even in this grouping there will be some room for disagreement, because a technology may be applied in ways that the designer did not consider.

Self-Care and Daily Living

Gaining the ability to bathe, dress, groom, and eat independently is one of the milestones of maturity. After learning to walk, potty training may be the most important landmark of infant development. For an adult with an acquired disability or age-related changes, losing these hallmarks of independence can be emotionally devastating, socially limiting, and possibly considered a reversion to the role of a child. Because of this, a great deal of effort in the field of occupational therapy has been applied to maintaining independence in the basic activities of daily living (BADLs).

Long before the appearance of an organized field of AT, occupational therapists were using dressing aids such as zipper pulls, buttonhooks, and sock aids. Similarly, therapists are generally perfectly willing to consider bath benches, long-handled sponges, and bathing mitts as fundamental tools in occupational therapy. The dressing, bathing, and grooming aids are all intended to allow a person with a disability to perform tasks that people without disabilities perform without aids. Hence, they all meet the definition of AT.

In the activity of dressing, occupational therapists routinely offer a wide range of assistive technologies. For clients who have difficulty with reaching, occupational therapists may provide dressing sticks, sock aids, or long-handled shoehorns. Because reaching shoes to tie them can be difficult, an occupational therapist may recommend or provide elastic shoe laces, slip-on shoes, or hook-and-loop fasteners. If the client has difficulty with fasteners, the occupational therapist may recommend adapted fasteners or may provide buttonhooks and zipper pulls. If the client cannot see colors but wants to be able to dress independently while avoiding colors that clash, the occupational therapist may provide tactile coding on the client's clothing, so that those items with two raised knots at the waistline can be worn together, but items with one knot should not be combined with items with three, for example.

For clients with difficulty in managing food and drink, occupational therapists have a wide range of assistive technologies available. One-handed eaters (individuals who have experienced stroke or amputation, for example) may have difficulty with cutting food or opening containers. The occupational therapist may provide a rocker knife (either a curved blade conventional knife or a variant on the Inupiat "ulu" knife (*Inupiat Style Ulu Knives*, 2008)) to allow the one-handed adult to cut a steak independently. High-sided plates may make scooping peas easier. Cups with large or adjustable handles may allow clients with limited hand function to lift their coffee to their mouths without spilling. For those who cannot lift a cup, long, flexible straws can give the client control during drinking.

When families are asked about the skills they find most important in maintaining a disabled or aging family member in the home, the most common responses are independence in bathing and toileting. To address these needs, occupational therapists commonly draw from a wide range of assistive technologies.

In bathing, one fundamental issue is the risk of falling. The assistive technologies that occupational therapists use to address such balance issues include tools such as grab bars, bath benches, and bath lifts. To assist washing distal portions of the body, occupational therapists recommend long-handled bath brushes and hand-held showers. For clients with limited hand function, a bath mitt or soap dispenser may enhance independence.

For toileting, an occupational therapist may recommend grab rails for balance and a raised toilet seat for assistance in standing from the toilet. In addition, however, occupational therapists may recommend devices to assist with hygiene, including custom toilet paper holders (for hygiene, not dispensing), bidet-like attachments, and adapted urinals.

To assist an individual in grooming, the occupational therapist may draw on another set of assistive technologies. These include adapted hairbrushes and combs for clients with limited grip and product dispensers for those with one hand or poor coordination. For those with limited grip or dexterity, adapted shaving and toothbrushing aids may be recommended. Some of these may be mass-market devices that are easier to use (e.g., electric shavers in place of manual razors), but others may have been designed specifically for individuals with disabilities (suction brushes and toothpaste dispensers).

While some, if not most, assistive technologies for self-care are easily understood, are available at low cost, and use relatively low technology, they are of great importance to the person who needs them. Other types of self-care technologies are more high-tech. Feeding machines are intended to pick up bite-sized quantities of food and deliver them to the user's mouth. Although these are conceptually quite straightforward, producing reliable devices has proven to be very challenging. An even greater challenge is posed by the field of rehabilitation robotics. In Japan and many parts of Europe, the number of individuals requiring assistance with daily living will soon outnumber the population able to provide it. To answer this need, research is being conducted to develop robots that will be able to assist with transfers, do light housework, and provide companionship. Functional service robots may be years away from the clinic but will be needed in the near future.

Instrumental Activities of Daily Living

Beyond the basic activities of daily living, occupational therapists must deal with the larger category of instrumental activities of daily living (IADLs). IADLs are those activities that go beyond basic self-care to managing oneself in the environment, including cleaning one's home, preparing meals, using the telephone, and managing one's money. As with the BADLs, occupational therapists rely on a wide range of assistive technologies to enable independence in daily living.

Many assistive technologies used to clean the home are adaptations or specialized versions of the same devices that are used by people without disabilities. A person who is not able to grasp and hold a duster or broom may find that adapted handles are beneficial. Replacing brooms with lightweight sweepers may also improve independence in cleaning. A "robot vacuum" such as Roomba[1] may be a novelty for a person without disabilities but will allow a person with limited endurance to be independent in cleaning her floors. Thus, for someone without disabilities, the device is not assistive technology, but for a person with a C-7 SCI or macular degeneration, it is.

Beyond the BADL of self-feeding, food management includes the larger area of meal preparation. While meal preparation is only a chore and survival skill for some, it is a highly valued activity for others. In either case, maintaining personal independence in meal preparation can be important to the health and well-being of the individual. As with dressing and grooming, occupational therapists can provide a wide range of assistive technologies that support independence in meal preparation. Such devices such as pan-holders allow a one-handed cook to stir food on the stove-top.

Some assistive technologies were developed for other purposes but can provide essential assistance to the cook with limited hand function. Consider, for example, the task of adding eggs to a recipe being prepared by a one-handed cook. If the cook has very good hand control, she or he might be able to learn one-handed cracking successfully. If the cook has less hand control, the adaptive technique of throwing an egg into a mixing bowl, then picking out the shell might be offered. A therapist who is aware of more alternatives may find solutions such as an "egg topper,[2]" which is designed to remove the top from soft-boiled eggs but can as easily remove the top of a raw egg, which can then be poured from the shell into the mixing bowl (Figure 18.7).

An individual with time management difficulties secondary to head injury may need some sort of reminder system. Historically, occupational therapists recommended appointment books in which the individual would write coming appointments, which

---

[1]iRobot, 8 Crosby Drive, Bedford, MA 01730; 781.430.3000.

[2]Sur la Table, http://www.surlatable.com/product/kitchen+%26+bar+tools/cooks+tools/egg+topper.do#

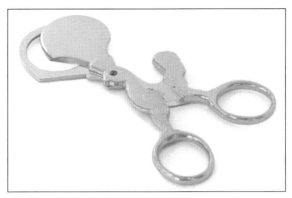

**Figure 18.7. The Egg Topper.
Image used with permission of Sur La Table, 5701 Sixth Avenue South, Suite 486, Seattle, WA 98108; 206-613-6002.**

would be looked up in the future. Electronic aids provided a more reliable reminder, as they did not depend on the client looking for an appointment at regular intervals. Unfortunately, the expensive and bulky systems developed for individuals with disabilities were neither particularly functional nor well accepted. When busy executives started using personal digital assistants, however, reminder systems became available that were small, convenient, and not stigmatizing. Modern cell phone technology allows options such as using the integrated appointment calendar of a cell phone to cue a person with mild cognitive impairments as well as providing an automatic or human-mediated service to call the client and provide reminders of coming appointments.

Devices for Work, Play, and Leisure

To a large extent, advanced assistive technology development has been driven by funding. Devices for self-care, both BADLs and IADLs, are often paid for by insurance providers and therefore have a relatively large market. Devices that enable employment are often funded by the Office of Vocational Rehabilitation and are therefore also prevalent. Devices for personal enjoyment, which is not considered "medically necessary" by many outside the field of occupational therapy, must often be paid for by the individual, so the market is much smaller, and the options are fewer, but hardly absent.

Assistive technologies to enable employment cover a wide range of applications. Most can be categorized as enabling access to and operation of tools, but the tools used in a job vary widely. In information processing, assistive technologies may allow access to telecommunications or computers. These technologies include telephones that allow calls to be made using voice, large buttons, or

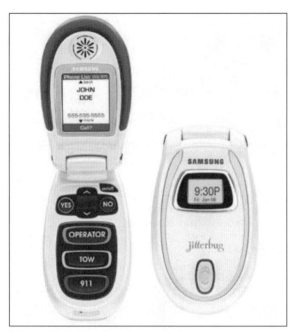

Figure 18.8. The Jitterbug cellphone.

operator assistance. Telephones are available that are hearing aid–compatible (sending signals directly to the user's hearing aid rather than depending on the speaker and microphone for the connection) or that use Braille displays.

As cellular telephones become smaller and gain features, they tend to become less and less usable by individuals with disabilities. The small displays on many cellular telephones can be difficult to see for a person with limited visual acuity. The small keyboards (especially those that provide a full QWERTY keyboard for texting) can be very difficult to operate for a person with limited hand control. Some adapted telephones, such as the Jitterbug[3] from Samsung, are available to meet some of the needs of those with age-related changes, but these do not yet provide access to a wide range of individuals (Figure 18.8).

Assistive technologies for information systems (computers) access are also diverse. For an individual who has difficulty with a conventional keyboard, assistive technologies are available to rearrange the keys to a more efficient pattern, make the keyboard larger or smaller, or change its behavior. The keyboard can be replaced by one or more switches, providing text input through scanning or Morse code. Some computers allow text input by voice, for those whose speech is more reliable than

their hands. For the person who has difficulty seeing the information display, the content can be made larger, can have increased or reduced contrast, or can be translated to sound (speech output) or touch (braille). Similarly, the sounds produced by information technology can be converted to lights "visual beep"), vibration, or even words (transcripts of audio tracks).

Job-related technologies for manufacturing and other technologies include modifications of conventional tools, innovative applications of existing tools, and custom tools and supports. Such assistive technologies are often highly specific, designed to enhance individuals' functions for very specific jobs. When these adaptations are highly successful, they may be provided to workers without disabilities as well. For example, a device that raised a bicycle to a level where it could be worked on by a person with limited ability to work near the floor was so successful that it became a widely used tool for workers without disabilities.

Seating, Positioning, and Mobility

Because individuals who need seating are also likely to require mobility aids, it is common to treat seating, positioning, and mobility as a single area of assistive technology. In fact, the three areas should be considered as overlapping but distinct areas of expertise, each with its own set of skills (Figure 18.9).

Seating

The area of seating includes wheelchair seating, which in clinical practice may be the primary focus

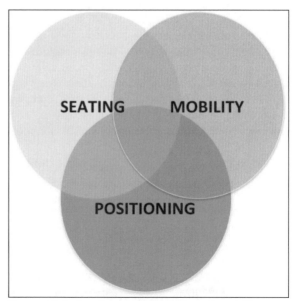

Figure 18.9. Seating, positioning, and mobility.

---

[3]Jitterbug Customer Service, P. O. Box 4428, Carlsbad, CA 92018; 1-800-733-6632.

of some practitioners. However, when considering seating for comfort, pressure management, or postural control, seating may also include accommodations to chair height at workstations or at tables for a person who is ambulatory. Many individuals who are able to walk independently or with mobility aids find rising from a too-low seat to be challenging. Providing a raised seat can be an important application of AT.

Positioning

Similarly, positioning is often an aspect of wheelchair provision, but individuals who require postural supports when seated in a wheelchair may also require aids when in bed, taking a shower, or when sitting in a favorite chair watching television. Positioning may include adjusting work surfaces for proper body alignment or providing prone-standers when a client is not seated.

Mobility

The broad area of mobility includes a wide range of assistive technology in addition to manual and powered wheelchairs (e.g., canes, crutches, walkers). Some of these overlap with seating and positioning. Some wheelchair users also require seating systems that provide pressure relief and postural support. Some people who use a cane or walker may require adapted seating when at the table. Some individuals may require only a mobility aid and no adaptive seating at all.

AT can be for other than ambulation. If a client requires an assistive device to move in bed, that is a type of mobility. Adaptations that allow driving or using mass transit also are considered examples of mobility technology. Just as in other areas of AT, the adaptations are those that allow the person with a disability to perform the same tasks (e.g., movement in bed, driving a car, riding a bus) that those without disability can do without the technology.

Environmental Adaptation and Control

The built environment (e.g., buildings, sidewalks, plazas) may be considered an environment within which a person performs a task or as an assistive technology that facilitates the task. For example, a person without disability might be able to walk from the house to the garage across the lawn and garden, while a person using a manual wheelchair might require a sidewalk. The sidewalk is part of the environment but also allows the person with a disability to perform a mobility task that the person without disability can do without it, qualifying it as AT.

Universal design has complicated AT while also improving the lives of people with disabilities. In cases where a person with a functional limitation is asked to perform a task—such as getting from the house to the garage—that does not make demands that the person cannot meet, no disability occurs. In that case, the sidewalk can be taken either as keeping a functional limitation from producing a disability or the assistive technology that enables the task.

One way to resolve this dual interpretation is to consider when an architectural feature is applied. If a building is designed and constructed to accommodate people with and without disabilities, it can be taken as an example of universal design, minimizing the need for assistive technologies. But if the architecture is a response to the needs of a specific individual with functional limitations, it may be considered an assistive technology.

Assistive technologies that can be applied to existing structures can be either superficial or structural. Lever-style bathroom fixtures and doorknobs, push-button door locks, and firm flooring may be designed into a building without significant structural changes and at relatively low cost. Widening doorways, installing ramps, or changing fixtures (e.g., sinks, tubs) in the bathroom require greater effort and are more expensive; these might be considered "moderate" levels of adaptation. Moving walls to expand a room, creating a new entryway, or building an extension onto a house are examples of "major" adaptations.

As the built environment becomes increasingly defined by electrical devices, the ability of a person to control the immediate environment can be limited. Electronic aids to daily living (EADLs) can be configured so the volitional actions available to an individual with a disability can control many aspects of the environment. To a person with an SCI, the ability to adjust the thermostat may be more than a matter of comfort—room temperature can be critical in controlling body temperature to maintain health and well-being. EADLs can be used to control lighting, open and close doors, operate appliances, and make a telephone call. Depending on the EADL unit, all of these functions can be controlled by voice, breath (sip and puff), a head movement, or any other action that the individual is able to do.

Orthotics and Prosthetics

Broadly speaking, an *orthotic* is a device that supports an existing ability, and a *prosthetic* device replaces an ability that has been lost. Using this broad definition, all of AT may be categorized as either orthotic or prosthetic; the Veterans Administration did exactly that at one time. However, within the field of rehabilitation, the terms orthotics and prosthetics have a special and restricted meaning.

In rehabilitation, an *orthosis* is a device that supports an existing body function that has been limited by injury or disease. An "ankle–foot orthosis" may be worn by an individual with a weak ankle to prevent toe-dragging during walking. Simple ring splints can provide joint protection for a person with swan-neck or boutonnière's deformity. A wrist-driven flexor hinge splint can provide a degree of pinch to a person who has lost the use of the finger flexors. In each case, the body segment remains, but its function has been impaired.

When a person has sustained the loss of a functional body part, whether through developmental abnormalities or secondary to a disease or injury, a *prosthetic device* may be required. Artificial legs, arms, and other body parts have been available throughout recorded history and provide a degree of functional restoration that reduces the effects of disability to some extent. Prosthetic devices generally focus on either maximizing cosmetic features (i.e., looking as much as possible like the body part they replace) or maximizing function, without regard for appearance.

In artificial legs, this difference is clearly shown in the difference between cosmetic feet and athletic feet. The award winning "Seattle Foot" was developed to improve walking and running for unilateral amputees, but is designed to look very much like a biological foot (Burgess, Hittenberger, & Lindh, 1983). It is formed with five toes, toenails, and can even be color matched to the skin tone of the wearer. By contrast, the Össur Flex-Foot Cheetah®[4] looks like (and is) a bent bar of carbon fiber, with no effort to look natural. However, it is such an effective tool for running that the International Association of Athletics Federations ruled that bilateral amputee Oscar Pistorius should not be allowed to complete against runners without a disability because the loss of his legs gave him an unfair advantage (Southern Methodist University, 2009).

In prosthetic arms, there is a similar division. The most commonly used prosthetic hand is probably the Hosmer–Dorrance voluntary-opening terminal device or hook (Fryer & Michael, 2002). This device makes no effort to look like a biological hand but provides a high degree of function. Myoelectric and electronic hands, conversely, are often designed to look natural but do not provide the fine pinch afforded by the hook (Keenan & Atkins, 2001). By contrast, the Otto Bock Electric Greifer[5] sacrifices "human appearance" to provide both fine pinch and strong grip as needed (Figure 18.10).

Communication

One key milestone in infant development occurs when a child becomes able to use language to communicate with others. From the first utterance of "mama" in the first year of life through learning to make a formal presentation, language development is key to functional living. But some people do not develop the ability to communicate fluently, and others lose this ability through disease or injury. Because of the importance of communication in daily life, assistive technology for communication is a diverse and active area.

Within assistive technology, communication systems span the range of simple alerting systems ("I need help") to the system that allows Stephen Hawking to advance theories about the nature of the universe. At the most basic, communication systems may be little more than call lights. An individual who cannot speak over distances may need a way to alert a caregiver to attend. The clinician may be involved in determining how the client will activate such a system and may train the client to use the system to call for help. More advanced systems may include several discrete messages ("I'm hungry" "I hurt." "I need to use the bathroom.") from which the client can select. A speech–language pathologist may determine the content and arrangement of the messages to be included. An occupational therapist may be involved in determining the way the client indicates which message is activated. In advanced systems, the individual may be able to draw on a core vocabulary of commonly used words and use a highly flexible system to generate an unlimited number of sentences.

Assistive technology for communication includes both the ability to produce casual, face-to-face language (usually, but not necessarily, spoken language) and long-distance communication. The technology for face-to-face communication ranges from the very simple to the very specialized and complex. A person who has experienced a head injury may have very rushed and difficult to

---

[4]Össur Americas, 27412 Aliso Viejo Parkway, Aliso Viejo, CA 92656; 800-233-6263.

[5]Otto Bock HealthCare GmbH, Max-Naeder-Str. 15, 37115 Duderstadt, Germany; (+49) 55 27 / 8 48-0.

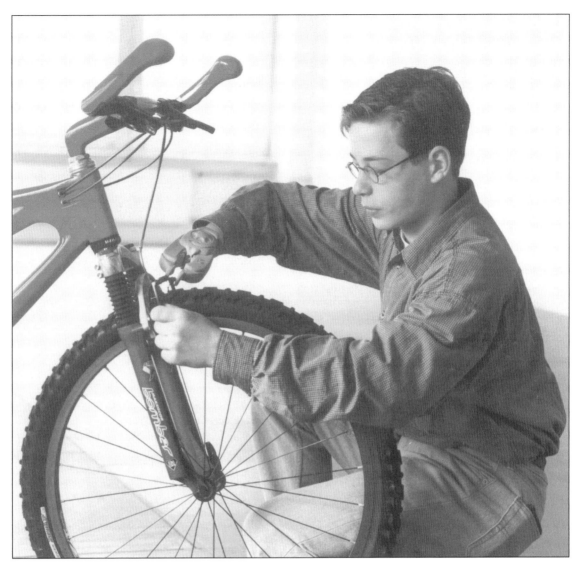

Figure 18.10. The Otto Bock Electric Greifer.
Source: Otto Bock Healthcare, Minneapolis, MN. Used with permission.

understand speech. If the person uses a "pacing board," moving a finger along a simple strip of wood or plastic with dividers spaced along it, he or she may have more intelligible speech. A pad of paper and a pencil can facilitate communication when one person in the conversation is hard of hearing or has a strong accent that is difficult for others to understand. Simple paper communication boards, which show the alphabet or common messages, can provide basic communication with very limited training required. Electronic AAC devices can allow a person who cannot verbalize to express any idea that he or she has but may require hundreds of hours of training before fluent communication is possible. Even after this training, the communication rates achieved by current technology remain very low.

Communication over distances can be in the form of telephone communication or written language. AT for telephone use may be as simple as providing amplification so that the sound from the handset can be heard by a person with impaired hearing. It might be as complex as a computer-mediated augmentative communication interface that allows a nonvocal person to call anyone with a standard telephone and communicate by voice. AT relay services can allow a deaf person who uses a TTY to type messages over the telephone to communicate with people who do not have a TTY through a "relay operator" who reads the typed message aloud and types spoken messages. Specially trained "speech-to-speech" relay operators can listen to the speech of a person with dysarthria and repeat what was said more understandably.

Role of the Clinician in AT Provision

The client should always be involved in selecting any AT device he or she will use. The current "client-centered" approach to service provision often is said to resemble a commercial transaction, where the client determines the desired technologies and services, and then acquires them. This model seems to play down the role of the clinician in the transaction. In fact, the role of the clinician remains vital. As noted earlier, the AbleData database lists over 22,000 currently available devices that are marketed as assistive technology. In addition, many devices not marketed as assistive technology may allow a person with a disability to perform tasks that they cannot manage otherwise . This presents such a huge range of choices to a client that careful decision making is very daunting. In many cases, the first assistive technology device that an individual must select will be chosen shortly after a disabling event, when the client's level of stress is very high, and many life-changing decisions must be made. Expecting the client to make careful decisions from among thousands of complex alternatives is unreasonable.

In the decision-making process, the therapist must act as an expert filter and present a small number of reasonable alternatives for the client to select from. Of hundreds of available dressing aids, a client who has difficulty tying his shoes may be interested in only the elastic shoe laces, slip-on shoes, and hook-and-fastener shoe closers. The advantages and disadvantages of each can be explored, and clients can decide which options they prefer. The decision is in the hands of the client, but the presentation of choices and information about options is the responsibility of the expert therapist.

Sources of Assistive Technology

Do-It-Yourself Assistive Technology

From the early days of the profession, occupational therapists have used splinting materials, wood, wire, and other craft materials to construct adaptive equipment for the specific needs of their clients. At times, this is because the exact device isn't readily available, or because the fabrication process can be part of a therapy program. In other cases, occupational therapists have created custom devices because funding for technology wasn't available, but the therapist's time could be billed. Before the age of the Internet, it may have seemed that there was no commercial value in the device that a specific client needed, so no company would invest in

commercializing a device when few clients would ever be found. Today, it is possible to create an online archive of "home-made" devices reaches millions, making the many "one-off" devices available to many other individuals.

One weakness of custom-made AT is that devices frequently need repair or maintenance that may be time consuming for the therapist who created it.

Commercial Assistive Technology Devices

Assistive technology devices are now available from a wide range of manufacturers and suppliers. While many of the ADL devices continue to be available through ADL catalogs, mainstream companies such as Sears,® Lowe's,® and Home Depot offer a wide range of home adaptation products directly to the consumer.

Internet search engines make it possible for the therapist to locate extremely specialized AT products. The advantage of Web searching is that new products become available to the therapist without the need to obtain new books or catalogs.

Some commercial AT is highly focused and is best suited to individuals with very specific needs. Other devices are more general and can be adjusted to accommodate a wide range of potential users. The role of the therapist in identifying commercial AT is to identify the device that most closely matches the needs of the individual, the demands of the task, and the requirements of the environment.

Role of the Occupational Therapist in Assistive Technology Provision

As noted earlier, there are over 22,000 products currently marketed as AT. Asking the client to make intelligent selections from the universe of available devices would assure poor decisions, abandoned devices, and unmet needs. It is the responsibility of the therapist, who has a thorough understanding of the client's skills and abilities and of the demands of his or her tasks and environments, to narrow the choices to a few from which the client can select. The therapist should tell the client or client's caregivers the likely functional outcomes of the technology, as well as any areas where it will not be useful. In this process, the therapist may obtain information from a number of sources beyond direct experience with the technologies.

Friends and Family of the Client

It is common for a client's friends and family to learn of to a new or unknown AT device or system, either by way of a friend, the media, or online. In many cases, these devices are inappropriate for the client, because they cannot meet the client's specific needs or are not yet commercially available. Some are even fraudulent. In some cases, however, the device will be appropriate for the client or another of the therapist's clients. When the family or a friend offers such assistance, the therapist should accept the information graciously, explain why it is not appropriate if that is the case, and express thanks for their help in keeping up with the rapidly changing AT market.

Assistive Technology Vendors

Many types of assistive technology are available through durable medical equipment vendors (DMEs). The representatives for such companies can often provide detailed information about the products in their catalog and assist with matching technology to the person and task.

While it is the vendor's job to know detailed information about the technology, it is not at all likely that he or she will have the detailed information about the client that the therapist has gathered through evaluation and daily contact. Additionally, while a vendor may have excellent information about the comparative advantages and disadvantages of the company's products, she or he is unlikely to be unbiased. It is as inappropriate to abdicate the AT decision to the vendor as it is to leave it entirely to the client. The occupational therapist should gather information from multiple vendors, make comparisons, and select the best product or mix of products. One of the skills of the advanced clinician is to integrate products from multiple vendors into a cohesive solution for the client.

Preferred Equipment Suppliers and Therapists as Vendors

In many settings, equipment may be supplied either directly by the therapist or from a preferred equipment supplier. This arrangement can simplify the decision process but may not meet the client's needs.

In some settings, especially in rural environments, the therapist will not have ready access to vendors to provide the equipment the clients need. A home health therapist might therefore keep a supply of commonly needed assistive devices on hand and bill the client directly. In other settings, using a preferred provider simplifies administration and allows the therapist to develop a strong relationship with the provider—rather than several weak relationships with several providers.

For the majority of clients, such relationships are perfectly adequate. However, the constant reliance on one source of equipment, whether from personal stores or from a preferred provider, can limit awareness of available solutions. Psychologist Abraham Maslow observed "When the only tool you have is a hammer, it is tempting to treat everything as if it were a nail" (Maslow, 1966). When the therapist routinely solves problems with a small set of assistive devices, there is a tendency to rely on those tools even when better solutions are available. Having a preferred provider is useful, but the therapist should not make him or her an exclusive provider. When the client's needs require a product not available from the preferred provider, the therapist must be ready to go to other providers as needed.

Prescriptions vs. Open-Market Purchases

Increasingly, assistive technologies are available through mass-market outlets. Products that are designed for individuals without a disability may also meet the needs of the client with a disability. Other products are sold specifically to meet the needs of customers with limited function, whether due to disability or aging.

As with almost all considerations in AT, mass-market devices have both advantages and disadvantages. When a device or adaptation is produced for the general market, the market size is usually substantially larger than that for devices intended for use by people with disabilities. Universally designed products or convenience aids can, therefore, often be purchased for a fraction of the cost of specialty products. This lowers the overall cost of care.

As noted earlier, products that are designed for individuals with disabilities often disclose the disability to the world. While some disabilities, such as tetraplegia or blindness, are generally readily observed, others, such as learning disability, are not. Moreover, in many cases, disability continues to carry a social stigma. Individuals with cognitive or learning disabilities may wish their limitations to remain private. When mass-market products become available that provide cognitive supports to busy and distracted executives, the same products can be used to provide support for individuals with cognitive limitations. The same product is used for the same purpose, and the need that is being supplied remains private.

The difficulty in providing mass-market products to individuals with disabilities stems from the current reimbursement system. Products that are medically necessary and identified as AT may be funded without challenge. Products purchased at the department or hardware store may not be recognized as serving a medical need and may not be reimbursed. If the product in question is a measuring cup with grippable handle, the cost may not be a significant issue. But if the product in question is a four-wheeler to allow a farmer with leg weakness access to his fields as an alternative to an all-terrain wheelchair, the issue might entail thousands of dollars of costs.

Training

The AT process does not end with the delivery of a product to the client. Most AT requires significant training to use effectively. Some assistive technologies function as appliances. Like eyeglasses (an assistive technology), the client simply applies the device, and it provides its assistance without requiring any conscious effort by the user. Other technologies are tools that are manipulated by the client to produce the desired result. This direct interaction with the device may require hundreds of hours to master. If the training is not supplied along with the device, the paucity principle suggests that the unassisted but ineffectual efforts seen before the technology was provided will require less overall energy, and the client will cease to use the device. Only when the adaptive techniques using the assistive technology require less effort than alternatives will the client continue to use and benefit from the technology.

AT is provided to enable specific tasks in specific environments. To the extent possible, the training should be provided in the environment where the device will be used. If access is not available, it may be possible to simulate the environment well enough for the training to be effective, although this compromises the fidelity of the training.

The training should include basic instruction in setting up the device and troubleshooting likely issues. While the client with profound physical disabilities will seldom be the person to set up the device, they are the sole constant in the setting, as attendants and caregivers change. For optimum independence, the client should be trained to direct another person to set up and adjust the device, and to ask the salient questions when the device is not working as expected. If these are done, the client will be able to direct other people in setting up the AT as needed.

Future of Universal Design, Assistive Technology, and Functional Independence

For the person with a disability, the world is a constantly shifting place. Parts of it that were once accessible become less so, and other parts that were inaccessible become more so. These changes often occur as new technologies become available, some of which enable and others of which disable. The introduction of self-cleaning ovens, for example, improved independence in IADLs for people with limited endurance, turning an arduous task into one that meant simply turning a few knobs on the range. At first, only high-end appliances had this feature, meaning individuals with disabilities had to spend more for their appliances. Now, many high-end appliances have smooth touch-panel controls that are impossible to use by touch alone. As a result, a blind individual can now purchase only a lower-end appliances that still use mechanical controls.

From the beginnings of AT, providing access to printed information to individuals with a wide range of disabilities has been an ongoing quest. The search for an effective page turner (one that works with all types of bound materials, from magazines to paperback books) has been so fruitless that asking "Has anyone found a good page-turner?" at the beginning of a presentation will be taken as a joke. Yet, for many years, all printed material has existed in electronic format that can generate a format that is accessible to a person who requires large print, who is blind, or who cannot turn pages. This should have ushered in a golden age of information access. However, most current electronic readers are designed with no thought of disability access. When a book is available to assistive technologies for conversion to voice, the publisher cannot sell the audiobook rights separately.

As business and culture have increasingly moved online over the past decades, the importance of computer access has changed from providing recreation to a requirement for work and education to a basic civil right, as it now is preferred for access to basic social services. New initiatives like "Raising the Floor" (2009) are seeking to ensure that basic access is available to everyone, regardless of disability, literacy, or age.

The role of the occupational therapist in this changing landscape will not change. Occupational therapists will work to help clients participate in meaningful activities. The tools available will change, as will some of the activities that clients find meaningful. In the early days of occupational therapy, basic handicrafts such as copper tooling, wood carving, and leather embossing were a part of everyday life and were key therapeutic activities. Today, those activities may be replaced by blogging, Web searching, and tweeting. For others, downhill skiing, sailing, or mountain climbing may continue to be important activities; with the help of occupational therapists and new generations of prosthetics and adaptive aids, these people can look forward to enhanced participation.

The problems occupational therapists will encounter will be the same as those they have faced in the past. On one hand, new technologies can be created recognizing that potential users have a range of sizes, skills, and limitations—universal design can make the world more accessible, and the need for occupational therapists to provide AT will decrease. On the other hand, when new structures, devices, and technologies are designed for only people without a disability—without considering accessibility— the need for therapists to perform careful assessment of the client, the task, and the environment, and to recommend technologies that enable independence, will remain.

Acknowledgment

This chapter revision started as a coauthorship with Roger Smith, whose busy schedule precluded his full participation in the process. The author acknowledges and thanks Roger for his work on the earlier editions of this chapter and in helping to form this chapter. However, any conceptual or factual errors are the sole responsibility of the author of this version.

Study Questions

1. What are the sources of AT information, and what is their value to the therapist and the client?

2. What is the role of the occupational therapist in a client-centered approach to AT provision?

3. How can a therapist balance the amount of effort applied to the various approaches to therapy (e.g., reduction of impairment, environmental adaptation, human assistance)?

4. Which environmental features in your practice area designed to improve access for individuals with disabilities do you use as well?

5. What is the paucity principal, and how does it apply to adaptive strategies in occupational therapy practice?

6. What are the advantages and disadvantages of using off-the-shelf, mass-market products as AT?

References

ABLEDATA. (2009). Retrieved July 1, 2009, from http://www.abledata.com

American Occupational Therapy Association. (2008). Occupational therapy practice framework: Domain and process (2nd ed.). *American Journal of Occupational Therapy, 62,* 625–683.

Americans With Disabilities Act of 1990, Pub. L. 101–336, 42 U.S.C. §12101.

Anson, D. (2001). Assistive technology. In L. W. Pedretti & M. B. Early (Eds.), *Occupational therapy: Practice skills for physical dysfunction* (5th ed., pp. 257–275). St. Louis, MO: Mosby.

Bailey, R. W. (1989). *Human performance engineering: Using human factors/ergonomics to achieve computer system usability* (2nd ed.). Englewood Cliffs, NJ: Prentice Hall.

Boston Athletic Association (2009a). *113th Boston Marathon.* Retrieved April 20, 2009, from http://www.bostonmarathon.org/BostonMarathon/113thMarathon.asp

Boston Athletic Association (2009b). *Top finishers.* Retrieved December 11, 2009, from http://www.bostonmarathon.org/2009/cf/public/TopFinishers.htm

Burgess, E. M., Hittenberger, S. M., & Lindh, D. (1983). The Seattle Prosthetic Foot: A design for active sports: Preliminary studies. *Orthotics and Prosthetics, 37*(1), 25.

Carlyle, T. (1833). *Sartor resartus.* Last accessed October 12, 2010, at http://digital.library.upenn.edu/webbin/gutbook/lookup?num=1051

Cook, A. M., & Hussey, S. M. (2002). *Assistive technologies: Principles and practice* (2nd ed.). Philadelphia: Mosby.

Cook, A. M., & Polgar, J. M. (2007). *Cook and Hussey's assistive technologies: Principles and practice.* St. Louis, MO: Mosby.

Fryer, C. M., & Michael, J. W. (2002). *Upper-limb prosthetics: Body-powered components.* Retrieved December 12, 2009, from http://www.oandplibrary.org/alp/chap06-01.asp

Inupiat style Ulu knives. (2008). Retrieved December 11, 2009, from http://www.ulu.com/gnpstore/cat3–1.htm

Keenan, D. D., & Atkins, D. J. (2001). Electric-powered prostheses. In L. W. Pedretti & M. B. Early (Eds.), *Occupational therapy: Practice skills for physical dysfunction* (pp. 945–946). St. Louis, MO: Mosby.

Kimbrough, P. (2008, June 13). *How Braille began.* Retrieved July 17, 2009, from http://www.brailler.com/braillehx.htm

Maslow, A. H. (1966). *The psychology of science: A reconnaissance.* Washington, DC: Regnery.

Merriam-Webster's Collegiate Dictionary. (10th ed.). (1996) Springfield, MA: Merriam-Webster.

Raising the Floor. (2009). *Putting the Web within reach of all those with disability, literacy, or aging-related barriers, regardless of their economic status.* Retrieved December 12, 2009, from http://raisingthefloor.net

Smith, R. O. (1991). Technological approaches to performance enhancement. In C. H. Christiansen (Ed.), *Occupational therapy: Overcoming human performance deficits.* Thorofare, NJ: Slack.

Southern Methodist University. (2009). *Oscar Pistorius: Amputee sprinter runs differently.* Retrieved December 12, 2009, from http://www.sciencedaily.com/releases/2009/06/090629132200.htm

Technology-Related Assistance for Individuals with Disabilities Act of 1988 as amended in 1994, Pub. L. 100-407 and Pub. L. 103-218 (U.S.C.).

Chapter 19

Environmental Adaptations: Foundation for Daily Living

MARGARET A. CHRISTENSON, MPH, OTR, FAOTA

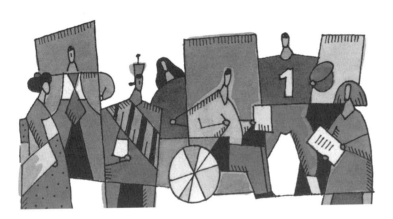

KEY WORDS

accessibility

accessible design

barrier-free design

functional capacity as a basis for design

home evaluation

home modifications

reverse mortgage

transgenerational design

universal design

visitability

HIGHLIGHTS

- The physical characteristics of a home can be either a barrier or a support to occupational performance.

- There are appropriate and effective environmental adaptations for any functional limitation to enhance occupational performance.

- Technological advances can increase the safety and function of a person who might have been unable to live alone prior to these supports.

- Universal design meets the occupational performance needs of people of all ages, sizes, and abilities by creating accessible and adaptive designs.

- There is a plethora of Web sites and resources available for home safety checklists, home modification ideas, adaptive solutions, and financing options.

Note. Portions of this chapter are reprinted with permission from *PresentEase: Compensations for Age-Related Sensory Changes*, M. A. Christenson, 4001 Stinson Boulevard, Suite 404, Minneapolis, MN: Lifease, Inc. Copyright © 2007, by Lifease, Inc.

OBJECTIVES

After reading this material, readers will be able to

- Discuss the legislation and movements that were the precursors to the Americans with Disabilities Act (ADA);

- Explain why ADA has only minimal effect on home design;

- Explain how functional capability can be used as a basis for design;

- List age-related adaptations for the sensory and physical changes of aging, and describe how compensating for these changes will benefit a wider population;

- Describe various home evaluations and ways they might be applied;

- Explain ways that home modifications may be financed for low-income households; and

- Discuss how a reverse mortgage can make it possible for people to obtain home modifications that enable them to continue living in their own home.

Our environment is a major component of living well and being able to care for ourselves. This is so fundamentally obvious that its significance is often overlooked. The environment should allow us to rest, do daily tasks, conduct work, move about, and play with as few limitations as possible. Yet the environment is a "hidden modality"—a treatment technique that is available but too often overlooked. The people using a space should be the major consideration in discussions of its design. This chapter discusses how one's environment relates to one's ability to carry out activities of daily living (ADLs) and how the environment can be adapted to changes that occur over time as a result of aging or disability.

Setting the Stage: Questions Asked When Building a New Home

Someone is building or remodeling a home must make many decisions:

- Where is the home, or where will it be located?
- How much will construction cost?
- How many people will live there? What are their ages?
- What work or hobbies need to be accommodated?

If an occupant of the home is in a wheelchair or has obvious visual difficulties, an additional set of questions must be answered: How wide must the doorways be? How will the person move over the threshold when entering the home? Can tactual markings be installed to help distinguish the function of various knobs, buttons, or switches?

When such questions are asked, the focus becomes compensating for a disability, entailing an entire set of specialized ideas and building approaches. When people with disabilities become segregated from the rest of society, however, accommodating a disability is sometimes perceived as less than desirable. Special terms in the design field sometimes contribute to this stigma; for example, terms such as *accessible, barrier-free, assistive technology,* and *assistive devices* all indicate designs and features considered outside the norm.

Historical Perspective

In the first half of the 20th century, civilians with disabilities were largely uncounted (and unassisted) by the government—after World War I, only about 2% of veterans with spinal cord injuries (SCI) survived more than 1 year. After World War II, the survival rate for veterans with SCI increased to 85%, an improvement that prompted major legislation to address the care of veterans. Subsequent amendments to that legislation broadened national recognition of people with disabilities and created rehabilitation benefits for civilians as well (Welch & Palames, 1995).

The polio epidemics of the early 1950s also drew further attention to the needs of civilians with disabilities. In 1954, the government allocated grant funds for research and demonstration projects on rehabilitation (Welch & Palames, 1995).

Legislative and scientific advances through the 1950s focused primarily on the clinical impairments of people with disabilities (Welch & Palames, 1995). In 1961, however, the American National Standards Institute (ANSI) published *A117.1—Making Buildings Accessible to and Usable by the Physically Handicapped.* The new voluntary standards described minimal requirements for eliminating major barriers that prevent people with disabilities from using buildings and facilities, including parking spaces, elevators, and toilet stalls. Unfortunately, as these recommendations were voluntary, they were often ignored and few changes were made (Welch & Palames, 1995).

During the mid-1960s, a national commission found that the greatest single obstacle to employment for people with disabilities was the physical design of the buildings and facilities they used. In response to those findings, Congress passed the Architectural Barriers Act of 1968 (P.L. 90-480). The act required that all buildings designed, constructed, altered, or leased with federal funds be made accessible. Following amendments in 1970 and 1976, the act began to have an effect on the accessibility of public buildings.

Public attitudes toward accessible building design have changed slowly. For significant change to occur, social and political perspectives on this issue must shift from a focus on overcoming the functional and vocational limitations of people who are labeled as "different" to emphasizing the environment's role in promoting full participation by everyone. This shift requires recognizing the role environment often plays in a person's disability (Hahn, 1988). One agent for change has been the disability rights movement, which had its roots in the civil rights movement and began to have its agendas recognized in legislation during the 1970s (Welch & Palames, 1995).

Sections of the Rehabilitation Act of 1973 (P.L. 93-112) provided the first regulatory definition of discrimination against people with disabilities. The act shifted disability issues from the realm of social services and therapeutic practice to the context of political and civil rights.

In 1975, Congress passed the Education for All Handicapped Children Act (P.L. 94-142), which mandated free, appropriate public education for children with disabilities. To accomplish "mainstreaming," public schools had to eliminate accessibility barriers.

In 1982, the Architectural and Transportation Barriers Compliance Board (ATBCB; 1982) issued its "Minimum Guidelines and Requirements for Accessible Design." The guidelines established the basis for the Uniform Federal Accessibility Standards (UFAS) issued jointly by the U.S. General Services Administration, U.S. Department of Defense, U.S. Department of Housing and Urban Development, and U.S. Postal Service. The Air Carriers Access Act (1986, P.L. 99-435) focused on expanding the rights of people with disabilities to participate in all aspects of society, in this case, the right to air travel.

In 1988, people with disabilities participated in lobbying for civil rights legislation, a process that resulted in Fair Housing amendments that included people with disabilities and families with children and the initial version of the Americans with Disabilities Act (ADA). An examination of the democratic tradition of equal rights was the focus (Welch & Palames, 1995).

ADA (P.L. 101-336) was passed in 1990. This legislation has been responsible for many positive changes for people with disabilities. The intent of the law is to extend civil rights protection to people with disabilities and to prohibit discrimination in employment, state and local government services, public transportation, telecommunications, and public accommodations (Perry, Jawer, Murdoch, & Dinegar, 1991). Many of the guidelines associated with ADA focus on accessibility and concentrate primarily on public buildings, including lobbies, dining rooms, restrooms, and admitting offices. It was hoped that through responsively designed environments and assistive technology, billions of dollars could be saved in institutional care that is largely underwritten by federal programs.

ADA has fostered public awareness that people with disabilities are not only people to be cared for but also viable members of and contributors to society. Today, places and products are being designed for use by a broad range of people, including those with disabilities.

Assistive Technology

Developing products to meet the needs of special populations is not a new concept to occupational therapists. Occupational therapy has been involved with providing assistive devices to clients almost from the inception of the profession. *Assistive technology (AT)* encompasses the research, development, and provision of services associated with assistive devices (Mann & Lane, 1995). The term also applies to devices created specifically to enhance the physical, sensory, or cognitive abilities of people with disabilities and to help them function more independently.

In the middle of the 20th century, AT emerged as one of the domains of rehabilitation engineering, a specialty that applies scientific principles and engineering methodologies to the problems of people with special needs. New engineering research centers sponsored by the Department of Veterans Affairs (VA) and other federal organizations addressed other technological problems of rehabilitation, including communication, mobility, and transportation. Now, decades later, ADA has helped awaken the American conscience to the fact that a broad sector of the population can benefit from more accessible and usable spaces and products.

Various terms have come into use to express such possibilities. *Accessibility* means free and normal movement throughout the environmental setting (Pirkl, 1994). An accessible environment minimizes obstacles and provides adequate, clearly defined cues for users with specific disabilities. The term *barrier-free* came into use during the 1950s as developing legislation responded to the demands of veterans and other people with disabilities and their advocates.

Early advocates of barrier-free design and architectural accessibility recognized the legal, economic, and social power of addressing the common needs of people with and without disabilities. As architects began to wrestle with the implementation of new standards, they realized that segregated accessibility features typically were more expensive to build or produce and were usually unsightly. They also noticed that many environmental changes made to accommodate people with disabilities actually benefited everyone. Today, architects and designers are beginning to recognize that many such features can be commonly provided, making them less expensive and stigmatized, and more attractive and marketable (Welch & Palames, 1995).

Perceptions of the scope of assistive devices also are changing. For example, some manufacturers have changed the marketing of their products. Nowhere is this approach better exemplified than with the way the OXO Company markets its "Good Grips" line of cooking tools. Promotional materials never mention the tools' usefulness for people with weak grasp. Rather, OXO's entire advertising has focused on the tools' ease of use and comfort. "Good Grips are designed by a fellow cook; they are easier to use, easier to hold, and easier to care for" (Farber, 1992). People like to hear "can-do" messages, and by evoking positive images, OXO's marketing approach directs consumers' attention to their products' universal appeal.

The therapist must be mindful, however, that just because a person needs a specific adaptation or adaptive product does not mean that he or she will purchase or use it. Most people who have difficulties with daily tasks still see themselves as active and healthy (Yeung, 2003). A primary reason people resist adaptations that are "assistive" in nature may be the desire to continue to be perceived as active and healthy. Indeed, using "assistive" to describe a device implies a need for help, even though many such devices actually promote greater independence. As a result of these perceptions, people often choose to "make do" until an overwhelming crisis forces them to adapt.

One way for these tools of living to become an accepted part of everyone's home is to change the focus from creating items that people "need" to items that they "want." The OXO example illustrates an approach that can be useful in marketing the benefits of assistive tools, particularly to older people. Also, because so many people prefer items that are attractive rather than utilitarian, the aesthetics of assistive devices and adaptive settings cannot be overlooked.

During the past 20 years, as people with disabilities have rebelled against being labeled "different," a movement to reduce the separation created by "special-needs" environments and products has taken hold. As professionals with and without disabilities in architecture, housing, interior design, medicine, nursing, physical and occupational therapy, and other allied fields have joined this movement, the trend toward greater inclusion has accelerated.

Universal Design

Pivotal to this change in thinking was the work of the late Ron Mace, an architect at the University of North Carolina. Mace coined the term *universal design*, and in 1988 he clarified the definition as "the concept of designing all products and the built environment to be aesthetic and usable to the greatest extent possible by everyone, regardless of their age, ability, or status in life."

Accessible or adaptable design codes and standards primarily have targeted people with mobility restrictions. By contrast, universal design has become an umbrella term that encompasses designs that meet the needs of a wide range of people. These include accessible and adaptive designs but target people of all ages, sizes, and abilities (Mace, 1988). Universal design integrates rather than segregates. It focuses on the widest possible applicability of products and spaces, does not restrict its focus to people with disabilities, and avoids potentially stigmatizing labels such as "special" or "different." Nonetheless, concepts of universal design have not been wholeheartedly embraced by the public. Some of that reluctance may come from the embedded notion that "universal design implies it could happen to me" (Leibrock & Terry, 1999).

Modifications that work for everyone and allow us to function at our maximum capacity can be seamless and totally inconspicuous. They may be as simple as an electronic switch or push button that allows us to automatically open and close a drape, a window, a door, or a garage door. Without the button, each of these tasks requires a different amount of strength and different uses of the body and hands. Some people may give no thought to opening a curtain, door, or window but find it challenging to open a garage door. Other people would find it difficult to open any of those items without assistive devices.

A variety of widely used tools and devices reduce physical effort and make everyday tasks easier for everyone. For example, no one relishes carrying garbage and trash to the curb for pickup, but the task has been made easier by the introduction of wheeled trash containers. Having used a wheeled container, few people prefer to return to lifting heavy trash cans. Labor-saving electrical devices also have become common; few kitchens lack an electric mixer, blender, toaster, microwave oven, and coffeemaker. The tasks these appliances perform make cooking considerably easier. These tools and devices make every home environment easier and more accessible.

Principles of Universal Design

With major funding provided by the National Institute on Disability and Rehabilitation Research of the U.S. Department of Education, the Center for Univer-

sal Design developed seven principles of universal design (Center for Universal Design, 1997). They cover a wide range of design disciplines, including environments, products, and communications, and provide criteria that can be used to evaluate existing designs, guide the design process, and educate designers and consumers on the characteristics of more usable products and environments (Table 19.1). The principles are intended to offer guidance so that designs will better meet the needs of as many users as possible.

Table 19.1. Principles of Universal Design

Principle 1

Equitable Use: The design is useful and marketable to people with diverse abilities.

Guidelines:
1a. Provide the same means of use for all users: identical whenever possible; equivalent when not.
1b. Avoid segregating or stigmatizing any users.
1c. Provisions for privacy, security, and safety should be equally available to all users.
1d. Make the design appealing to all users.

Principle 2

Flexibility in Use: The design accommodates a wide range of individual preferences and abilities.

Guidelines:
2a. Provide choice in methods of use.
2b. Accommodate right- or left-handed access and use.
2c. Facilitate the user's accuracy and precision.
2d. Provide adaptability to the user's pace.

Principle 3

Simple and Intuitive Use: Use of the design is easy to understand, regardless of the user's experience, knowledge, language skills, or current concentration level.

Guidelines:
3a. Eliminate unnecessary complexity.
3b. Be consistent with user expectations and intuition.
3c. Accommodate a wide range of literacy and language skills.
3d. Arrange information consistent with its importance.
3e. Provide effective prompting and feedback during and after task completion.

Principle 4

Perceptible Information: The design communicates necessary information effectively to the user, regardless of ambient conditions or the user's sensory abilities.

Guidelines:
4a. Use different modes (pictorial, verbal, tactile) for redundant presentation of essential information.
4b. Provide adequate contrast between essential information and its surroundings.

4c. Maximize "legibility" of essential information.
4d. Differentiate elements in ways that can be described (i.e., make it easy to give instructions or directions).
4e. Provide compatibility with a variety of techniques or devices used by people with sensory limitations.

Principle 5

Tolerance for Error: The design minimizes hazards and the adverse consequences of accidental or unintended actions.

Guidelines:
5a. Arrange elements to minimize hazards and errors: most used elements, most accessible; hazardous elements eliminated, isolated, or shielded.
5b. Provide warnings of hazards and errors.
5c. Provide fail-safe features.
5d. Discourage unconscious action in tasks that require vigilance.

Principle 6

Low Physical Effort: The design can be used efficiently and comfortably and with a minimum of fatigue.

Guidelines:
6a. Allow user to maintain a neutral body position.
6b. Use reasonable operating forces.
6c. Minimize repetitive actions.
6d. Minimize sustained physical effort.

Principle 7

Size and Space for Approach and Use: Appropriate size and space is provided for approach, reach, manipulation, and use regardless of user's body size, posture, or mobility.

Guidelines:
7a. Provide a clear line of sight to important elements for any seated or standing user.
7b. Make reach to all components comfortable for any seated or standing user.
7c. Accommodate variations in hand and grip size.
7d. Provide adequate space for the use of assistive devices or personal assistance.

Source. Connell, B. R., Jones, M., Mace, R., Mueller, J., Mullick, A., Ostroff, E., et al. (1997). *The principles of universal design.* Raleigh, North Carolina State University, Center for Universal Design. Used with permission.

A Convergence of Design Trends

Although they evolved from different starting points, universal design and assistive technology often converge in practice. AT attempts to meet the specific needs of individuals; universal design strives to integrate people with disabilities into mainstream society, laying a foundation on which environments and products meet the needs of a broad segment of society. At the intersection of the two disciplines, products and environments are neither clearly universal nor clearly assistive; rather, they have characteristics of both types of design. An attractive, properly placed grab bar, for example, acts as an assistive device to help a person get in or out of a bathtub. When towels are hung on it, it blends into the decor and becomes another component of universal design (Figure 19.1).

Professionals in many fields come together to wrestle with this task of creating environments that everyone may use to the greatest extent possible. The potential benefits of this cooperation seem exciting but are often unrealized. Consider the collaboration between interior designers and occupational therapists. Designers can learn much from occupational therapists' understanding of the functional needs caused by disability and aging. At the same time, occupational therapists and their clients can benefit from designers' expertise in creating products and environments that work well, are safe, and are attractive for users.

Sometimes conflicts occur. When curb cuts were first introduced, little thought was given to the difficulty they might present for people with visual problems. The focus was strictly on making sidewalks wheelchair accessible. Before the advent of curb cuts, people with severe visual impairments had used the tactual cue of feeling the edge of the curb with their canes. With no curb, this cue was lost.

In response, curb cuts evolved to include textured surfaces on the slope of the cut to restore a tactual cue. This was an improvement, but people with partial sight and who did not use canes still needed a cue to alert them that the end of the curb had been reached. To accommodate this need, color contrast has now been incorporated into the textured slope (Christenson, 1999).

Functional Performance as the Framework for Design

When a living space is built or a tool is made for performing a task, it makes sense that the design of the space or tool should allow as wide a range of people as possible to accomplish the desired task. Because designers, contractors, and manufacturers do not always understand specialized needs, however, environmental features and products often are created that do not work for everyone. A design framework needs to be created that provides guidelines for making products and spaces usable by as many people as possible. To focus this effort, there must be a group for whom

- A well-designed space or tool allows them to function at their maximum capacity;
- The performance components lost or impaired include physical, sensory, and cognitive capabilities;
- Addressing multiple functional needs will allow more activities to be possible in the setting; and
- Modifications allow tasks to be done relatively easily, so that any continued difficulties clearly arise from intrinsic problems directly related to the person's diagnosis or condition rather than from deficiencies in the environment.

The population of older adults constitutes such a group. When features of products or built environments maximize physical, sensory, and cogni-

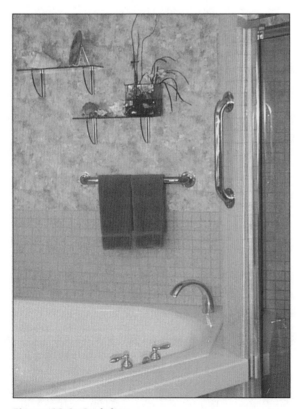

Figure 19.1. Grab bar.

tive capabilities, we are on the road to universal design. Developing adaptations for these age-related changes will create a broad base of tools and environments that are usable by a wide range of people.

Transgenerational Design

Basing design on the compensations needed by an older population is not a new idea. Introduced almost 20 years ago by James Pirkl, *transgenerational design* uses age-related needs as a basis for design. Transgenerational design is the practice of making products and environments compatible with aging-associated physical and sensory impairments that limit activities. It insists that "products and environments be designed at the outset to accommodate a transgenerational population, which includes the young, the middle-aged, and the elderly, without penalty to any group" (Pirkl, 1994, p. 228). Examples of transgenerational design are no-step thresholds at entry doors and placement of handrails on both sides of a staircase.

Visitability

In an attempt to incorporate some of the benefits of universal design info single-family housing, the concept of *visitability* took root in the suburbs of Atlanta in 1986. Visitability seeks to ensure basic access for people with disabilities in newly constructed private homes. Importantly, visitability applies for all homes, not just those for people with special needs. The rationale is that no one should be barred from visiting a home because of the structure's inaccessible design.

The Inclusive Home Design Act (H.R. 1408), discussed in various congressional committees, calls for "basic access"—at least one step-free entrance, wider interior doors, and a bathroom everyone can get into and use—in all homes built or otherwise assisted with federal assistance. The bill is the latest effort of the burgeoning visitability movement in the United States.

Visitability features include no-step entrances, hallways at least 36 inches wide, and one bathroom with a 32-inch doorway in each home or apartment. An advantage of visitability features is that they remove barriers for many groups of people, not just older adults; they work just as well for a child's school friend who may have a disability, parents, aging grandparents, anyone with a broken leg, users of wheeled luggage, parents with strollers, and people with wheelchairs. Visitability allows a home to welcome all people (Clause, 2002). (More information about visitability is available at www.concretechange.com, the movement's founding organization.)

Designing for Children

Children with physical disabilities that affect mobility, stability and balance, hand and arm functions, and other capabilities share some of the same needs as adults with disabilities. They also benefit from no-threshold entrances, automated openers, and ease-of-use items. Significantly, the needs of children with physical disabilities change as they progress through the major developmental stages; infancy, toddler, preschool, school age, adolescence, and early adulthood each bring different challenges and demands. Spaces designed and built with considerable flexibility work best. Major concerns in addition to accessibility include limiting damage from wheelchairs, controlling access to danger zones, and solving toileting problems. The home design also must consider the child's needs for independence, socialization, and privacy (Olsen, Hutchings, & Ehrenkrantz, 2000).

Adaptations for children with disabilities involve smaller scales but often feature additional components to accommodate caregivers. For example, carrier seating that brings a child to eye level with peers aids in socialization. In the bathroom, a bath chair should be of the correct proportions. A reclining bath chair is appropriate for children who are unable to maintain balance.

The needs and desires of other family members also must be considered. A properly designed home makes tasks easier for all family members. For example, if the child with a disability is unable to bathe independently, a raised bathing and changing table can eliminate the need for caregivers to bend when they bathe or assist the child with bathing (Olsen et al., 2000).

Of particular interest to occupational therapists are Olsen's design suggestions for children with sensory integrative disorders. Olsen describes such children as either "avoiders" or "seekers." For children who generally try to avoid sensory stimuli, the sight of a vacuum cleaner may cause panic because they associate the loud noise from the vacuum with pain. These children also may avoid other stimuli, such as rough materials. By contrast, seekers do not respond to sensory stimuli presented to them, so they tend to seek greater tactual contact. Design suggestions for the homes of seeker children include lots of texture, such as rock walls, rattan chairs, pillows, and carpeting. Seekers will enjoy the vestibular stimuli afforded by a front porch swing. Homes of avoider children could include small prints, less dramatic color, and smooth flooring. A recessed nook with a curtain for privacy provides a perfect hideaway for an avoider. White boards can offer beneficial outlets for all children (Olsen et al., 2000).

Baby Boomers: Becoming the Older Population

Throughout their lives, the Baby Boom generation has been a driving force for change in the United States and other industrialized societies. The baby boomers are now reaching the age of 65 and officially joining the population of older adults. If they affect society's attitude on aging as much as they have affected other trends, the idea that an older person must be seen as a person first, and then as someone who is old, will doubtless become society's standard (Comfort, 1990).

As Baby Boomers reach their older years, the standards that have been established to determine appropriate design criteria will likely change. In the past, recommended dimensions have been based on the measurements of 18-to-25-year-old male military personnel. The standards were based on this group because, some time ago, the federal government committed the necessary resources to compile the data it needed to properly equip and clothe its military personnel. Because few comparable civilian studies existed, the anthropometric measurements of these young men were extrapolated to the population at large (Panero & Zelnik, 1979). As the U.S. population shifts in age, however, the measurements will likely cease to be the basis for design criteria.

Focusing on the functional needs of the older population has a sound basis. In the United States, 70 million people are older than 50 years of age, a group that represents 25% of the adult population (U.S. Census Bureau, 2007). Older adults continue to be the fastest growing demographic group.

The United States is not alone in its recognition that the needs of older adults should play a key role in the development of new approaches and techniques for designing products and environments. In 1999, the Centre for Applied Gerontology at the U.K.'s University of Birmingham was established to gather information about what older people think about the products of modern industry, what their unmet needs are, and how industry can best provide for these needs. The Centre's motto is "Design for the young and you exclude the old; design for the old and you include the young" (University of Birmingham, Centre for Applied Gerontology, 1999). Coined by the late Bernard Isaacs, this motto reflects the philosophy of people everywhere who seek to make environments more accessible and products more usable by a much wider segment of the population.

Older adults tend to have not one severe disability, but many minor ones. They may have impairment of mobility, vision, hearing, strength, dexterity, balance, and memory to different degrees. They may neither need nor want specially designed products, but they may both need and want some modifications of existing products to make them easier to use. Widening the appeal of future products and environments for this market also will mean making them aesthetically pleasing.

Modifications for Age-Related Changes

Modifications for common age-related changes can be categorized as physical, sensory, and cognitive. This section provides a few examples of specific applications and considerations in each category. Many additional possibilities exist. Occupational therapists must incorporate this knowledge so that they can find and recommend products and environments that go beyond meeting the basic needs of the client. "Being an occupational therapist is more than being a clinician. It is about scanning your environment and determining how your present skills, combined with clinical knowledge, can meet the needs of a population" (Yeung, 2003).

Age-Related Physical Changes

The physical challenges that result from aging can be grouped into 10 areas:

1. Stability
2. Mobility
3. Carrying items
4. Climbing stairs
5. Sitting
6. Rising
7. Bending
8. Reaching
9. Grasping
10. Pinching.

Injuries or illness at any age can cause similar challenges. Modifications can be suggested to address each type of age-related physical concern.

Maintaining Stability and Mobility

Stability is the ability to stand upright and move about without losing one's balance. The degree of a client's problem with stability determines the kind and amount of support used or needed. *Mobility* is the capacity to move over a variety of surfaces by walking or rolling; it includes lifting the foot up and over a rise or an obstacle. Surface resistance, degree of incline and, for people with wheelchairs, the turning radius of the wheelchair are factors in mobility. These features and strategies related to stability and mobility should be considered:

- A front entry door should have no threshold and a protected overhang. A small wood or metal wedge-type ramp can be placed over an existing threshold. Similar inserts can be used for sliding doors.
- When ramps are needed, they should have a 1:20 pitch (the ramp must extend 20 ft for each foot of elevation).
- Nonslip wood, vinyl, or limestone floors provide surfaces that are easy to roll on.
- Removing scatter rugs from smooth floors or using nonslip material between the floor and rug enhances safety (Figure 19.2).
- Outdoors, ground surfaces should be kept free of ice, snow, moss, and wet leaves to prevent slipping.
- Ice grippers worn on shoe bottoms can reduce the possibility of slipping.
- Moss inhibitors can be applied to walkways.
- Stable furniture and handrails provide support. Handrails should contrast in color with the wall, have a diameter of 1.25 in. to 1.50 in., and be placed no more than 1½ inches from the wall. In ramped areas, an additional lower rail helps people with wheelchairs pull themselves along.
- For wheelchair access, doorways need a minimum width of 32 inches. If more clearance is needed, an offset hinge will add 2 inches. Ideally, doors should be 36 inches wide. Wheelchairs require a turning radius of 5 feet; motorized chairs require a turning radius of up to 7 feet.
- In bathrooms and kitchens, floor coverings should extend to the back wall under the sink so that people with wheelchairs can access the sink, counter, or cooktop.

Grab bars should be installed for use when entering and exiting bathtubs so that clients will not use unsafe towel bars for support. Grab bars must be mounted into studs, into 2 inches by 6 inches supports placed between the studs, or on wall surfaces covered with ¾ in. plywood. Mounted plywood will allow the grab bars to be installed at any point on the wall. A patented fastener called the WingIt (www.wingits.com) also can be used to install grab bars on walls without structural backing.

- Towel bars are not sufficiently sturdy to be used as grab bars, but grab bars can be used as towel bars. Available in a variety of colors and

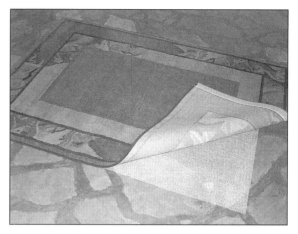

Figure 19.2. Nonslip rug pad.

textures, grab bars can be attractive bathroom accessories. If a grab bar is also used as a towel holder, the number of towels hung on the bar should be limited to preserve an open place for the client to grasp. A vertical grab bar should be installed for support when exiting a tub.
- Curbless showers allow access for a shower chair (Figure 19.3). Doors on curbless showers should be installed with a tight seal on the door. A long, narrow shower built with glass blocks and a sloped floor to drain eliminates the need for a shower door. The drain should be located toward the back of the shower floor with a drop to the drain of no less than 1.25 inches.

Public buildings present distinct challenges. Elevators are not always easily available to people with wheelchairs.

- A mechanism that accommodates people moving between floors is the Travelator, an angled escalator without steps (Figure 19.4). The surface of the Travelator is smooth, which allows wheeled luggage, strollers, or wheelchairs ease of movement from one floor to another.

Carrying Items

Carrying is the ability to lift an item and move it from one place to another. A variety of carts, trolleys, and other wheeled devices can help older people move items at home. For example, a small plant trolley on casters can be used to move heavy trash bags or boxes from one area to another.

Climbing Stairs

Climbing stairs requires a combination of endurance, balance, and leg strength, as well as arm and hand strength to use handrails.

- In public buildings, handrails on stairways often have a horizontal extension to provide

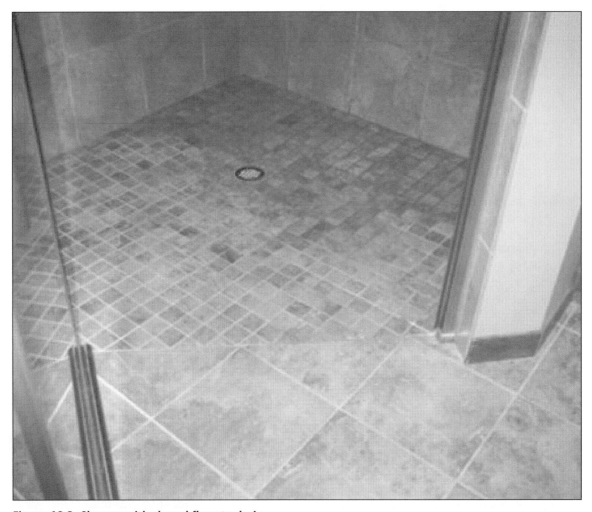

Figure 19.3. Shower with sloped floor to drain.

support on the landings. This feature should be included in the home.

- Stair gliders provide a means for a person with limited climbing ability to move between floors. Some gliders are designed with tracks that go around landings.

When a new home is built, placing identical closets one above the other on each floor can make future installation of a home elevator much easier. The dimensions of the closets should reflect the fact that most elevators are deeper than they are wide.

- Additional closet space on the bottom floor can be converted to a mechanical room.

Sitting and Rising

Sitting and rising are the combined capabilities of getting up or down from a raised surface such as a bed, toilet, or couch and standing up from the floor, a

tub bottom, the ground, and so forth. Designers should consider both the amount of support needed and how that support can be obtained, such as by providing handholds to grasp or stable surfaces to lean on.

- Chairs should have wide, solid arms; provide good neck support; and allow ample space under the chair for an older person to place his or her feet for ease in getting up and down.
- Chairs with a sled base are easier to move but compromise safety because canes or walkers can become caught between the base and the area under the chair.
- Tables that are high enough to accommodate wheelchairs can be uncomfortable for non-wheelchair users because they must have at least 29 inches of clearance from the floor to allow space for wheelchair arms. As a result, ambulatory residents and residents in wheelchairs

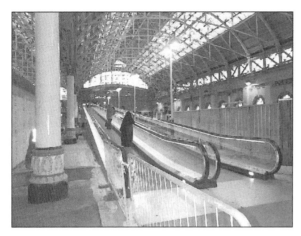

Figure 19.4. Travelator.

tend to sit at separate tables—an example of how environments can separate people rather than bring them together. One way to provide common table seating at mealtimes is to insert a leaf into a square table. The person with a wheelchair can be seated in front of one of the apronless leaves.

• Round pedestal tables also can be problematic because wheelchair foot pedals often touch the pedestal, preventing the person from pulling up closely enough to use the table. Tables with legs work better and are more stable. They often are discouraged in long-term-care facilities, however, because the table legs can become nicked by the foot pedals.

• Higher toilets make it easier for some older people to sit down or get up but can create problems for shorter people. It may be preferable to leave the toilet at the lower height but add grab bars. If the toilet is positioned next to a wall, one grab bar can be installed on the wall and a fold-down grab bar installed on the opposite side. If the toilet is not near a wall, fold-down grab bars can be used on each side. If placement of a grab bar is not possible, a grab pole may be installed.

• Former tub bathers who need bath chairs will benefit from transfer benches that have an extension over the side of the tub.

• Replacing a shower door with a shower curtain allows maneuvering room when getting in and out of the tub and while bathing. A two-paneled curtain that draws toward the middle will close around the bench, reducing water splashes on the floor.

• Showers may be adapted with handheld shower devices.

Bending and Reaching

Reaching is the extension of the arms and hands away from the body at or above shoulder level, at or below knee level, or away from the body directly in front or to the side. *Bending* is the ability to lean forward and bring the shoulders and arms down to the level where the hips would be when standing. The definitions of bending and reaching include the ability to use these motions to complete tasks. Bending and reaching in the kitchen can be facilitated by several design features:

• Installing open shelves instead of cupboards will make it easier to reach items.
• Revolving corner shelves can make accessing items in corner cupboards easier.
• Installing pullout shelves in place of stationary shelves can eliminate some of the need for bending.
• A raised dishwasher reduces the need to bend. If the appliance is placed under a counter, 6 inches to 8 inches is usually the maximum it can be raised (Figure 19.5). If it is built into a cabinet, it often can be raised up to 18 inches. The additional height allows a person in a wheelchair to reach to the back of the dishwasher; it also is beneficial for anyone standing to load or unload it

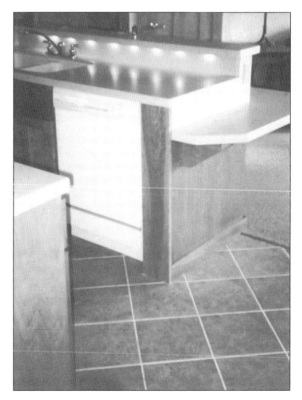

Figure 19.5. Raised dishwasher.

- Reaching over burners to get at the back controls of stoves is dangerous. Appliances that have control knobs at the front are preferred. Recent safety innovations include knob covers that can prevent small children from turning the knobs. Alternatively, the knobs can be removed when the stove or cooktop is not being used.
- Elsewhere in the house, lowering the rods in bedroom closets or placing them in the open in the bedroom makes accessing clothing easier.
- Shoes can be stored for easy retrieval on a bedroom closet shelf.
- In the laundry room, washers and dryers with front controls can be raised by placing the appliances on a platform.
- A long-handled dustpan can reduce the need to bend when sweeping.
- Varieties of reachers or grabbers are marketed through many sources.

Grasping and Pinching

Grasping is the ability to move the hand into a variety of positions and to manipulate an object with one or both hands. Manipulation requires adequate strength to grasp, release, or squeeze the object. *Pinching* is the ability to bring the thumb and fingers in opposition and requires adequate strength to remove or close objects such as bottle caps or to pick up small items. A criterion for making a decision about an assistive device is whether it can be manipulated easily with a closed fist without the need for grasping or pinching.

A number of accommodations and devices can help older adults maintain independence in tasks that involve grasping or pinching.

- Rocker-style light switches may be turned on with the fist, palm, or even the elbow.
- Stable lamps with rocker switches near the base are available.
- Lamps can be converted to touch-control lamps by plugging them into a control unit that is then plugged into the electrical outlet. Both types of switches eliminate the need to reach overhead or fumble for the lamp switch.
- Lever door handles are much easier to turn than door knobs because they virtually eliminate the need for grasping.
- The backs of door handles should be filled or enclosed because an open back often has a rough, uncomfortable surface.
- Similarly, lever faucets require less grasping ability than do round knobs.

- Lever-handled shower controls that allow temperatures to be preset are easy to operate.
- In the kitchen, glassware styles can facilitate or hamper hand function. Textured plastic drinking glasses will not slip out of a person's hands as easily as smooth plastic or glass styles.

Age-Related Sensory Changes

Age-related sensory changes affect a person's vision, taste, smell, touch, temperature, hearing, and balance.

Vision

Low vision concerns can include difficulties with acuity, accommodation, lighting, glare, sight recovery, color perception, depth perception, and upward gaze. Aging results in decreased *visual acuity,* the ability to see objects clearly. This occurs when

- The eyeball develops internal structural changes, small opacities, and vascularities;
- The muscles that surround and control the eye change;
- The lens of the eye becomes less elastic and gradually thickens at its center; or
- The changes collectively generate a scattering of light that blurs the retinal image.

A number of accommodations can improve visual acuity and also support the older person whose visual acuity is diminishing.

- Major color contrasts can enhance acuity in distinguishing signs and symbols; cups, dishes, utensils, and table settings; and telephone or other appliance controls.
- In long-term-care settings, handrails should contrast with wall colors.
- In dining rooms, trays and tables should contrast, and dishes and napkins should contrast with the trays.
- Controls on appliances, telephones, and kitchen tools should have large numbers in contrasting colors from the background.
- Bath towels, bedspreads, and carpets also should be in contrasting colors.

Presbyopia

Sometimes called "far-sightedness," *presbyopia* is a decrease in the eye's ability to accommodate and differentiate details, leading to diminished ability to focus on objects that are close at hand. Presbyopia occurs because the lens of the eye becomes less elastic with age, and the ciliary muscle is less able to adjust the curvature of the lens. Initially, corrective lenses for near vision will rectify difficulties in reading fine print, but correction may not be possible in later stages. When bifocal lenses no longer compensate for the inability to read fine print, switching to large-print newspapers, books, and magazines can be helpful. Published material increasingly is available in electronic and digital media. Magnifiers can meet a variety of needs; they can be worn around the neck or handheld, and they come in lighted and nonlighted variations, including magnifying mirrors in the bathroom.

With aging, the lens of the eye gradually thickens and becomes less transparent, admitting less light to the retina. The pupil also becomes smaller. Both changes reduce the ability of the eye to function in low light. At 80 years of age, a person needs approximately three times more light to read than he or she did at 15–20 years of age. There are many adaptations and adjustments that may be helpful.

- Window treatments can be adjusted to help control levels of sunlight.
- Many types of light bulbs and lamp designs also are available to enhance artificial illumination (e.g., angled shades project direct light straight downward, and fixtures with incandescent bulbs create diffused light).
- Positioning lamps to direct light below eye level can be helpful (e.g., strip lighting can be placed under cabinets to provide task lighting; Figure 19.6).
- Night-lights and small, portable lights like those available on key chains can also be invaluable.

Most standard lamps and shades are designed for use with bulbs rated at 60 watts. Be sure to select light bulbs of the appropriate type and wattage for the lamp. Using high-wattage bulbs in fixtures that are not designed to handle them can create a risk of fire.

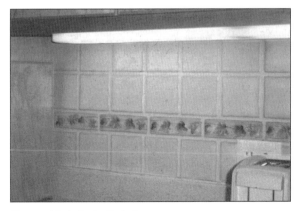

Figure 19.6. Strip lighting.

Glare

Glare is a painful and often disorienting problem caused by too much illumination. *Direct glare* occurs when light floods the eye directly from its source. *Indirect glare* arises when the light reflects into the eye after rebounding off of another surface. To reduce the problem with direct glare, position seating so that the older person does not have to look directly into sunlight and consider torchiere lamps, which provide a source of indirect lighting.

To reduce indirect glare, use lightly buffed flooring rather than flooring that is shiny.

Color Perception and Depth Perception

With increasing age, the lens of the eye takes on a yellowish color that alters the quality of light entering the pupil. The perception of green, blue, and purple hues can become problematic. Differences among pastel shades often become impossible to detect, and dark shades of navy, brown, and black can become indistinguishable except in intense light. Changes in color perception should be considered when choosing contrasting colors to enhance visual acuity. Care must also be taken with medications, because many medications have similar colors and may be difficult for the older person to distinguish.

Depth perception depends on brightness and contrast. Therefore, any age-related process that affects the amount of light reaching the retina also will affect a person's depth perception. Again, contrasting colors can help with age-related changes in depth perception.

- From a distance, any item that contrasts with its background will be easier to perceive (another reason why seating should contrast with the color of the floor).
- Providing color contrast between the edge of the bathtub, the floor, and the inside of the tub enhances safety by providing stronger visual cues.
- In long-term-care facilities, pictures, objects, and signs should be large and positioned about 20 ft. apart so that they can be easily distinguished. Highlight the edges of steps, particularly top and bottom steps. Outdoor steps or stairs leading to a basement can be marked with tape or paint. On carpeted stairs, place stair lights along the steps, with switches at both the top and bottom of the stairs.
- Carpet or rug colors and patterns also should be selected to minimize confusion. To an older person, sections of markedly darker color on a floor may appear recessed, which

may prompt the person to try to step down. Lighter patterns may appear elevated, causing the person to attempt to step up.

In an older person, the amount of time required for the eye to adjust when moving from a dark area into a light area or vice versa is markedly increased. Light intensity also affects adjustment time. The greater the contrast, the more time that is required. For those reasons, objects should not be placed in entryways, and lighting should be designed to avoid sudden changes in light levels. Areas should be illuminated before anyone steps inside.

Upward Gaze

The ability to see items that are placed above eye level often becomes limited as people age. This may be caused by multiple reasons, including increased age; the failure of the eyelid to open as widely as when the person was younger; a forward inclination of the head, reflecting weakened neck muscles; or a forward tilt of the entire upper body because of osteoporosis. To offset difficulties with upward gaze, place important signage, like directional signs or numbers, within the person's field of vision. Ideally, signs should be placed about 3½ feet to 5 feet above the floor. In some situations, placing directional signs on the floor itself may be helpful.

Taste and Smell

A person's taste buds distinguish sweet, salty, bitter, and sour flavors. The taste buds for those flavors are located from front to back on the tongue, and they lose sensation in that order (i.e., the first taste buds to lose their sensitivity are the sweet taste buds). Two-thirds of our response to taste lies in our sense of smell. Food aromas can change mere acceptance into appreciation of flavor. The sense of smell affords both protection and pleasure and often generates associations with past experiences.

Older adults may lose sensitivity to body and household odors. A reduced ability to smell smoke or gas fumes can become a safety concern, as can difficulty in distinguishing spoiled food. Visual signaling devices can be installed to enhance smoke detectors and natural gas leak detectors for older people who also have difficulty with hearing. Other helpful accommodations related to smell include reprinting expiration dates on food packaging with a marking pen using large numbers or labeling refrigerator shelves for each week of the month and placing food on the designated shelves. Check perishable items every 2 weeks to be sure expired items are being discarded.

Tactual and Temperature Cues

Sensory input conducted through the skin is subdivided into the touch and the tactual systems. Touch provides awareness and allows for protective responses. Tactual perception also involves kinesthetic senses, which provide information about the location of limbs in space, and is instrumental to interactions with the environment, For example, touching a door provides a pressure sensation, but feeling the door move gives other important information necessary for moving in the environment and thus has implications for environmental design, particularly when vision is compromised. Temperature sensitivity also decreases with age. Because an older person's responsiveness to heat and cold is diminished, accidental scalding is a danger. Settings for hot water heaters should not exceed 120 degrees.

Hearing

As people age, their ability to hear high-frequency sounds and sounds in general diminishes. Hearing aids have been developed that amplify sound at different frequencies, but many hearing aids also transmit confusing background noise. Many signaling devices are available to alert people with hearing impairments to sounds in the environment. In-depth information about hearing loss and hearing aids can be obtained from the National Institute on Deafness and Other Communication Disorders (see www. nidcd. nih.gov).

Older people may find that hearing consonants is more difficult than distinguishing between vowel sounds. When speaking to an older person with hearing impairment, it can be helpful to

- Move closer to the person,
- Speak more slowly,
- Allow a longer separation between words,
- Use a slightly louder voice, or
- Consciously lower vocal tone.

Carpeting in corridors and other noisy areas helps reduce distracting ambient noise. Acoustical panels placed around small groupings of tables in a dining room also can make it easier for older adults to hear each other when conversing (Figure 19.7).

Kinesthesia

Kinesthesia, the position sense of muscles, tendons, and joints, includes *proprioceptive* and *vestibular* input and is affected by aging. Proprioception is discussed under "balance" in the modifications for age-related physical changes section of this chapter. Vestibular input relates to the way a portion of the

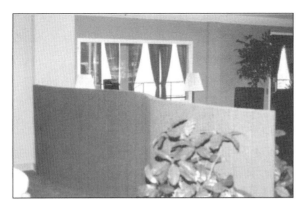

Figure 19.7. Partition.

inner ear helps a person determine the position of his or her head in space. With age, this internal orienting mechanism can become less reliable.

Problems with kinesthesia can contribute to difficulties with falls and, in subtle ways, with a person's sense of orientation in space. Environmental adaptations can compensate for certain losses in these senses (Birren & Schaie, 1977). For example, when a person's detection of vertical movement has become compromised, signage or other cues indicating the location of the floor must be obvious when he or she gets off an elevator.

Age-Related Cognitive Changes

Specific interventions are crucial for clients with dementia as well as their caregivers. Everyone, however, can benefit from adaptations that assist memory, such as automatic shut-off switches on small appliances and effective directional cues in corridors.

People with dementia often experience certain sensory and physical changes, but in dealing with the specific manifestations related to the dementia, other age-related changes often are overlooked. Before specific environmental adaptations are made for people with dementia, the environment should be assessed and changes made that compensate for general age-related changes. When modifications for age-related changes are made, behaviors associated with cognitive difficulties often are reduced. When modifications or additions to the environment reduce problematic behavior, they also make the role of the caregiver easier.

Adaptations recommended for people with dementia include

- Safety awareness,
- Way finding,
- Reducing confrontation,
- Visual cues,

- Promoting memory and reminiscing,
- Medication management,
- Providing reassurance and support,
- Avoiding confrontations,
- Creating a calm environment, and
- Addressing wandering.

Basic Safety Issues

Always the first consideration in any home modification, basic safety includes the security of the person as well as general security from outside forces. Trim foliage near windows and add prickly bushes, such as holly, fire bush, roses, Russian olive, bougainvillea, or similar plantings to eliminate hiding places. Always select nonpoisonous plants for outdoor and indoor locations. In the kitchen, remove flammable items that might be placed on the stove or stored in the oven. If possible, select appliances with automatically timed shutoff switches.

Orientation

Everyone relies on signs and landmarks to find one's way through unfamiliar territory. For the person with cognitive difficulties, consistent cues become crucial and should be thoughtfully incorporated into the daily environment. For example, in long-term-care facilities, landmarks (any building design, item, or picture that helps identify a specific place) should be placed in conspicuous places on the corridor walls, where they can be used for cuing. Such signage might include the barber shop, coffee shop, library, and so on. Interior landmarks may include specific items, such as a grandfather clock, an interior mailbox, or a mural. Ideally, large pictures should be of familiar scenes. All landmarks should have distinctive, easily recognized colors and offer good contrast with the surroundings.

In multifloor residences, determining which floor one is on can be challenging, particularly to someone with cognitive or kinesthetic challenges. From inside an elevator, the space immediately outside the elevator should appear markedly different on each floor. Signs by the doors of residents' rooms should be positioned at their eye level, should provide effective contrast between the numbers or letters and the background colors, and have numbers at least 2 inches high. It also can be helpful to provide space on the signs for small personal mementos or allow wall space on which such mementos can be placed.

Importance of Visual Cues

Beyond adapting for age-related visual changes, arrangement of items helps the person with dementia with activities of daily living. Planning and organizing the environment with this in mind can reduce some frustrations. For example, grouping items that are used together in the same place, such as placing a shirt and pants for one outfit on the same hanger, can help with functioning. Similarly, a person's toothbrush and toothpaste can be grouped on a vanity counter, a water glass and water pitcher can be grouped on a table, and so forth. Another strategy is to put clothing of one type in a drawer, which can be labeled if the person still understands the meaning of written words. A third strategy may be to place clothing in open baskets, where it can be readily seen.

Products and ideas that compensate for short-term memory loss can be helpful. Some items also may stimulate long-term memory. To help clients with orientation to people, time, and place, photo albums with labels of people and places can stimulate long-term memory. Maps can be given to residents to use to show where they were born or where significant events in their life took place. A calendar on which days are marked off can help orient a person in time. Sometimes clients will retain the meanings of certain symbols, such as flags or items of ethnic significance. Such items can be used to elicit discussion.

People with cognitive difficulties such as dementia may have problems with taking (and not taking) medications. Consider a variety of tools and techniques to ensure proper adherence to medication regimens, from simple reminders and organizers to measures designed specifically to prevent overmedication.

Reassurance and Support

Products and measures that provide reassurance to clients with dementia can increase both client and caregiver peace of mind. Interventions may be as simple as compiling information about where to go, or whom to call for information, or establishing procedures to ensure that help will be available in an emergency. People and technology can help in preparing emergency plans. For information about the emergency response system, the best source is the client's local hospital. Soon, cell phone technology will help monitor people with dementia. Telephones in which picture inserts replace the speed dial buttons provide photo cues and links to significant people when programmed numbers might be forgotten.

Each person with dementia may respond differently to a set of circumstances. It is possible to identify and avoid many situations that might lead to major confrontations—that might escalate to what

are referred to as "catastrophic reactions," that is, a severe emotional and behavioral response to a situation that can include anger, fear, agitation, screaming, aggression, weeping, or other reactions. Attempting to view the environment from the perspective of the client can be helpful. When a potential problem is identified, it can often be solved, as in the following examples:

- Some clients inappropriately remove their clothes. In response, caregivers often reverse regular clothing to make it more difficult to remove. Doing so, however, may be irritating to the client, exacerbating the problem because the clothing will not fit properly. Instead, caregivers should purchase comfortable clothing designed with zippers in back.
- If a client attempts to crawl over bedrails (if present), risking a dangerous fall, his or her mattress can be placed on the floor. It may be necessary to obtain a waiver to do this. Additional precautions might need to be put in place to prevent wandering.
- If the client uses objects for different purposes (e.g., mistaking a water fountain for a urinal or a wastebasket for a toilet), they can be removed or changed. For example, rather than have the client walk to the water fountain to get a drink and risk becoming confused, a plastic pitcher of water and glasses can be placed in a nearby place.
- The client's inability to discern noncontrasting colors may permit camouflaging doors to storage and linen closets by making the signs and the wall the same color.
- Magnetic locks can be installed on doors to cupboards where harmful or fragile items are kept, so the door remains locked until a magnet is placed on the door opposite the lock to release the catch mechanism.
- The environment can be designed with calming colors and tranquil motifs.
- Moving water has a calming effect. If an artificial pond or stream will be part of the landscaping, the depth of the stream should be less than 1 inch, and pebbles should be embedded in the concrete bed. Large, immovable stones also may be added.

Movement and Wandering

The client with dementia often has an ingrained need for movement that may play itself out as wandering. Providing a place where the client can expend excess energy, therefore, can be beneficial. Ideally, an enclosed, safe, outdoor area will allow the

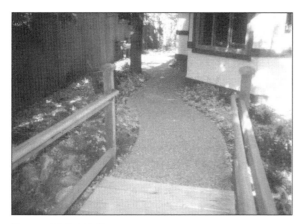

Figure 19.8. Walkway.

client to move about freely. A circular path is best, with no dead ends or points where decisions must be made about which way to go. The walkway shown in Figure 19.8 goes around the house to another door.

The Alzheimer's Association makes available a variety of person identifiers, including pendants, bracelets, key chains, and clothing labels. Identification is available for caregivers as well as for the person with dementia.

Home Evaluations

When chronic health conditions or disability coexist with age-related changes, the therapist must work with the client or family to identify the specific home modifications needed. To accomplish this task, a thorough home evaluation is crucial to determine the best course of action. The evaluation provides a means of communicating with the client and incorporating his or her specific wants and desires. The needs of caregivers, if any, should also be considered in a final plan that can grow and change with the needs of the client and the family (Duncan, 2002, 2003).

The occupational therapist is a valuable member of the assessment team taking part in the home evaluation. His or her expertise can lead to an assessment that more thoroughly accounts for the complexities of the client's functional concerns. Many client homes were built more than 40 years ago and do not compensate for lifestyle changes. Most were built without universal design principles, so they have features such as steep stairs, poor lighting, raised thresholds, and doorknobs.

The type of home evaluation depends on several factors, including time and funding available; detail required; expertise of the builder, remodeler, or designer; and client diagnosis, health complications, and prognosis. To encompass as many of these factors as possible, the ideal home assessment

team includes the building contractor, designer, occupational therapist, client, and the client's family, as appropriate (Duncan, 2002).

Performing a home evaluation historically has been a part of occupational therapy practice, and many therapists have created their own forms. Most home evaluations available from involved organizations ask questions about the home but not about the client—making the occupational therapist's unique insight into the client's needs all the more important.

The resources in the following section offer readers additional ideas for home evaluation.

Home Environment Checklists

Home safety checklists and universal design guides have been developed by a variety of organizations, primarily for consumers but also useful to therapists. Many are free of charge on the Internet; others are available for a small fee. They vary in length and content, and include safety tips; home modification ideas; and often, rationales for those ideas.

The Accessible Home

The Accessible Home is a pocket-sized checklist for people buying or remodeling a home. It provides information about which features need to be addressed immediately to make it accessible and which might be considered in the future. It lists useful information about areas of the home, which items should be considered, and why. Each of the recommendations is followed by the rationale for the suggestion (Lasoff & Lorentzen, 2003).

Web Site Resources

1. *Older Consumers Safety Checklist.* In 1981, the U.S. Consumer Product Safety Commission (CPSC) developed this checklist. Research had estimated that over 622,000 people older than age 65 were treated in emergency rooms for injuries associated with everyday products. Reasoning that many of these injuries resulted from hazards in the home that are easy to overlook and that finding and fixing some of them would prevent many injuries, CPSC developed the checklist to help spot possible home safety hazards. The result was the creation of the checklist which is available at www.cpsc.gov/cpscpub/pubs/705.pdf.
2. *AARP.* AARP offers free material on www.aarp. org under "Home Modifications," including *Home Modification: Your Key to Comfort, Safety, and Independent Living* and *Taking Steps to Prevent Falling Head Over Heels.*

3. *Practical Guide to Universal Home Design.* This guide, created by East Metro Seniors Agenda for Independent Living of St. Paul, Minnesota, lists common-sense features that can make a home safer and more pleasant (see SAIL, 2002, or www.lifease.com). Including these features in a home when it is built can make future changes unnecessary. The checklist gives options room by room; we hope that many of the ideas will become standard in the future, just as safety and energy-efficiency features have become in recent years.

4. *Rebuilding Together®* produces a checklist that focuses on accessibility issues. *Home Modifications Assessment and Solutions Checklist* (2007) identifies accessibility issues and fall hazards and prioritizes work tasks. See www.rebuildingtogether.org.

5. *Gerontological Environmental Modifications* (2005) is a downloadable checklist providing a comprehensive, walk-through guide to the environment. It poses questions about various potential obstacles and hazards and includes questions for a return visit to indicate if the problem has been corrected. See www.cornellaging.org/gem.

6. *LivAbility Falls Prevention Checklist and Resource Guide.* In 2010, a new checklist and free resource guide will be available at www.lifease.com, providing information and Internet sites for solutions that can reduce falls. After assessing a person's functional abilities and the potential problem areas in the home, it recommends solutions. It is being developed as a collaboration between the Minnesota Falls Prevention Initiative and Lifease.®

7. *Minnesota Falls Prevention Initiative.* One-page fall prevention fact sheets are available at www.mnfallsprevention.org. An additional in-depth home safety checklist is available at www.minnesotasafetycouncil.org. Check other states for their Falls Prevention Initiative programs.

Financing Home Remodeling

A person's home is usually the most important investment he or she makes. Using home equity, or cashing in a long-term home investment while continuing to live in the home can be ways to pay for necessary home modifications. For people with low incomes, there may be grants and loans or other types of funds available.

Housing and Community Development Grants

The Community Development Block Grant (CDBG) program and the HOME block grant program developed by the U.S. Department of Housing and Urban Development (HUD) are two of the more significant nationwide sources of funding for accessibility remodeling. CDBG covers a broad range of activities, one of which is housing rehabilitation. HOME finances housing construction and rehabilitation activities only.

In CDBG, larger communities receive part of a state's share in each program as a direct award and select their own priorities. A state agency typically receives the balance of a state's allocation for each program and either makes it available to smaller communities through a competitive application process or uses the resources to extend existing programming.

Section 504 Loans/Grants are available in rural areas. Funds are allocated for low-income households for the removal of health and safety hazards. The community must have a population of less then 20,000. Loan length is from 10 to 20 years, and interest is at 1% for people who will be able to repay it. Grants with a lifetime maximum of $7,500 are available for homeowners over 62 who do not qualify for a Section 504 loan. In the latter case, if the home is sold within 3 years of receiving the assistance, the loan must be repaid.

These loans are available from the U.S. Department of Agriculture, and more information is available at www.usda.gov/services.html. Local Rural Development offices process Section 504 loan/grant applications. Their Web sites are http://www.rurdev.usda.gov/rhs/common/indiv_intro.htm and www.rurdev.usda.gov/recd_map.html.

Funds From Organizations

Many types of organizations provide funds for housing renovations for people with disabilities, including local community groups, religious organizations, building supply companies, housing rehabilitation agencies, and neighborhood associations or planning councils. Public agencies, foundations, and other donors may provide funds that are administered through housing and community development agencies (Sprague, 2009).

Social Services and Health Waivers

When a person's medical condition requires accessibility modifications for health and safety or to enable the person to live independently at home, *medical assistance waivers* may provide funds. This option is for people who would be institutionalized if changes were not made. Information on waivers is available from the state or local department of human services.

Veterans Specialty Housing Grants

If a U.S. veteran has major service-related disabilities, grants from the VA are available to build or purchase an accessible home or to remodel the home the veteran currently owns. In 2006, Congress approved legislation providing grants of up to $14,000 to modify family members' homes when severely disabled veterans temporarily or permanently reside with them. For information about eligibility, contact the VA field office where the veteran's records are located. The VA website is www.va.gov. The VA also offers home improvement loans to assist veterans with nonservice-related disabilities.

Vocational Rehabilitation Centers and Independent Living Centers Resources

If a person cannot function at home, it also may be impossible for him or her to work. Vocational rehabilitation centers provide advocacy, skills training, counseling, information, and referral services. Some staff members have expertise in home assessment, construction, and financing.

Worker's Compensation

Compensation for work injuries may include home modifications. To be eligible for compensation, the alterations must be required for the person to function.

Crime Victims' Services

Crime victims, their family members, and dependents may qualify for home modifications funding. Maximum awards are $50,000. For more information, see www.ojp.state.mn.us/mccvs/FinancialHelp/index.htm

Civic, Advocacy, Trade Groups Projects

Many community groups provide money, volunteer labor, or materials for home accessibility projects. Local options vary greatly but might include

- Organizations raising funds from certain types of gambling;
- Civic groups, churches, and synagogues;
- Community groups that dedicate a period of time to home repair projects;
- Groups that work on repair projects for low-income households; and
- Building industry product retailers or professionals, advocacy agencies, and vocational technical schools.

Private Loans

Refinancing a home mortgage may provide additional funds for remodeling. The lender evaluates factors relating to repayment and property value to determine whether and how much it will lend. If the homeowner has other outstanding loans, they may be consolidated into the new mortgage.

Long-term care insurance may pay for home accessibility features. It supplements health care insurance and provides both institutional and in-home coverage. A benefit for accessibility modifications can be included.

Equity is the difference between the purchase price of a home and its current value. An *equity line of credit* is like a credit card, making loans available up to a certain amount, based on equity in the home. Amounts can be paid back in a lump sum or in periodic payments.

A *reverse mortgage* is a loan used primarily by older Americans to convert the equity in their homes into cash. In a reverse mortgage, the payment stream is "reversed." Instead of a homeowner making monthly payments to a lender, as with a regular mortgage or home equity loan, the lender makes regular payments to the homeowner in return for a share of the equity in the home. While a reverse mortgage loan is outstanding, the homeowner continues to hold the title to the home.

To qualify for a reverse mortgage, a person must be at least 62 years of age and own his or her home. No income or medical requirements are involved. A person may be eligible for a reverse mortgage even if he or she owes money on a first or second mortgage. The most popular way to receive the proceeds is through a line of credit. Other homeowners may select a lump sum or fixed monthly payment (National Reverse Mortgage Lenders Association, 2002).

The size of the reverse mortgage depends on age when applying, the type of mortgage, the value of the home, the amount of any outstanding debts against it, current interest rates, and neighborhood market conditions. The costs associated with getting a reverse mortgage are similar to those for regular mortgages.

The money provided by a reverse mortgage is tax-free. It does not affect regular Social Security benefits, but it may affect certain other types of government aid, such as Medicare. Specific information is available from local Area Agency on Aging offices (see www.eldercare.gov). A meeting with an approved financial counseling agency must precede the application for a reverse mortgage. HUD has posted a list of approved counseling agencies by state at http://portal.hud.gov/portal/page/portal/HUD.

Tax Benefits

Some, but not all, accessibility modifications installed in an existing home may qualify as a personal income tax itemized deduction when the accommodations are for a resident with a disability. The IRS distributes resource booklets with information on medical capital deductions (see www.irs.gov).

A portion of capital expenses is deductible for a home used for business. The business can also deduct improvements needed to make it accessible. The same design standards are used as those for public and commercial space.

Some states offer a sales tax exemption on materials purchased for installing stair glides, platform lifts, or elevators. A physician must authorize the need for these features.

If an older home is having accessibility improvements made that will increase the value of the home, a portion of that increase may be excluded from the property value of that home. There is a time limit on the exclusion. Check with the local government for more details.

Summary

Adapting the home to create an environment where people can remain independent for a much longer period of time is not only doable, but the results can be an environment that is attractive and create a place where nearly anyone would like to live. The ideas and resources in this chapter will help the occupational therapy practitioner to look at the home environment in a new way.

Box 19.1. Case Study: Mr. C.

Mr. C. developed a neurological condition that created severe pain in his lower right leg and mobility difficulties including the use of stairs. He had limited arm range of motion, particularly above his shoulders. He was forced to retire and spent his day lying on a bed that had been placed in the family room.

The family home consisted of multiple levels. The family room was the only living space on the ground level and the entrance was from the garage. A laundry room with a sliding door adjoined the family room. A small bathroom with a shower was located on the other side of the laundry room. Mr. C. was not able to stand up to shower.

To provide room for Mrs. C. to help her husband shower the door between the bathroom and laundry was removed. A shower chair was placed in the shower but to allow Mr. C. to sit it was necessary to also remove the shower door. Because of his limited range of motion, he could not use a handheld shower himself. Mrs. C. donned a raincoat and assisted him with his shower.

The couple's children were married, and two of them lived in the same city. Including Mr. C. in family gatherings was virtually impossible because he could not go to either the living room or the basement entertainment area, and meeting in the family room was too crowded. Therefore, Mr. C. could not be a part of the family activities. Not only had his life been compromised by his disability but that of the entire family as well. They determined that finding a home to remodel would be the best solution.

A home in the area was purchased, and extensive remodeling began. In the planning process, it was decided to incorporate a universal design perspective in the home design, and the furniture that was purchased. These included the single-level home, wide doorways and hallways, sturdy furniture, dining room chairs with arms, raised dishwasher, raised dryer, no-threshold entry, decorator grab bars, rocker light switches, and lever door handles. All these features are inconspicuous and added to a sense of openness and increased the home's ease of use. The outdoors has a deck off of the great room and the laundry room. A walkway goes around the house with ramped areas and handrails to the decks.

The new home provided ample room for Mr. C. to move about both walking and in a wheelchair when necessary. The bathroom included an open "wet room" and a stationery shower seat with a regular shower that allowed him to once again be independent in bathing.

Mr. C. had a change in medications; received pain management interventions; and because of his poor physical condition, underwent an intensive period of rehabilitation, including both occupational and physical therapy. He was once again able to walk and no longer limited to only lying on a bed. The floor plan of the home with its wide hallways and handrails, open great room with stable furniture allowed Mr. C to continue to gain independence. The exterior also promoted exercise outdoors. Family gatherings once again included him.

Any limitations he now experiences are an integral part of his disease process, but the home environment presents no obstructions to his independence. Mr. C. maintains the design of the house was significant in his recovery.

Study Questions

1. Which group was the initial driving force behind legislation in the United States that focused on people with disabilities?
2. What are 3 essential components in visitability?
3. What is the ADA, and when was it passed?
4. What are the 7 principles of universal design, and what do they mean?
5. What modifications will adapt a home for a client with age-related physical changes?
6. What are 5 modifications that will adapt a home for a client with age-related sensory changes?
7. What are 3 modifications that will adapt a home for a client with cognitive issues?
8. What resources are available for financing modifications to a home?

References

AARP. (1995). *Does yourhome meet your reeds? A checklist, universal design: Home modifications*. Retrieved October 8, 2003, from www.aarp.org

Air Carriers Access Act of 1986, Pub. L. 99–435, 100 Stat. 1080, 49 U.S.C. ß 41705.

American National Standards Institute. (1961). *Making buildings accessible to and usable by the physically handicapped*. Washington, DC: Author.

Americans With Disabilities Act of 1990, Pub. L. 101–336, 42 U.S.C. ß 12101.

Architectural Barriers Act of 1968, Pub. L. 90–480.

Architectural and Transportation Barriers Compliance Board. (1982). Minimum guidelines and requirements for accessible design—Architectural and Transportation Barriers Compliance Board. Final rule. *Federal Register, 47*(150), 33862–33893.

Birren, J., & Schaie, K. (1977). *Handbook of the psychology of aging*. New York: Van Nostrand Reinhold.

Center for Universal Design. (1997). *Principles of universal design*. Retrieved November 2, 2009, from http://www.design.ncsu.edu:8120/cud/

Christenson, M. A. (1999). Embracing universal design. *OT Practice, 4*(9), 12–15, 25.

Clause, A. (2002). *Eleanor Smith looks to affect Concrete Change*. Retrieved October 31, 2003, from http://www.goshen.edu/news/bulletin/02June/eleanor_smith.php.

Comfort, A. (1990). *Say yes to old age: Developing a positive attitude toward aging*. New York: Crown.

Duncan, S. (2002). *Up close and personal: Part 2 of the ABC's of adaptability*. Seattle, WA: ADAptations.

Duncan, S. (2003). Universal design is good design for everyone. *Housing Washington*, pp. 8–9.

Education for All Handicapped Children Act of 1975, Pub. L. 94–142, 20 U.S.C. § 1400 *et seq.*

Farber, S. (1992). New York: OXO International.

Gerontological Environmental Modifications. (2005). *Environmental modifications*. Retrieved October 25, 2003, from www.cornellaging.org/gem

Hahn, H. (1988). The politics of physical differences: Disability and discrimination. *Journal of Social Issues, 44*(1), 21–113.

Inclusive Home Design Act of 2009, H.R. 1408, retrieved November 29, 2009, from http://www.govtrack.us/congress/bill.xpd?bill=h111-1408

Lasoff, S., & Lorentzen, L. (2003). *The accessible home*. Minneapolis, MN: Fairview Press.

Leibrock, C. A., & Terry, J. E. (1999). *Beautiful universal design*. New York: John Wiley & Sons.

Mace, R. (1988). *Housing for the lifespan of all people*. Washington, DC: U.S. Department of Housing and Urban Development.

Mann, W. C., & Lane, J. P. (1995). *Assistive technology for persons with disabilities*. Bethesda, MD: American Occupational Therapy Association.

National Reverse Mortgage Lenders Association. (2002). *Just the FAQs: Answers to common questions about reverse mortgages*. Washington, DC: Author.

Olsen, R. V., Hutchings L., & Ehrenkrantz, E. (2000). *A house for all children*. Newark: New Jersey Institute Press.

Panero, J., & Zelnik, M. (1979). *Human dimension and interior spaces*. New York: Whitney Library.

Perry, L. G., Jawer, M. A., Murdoch, J. R., & Dinegar, J. C. (1991). *BOMA International's ADA compliance guidebook: A checklist for your building*. Washington, DC: Building Owner's and Manager's Association.

Pirkl, J. J. (1994). *Transgenerational design: Products for an aging population*. New York: Van Nostrand Reinhold.

Rebuilding Together. (2007). *Home modifications assessment and solutions checklist*. Retrieved November 18, 2009, from www.rebuildingtogether.org

Rehabilitation Act of 1973, Pub. L. 93–112, 29 U.S.C. § 701 *et seq.*

SAIL. (2002). *Practical guide to universal home design*. St. Paul, MN: East Metro Seniors Agenda for Independent Living.

Sprague, D. (2009). *Financial resources for low income households*. Retrieved November 19, 2009, from www.lifetimehome.us

U.S. Census Bureau. (1999). *Federal Interagency Forum on Age-related Statistics. Data base news in aging*. Washington, DC: Author.

U.S. Consumer Product Safety Commission. (1981). *Safety for older consumers home safety checklist*. Washington, DC: Author.

University of Birmingham, Centre for Applied Gerontology. (1999). Retrieved October 15, 2003, from www.gerontology.bham.ac.uk

Welch, P., & Palames, C. (1995). *A brief history of disability rights legislation in the United States: Strategies for teaching universal design*. Boston: Adaptive Environments Center.

Yeung, Y. (2003). Educating older adults in AT. *OT Practice, 8*(15), 12–15.

Chapter 20

Therapeutic Partnerships: Occupational Therapy and Home-Based Care

MARGARET A. PERKINSON, PHD; CLAUDIA L. HILTON, PHD, OTR/L, SROT, FAOTA; KERRI MORGAN, MSOT, OTR/L; AND MONICA PERLMUTTER, MA, OTR/L

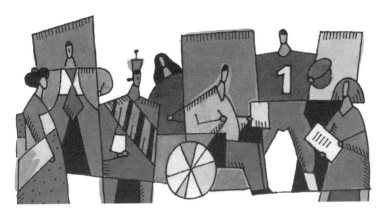

KEY WORDS

ethnographic approach

explanatory model of illness

family caregiver

family-centered care

personal assistance services

personal care attendant

HIGHLIGHTS

- Family caregivers play a key role in developing daily living strategies, serve as gatekeepers to the health and social services providers, and assist with decision making when a client is unable manage his or her health care independently.

- Family-centered approaches are used across the lifespan and focus on a collaborative relationship wherein the client, family, and therapist participate in the evaluation and intervention-planning processes, and decisions made by the family are respected.

- Use of an explanatory model will provide the therapist with insight into the client's and family's beliefs and knowledge of the illness and guide assessment and intervention.

- Many different caregiver assessments are available, including informal interviews and observations as well as standard measures such as the Functional Behavior Profile, the Burden Interview, and the Memory and Behaviors Problems Checklist.

- Occupational therapy intervention is enhanced by caregivers who can help clients voice their concerns, give the therapist tips for interacting with the client, and provide insight regarding how receptive the client may be to a given treatment plan.

- The role acquisition, role enactment, and role disengagement and re-engagement stages of caregiving bring different challenges and needs to the client and family member and should be considered as treatment plans are developed.

- Occupational therapists can be instrumental in helping clients learn to hire and manage personal care attendants.

OBJECTIVES

After reading this material, readers will be able to

- Understand the scope of formal and informal caregiving services currently provided;

- Describe the characteristics of a family-centered approach to occupational therapy practice;

- Define an explanatory model of illness;

- Explain the impact of the HIPAA Privacy Rule on communication between occupational therapists and family members;

- Identify the family caregiver's values, needs, and priorities as part of the occupational therapy evaluation process for any patient or client;

- Describe the contributions a family caregiver can make to the planning and implementation of treatment;

- Identify the three stages of a caregiving career and the ways in which the occupational therapist can work with the family caregiver at each stage; and

- Recognize the occupational therapist's role in working with a person to develop the IADL skills of an attendant care manager.

Family caregivers frequently play a pivotal role in developing daily living strategies for people with disabilities. They represent the major proportion of the long-term care workforce in the United States (Wolff & Kasper, 2006). In addition to assisting with activities of daily living (ADLs), family caregivers act as gatekeepers to the health and social services system for relatives requiring more extensive assistance. For people who cannot manage health decisions alone, family caregivers usually interpret the illness, decide how symptoms should be managed, and eventually decide when and how professional health care providers should become involved.

Family caregivers are most often informal (i.e., unpaid relatives), although that is not universally the case (Family Caregiver Alliance, 2007; LaPlante, Harrington, & Kang, 2002). Formal caregivers are paid personal care attendants who are directly employed by the person or family requiring assistance.

This chapter explores how occupational therapists can best work with formal and informal care providers to people with disabilities.

Importance of Family Care Providers

Approximately 10.3 million people ages 18 or older who live in communities (not in institutions) experience difficulty in completing daily activities. Of these, approximately, 4.6 million need assistance with ADLs—dressing, bathing, toileting, grooming, transferring, feeding, meal preparation, and light household work. Over 9 million also require assistance with instrumental activities of daily living (IADLs), for example, taking medications, visiting health care facilities, and shopping (Center for Personal Assistive Services, 2009).

Family caregivers are the major source of care for people with disabilities (Stone & Newcomer, 2009). In the United States, approximately 80% of noninstitutionalized adults who require long-term care receive it entirely from informal caregivers (Thompson, 2004). The estimated value of family caregiving services is $306 billion, nearly twice the amount spent on formal home care and nursing home services combined ($158 billion; Arno, 2006). Although most recipients of home care are elderly, more than one-third are younger than 60 years of age (Marks, 1996). Family members provide care for people who have a variety of physical or mental disabilities or chronic conditions, ranging from cerebral palsy and Down syndrome to cancer, HIV/AIDS, diabetes, dementia, arthritis, multiple sclerosis, and heart disease.

Changes in the health care scene make the role of the family in caregiving more important now than ever before. Changes in Medicare's reimbursement policies have resulted in the discharge of patients to the community earlier in their recovery (Wolff & Kasper, 2006), putting greater responsibility on the family to provide post-hospital care. Higher survival rates for previously fatal injuries and conditions, the AIDS epidemic, and policies favoring deinstitutionalization also contribute to the increase in home care (Baum & LaVesser, 1994).

Perhaps most significant in the rise in family caregiving, however, is the rapidly growing number of older adults. In 1900, people older than 65 years of age represented only 4% of the U.S. population. By 2007, this group had grown to 37.9 million, or 12.6%, and by 2030 they are projected to represent 70 million, or almost 20% of the total population (Harrington, Ng, Kaye, & Newcomer, 2009; U.S. National Center for Health Statistics, 2009).

The oldest of the old (those ages 85 or older) represent the fastest growing segment of the population, projected to grow from 4.2 million in 2000 to 5.7 million in 2010, an increase of 36% in 10 years (Administration on Aging, 2008). Aging does not inevitably lead to disability, and most older adults do not require help with ADLs. Nevertheless, activity limitations tend to increase over time as a result of underlying disease states (U.S. National Center for Health Statistics, 2009).

The need for assistance with ADLs increases with age; less than 3% of people younger than 65 years of age require help with ADLs, compared to 3.2% of people 65–74 years of age, and 8.6% of people ages 75 or over (U.S. National Center for Health Statistics, 2009). Most adults with disabilities continue to live in the community. They are able to do so because of the informal care they receive from family members (Schultz & Martire, 2004). Caregivers' attributes, such as level of perceived burden and self-rated health, are important predictors of early institutionalization of people with disabilities (Gaugler, Kane, Kane, Clay, & Newcomer, 2003; Schultz & Matire, 2004).

Research on family caregiving shows that maintaining people with disabilities in the community is challenging (Pruchno, 1999; Roth, Perkins, Wadley, Temple, & Haley, 2009). Family caregiving can be disruptive and stressful and can have significant negative effects on the mental and physical health of care providers (Pinquart & Sorenson, 2003). Family caregiving also can provide positive and uplifting experiences (Beach, Schultz, Yee & Jackson, 2000; Ohaeri, 2003). As a group, caregivers do not receive sufficient support from family and friends, and health and social services providers generally do not offset this need for assistance (Aneshensel, Pearlin,

Mullan, Zarit, & Whitlatch, 1995; Bookman & Harrington, 2007). How can occupational therapists more effectively aid family caregivers; that is, how can they ameliorate the negative aspects of providing care and enhance its positive dimensions?

Parent as Caregiver

Families are the first and most important source of stability in a child's life. They typically hold primary responsibility for making decisions about their children (Erwin & Brown, 2003). Good quality of life for the family will result in positive outcomes for the child. Therefore, families must be recognized as equal partners in providing services to their children with disabilities. Factors that contribute to parental stress and support parental effectiveness are discussed below.

Parental Stress

Parental stress has been examined in many studies of parents of children with disabilities. Behavioral problems or regulatory problems are commonly associated with increased parental stress (Anderson, 2008; Davis & Carter, 2008; Eisenhower, Baker, & Blacher, 2009; Ketelaar, Volman, Gorter, & Vermeer, 2008). They can lead to marital problems and feelings of depression and incompetence. Maladaptive behaviors, poorer health, and greater social impairment also contribute to less positive mother–child relationships, less maternal involvement in the child's education, and compromised ability to parent effectively (Anderson, 2008; Benson, Karlof, & Siperstein, 2008; Orsmond, Seltzer, Greenberg, & Krauss, 2006). Single parents and parents in poor health report significantly higher levels of stress than other parents (Anderson, 2008).

Sleep disruptions, a common problem faced by parents of children with chronic illness, can lead to poor sleep quality, depression, and anxiety (Meltzer & Moore, 2008). A study that examined responses of parents of adolescents with burns found a higher incidence of mental health problems and cardiovascular health problems than a control group in the first 2 years after the incident (Dorn, Yaermans, Spreeuwenberg, & van der Zee, 2007). In another study, mothers of children with developmental disabilities reported a sense of isolation, depression, and the feeling of being overwhelmed (Parish, 2006). In a study of mothers of children with Asperger syndrome, stress levels were positively correlated with the levels of sensory sensitivities observed in the children (Epstein, Saltzman-Benaiah, O'Hare, Goll, & Tuck, 2008).

Community Issues

Difficulties in securing care for their children and the lack of coordination of care among service providers were identified as stress factors for parents (Parish, 2006; Law et al., 1999). In addition, a lack of transition planning and the drastic decline of services available once the children become adolescents were identified as barriers faced by mothers and their children with disabilities (Parish, 2006).

Supports

Support from extended families and families with high levels of involvement and cohesion was correlated with significantly less stress for mothers of children with disabilities (Anderson, 2008; Parish, 2006). Support from peers without disabilities was also identified as a factor related to lower stress. Mothers identified respite care, summer programs, after-school care, and training services funded by Medicaid as critical supports for managing family life (Parish, 2006). In addition, and perhaps contrary to popular opinion, working mothers reported finding emotional and psychological benefits from continuing to work (Parish, 2006).

Use of Routines

Daily routines provide opportunities for mothers to facilitate their children's development (Kellegrew, 1998, 2000). Routines constructed by mothers of young children with disabilities are based on the mother's available time, her values, and her anticipation of the child's future needs.

Consideration of parental stress, supports, and routines is helpful when completing an assessment and developing an intervention plan for a child, because they will help the therapist better understand the abilities and limits of the parent. In this way, the therapist will be better able to prioritize goals in order to achieve an optimal level of care for the child.

Therapist–Family Caregiver Relationship

According to the *Occupational Therapy Practice Framework* (American Occupational Therapy Association [AOTA], 2008) (hereinafter the *Framework*), both the person referred for therapy and the people supporting or caring for that person may be considered clients. The expanded scope of the concept *client* raises a number of issues that affect the therapist's role. As noted above, family caregivers typically experience significant stress, which often leads to physical and mental distress (Berg-Weger, Rubio, & Tebb, 2000). Signs of depression, such as

emotional exhaustion, listlessness, inability to sleep (or sleeping too much), loss of appetite, loss of interest in favorite activities, and feelings of guilt or sadness are signals that the family member requires some form of intervention (Morris & Gainer, 1997; Navaie-Waliser et al., 2002). Suggestions for coping with stress, such as time management techniques and the use of respite care, may help family members who are approaching caregiving burnout.

Although the caregiver-as-client approach is useful in certain situations, it still defines the relationship between the occupational therapist and family member as one between an expert and a person in need. This type of relationship implies an imbalance of power in which the client is expected to defer to the authority of the expert (Lawlor & Mattingly, 1998; Perkinson, 1992). By definition, clients have a dependent status; they are encouraged to rely on experts to define their problems, assess the causes of those problems, and determine the proper treatments. Clients are expected to comply with the plans proposed by experts and provide little active input into solutions. Such relationships, however, frequently lead to "unilateral dependency" (Estes & Binney, 1991), in which clients give up their responsibility to be actively involved in decision making and passively accept the expert's advice.

A different model of care, based on a philosophy of "helping people to help themselves," emphasizes the development of self-reliance and empowerment. Advocates of this model encourage clients to take an active role in resolving their problems and meeting their needs. The goal is to encourage caregivers and people with disabilities to discover and develop their own strengths and talents, thus improving their likelihood of success in dealing with their situations (Perkinson, 1992).

Therapists using this model see people with disabilities and their family members as partners in care and work to develop a collaborative therapeutic relationship. The result is a "therapeutic alliance" based on mutual understanding, respect, and cooperation among the therapist, the family members, and the client or patient (Brown, 1998). The trend toward a family-centered partnership approach has evolved throughout the field, from pediatric to geriatric occupational therapy (Baum, 1991; Case-Smith & Nastro, 1993; Hasselkus, 1991). It is the fundamental intervention model promoted in the Education for All Handicapped Children Act Amendments of 1986 (P.L. 99-457, p. 677; Schultz-Krohn, 1997).

Family-centered care acknowledges that family members know their relatives in ways that the therapist does not and that they often are well qualified

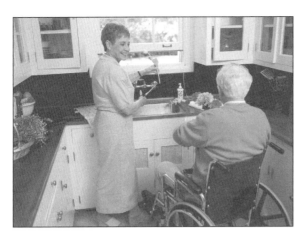

Figure 20.1. Family-centered caregiving is a philosophy that encourages partnerships between therapists and family members. It recognizes that family members bring important knowledge and are essential to the caregiving process.
Photo © PhotoDisc, Inc. Used under license.

to join in making decisions regarding their relative's care (Law, 1997; Perkinson, 2002; see Figure 20.1). Unlike health care professionals, who come and go, family members are a permanent and vital part of the life of a person with disabilities (Weinstein, 1997). With family-centered care, the focus is on the care recipient as part of a family (rather than on the care recipient alone). Rather than use their professional expertise to control and direct intervention, therapists provide information, knowledge, and options to the family and respect the decisions made by the family (Allen & Petr, 1998). In a collaborative relationship, the client, family and therapist participate in the evaluation, problem-solving, and decision-making processes. The family contributes to the process of determining the extent, type, and priorities of therapy. The traditional therapist-as-expert thinking is supported by a strict medical model but may affect the caregiver in ways the therapist does not anticipate (Case Study 20.1).

Multiple issues affect family-centered therapy. Family members' involvement in health care decision making typically occurs and escalates with low or diminished client capacities (i.e., with children or adults with cognitive impairments). Especially in cases of adults with declining cognitive ability. Determining who should be included in their health and research decisions and when to do so are open to multiple interpretations (Saks et al., 2008). Issues of client privacy and autonomy assume critical importance. Occupational therapists should be aware of the Health Insurance Portability and Accountability Act (HIPAA) of 1996 (P.L. 104-191) and its impact on communication with caregivers. Information provided by the U.S. De-

partment of Health and Human Services [DHHS], Office for Civil Rights (2006) states that HIPAA Privacy Rule (45 CFR 164.510b) permits covered entities to share information that is directly relevant to the involvement of a spouse, family members, friends, or other persons identified by a patient, in the patient's care or payment of health care (p. 57). The HIPAA Privacy Rule allows parents, a child's personal representative, or a recognized proxy the right to information regarding their relative's medical care. Exceptions include "when the minor is the one who consents and consent of the parent is not required under state law," when "the minor obtains care at direction of the court," or when "the parent agrees that the minor and the health care provider may have a confidential relationship" (DHHS, 2006, p. 56). The guidelines suggest that, ideally, the patient should have the opportunity to agree to discuss their care with family members or other involved persons. Some hospitals and clinics require written consent before health professionals can discuss medical information with caregivers, but this is not required by HIPAA regulations (DHHS, 2006). Various methods to assess the capacity to appoint a proxy for research consent have been suggested (Kim & Appelbaum, 2006). Recent research on lack of agreement between older adults and their adult children in regard to perceptions of the parents' psychosocial preferences, health status, and desired medical treatment further complicate the dynamics of health care decision making (Carpenter, Kissel, & Lee, 2007; Roberto, 1999; Whitlatch & Feinberg, 2003; Whitlatch, Piiparinen, & Feinberg, 2009).

A collaborative partnership represents a fundamental shift in the way therapy is defined and delivered (Toth-Cohen, 2000). Lawlor and Mattingly (1998) noted that this model presents challenges for the therapist, such as understanding issues confronting the person with disabilities and his or her family from the family's point of view and sharing decision-making power. The following section suggests ways to deal with some of those issues to achieve an effective partnership with family caregivers.

First Steps Toward Partnership With Family Caregivers: Assessment Issues

An effective partnership between caregivers and therapists depends upon a shared view and understanding of the illness or disability involved and how it should be treated (Hasselkus, 1988; LeNavenec & Vonhof, 1996). The first step toward achieving that goal is to identify the *explanatory model* of illness held by the client and the caregiver.

Case Study 20.1. Carrie—Medical Model Applied to Dealing With a Family Caregiver

Twelve-month-old Carrie was diagnosed with cerebral palsy, moderate right hemiplegia. She was referred for early intervention services, including occupational therapy. Carrie was living with her mother, father, and three older siblings in a one-story, ranch-style house on a farm owned and operated by her parents and grandparents.

Even with years of experience parenting Carrie's two brothers, ages 5 and 7 years, her mother was having tremendous difficulty dealing with Carrie's needs and emerging developmental delays. At the time of referral, Carrie was not using her right hand at all, was demonstrating asymmetrical posture, and used scooting in a sitting position as her primary means of mobility. Her drooling and difficulty handling table foods made mealtimes difficult. The occupational therapist assigned to the case quickly established a home program emphasizing neurodevelopmental treatment techniques to address the identified motor difficulties. Although she could find time in her schedule to see Carrie only once a week, the therapist spent considerable time teaching the home program she had designed to Carrie's mother.

Carrie began to show progress, so the occupational therapist was greatly surprised when the mother informed her that she was no longer in need of occupational therapy services through the early intervention agency. Instead, she was going to drive 50 miles roundtrip to the nearest children's hospital to have Carrie receive outpatient occupational therapy services twice a week.

An interview with the family at this time revealed some interesting information. It was learned that, although the occupational therapist had always been professional and friendly, she was always rushed and seemed never to ask Carrie's mother for her opinion of what was needed. The home program instructions were always written out and reviewed, but the tasks involved were more complicated and took more time than the mother thought she could handle. She reported feeling inadequate and guilty that she could not accomplish everything, frustrated with her attempts, and angry with the therapist for not being aware of her difficulties. When routinely asked "How are you doing with the exercises?" she felt chastised for not doing more. She also had mixed feelings about the direction the therapy was taking. She agreed that Carrie's motor skill development was important, but what really worried her was that Carrie was not getting enough nutrition because of her feeding difficulties, and she just wanted to have a pleasant mealtime with the entire family. Finally, she believed that more therapy on a regular schedule was desirable and that she could handle the drive better than she could handle being a surrogate therapist for her daughter.

Case Analysis: What Should Have Happened?

Had the occupational therapist approached this case from a family-centered perspective, the results may have been different. On the first visit, a family interview could have identified and ranked family strengths, needs, and goals. Collaborating with the family on an ongoing basis most likely would have moved things along a different course, resulting in progress for Carrie and better satisfaction for her mother and the family.

Explanatory models are sets of beliefs and knowledge that people use to explain sickness and treatment. The models provide a way of thinking about illness that influences its meaning and guides choices among various therapies (Kleinman, 1988; Krefting & Krefting, 1991). An explanatory model can include beliefs about an illness's cause, seriousness, and prognosis; the possibility of a cure; the appropriate treatment; and legitimate sources of help. The model influences whether a person even recognizes or believes a problem exists. The explanatory model underlies decision making about the illness, guiding decisions about treatment and help-seeking and defining sources of help and caregiving goals.

People understand the health care information and messages they receive within the context of their own beliefs. In effect, information and suggestions from the therapist are filtered through the explanatory models of both the person with disabilities and the caregiver. Aspects of the message that are most compatible with a person's explanatory model are more likely to be heard, accepted, and remembered. Elements of the message that conflict with the model are more likely to be tuned out or dismissed. For example, if a family caregiver of a cardiac patient sees the heart as a machine that has been fixed by the patient's bypass surgery, the caregiver may believe that the heart problem has been resolved and treatment is over. The caregiver may not understand the need for ongoing attention to lifestyle changes, such as modification of diet or maintenance of a permanent exercise plan. Therapists need to recognize the role of the caregiver's health beliefs and how these beliefs affect their behavior.

To develop a collaborative partnership with the family, the therapist must identify the caregiver's explanatory model (and the explanatory model of the person with disability) and recognize potential points of conflict or differences in understanding between them and the therapist's explanatory model. In conducting the initial assessment, the therapist might include questions to elicit the caregiver's explanatory model (as well as that of the person with disabilities, when appropriate). Therapists might include some or all of the following questions, depending on the level of sensitivity of particular questions in a given case:

- What worries you the most about this illness or condition?
- What do you think caused the problems of the person with disabilities?
- Why do you think this illness happened at this particular time?
- How serious do you think this illness or condition is?
- What kind of treatment would you like your family member to receive?
- What are the most important results you expect to achieve with treatment? (Kleinman, 1980; Krefting & Krefting, 1991).

During the initial assessment, the therapist also should determine the meaning of the caregiving role to the family member and how he or she makes sense of caregiving experiences. Additional questions might include the following:

- What motivates you, and what is the significance of caregiving to you?
- What influences how you provide daily care?
- What do you find most burdensome about caregiving?
- What do you find most satisfying about caregiving?
- What are your major concerns? (Gubrium & Sankar, 1990; Hasselkus, 1988, 1989).

The assessment should include a joint evaluation by the caregiver and therapist of the family's problems and resources in addressing caregiving needs. The caregiver and therapist can then collaborate on the basis of the joint assessment to develop goals and procedures that are acceptable to all the people involved.

Additional assessment tools are available to obtain essential information on clients and family caregivers. The Canadian Occupational Performance Measure (COPM; Law et al., 1998) is a useful assessment to establish occupational profiles of people with disabilities as well as their caregivers (AOTA, 2008). This tool is an interview-based assessment that asks the person with disabilities or the family member to identify problem areas and priorities for intervention. Another tool, the Functional Behavior Profile (Baum, Edwards, & Morrow-Howell, 1993), asks caregivers to report the frequency of various behaviors that they have observed during recent interactions with the person with disabilities and provides valuable information for case planning. The Burden Interview (Zarit, Reever, & Bach-Peterson, 1980) and the Memory and Behavior Problems Checklist (Teri et al., 1992) provide therapists with insight into the factors that contribute to feelings of burden in family members.

If the occupational therapist has limited time for assessment and productivity standards are an issue, caregiver evaluations may be sent home for the family member to complete. Caregiver evaluation can be prioritized to focus on the client's and caregiver's primary concerns, such as ability to use the telephone or to transfer safely to the toilet. Occupational therapists may require extra time to establish rapport with the client and family before addressing some of the more sensitive questions related to caregiving.

The therapist may supplement traditional assessment techniques with an ethnographic approach to information gathering about caregiving. Ethnographic methods offer ways to understand the caregiver's perspective and techniques to achieve a joint appraisal of the situation and the client's needs (Gitlin, Corcoran, & Leinsmiller-Eckhardt, 1995; Hasselkus, 1990, 1997). Using an ethnographic approach, the therapist attempts to understand a way of life as it is viewed by another person (in this case, the family caregiver). An ethnographic interview focuses on values, meanings, beliefs, and how the person providing the information makes sense of his or her situation. Conducting the interview in a nonjudgmental manner, the therapist suspends his or her own beliefs and values as to the appropriate course of treatment in an attempt to discover what actually drives client and caregiver perceptions and behaviors (Gitlin et al., 1995). The interview is semistructured; it consists of open-ended questions and appropriate probes with which the therapist attempts to elicit and understand the caregiver's (or, when appropriate, care recipient's) point of view.

The questions used to elicit caregivers' explanatory models, discussed above, is one example of the ethnographic interview. Another relevant example is the semistructured interview designed to discover the level of knowledge and comfort of family members or principal caregivers with their role (Weinstein, 1997). Weinstein's semistructured interview format invites caregivers to

- Identify their opinions, personal goals, and needs;
- Describe their perceptions of the care recipient's problem;
- Describe a typical day at home;
- Describe the effect of the situation on themselves and other members of the family; and
- Identify what kind of information they personally would like from the occupational therapist.

This type of interview can lay the groundwork for establishing the collaborative partnership that is central to the philosophy of family-centered care. As the therapist takes the time to understand the caregiver's perspective (including the meaning ascribed to caregiving, how care is provided in the home, and what is perceived as problematic), the therapist also builds rapport with the family member. This rapport establishes a measure of trust and enhances the level of comfort with future discussions in which the therapist can share perspectives on the caregiving situation (Hasselkus, 1997).

After identifying the caregiver's views and his or her understanding of the care recipient's condition and needs, the therapist may want to discuss any differences in perspective that could lead to misunderstandings or points of disagreement. Respect for the caregiver's and care recipient's points of view should always be maintained during this process.

Often, family caregivers and the therapists use different explanatory models for the condition of the person with disabilities. Medical anthropologists have developed a therapeutic approach to enhance cross-cultural communication between patients and health care providers (Berlin & Fowkes, 1983) that could be useful when this occurs. Structured around the acronym *LEARN,* this set of guidelines helps therapists and family caregivers with initially different points of view to "get on the same wavelength" and take the first step toward developing a therapeutic alliance. The steps of the LEARN approach are as follows:

- *Listen* with sympathy and understanding to the caregiver's perception of the illness and caregiving situation. After the family caregiver's perspective has been recognized and

good rapport has been developed with the caregiver, the therapist can then share a personal point of view.
- *Explain* the therapist's perceptions of the problem.
- *Acknowledge* and review the areas in which the therapist and the caregiver agree, and work to resolve major conceptual conflicts.
- *Recommend* a treatment plan that involves both sides as full partners in deciding what to do.
- *Negotiate* to reach a treatment plan that is agreeable to all parties and that takes the perspective of each person (the person with disabilities, the caregiver, and the therapist) into account.

The ethnographic approach and the LEARN techniques can help therapists work with family caregivers to develop treatment strategies that fit the values and beliefs of each member but remain rooted in the theory and practice of occupational therapy. Viewing the family caregiver as a partner and taking values and beliefs of the family into account will increase the likelihood that the jointly developed treatment plan will be successfully integrated into family routines (Corcoran & Gitlin, 1992; Gitlin, 1993). In acknowledging the family caregiver as a partner who has much to contribute, the therapist encourages the family to assume and maintain responsibility for long-term care.

What Family Caregivers Can Contribute to Occupational Therapy Intervention

A family caregiver has much to contribute as a partner in the planning and execution of the treatment process (Perkinson, 2002). As a mediator between the person with disabilities and the therapist, the family caregiver can

- Help the family member with disabilities voice his or her own needs and concerns,
- Communicate those needs and concerns to the therapist, and
- Communicate or clarify treatment plans and goals to the family member with disabilities.

To the extent possible, the family member should negotiate with the client the nature and level of his or her involvement in the caregiving role. Therapists may assist in this process, if necessary, with sensitivity toward the needs and perspectives of all involved. Preservation of the client's sense of control and empowerment should be a priority in this negotiation. However, as mentioned, family members may disagree among themselves, with the client, or both in their perceptions of the client's situation and preferences and in regard to appropriate treatment and goals. This diversity of perspectives represents one of the major barriers to achieving true client- or family-centered care (Kyler, 2008; Sumsion, 1999). Therapists should be sensitive to such situations. To avoid taking sides, the therapist should conduct assessments, including the questions in Table 20.1, with the client first, if possible, and then, with the client's permission, ask the caregiver to confirm or add to the client's responses, maintaining a tone of support for the client at all times.

Although there are potential pitfalls, family caregivers typically have a wealth of information that can help therapists better understand the client, the needs, and how best to address them (Perkinson, 2003). Caregivers often are attuned to the nuances of behavior and physical states of family members with disabilities. The caregiver knows what is "normal" and can help the therapist define realistic treatment goals. Caregivers also can advise the therapist of significant changes in the health status of clients. A caregiver typically has knowledge of the person's ability to perform self-care tasks that may affect treatment plans.

The family caregiver can give the therapist tips for interacting with the person with disabilities and for interpreting his or her reactions to the therapist or to treatment suggestions. Caregivers often can sense how receptive the family member will be to a given treatment plan and may suggest ways to present the plan to maximize the likelihood that the client will accept it. For example, the caregiver might present the

Table 20.1. Checklist of Information About the Client to Assist in Planning Caregiver Intervention

Information Category	Information Caregivers May Provide
Client characteristics	• What significant background information about the care receiver will help the therapist know the client as a person and better understand the care receiver's behavior and moods? For example, information on the care receiver's past occupation, hobbies, interests, significant life events, memberships in clubs or organizations, and travels will help the practitioner interact with the client on a more personal level. • What are known motivators (i.e., what pleases or excites the client)? • Does the client have particular idiosyncrasies (e.g., unusual modesty, aversion toward noise)? • What fears does the client have (e.g., fear of confined spaces, crowds, or being left alone)? • What special activities can be used to deal with emotions? When the client is upset or stressed, what are the habitual or effective ways of dealing with this (e.g., calming music, being left alone, diverting attention, touch, massage)? Is the client receptive to trying new routines, or does he or she prefer an established pattern of activity? • What are the client's known allergies, pet peeves, and emotional triggers? • How well does the client typically cope with stress?
Activities of daily living/ Instrumental activities of daily living	• Does the client prefer a shower or a bath? • When is bathing preferred? • Are there bathing accessories that are customarily used (e.g., bath oils, loofah mitts, sponges, scrubbers, brushes)? • What dressing and grooming preferences does the client have (e.g., hairstyles, type of perfume or cologne, body lotions, clothing styles and colors, aversive reactions to fabrics)? • What are the client's food preferences and eating habits (e.g., eating a large breakfast, snacking throughout the day)? • Can the family caregiver assist in maintaining the client's proper diet or nutritional needs during meal preparation? • Can the family member identify a suitable bathing assistant with whom the client can be comfortable?
Leisure	• What are the client's favorite types of exercise or physical activity? • Is the client motivated to pursue an exercise program? • Does the client like to read the paper and/or magazines? Does he or she have favorite television programs? • Does the client have favorite hobbies or other pastimes (e.g., board games, crossword puzzles)?
Social participation	• Does the client call friends and relatives regularly? • Does the client regularly receive and send mail or e-mail?

plan to the care recipient or, to the extent possible, enlist him or her in development of the plan (enhancing the family's investment in it). Table 20.1 offers a checklist of useful client-related information that family members can share with the therapist to optimize intervention planning. Family caregivers also can assist in motivating people with disabilities by encouraging them to cooperate with the treatment plan.

Occupation is a critical factor in determining quality of life, no matter how ill a person may be or what disabilities he or she may have (Baum, 1995). With their knowledge of the family member's past history and preferences, family caregivers can play a vital role in identifying meaningful tasks and engaging the person with disabilities in those activities. They can also help identify the person's abilities and limits, what tasks or activities frustrate the person, and what tasks or activities give him or her satisfaction. This information helps the therapy team set realistic, appropriate, and challenging goals. Identifying and incorporating the preferences of the person with disabilities into the treatment plan should significantly improve his or her quality of life and the probability that he or she will find the plan acceptable. As the treatment plan is carried out, the family caregiver also can assist in its evaluation and modification by giving feedback to the therapist about what is working and what should be changed.

What Family Caregivers Need at Key Stages of the Caregiving Process

As research on family caregiving has expanded to include longitudinal studies, researchers have begun to develop the outlines of various stages of the caregiving career (see Table 20.2, containing stages modified from Aneshensel et al., 1995). Those stages include role acquisition, role enactment, role disengagement, and role re-engagement. Each stage brings different challenges and needs on the part of the person with disabilities and the caregiver. The family-centered treatment plan should take into account these stage-related needs (see Case Study 20.2). Although the stages were extrapolated from populations of caregivers for adults with impairments (especially in cognitive function), many points are relevant to caregivers for young clients as well.

Role Acquisition Stage

Role acquisition occurs at the onset of the condition or illness or when the family member first assumes the role of caregiver. During this stage, the person with disabilities and the caregiver must learn to adjust to the new situation and plan for the future. The family caregiver typically has little knowledge about the illness, unless it tends to run in the family or the family caregiver has had experience in the health care field. Therapists can assist caregivers in this stage by providing information to help the family understand the illness, its possible causes, the various options for treatment, and what typically lies ahead.

The initial stage of a major illness represents a significant life transition for both the person with disabilities and his or her family caregiver. It often requires considerable adjustments in life goals, relationships, daily activities, and routines. Emotional support is essential at this stage (Meuser & Marwit, 2001; Pinquart & Sorenson, 2003), and the therapist may consider linking the family to appropriate counseling services. Interaction with family members and caregivers of people with similar

Table 20.2. Stages and Needs of the Caregiving Career

Stage	Family Challenges	Practitioner Role
Role acquisition	Must adjust to new demands Must learn about illness and what lies ahead	Provides information and reassurance Helps family anticipate future needs
Role enactment	May need training in direct care skills and behavioral management May need advice about institutional placement or community resources	Provides training as needed, such as in the use of assistive devices and transfer skills Provides information on placement options and resources
Disengagement	Adjustment to death of care receiver Adjustment to social isolation and burnout	Assists family with transition Makes referrals to resources that can help with grief or readjustment

Case Study 20.2. Mrs. Kannon—Stages of Caregiving

Background

Mrs. Kannon is an 84-year-old woman with macular degeneration (AMD), dementia, and depression. She experienced complete loss of her hearing at age 13. Her primary caregiver is her daughter, Carol.

Occupational Profile

Mrs. Kannon raised two children and enjoyed a happy 40-year marriage before her husband passed away. She liked to garden and read, was active in her church, and loved to travel throughout her adult life.

Carol is 66 years old and lives with her husband; she is a retired librarian. She loved to decorate her home, do cross-stitch, and attend Bible study classes. Carol is in relatively good health, although she has intermittent low back pain.

Role Acquisition Stage

Mrs. Kannon began to experience memory problems about the same time she began to lose her central vision due to AMD. She had difficulty remembering to pay her bills and forgot the names of acquaintances at church. Mrs. Kannon lived in her home of 60 years in a Kansas City suburb. Her daughter, Carol, lived in Chicago, and Mrs. Kannon's son, John, lived in Los Angeles. Carol began to visit her mother more frequently to accompany her mother to doctor's appointments and assist with transportation to the grocery store. Mrs. Kannon decided that this would be a good time for her daughter to assume power of attorney in case this was needed in the future. Mrs. Kannon and her daughter also revisited her advance directive and updated her will with the assistance of an attorney. In addition, they visited the local Low Vision Resource Center.

Role Enactment Stage

After a year or so of Carol making regular trips to help her mother, Mrs. Kannon began to have increased confusion and memory loss. Their neurologist indicated it was likely that she had Alzheimer's disease (AD). She required more support from her daughter to plan meals and clean the house and was no longer able to monitor her financial needs. One weekend, Mrs. Kannon went out to get the mail and wandered off. This event prompted Carol to ask her mother to move to Chicago to live with her and her husband. Mrs. Kannon was very reluctant, but agreed.

Mrs. Kannon was able to participate in all of her self-care but needed supervision for cutting food, retrieving clothes, and bathing. Carol attempted to involve her mom in household chores and activities, but as Mrs. Kannon's cognitive status declined she was less able to participate.

Carol consulted the local Alzheimer's Disease Foundation and acquired information regarding making her home safe for her mother; Carol was still very concerned about her mother's wandering. In addition, she consulted an occupational therapist who specialized in low vision. The therapist administered the COPM to Mrs. Kannon and her daughter, which revealed that Mrs. Kannon had difficulty using her computer and TTY telephone and was no longer able to read standard print and to garden. The therapist provided recommendations regarding self-care concerns, such as grab bars for the shower and toilet to increase safety and independence. Additional locks for the front and back doors were suggested to reduce wandering risk. Lighting was improved in key areas of the home and large, bold keyboard labels were applied to the TTY telephone. Various adaptive strategies were recommended so Mrs. Kannon could pursue her leisure interests.

The occupational therapist also conducted an informal caregiver interview and administered the Memory and Behavior Problems Checklist. These caregiver assessments indicated that Carol was feeling overwhelmed with caring for her mother. Carol expressed frustration with her mother's repetitive behaviors, need for constant reminders, and the lack of available medical treatment to help her mother. Carol indicated she was grieving the loss of the mother she had always known and stated "Alzheimer's disease stole my mother." She expressed the need for a companion to stay with her mother so she could run errands and attend her Bible study class. Carol indicated growing resentment toward her brother, because she was bearing the majority of the responsibility for her mother's care. The therapist contacted the local deaf communication program that had students who might be able to provide respite services. The therapist also provided resources re: the local Alzheimer's Association, a support group, and an online chat room for caregivers of persons with AD. Carol and the therapist discussed ways of approaching her brother and determining how he might be able to take on some of the responsibilities.

Mrs. Kannon lived with her daughter and son-in-law for 2 years. During this time, a companion stayed with Mrs. Kannon two mornings per week, allowing Carol to attend Bible study classes and run errands. Mrs. Kannon's son, John, made 2–3 trips to Chicago per year so that Carol and her husband could travel. As Mrs. Kannon's cognitive abilities further declined, it

(Continued)

Case Study 20.2. Mrs. Kannon—Stages of Caregiving *(cont.)*

became evident that she would be better cared for in a nearby nursing home setting. This difficult transition for Mrs. Kannon and her children was made easier with the support of the occupational therapist, social worker, and nursing home staff. Mrs. Kannon visited her mother daily and, over time, developed a collaborative relationship with the nursing home staff.

Role Disengagement

Mrs. Kannon passed away after living in the nursing home for 5 months. Carol and her brother experienced a significant sense of loss. Carol found that she had become somewhat socially isolated and had to slowly rebuild her connections with her friends and volunteer activities. She attended several bereavement support group sessions, and the occupational therapist at the nursing home talked with her about identifying her priorities and re-structuring her weekly routine.

---

conditions through support groups or peer counseling programs can be especially helpful. Peer caregivers can share strategies for dealing with everyday issues, including managing ADLs, and provide encouragement rooted in empathy (Perkinson, 1995).

Therapists can provide much assistance at this stage by helping the family take steps to prevent future problems. They can help identify potential legal and financial issues, such as the need to obtain durable powers of attorney for asset management and health care (if the family has not already addressed these issues). Therapists also can provide general information and referrals to legal or financial planning sources for help with other issues, such as advance directives, wills, and arrangements, to anticipate increased medical costs (Baum, 1991; Overman & Stoudemire, 1988).

Role Enactment Stage

Following role acquisition, the role enactment stage encompasses most of the caregiving experience. It includes the provision of home care and, in some cases, the decision for institutional placement. During this stage, family caregivers require continued education about the nature of the illness or condition of the person with disabilities, including its expected trajectory. Caregivers also may benefit from training in direct-care skills, especially those relating to helping the person with disabilities perform self-care tasks. Topics of interest might include safely transferring or bathing the person with disabilities, learning to cue various ADL and IADL tasks, and setting up routines to promote the highest level of performance (Baum, 1991; Schulz, 2000; Sorenson, Pinquart, & Duberstein, 2002).

Therapists can also instruct the caregiver in the use of relevant assistive devices and conduct home assessments to suggest various environmental interventions that may make the home safer (Gallagher-Thompson, 1994; Gitlin, Corcoran, Winter, Boyce, & Hauck, 2001; Heagerty & Eskenazi, 1994).

When appropriate, coaching in behavior management techniques may be especially helpful to caregivers in dealing with disruptive behaviors (Teri et al., 2003; Zarit & Teri, 1991). In some cases, such as the advanced stages of Alzheimer's disease or other forms of dementia, family caregivers may benefit from instruction in communication techniques. A growing literature suggests ways to preserve identity and personhood for people with severe cognitive impairments and ways to communicate with them more effectively (Leibing, 2006; McLean, 2007; Perkinson, 1999; Sabat & Harre, 1992).

Family caregivers may benefit from instruction in stress management (Steffen, 2000) and time management. They may need help in setting limits, developing realistic standards, and prioritizing goals (Aneshensel et al., 1995). Caregivers also may require help in dealing with changing family dynamics. Disagreements among family members often emerge as a result of differences in perceptions of the illness or condition and methods for managing it. Conflicts may arise in determining who will assume responsibility for tasks previously performed by the person with disabilities and how the additional work and costs of caregiving will be shared. Caregivers also may need guidance on how to explain the family member's illness or condition to extended family and friends in such a way that they maintain continued supportive relations (Fortinsky & Hathaway, 1990).

Family caregivers often are unaware of available community resources and how to access them (Morris & Gainer, 1997). Therapists should develop a resource file to identify relevant resources, including payment sources. Such resources would include programs offering training and support, such as classes in caregiving and health education, support groups, e-mail discussion groups, and 24-hour hotlines. The therapist can identify a number of useful health newsletters, Web sites, and publications on caregiving, such as *The 36-Hour Day* (Mace & Rabins, 2006).

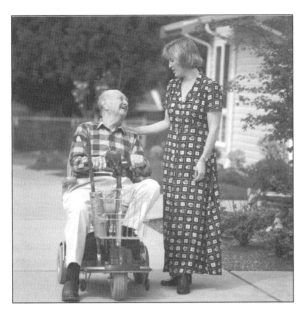

Figure 20.2. Occupational therapists can advise family caregivers on strategies to promote the well-being of their loved one while coping with stress and avoiding burnout. Photo © PhotoDisc Inc. Used under license.

Therapists can provide advice to family caregivers regarding in-home services that offer help with self-maintenance tasks, such as home health aides who can help with bathing, dressing, grooming, and transfers (Figure 20.2). Homemaking services can be hired to help with specific household chores like cleaning, laundry, or even shopping. Nutritionists can instruct caregivers in special nutritional needs, and agencies providing home-delivered meals can help meet them. Occupational therapists can work with physical therapists and exercise or rehabilitation programs to develop and maintain individualized exercise regimens based on preferred occupations of persons with disabilities (Gitlin et al., 2009; Perkinson, 2008).

Family caregivers must recognize the stressful nature of their role and take active steps to prevent burnout (Figure 20.3; Gitlin et al., 2003). Therapists can assist caregivers by encouraging self-care and discussing community sources of respite care, such as

- Adult or child day care programs,
- Extended overnight respite programs (offered by some nursing homes and assistive living facilities), and
- Informal support systems that can provide respite (e.g., the caregiver's support systems of family and friends).

In addition to learning how to access community services and programs and to locate appropriate

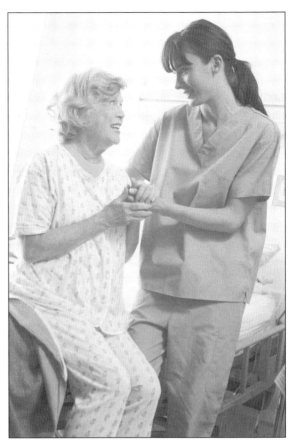

Figure 20.3. When caregiving burdens become too great for family members, therapists can assist in exploring alternative care options or can recommend temporary respite care. Photo © PhotoDisc Inc. Used under license.

sources of payment for these services, caregivers also can benefit from instructions on how to work effectively with health providers (Perkinson, 2002). The following section offers suggestions for caregivers working with formal personal care attendants, a type of health provider especially relevant for people with disabilities requiring outside assistance with ADLs.

Caregiving and Personal Care Attendants

Occupational therapists can play an important role in helping persons with disabilities coordinate personal assistance services. *Personal assistance services (PAS)* are defined as "a range of human and mechanical assistance provided to persons with disabilities of any age who require help with routine activities of daily living . . . and health maintenance activities" (Doty, Kasper, & Litvak, 1996).

Formal personal assistance is provided by home health care agencies, government employees, centers for independent living, or providers hired by the individual in need of help. An estimated 13.6 percent of personal assistance hours received by people with a disability are formal personal assistance (LaPlante et al., 2002). Many factors, including living alone (Tennstedt, McKinlay, & Kasten, 1994), increase the likelihood that a person with a disability requires formal PAS. Old age (LaPlante et al., 2002), low economic status (Kennedy, 1997), female gender (LaPlante et al., 2002), African-American ethnicity (LaPlante et al., 2002), and severity of medical condition (Agree, 1999) are also indicators.

PAS are associated with the Independent Living (IL) Movement, which began in the early 1970s (DeJong & Wenker, 1983). The concept is to allow people with disabilities to live as they choose in their communities rather than confining them to institutions. Services provided by personal care attendants enable people with severe disabilities to live independently within the community. The Olmstead Supreme Court decision (*Olmstead v. LC*, 1999) directed states to provide necessary support for people with disabilities who are able and willing to live and participate in community settings. As a result, state and federal programs have begun to reduce barriers to community living for such individuals. The Medicaid Home and Community-Based Waiver programs provide paid PAS to individuals with disabilities who meet the state's income eligibility criteria. The purpose of these and other PAS programs is to help people with a disability increase their ability to engage in activities that are difficult or impossible for them to do alone (Doty et al., 1996; Litvak, Zukas, & Heumman, 1987).

A person with a disability who seeks formal PAS has two options: agency-provided services or consumer-directed services. Traditionally, the person with a disability would be referred to a company or agency to arrange the necessary assistance. Agencies hire, train, evaluate, and pay their own employees, whom they assign to new clients. The person with a disability must accept the attendant provided by the agency, without any certainty that the attendant is reliable, friendly, or efficient. The consumer has little choice in hiring, firing, or asserting control over the person sent by the agency (Batavia, 1996; Schopp et al., 2007).

The shift toward the IL model in the disability community prompted a greater emphasis on consumer control and direction of PAS delivery. Under this model, the person with disabilities determines the services needed; their frequency and duration; and the selection, training, and retention of personal care attendants (DeJong & Wenker, 1983;

Doty et al., 1996; Flanagan & Green, 1994; Scherzer, Wong, & Newcomer, 2007; Shapiro, 1993). The person with disabilities (or, sometimes, the family caregiver) is responsible for actively recruiting, selecting, managing, and directing the personal care attendants or other service providers (Batavia, DeJong, & McKnew, 1991).

Occupational therapists play a crucial role in working with the person with a disability to identify tasks that can be adapted and performed independently and tasks that will need to be completed with a personal attendant. Early in the course of rehabilitation, the therapist should help both the person with disabilities and his or her family begin the process of identifying specific PAS needs. This process starts with clarifying needs and expectations regarding relationships, work, and family. Encouraging the client to become assertive and to discuss his or her personal care needs facilitates this process. Consider the following questions in relation to specific ADLs:

- What does the person with the disability value more—independence in performing a specific task, or conserving energy and time for other tasks?
- Who should provide assistance for this task?
- What does the person with disabilities expect or want from the attendant?
- Should a person with disabilities struggle for more than an hour getting dressed alone?
- If so, how much energy will be left for other tasks during the rest of the day?

Some clients will find it important to perform self-care tasks independently. Others find that the challenges of work and the pleasures of family or other relationships are enhanced when they receive assistance from someone whom they have personally chosen and trained to help with self-care and other daily requirements.

Once the need for a personal care attendant has been established, the responsibility of the occupational therapist includes helping the person with disabilities and his or her family develop skill as an "attendant manager." The exercise of this skill can be considered an IADL. The relationship between people with disabilities and their attendants has been described as an employer–employee relationship (Lindley, 1995). Lack of management skills may be one of the most common problems encountered by the person with a disability in dealing with a personal care attendant. Necessary management skills related to personal care attendants include the ability to communicate expectations in terms of standards of performance, provide appropriate and timely feedback, and terminate employment when necessary (Opie & Miller, 1989). People with disabilities also must have the knowledge and communication skills necessary to train personal care attendants to complete the necessary tasks.

Recruitment, selection, and retention of PAS attendants can be difficult. Attendant turnover is a critical problem for PAS consumers. High turnover often can be attributed to employment disincentives such as low pay, few benefits, and lack of job status (Ulicny, Adler, & Jones, 1990). Under the IL model, occupational therapists typically are not directly involved with this aspect of PAS. They can, however, help the person with disabilities think through specific issues (Ulicny & Jones, 1985), such as how personal attendant chores should be defined and the times of day at which assistance will be needed. For example, a person who must leave for work early in the morning might need assistance with minimal self-care tasks (e.g., washing, dressing, brushing teeth). More time-consuming tasks (e.g., bowel care, showering) can be scheduled for the evening, when time is not at a premium. Similarly, housekeeping and environmental management tasks can be organized into specific time slots. For example, meals may be prepared ahead of time, cleaning tasks interspersed with cooking, and laundry started in the morning and finished in the evening.

Ulicny and Jones (1985) proposed using performance checklists to outline certain job tasks for the attendant. Specific work routines can be outlined to identify the frequency of the task, the materials needed to support it, and the setup. Checklists provide specific instructions and help the employer monitor, evaluate, and provide feedback on the attendant's performance. Once training has been completed, checklists can be used for continued supervision. Checklists also can be used during interviews to help a prospective employee know what will be expected of him or her. The process for developing a checklist is straightforward. First, self-care tasks that require assistance are defined. Then the identified tasks are analyzed to develop a written list of procedures to support and accomplish each one.

Another suggestion that can help potential employers of personal care attendants is to write an employment contract (De Graff, 1988). A contract can outline in great detail all the tasks to be performed and specify the expectations and obligations of both the attendant and the employers. Contracts cover items such as the hourly rate, the pay rate for portions of an hour worked, if and what the attendant will be paid if work is cancelled, expectations if the attendant cancels, and any other potential problems. Occupational therapists should be aware of local community resources that can help employ and manage personal care attendants.

The therapist should be able to inform people with disabilities requiring PAS about these resources. For example, many centers for independent living have PAS programs that can help recruit, interview, train, and provide funding options for personal care attendants. Local colleges may have a service program for students with disabilities or even a personal care attendant pool. Community organizations, such as the local Spinal Cord Injury Association chapter, American Heart Association, Multiple Sclerosis Society, and local rehabilitation centers also may provide resources for people with disabilities requiring PAS. Finally, hiring through a home health agency may provide convenience and a higher level of training in exchange for some control, especially in terms of choice of providers.

For many people with disabilities, formal PAS are a vital part of living independently in their communities. Occupational therapists play an important role in determining the need for PAS, training people with disabilities to manage their attendants, and providing information on available resources.

Caregiving Options in Residential Facilities

If the demands of caregiving exceed the abilities and resources of family care providers, even with the help of in-home and community services, the therapist can identify various residential options for placement of the person with disabilities. These might include assisted living facilities, group homes, continuing care retirement communities, hospice, or nursing homes. The therapist, working with the client's physician, social worker, and physical therapist, can review the advantages and disadvantages of each option and suggest the level of care most appropriate for the care receiver. The therapeutic team also can offer suggested criteria for evaluating and selecting a residential facility.

Placement of a loved one in an institutional setting represents a difficult transition for the family caregiver and the person with disabilities. Many family members prefer to remain involved in their relative's care but are unsure what they could do or will be allowed to do (Perkinson, 2003). A growing body of evidence shows that family involvement in nursing home care is linked to lower levels of depression among family caregivers and higher life satisfaction among nursing home residents whose family caregivers remain involved (Bowers, 1988; Brody, Dempsey, & Pruchno, 1990).

Therapists can assist family caregivers at this stage of their caregiving career by helping them learn to negotiate the nursing home system. They can identify daily routines within the facility, suggest how to voice concerns effectively to nursing home staff and administrators, and outline strategies to help the person with disabilities adjust to life in his or her new setting (Perkinson, Rockemann, & Mahan, 1996).

For safety reasons, family members of nursing home residents generally are discouraged from assisting in the more physically demanding tasks of self-care such as toileting, transferring, or bathing. Family members may be encouraged, however, to help with ADLs such as grooming and feeding. In addition to helping with these kinds of tasks, family members continue to offer companionship to their relative and, when necessary, may act as advocates (Perkinson, 2003). Family members also can help make the nursing home (or other residential care facility) feel more like home, personalizing their relative's room with furniture from the previous home, decorations, photographs, and other items that hold special significance. They also can serve as a conduit to the outside world, helping the resident maintain ties to friends, relatives, and clubs or organizations, and keep abreast of local, national, and international news and cultural events.

Final Stage: Role Disengagement and Re-engagement

As death approaches, the caregiver can play a critical role in assisting the dying person to engage in the final stages of personal development (Erikson, Erikson, & Kivnick, 1994). The caregiver can encourage and support a life review, a recollection of the meaningful occupations of a life, and a coming to terms with that life (Butler, 1974; Haight et al., 2003; Haight, Coleman, & Lord, 1995). Occupational therapists, especially those who work in hospice or palliative care settings, can assist in this process (Hasselkus, 1993; Jacques & Hasselkus, 2004; Pizzi & Briggs, 2004; Rahman, 2000).

The death of the person with disabilities signals the final stage of the caregiving career, during which the family member must deal with bereavement and loss. The family caregiver typically undergoes a period of adjustment in which he or she must disengage and come to terms with the end of the caregiving role. Caregiving during the later stages of an illness often is all-consuming, and caregivers frequently cut out social activities and neglect friendships as they attempt to address the ever-growing needs of the family member with dis-

abilities. When the person dies, the caregiver often finds himself or herself socially isolated. In addition to emotional support, he or she may need help developing new activities to restore balance to a life long structured around the caregiver role (Aneshensel et al., 1995; Mullan, 1992; Strang & Koop, 2003). For some, the caregiving role may have become an integral part of their self-identity. These people may benefit from involvement in the occupation of caregiving in other forms, perhaps as a volunteer assisting other people with disabilities. Occupational therapists can help find replacements for the caregiver role and help make the transition to a new phase of life.

Summary

Family-centered caregiving has limits. Some families may be uncomfortable with various levels of participation in decision making and prefer to remain in the passive role traditionally assigned them by the health care system (Weinstein, 1997). With family-centered care, family caregivers should be able to select their own levels of involvement. This level may vary according to the ability of the person with disabilities to participate in decision-making, the type of services available, the caregivers' comfort level with their own opinions, and their experiences as providers of care. They should not be pressured into taking on more than they can handle. Some family members may lack the necessary skills or knowledge to act as partners in the therapeutic relationship. Some practice environments may simply not support the implementation of a family-centered model.

To overcome these obstacles, various strategies can be implemented. One possibility is simply to make a personal commitment as a therapist to implement a more family-centered approach to intervention (Weinstein, 1997). Therapists can schedule in-service training on the topic to share ideas for increased collaboration with families. They also can encourage family participation in the treatment process by modeling appropriate behaviors and recognizing that family resistance may need to be overcome gradually. To incorporate family-centered approaches into existing service delivery systems, these concepts should be taught in educational programs for occupational therapists. Expanding the family-centered model into practice with people at all stages of the life cycle should be a priority.

Finally, therapists should be mindful that the legal and ethical issues of care do not disappear when family-centered approaches are used. Personal safety issues take priority over family preferences.

Occupational therapists will always be challenged to balance the best interests of the person with disabilities, respect for the family as a unit, and their own professional expertise in any situation (Allen & Petr, 1998).

Study Questions

1. What are 4 reasons why the number of families providing care to family members has grown significantly in recent years?

2. What are the differences between the medical model and family-centered approaches to working with caregivers?

3. Imagine yourself in the role of caregiver to an elderly relative or a child with special needs. Describe your explanatory model of the illness. How might your model differ from someone else's model of the same illness? Consider role-playing an interview session with a peer.

4. What is an assessment tool that would be useful in identifying a family caregiver's values, needs, and priorities to use in a collaborative approach to intervention? Practice completing this assessment with a peer or client.

5. What are methods of including the person with disabilities in a family-centered caregiving approach and ways for the person to maintain as much control as possible?

6. Matthew is a 6-year-old boy with cerebral palsy who requires significant assistance with self-care and play activities. What factors may contribute to the stress that his parents experience, and what support can you offer to alleviate this stress?

7. A 35-year-old woman who was diagnosed with multiple sclerosis in her late 20s is referred to you for home health occupational therapy assessment and intervention. She lives with her mother and father. At what stage of their caregiving career are her parents, and how will you include them in your assessment and treatment plan?

8. You have been working with a young man who sustained a spinal cord injury and is an inpatient in a rehabilitation unit. He is ready for discharge to home and needs to consider hiring a personal care attendant. How would you plan a treatment session during which you will assist him with developing the IADL skill of attendant care manager?

References

Administration on Aging. (2008). *A profile of older americans: 2008.* Washington, DC: U.S. Department of Health and Human Services.

Agree, E. M. (1999). The influence of personal care and assistive devices on the measurement of disability. *Social Science and Medicine, 48,* 427–444.

Allen, R. I., & Petr, C. G. (1998). Rethinking family-centered practice. *American Journal of Orthopsychiatry, 68*(1), 4–15.

American Occupational Therapy Association. (2008). Occupational therapy practice framework: Domain and process (2nd ed.). *American Journal of Occupational Therapy, 62,* 625–683.

Anderson, L. (2008). Predictors of parenting stress in a diverse sample of parents of early adolescents in high-risk communities. *Nursing Research, 57,* 340–350.

Aneshensel, C. S., Pearlin, L. I., Mullan, J. T., Zarit, S. H., & Whitlatch, C. J. (1995). *Profiles in caregiving: The unexpected career.* San Diego, CA: Academic Press.

Arno, P. S. (2006, January). *Economic value of informal caregiving: 2004.* Paper presented at the Care Coordination and the Caregiver Forum Department of Veteran Affairs, National Institutes of Health, Bethesda, MD.

Batavia, A. I. (1996). Health care, personal assistance, and assistive technology: Are in-kind benefits key to independence or dependence for people with disabilities? In J. L. Mashaw et al. (Eds.), *Disability, cash benefits, and work.* Kalamazoo, MI: W. E. Upjohn Institute for Employment Research.

Batavia, A. I., DeJong, G., & McKnew, L. B. (1991). Toward a national personal assistance program: The independent living model of long-term care for persons with disabilities. *Journal of Health Politics, Policy, and Law, 16*(3), 523–545.

Baum, C. M. (1991). Addressing the needs of the cognitively impaired elderly from a family policy perspective. *American Journal of Occupational Therapy, 45*(7), 594–606.

Baum, C. M. (1995). The contribution of occupation to function in persons with Alzheimer's disease. *Journal of Occupational Science: Australia, 2*(2), 59–67.

Baum, C., Edwards, D. F., & Morrow-Howell, N. (1993). Identification and measurement of productive behaviors in senile dementia of the Alzheimer type. *The Gerontologist, 33*(3), 403–408.

Baum, C., & LaVesser, P. (1994). Caregiver assistance: Using family members and attendants. In C. H. Christiansen (Ed.), *Ways of living: Self-care strategies for special needs* (pp. 453–482). Rockville, MD: American Occupational Therapy Association.

Beach, S. R., Schulz, R., Yee, J. L., & Jackson, S. (2000). Negative and positive health effects of caring for a disabled spouse: Longitudinal findings from the caregiver health effects study. *Psychology and Aging, 15*(2), 259–271.

Berlin, E. A., & Fowkes, W.C. (1983). A teaching framework for cross-cultural health care. *Western Journal of Medicine, 139*(6), 934–938.

Benson, P., Karlof, K., & Siperstein, G. (2008). Maternal involvement in the education of young children with autism spectrum disorders. *Autism, 12,* 47–63.

Berg-Weger, M., Rubio, D. M., & Tebb, S. S. (2000). Living with and caring for older family members: Issues related to caregiver well-being. *Journal of Gerontological Social Work, 33*(2), 47–62.

Bookman, A., & Harrington, M. (2007). Family caregivers: A shadow workforce in the geriatric health care system? *Journal of Health Politics, Policy, and Law, 32*(6), 1005–1041.

Bowers, B. J. (1988). Family perceptions of care in a nursing home. *The Gerontologist, 28*(3), 361–368.

Brody, E., Dempsey, N., & Pruchno, R. (1990). Mental health of sons and daughters of the institutionalized aged. *The Gerontologist, 30,* 212–219.

Brown, P. J. (1998). *Understanding and applying medical anthropology.* Mountain View, CA: Mayfield.

Butler, R. (1974). Successful aging and the role of the life review. *Journal of the American Geriatrics Society, 22,* 529–535.

Carpenter, B. D., Kissel, E. C., & Lee, M. M. (2007). Preferences and life evaluations of older adults with and without dementia: Reliability, stability, and proxy knowledge. *Psychology and Aging, 22*(3), 650–655.

Case-Smith, J., & Nastro, M. A. (1993). The effect of occupational therapy intervention on mothers of children with cerebral palsy. *American Journal of Occupational Therapy, 47,* 811–817.

Center for Personal Assistive Services. (2009). *Disability prevalence in the U.S.* San Francisco: University of California.

Corcoran, M. A., & Gitlin, L. N. (1992). Dementia management: An occupational therapy home-based intervention for caregivers. *American Journal of Occupational Therapy, 46*(9), 801–808.

Davis, N. O., & Carter, A. S. (2008). Parenting stress in mothers and fathers of toddlers with autism spectrum disorders: Association with child characteristics. *Journal of Autism and Developmental Disorders, 38,* 1278–1291.

DeJong, G., & Wenker, T. (1983). Attendant care. In N. M. Crewe & I. K. Zola (Eds.), *Independent living for physically disabled people* (pp. 157–170). San Francisco: Jossey-Bass.

Dorn, T., Yaermans, J. C., Spreeuwenberg, P. M., & van der Zee, J. (2007). Physical and mental health problems in parents of adolescents with burns—A controlled, longitudinal study. *Journal of Psychosomatic Research, 63,* 381–389.

Doty, P., Kasper, J., & Litvak, S. (1996). Consumer-directed models of personal care: Lessons from Medicaid. *The Milbank Quarterly, 74*(3), 377–409.

Education for All Handicapped Children Act Amendments of 1986, Pub. L. 99-457, U.S.C. § 1401, Part H, Section 677.

Eisenhower, A. S., Baker, B. L., & Blacher, J. (2009). Children's delayed development and behavior problems: Impact on mothers' perceived physical health across early childhood. *Social Science and Medicine, 68,* 89–99.

Epstein, T., Saltzman-Benaiah, J., O'Hare, A., Goll, J. C., & Tuck, S. (2008). Associate features of Asperger syndrome and their relationship to parenting stress. *Child: Care, Health, and Development, 34,* 503–511.

Erikson, E., Erikson, J., & Kivnick, H. (1994). *Vital involvement in old age: The experience of old age in our times.* New York: W. W. Norton.

Erwin, E. J., & Brown, F. (2003). From theory to practice: A contextual framework for understanding self-determination in early childhood environments. *Infants and Young Children, 16,* 77–87.

Estes, C., & Binney, E. (1991). The biomedicalization of aging: Dangers and dilemmas. In M. Minkler & C. Estes (Eds.), *Critical perspectives on aging: The political and moral economy of growing old* (pp. 117–134). Amityville, NY: Baywood.

Family Caregiver Alliance. (2007). *Family caregiving: State of the art, future trends. Report from a national conference.* San Francisco: National Center on Caregiving at Family Caregiver Alliance.

Flanagan, S., & Green, P. (1994). *Consumer-directed personal assistant services: Key operational issues for state CD–PAS programs using intermediary service organizations.* Cambridge, MA: SysteMetrics, MEDSTAT Group.

Fortinsky, R. H., & Hathaway, T. J. (1990). Information and service needs among active and former family caregivers of persons with Alzheimer's disease. *The Gerontologist, 30,* 604–609.

Gallagher-Thompson, D. (1994). Direct services and interventions for caregivers: A review of extant programs and a look to the future. In M. H. Cantor (Ed.), *Family caregiving: Agenda for the future* (pp. 102–122). San Francisco: American Society for Aging.

Gaugler, J. E., Kane, R. L., Kane, R. A., Clay, T., & Newcomer, R. (2003). Caregiving and institutionalization of cognitively impaired older people: Utilizing dynamic predictors of change. *The Gerontologist, 43,* 219–229.

Gitlin, L. N. (1993). Therapeutic dilemmas in the care of the elderly in rehabilitation. *Topics in Geriatric Rehabilitation, 9,* 11–20.

Gitlin, L. N., Belle, S. H., Burgio, L. D., Czaja, S. J., Mahoney, D., Gallagher-Thompson, D., et al. (2003). Effect of multi-component interventions on caregiver burden and depression. The REACH multisite initiative at 6-month follow-up. *Psychology and Aging, 18*(3), 361–374.

Gitlin, L. N., Corcoran, M., & Leinsmiller-Eckhardt, S. (1995). Understanding the family perspective: An ethnographic framework for providing occupational therapy in the home. *American Journal of Occupational Therapy, 49*(8), 802–809.

Gitlin, L. N., Corcoran, M., Winter, L., Boyce, A., & Hauck, W. W. (2001). A randomized, controlled trial of a home environmental intervention: Effect on efficacy and upset in caregivers and on daily function of persons with dementia. *The Gerontologist, 41,* 4–14.

Gitlin, L. N., Winter, L., Earland, T. V., Herge, E. A., Chernett, N. L., & Piersol, C. V. (2009). The tailored activity program to reduce behavioral symptoms in individuals with dementia: Feasibility, acceptability, and replication potential. *The Gerontologist, 49*(3), 428–439.

Gubrium, J. F., & Sankar, A. (1990). *The home care experience: Ethnography and policy.* Newbury Park, CA: Sage.

Haight, B. K., Bachman, D. L., Hendrix, S., Wagner, M. T., Meeks, A., & Johnson, J. (2003). Life review: Treating the dyadic family unit with dementia.

Clinical Psychology and Psychotherapy, 10(3), 165–174.

Haight, B. K., Coleman, P., & Lord, K. (1995). The linchpins of a successful life review: Structure, evaluation, and individuality. In B. K. Haight & J. D. Webster (Eds.), *The art of science and reminiscing: Theory, research, methods, and applications* (pp. 179–192). Washington, DC: Taylor & Francis.

Harrington, C., Ng, T., Kaye, H. S., & Newcomer, R. (2009). Medicaid home and community-based services: Proposed policies to improve access, costs, and quality. *Public Policy and Aging Report, 19*(2), 13–18.

Hasselkus, B. R. (1988). Meaning of family caregiving: Perspectives on caregiver/professional relationships. *The Gerontologist, 28,* 686–691.

Hasselkus, B. R. (1989). The meaning of daily activity in family caregiving for the elderly. *American Journal of Occupational Therapy, 43,* 649–656.

Hasselkus, B. R. (1990). Ethnographic interviewing: A tool for practice with family caregivers for the elderly. *OT Practice, 2,* 9–16.

Hasselkus, B. R. (1991). Ethical dilemmas in family caregiving for the elderly: Implications for occupational therapy. *American Journal of Occupational Therapy, 45,* 206–212.

Hasselkus, B. R. (1993). Death in very old age: A personal journey of caregiving. *American Journal of Occupational Therapy, 47*(8), 717–723.

Hasselkus, B. R. (1997). Everyday ethics in dementia care: Narratives of crossing the line. *The Gerontologist, 37,* 640–649.

Heagerty, B., & Eskenazi, L. (1994). A practice and program perspective on family caregiving: Focus on solutions. In M. H. Cantor (Ed.), *Family caregiving: Agenda for the future* (pp. 35–48). San Francisco: American Society for Aging.

Health Insurance Portability and Accountability Act of 1996, Pub. L. 104–191, 110 Stat. 136.

Jacques, N. D., & Hasselkus, B. R. (2004). The nature of occupation surrounding dying and death. *Occupation, Participation and Health, 24*(2), 44–53.

Kellegrew, D. (1998). Creating opportunities for occupation: An intervention to promote the self-care independence of young children with special needs. *American Journal of Occupational Therapy, 52,* 457–465.

Kellegrew, D. (2000). Constructing daily routines: A qualitative examination of mothers with young children with disabilities. *American Journal of Occupational Therapy, 54,* 252–259.

Kennedy, J. (1997). Personal assistance benefits and federal health care reforms: Who is eligible on the basis of ADL assistance criteria? *Journal of Rehabilitation, 63*(3), 40–45.

Ketelaar, M., Volman, M. J. M., Gorter, J. W., & Vermeer, A. (2008). Stress in parents of children with cerebral palsy: What sources of stress are we talking about? *Child: Care, Health, and Development, 34,* 825–829.

Kim, S. Y. H., & Applebaum, P. S. (2006). The capacity to appoint a proxy and the possibility of concurrent proxy directives. *Behavioral Sciences and the Law, 24,* 469–478.

Kleinman, A. (1980). *Patients and healers in the context of culture.* Berkeley: University of California Press.

Kleinman, A. (1988). *The illness narratives: Suffering, healing, and the human condition.* New York: Basic Books.

Krefting, L., & Krefting, D. (1991). Cultural influences on performance. In C. Christiansen & C. Baum (Eds.), *Occupational therapy: Overcoming human performance deficits* (pp. 101–124). Thorofare, NJ: Slack.

Kyler, P. (2008). Client-centered and family-centered care: Refinement of the concepts. *Occupational Therapy in Mental Health, 24*(2), 100–120.

LaPlante, M. P., Harrington, C., & Kang, T. (2002). Estimating paid and unpaid hours of personal assistance services in activities of daily living provided to adults living at home. *Health Services Research, 37*(2), 397–415.

Law, M. (1997). *Client-centered occupational therapy.* Thorofare, NJ: Slack.

Law, M., Baptiste, S., Carswell, A., McColl, M. A., Polatajko, H., & Pollack, N. (1998). *Canadian occupational performance measure* (3rd ed.). Toronto, Ontario: CAOT Publications.

Law, M., Haight, M., Milroy, B., Willms, D., Stewart, D., & Rosenbaum, P. (1999). Environmental factors affecting the occupations of children with physical disabilities. *Journal of Occupational Science, 6,* 102–110.

Lawlor, M. S., & Mattingly, C. F. (1998). The complexities embedded in family-centered care. *American Journal of Occupational Therapy, 52*(4), 259–267.

Leibing, A. (2006). Divided gazes: Alzheimer's disease, the person within, and death in life. In A. Leibing & L. Cohen (Eds.), *Thinking about dementia: Culture, loss, and the anthropology of senility* (pp. 240–268). New Brunswick, NJ: Rutgers University Press.

Le Navenec, C., & Vonhof, T. (1996). *One day at a time: How families manage the experience of dementia.* Westport, CT: Greenwood.

Lindley, J. (1995). *Finding and keeping an attendant.* Puyallup, WA: Center for Independence.

Litvak, S., Zukas, H., & Heumann, J. E. (1987). *Attending to America: Personal assistance for independent living. A survey of attendant services in the United States for people of all ages with disabilities.* Berkeley, CA: World Institute on Disability.

Mace, N. L., & Rabins, P. V. (2006). *The 36-hour day* (4th ed.). Baltimore: Johns Hopkins University Press.

Marks, N. F. (1996). Caregiving across the lifespan: National prevalence and predictors. *Family Relations, 45,* 27–36.

McLean, A. (2007). *The person in dementia: A study of nursing home care in the U.S.* Peterborough, Ontario: Broadview.

Meltzer, L. J., & Moore, M. (2008). Sleep disruptions in parents of children and adolescents with chronic illnesses: Prevalence, causes, and consequences. *Journal of Pediatric Psychology, 33,* 279–291.

Meuser, T., & Marwit, S. (2001). A comprehensive, stage-sensitive model of grief in dementia caregiving. *The Gerontologist, 41,* 658–670.

Morris, A., & Gainer, F. (1997). Helping the caregiver: Occupational therapy opportunities. *OT Practice*, 36–40.

Mullan, J. T. (1992). The bereaved caregiver: A prospective study of changes in well-being. *The Gerontologist*, *32*(5), 673–683.

National Center for Health Statistics. (2008). *Health, United States, 2008*. Hyattsville, MD: U.S. Department of Health and Health Services.

Navaie-Waliser, M., Feldman, P., Gould, D., Levine, C., Kuerbis, A., & Donelan, K. (2002). When the caregiver needs care: The plight of vulnerable caregivers. *American Journal of Public Health, 92*, 409–413.

Ohaeri, J. U. (2003). The burden of caregiving in families with a mental illness: A review. *Current Opinion in Psychiatry, 16*(4), 457–465.

Olmstead v. L.C., 527 U.S. 581 (1999).

Opie, N. D., & Miller, E. L. (1989). Personal care attendants and severely disabled adults: Attributions for relationship outcomes. *Archives of Psychiatric Nursing, 3*, 205–210.

Orsmond, G., Seltzer, M. M., Greenberg, J. S., & Krauss, M. W. (2006). Mother–child relationship quality among adolescents and adults with autism. *American Journal of Mental Retardation, 111*, 121–137.

Overman, W., & Stoudemire, A. (1988). Guidelines for legal and financial counseling of Alzheimer's disease patients and their families. *American Journal of Psychiatry, 145*(12), 1495–1500.

Parish, S. L. (2006). Juggling and struggling: A preliminary work-life study of mothers with adolescents who have developmental disabilities. *Mental Retardation, 44*, 393–403.

Perkinson, M. A. (1992). Maximizing personal efficacy in older adults: The empowerment of volunteers in a multipurpose senior center. *Physical and Occupational Therapy in Geriatrics, 10*(3), 57–72.

Perkinson, M. A. (1995). Socialization to the family caregiving role within a continuing care retirement community. *Medical Anthropology, 16*, 249–267.

Perkinson, M. A. (1999). Family and nursing home staff's perceptions of quality of life in dementia. In R. Rubinstein, M. Moss, & M. Kleban (Eds.), *The many dimensions of aging* (pp. 116–128). New York: Springer.

Perkinson, M. A. (2002). *Nurturing a family partnership: Alzheimer's home care aide's guide*. Washington, DC: AARP Andrus Foundation.

Perkinson, M. A. (2003). Defining family roles within a nursing home setting. In P. B. Stafford (Ed.), *Gray areas: Ethnographic encounters with nursing home culture*. Santa Fe, NM: School of American Research Press.

Perkinson, M. A. (2008). Negotiating disciplines: Developing a dementia exercise program. *Practicing Anthropology* (Special issue on Anthropology and Occupational Therapy), *30*(3), 10–15.

Perkinson, M. A., Rockemann, D., & Mahan, L. (1996). *Families in nursing homes manual*. Washington, DC: AARP Andrus Foundation.

Pinquart, M., & Sorensen, S. (2003). Differences between caregivers and noncaregivers in psychological health and physical health: A meta-analysis. *Psychology and Aging, 18*(2), 250–267.

Pizzi, M., & Briggs, R. (2004). Occupational and physical therapy in hospice: The facilitation of meaning, quality of life, and well-being. *Topics in Geriatric Rehabilitation, 20*, 120–130.

Pruchno, R. A. (1999). Caregiving research: Looking backward, looking forward. In R. Rubenstein, M. Moss, & M. Kleban (Eds.), *The many dimensions of aging* (pp. 197–213). New York: Springer.

Rahman, H. (2000). Journey of providing care in hospice: Perspectives of occupational therapists. *Qualitative Health Research, 10*(6), 806–818.

Roberto, K. A. (1999). Making critical health care decisions for older adults: Consensus among family members. *Family Relations, 48*, 167–175.

Roth, D. L., Perkins, M., Wadley, V. G., Temple, E. M., & Haley, W. E. (2009). Family caregiving and emotional strain: Associations with quality of life in a large national sample of middle-aged and older adults. *Quality of Life Research, 18*(6), 679–688.

Sabat, S. R., & Harre, R. (1992). The construction and deconstruction of self in Alzheimer's disease. *Aging and Society, 12*, 443–461.

Saks, E. R., Litt, M., Dunn, L. B., Wimer, J., Gonzales, M., & Kim, S. (2008). Proxy consent to research: The legal landscape. *Health Policy Law and Ethics, 37*, 37–92.

Scherzer, T., Wong, A., & Newcomer, R. (2007). Fiscal management services in consumer-directed programs. *Home Health Care Services Quarterly, 27*(1), 29–42.

Schopp, L. H., Clark, M. J., Hagglund, K. J., Sherman, A. K., Stout, B. J., Gray, D. B., et al. (2007). Life activities among individuals with spinal cord injury living in the community: Perceived choice and perceived barriers. *Rehabilitation Psychology, 52*(1), 82–88.

Schultz-Krohn, W. (1997). Early intervention: Meeting the unique needs of parent–child interaction. *Infants and Younger Children, 10*, 47–60.

Schulz, R. (Ed.). (2000). *Handbook on dementia caregiving: Evidence-based interventions for family caregivers*. New York: Springer.

Schulz, R., & Martire, L. M. (2004). Family caregiving of persons with dementia: Prevalence, health effects, and support strategies. *American Journal of Geriatric Psychiatry, 12*(3), 240–249.

Shapiro, J. (1993). *No pity: People with disabilities forging a new civil rights movement*. New York: Times Books/Random House.

Sorensen, S., Pinquart, M., & Duberstein, P. (2002). How effective are interventions with caregivers? An updated meta-analysis. *The Gerontologist, 42*(3), 356–372.

Steffen, A. M. (2000). Anger management for dementia caregivers: A preliminary study using video and telephone interventions. *Behavior Therapy, 31*, 281–299.

Stone, R., & Newcomer, R. (2009). Advances and issues in personal care. *Clinics in Geriatric Medicine, 25*(1), 1–9.

Strang, V. R., & Koop, P. M. (2003). Factors which influence coping: Home-based family caregiving of persons with advanced cancer. *Journal of Palliative Care, 19*(2), 107–114.

Sumsion, J. (1999). A neophyte early childhood teacher's developing relationships with parents: An ecological perspective. *Early Childhood Research and*

Practice, 1(1). Retrieved August 27, 2010, from http://ecrp.uiuc.edu/v1n1/sumsion.html

Tennstedt, S., McKinlay, J., & Kasten, L. (1994). Unmet need for formal support services among home health client. *Social Science and Medicine, 38*, 915–924.

Teri, L., Gibbons, L. E., McCurry, S. M., Logdon, R. G., Buchner, D. M., Barlow, W. E., et al. (2003). Exercise plus behavioral management in patients with Alzheimer's disease: A randomized controlled trial. *JAMA, 290*(15), 2015–2022.

Teri, L., Truax, P., Logdon, R. G., Uomoto, J., Zarit, S. H., & Vitaliano, P. P. (1992). Assessment of behavioral problems in dementia: The Revised Memory and Behavior Problems Checklist. *Psychology and Aging, 4*, 622–631.

Thompson, L. (2004). *Long-term care: Support for family caregivers* [Issue Brief, Long-Term Care Financing Project]. Washington, DC: Georgetown University.

Toth-Cohen, S. (2000). Role perceptions of occupational therapists providing support and education for caregivers of persons with dementia. *American Journal of Occupational Therapy, 54*(5), 509–515.

Ulicny, G., Adler, A., & Jones, M. L. (1990). Training effective interview skills to attendant service users. *Rehabilitation Psychology, 35*(1), 55–66.

Ulicny, G., & Jones, M. L. (1985). Enhancing the attendant management skills of persons with disabilities. *American Rehabilitation, 2*(2), 18–20.

U.S. Department of Health and Human Services, Office of Civil Rights. (2006). *Regulation text: CFR parts160, 162, and 164*. Washington, DC: Author.

U.S. National Center for Health Statistics. (2009). *Health, United States*. Available online at http:/www.cdc.gov/NCHS/HHS.htm.

Weinstein, M. (1997). Bringing family-centered practices into home health. *OT Practice, 2*(7), 35–38.

Whitlatch, C. J., & Feinberg, L. F. (2003). Planning for the future together in culturally diverse families: Making everyday care decisions. *Alzheimer's Care Quarterly, 4*(1), 50–61.

Whitlatch, C. J., Piiparinen, R., & Feinberg, L. F. (2009). How well do family caregivers know their relatives' care values and preferences? *Dementia, 8*, 223–243.

Wolff, J. L., & Kasper, J. D. (2006). Caregivers of frail elders: updating a national profile. *The Gerontologist, 46*(3), 344–356.

Zarit, S. H., Reever, K. E., & Bach-Peterson, J. (1980). Relatives of the impaired elderly: Correlates of feelings of burden. *The Gerontologist, 20*, 649–655.

Zarit, S. H., & Teri, L. (1991). Interventions and services for family caregivers. *Annual Review of Gerontology and Geriatrics, 11*, 287–310.

Glossary

A

ABLEDATA: An Internet directory that provides a searchable database of assistive technology and rehabilitation devices (see www.abledata.com)

Accessibility: Free and normal movement throughout the environmental setting

Accessible design: Products and environments designed and constructed to be readily accessible to and usable by people with disabilities

Acquisition: The initial learning phase of an activity where learners may not be able to perform the target skill at all or may perform with limited competence

Activities of daily living (ADLs): Areas of occupation that include activities oriented toward taking care of one's own body. Also referred to as basic activities of daily living (BADLs) and personal activities of daily living (PADLs)

Activity limitation: Loss or limitation of opportunities to take part in the life of the community on an even level with others

Adaptive: Pertaining to adjustments or alterations necessary for function

Adaptive equipment: Devices or materials used to allow engagement in an occupation for people with impairment in the performance skills, patterns, and/or client factors needed to complete the targeted occupation; these may include modifications to existing equipment, such as seat inserts, or the use of new devices or materials, such as use of reachers

Adaptive strategies: Actions taken by an individual to accomplish a task or meet an environmental demand; may involve equipment, techniques, or routines

Age appropriate: Suitable or proper for a person of a given age

Allostatic load: A composite measure of the cumulative physiological burden of stressors in life

Alzheimer's dementia (AD): A progressive, degenerative disease of uncertain causes that manifests itself in damage to the brain

Alzheimer's dementia stages: The three stages of cognitive decline described as mild, moderate, and severe; used to describe and predict behaviors that are expected to emerge during the course of the disease that may span 17 years

Analysis of occupational performance: The step in the evaluation process during which the client's assets, problems, or potential problems are specifically identified, preferably in context in order to identify barriers and resources to occupational performance; skills and patterns of performance, contexts, activity demands, and client factors are considered, but not all may be individually assessed; desired (target) outcomes are identified

Ankylosing spondylitis (AS): A chronic systemic disease in which the primary sites of inflammation are the ligamentous, capsular, and tendinous insertions into the bone; primarily involving the sacroiliac, spinal apophyseal, and axial joints

Antecedent events: Circumstances, activities, or conditions that precede a given poin in time

Aphasia: Absence or impairment of the ability to communicate through speech, writing, or signs due to dysfunction of brain centers

Apraxia: Inability to perform purposive movements although there is no sensory or motor impairment

ASIA Impairment Scale: Defines the level of injury as the last caudal segment with intact motor and sensory innervations; also referred to as the International Standards for Neurological and Functional Classification of Spinal Cord Injury

Assertive community treatment: Originated in Madison, Wisconsin, and called the PACT program (Program of Assertive Community Treatment); offers full-support case management services in the community with a team whose expertise informs the group decision making; teams work with the community and families as a collaborative process

Assessment: The use of specific tools in the evaluation process

Assistive devices: Equipment or devices used to increase, maintain, or improve performance of occupations

Assistive technology (AT): Any of a broad category of devices to assist with the performance of tasks required in everyday living

Assistive technology device: A commercial, custom fabricated, or homemade device used to assist in the performance of tasks involved in everyday living

Ataxia: Inability to perform coordinated muscle movements

Augmentative and alternative communication (AAC): Sytems employed with the purpose of enhancing or enabling communication abilities

Autograft: A graft of tissue taken from a different area of the person receiving the graft

Autonomic dysreflexia: A reflex action of the autonomic nervous system in response to noxious stimuli, such as a distended bladder, bladder irritation, painful stimuli, and visceral distention; a phenomena seen in people with spinal injuries above the C4–C6 level. Symptoms may include pounding headache, anxiety, perspiration, flushing, chills, nasal congestion/paroxysmal breathing, hypertension, and bradycardia; a medical emergency and life-threatening

B

Barrier-free design: Similar to accessible design but refers primarily to the environment

Baseline data: Level of a client's performance as measured before instruction begins

Biological citizenship: An emerging philosophical and political concept of individual and collective rights, values, identities, and obligations associated with one's status as a living being and the condition of one's body

Biopower: A term originating with French philosopher Michel Foucault that pertains to the efforts of nation states to influence groups through the regulation of customs, habits, health and reproductive practices, family, blood banks, and policies to engender well-being

Biscapular abduction: The movement of both shoulders forward and laterally creating a condition where the scapulae are separated and the pectoralis major muscles are squeezed together. This movement is used for mechanical control of mechanical upper extremity prostheses. The motion, along with humeral flexion, produces cable tension that operates the terminal device

Body-powered prosthesis: The terminal device and/or elbow unit on the prosthesis operated by upper-extremity or upper-quadrant voluntary muscle movements

Boutonnière deformity: A deformity caused by disruption of the extensor apparatus at the proximal interphalangeal joint level resulting in proximal interphalangeal joint flexion and distal interphalangeal joint hyperextension when active finger extension is attempted

Boutonnière precautions: Avoidance of composite active flexion of the fingers with deeper partial or full-thickness dorsal hand burns; instead, isolated MP flexion is combined with IP joint extension to avoid stress to a possibly compromised extensor tendon mechanism

Braille: A system of reading and writing using a configuration of six raised dots in a rectangular pattern resembling a muffin pan

Brain cortex lobes: The part of the nervous system that is most significantly damaged by Alzheimer's disease (AD) and traumatic brain injury (TBI); the four main structures of the brain that are commonly affected by AD and TBI are the frontal, parietal/ temporal/ and occipital lobes

C

Case management: A service that assists clients in negotiating for services that they both need and want

Cataracts: An opacity/or cloudiness of the normally clear lens inside the eye

Central vision loss (CVL): The loss of central or straight-ahead vision

Cerebral palsy: A disability resulting from a non-progressive lesion of the central nervous system originating before/ during or shortly after birth that manifests as a muscular in-coordination; intellectual, sensory} speech, seizure, and behavioral disorders may also be present

Chronic disability: Any condition which results in continuing or persistent limitations in activity and therefore threatens diminished participation in aspects of life viewed as necessary or valuable to the client

Chronobiology: The study of physiological rhythms (body clocks) and their effect on function

Client-centered occupation-based approaches: Occupational therapy interventions and models that emphasize participation in roles and activities as the primary goal of care and engender the active participation of clients in the goal-setting process

Clubhouse Model: Also known as the Fountain Clubhouse Model in which people with serious mental illness join together to support one another as they adjust to community living and help one another find jobs; people join as "members" and work side-by-side with staff to run the psychosocial clubhouse and the many programs offered

Cognitive rehabilitation: Interdisciplinary interventions designed to remediate or compensate for cognitive function, activities, and participation; use of cognitive and behavioral learning strategies to design programs for AD and TBI

Community support program (CSP): A model of psychosocial intervention in which the mental health practitioners go to where the client lives and works to provide the needed services

Compassion: A quality among caregivers of feeling kindly when faced with another person's sufferings and responding willingly and helpfully to their needs

Compensatory: Finding a new way to accomplish a task when performance capabilities are limited; occurs through modifying the task or environment

Consequences: The events (planned or unplanned) following a target response

Co-occurring disorders: Disorders that coincide with a certain condition; *dual diagnosis* and *comorbidity* are terms with similar meanings

Correlation: The extent to which two or more variables or tests are related statistically (i.e., they covary or change together)

Core affect: A basic psychological state defined by dimensions of pleasure and activation

Correlation: The extent to which two or more variables or tests are related. An index of the degree to which two phenomena are related, expressed as a value from 0 to 1. The sign before a correlation coefficient indicates the direction of a relationship. Phenomena may be correlated directly or positively, in which when one changes, the other changes a proportionally in the same direction. They may also be correlated negatively or inversely. In this case, they change in opposite directions. That is, as the value of one goes up, the value of the second goes down, or vice versa

D

Desynchronosis: The physiological state of disentrainment between the body and the environment illustrated by jet lag

Developmental disabilities: Severe, chronic disabilities of a person that is attributable to a mental or physical impairment or combination of mental and physical impairments; developmental disabilities are manifested before the person attains age 22; are likely to continue indefinitely; result in substantial functional limitations in three or more of the following areas of major life activity: self-care, receptive and expressive language, learning, mobility, self-direction, capacity for independent living, or economic self-sufficiency; and reflect that person's need for a combination and sequence of special, interdisciplinary, or generic care, treatment, or other services that are individually planned and coordinated

Diabetic retinopathy: A condition that affects the retinas of some individuals who are diabetic; diabetes may cause hemorrhages or blood vessel changes that affect the retina and thus interfere with vision

Disability: Impairment, activity limitation, and participation restriction

Disarticulation: Amputation occurring through a joint, lower extremity, wrist, elbow, or shoulder

Disease: A pathological or disordered condition of a part, organ, or system of an individual (or organism) resulting from various causes, such as infection, genetic defect, or environmental stress, and identifiable by a designated group of signs or symptoms

Donor site: Area from which the upper layer of the skin is taken for a skin graft

Dysarthria: Difficult and defective speech due to impairment of the tongue or other muscles essential for speech

Dysphagia: Inability to swallow or difficulty in swallowing

E

Eccentric viewing: A means of locating and using the area of best visual function on the retina of a person with macular degeneration or a central vision loss

Ectropion: The turning outward or eversion of the eyelids or lips due to skin contractures

Electronic aids to daily living (EADLs): Devices that enable operation or manipulation of one or more electronic appliances, such as televisions, radios, CD/DVD players, lights, and fans, using voice activation, switch access, computer interfaces, and or other adaptations. Also known as ECU (Environmental Control Units)

Electronic documentation: The of digital technologies to record interactions (evaluations, progress notes and summaries) for clients

Electronic prosthesis: A prosthesis that uses a combination of electronic circuitry (e.g., microprocessor) and physiological processes (e.g., EMG signals) for functional control

Embodiment: The subjective experience of one's own body, which is different from the objective or scientific picture of a body in physiological terms. The specific ways people experience themselves as embodied thus become important ways for understanding knowledge and experience

Empathic witnessing: The process of recognizing feelings of distress and their causes in clients in order to better understand relevant contexts and situations prior to planning intervention

Empowerment models: Also referred to as *consumer/survivor models*, in which consumers have much greater control over services and may actually provide them

Energy conservation: Using daily strategies that minimize fatigue, conserve energy, enhance safety, and foster adequate stability

Engagement: State of being involved with occupations that are meaningful to the person

Environmental factors: Social attitudes, architectural characteristics, legal and social structures, as well as climate, terrain, and so forth

Epidermis: The outermost layer of the skin

Eschar: Nonviable, slough of necrotic tissue produced by a burn

Ethnographic approach: The attempt to understand another way of life from the informant's point of view; focuses on values, meanings, beliefs, and how the informant makes sense of his or her situation

Evaluation: An ongoing process of collecting and interpreting data necessary for planning intervention

Existential anxiety: An unconscious fear about loss of physical capabilities that abie-bodied people often experience when in contact with people with disabilities

Explanatory model of illness: A set of beliefs and knowledge; explanations of sickness and treatment, which provide a conceptual framework to give meaning to a particular illness experience and guide choices among various therapies

Extended care network: The group of individuals who have an interest in a client's well-being, including employers, group home supervisors, guardians, and others

F

Family caregiver: Any family member providing unpaid care to a person who, because of a physical, cognitive, or psychological impairment, would not be able to care for himself or herself

Family-centered care: A term used to describe a constellation of beliefs, values, and treatment approaches that recognizes the role of family members as full collaborators on the health care team

Fibromyalgia (FM): A chronic and painful disorder characterized by widespread discomfort and tenderness at anatomically defined points that are thought to be influenced by the neuroendocrine, biorhythmic, and nociceptive systems

Flourishing: Thriving in a manner that enables a continued sense of personal growth and life satisfaction

Fluency: Phase of learning that concerns improving the accuracy, quality, and speed of performance

Frontal Lobe: The portion of the brain positioned anterior to (in front of) the parietal lobes and above and anterior to the temporal lobes. It is separated from the parietal lobe by the primary motor cortex, which controls voluntary movements of specific body parts. The frontal lobe is associated with reward, attention, long-term memory, planning, and motivation

Full-thickness burn: A burn that extends through and causes necrosis of all three layers of the skin

Functional capacity as a basis for design: A decision framework that provides guidelines for the applicability of all products and home modifications based on the identified sensory, physical, and cognitive changes of aging

Functional effects on sexual activity: The effects of a disability that may impede sexual activity

Functional mobility: The use of wheeled devices such as strollers, transport chairs, or wheelchairs to enable transportation if disability restricts it

G

Generalization: Phase of learning that is concerned with how a skill is performed and improved under changing conditions (e.g., location, materials, time, task variation)

Glasgow Coma Scale (GCS): A commonly used scale for measuring the severity of brain injury at the onset of the brain trauma, consisting of a point scale used to rate eye opening and motor and verbal responses; based on the duration of prolonged unconsciousness or deep sleep

Glaucoma: A leading cause of blindness in the United States, causes damage to the optic nerve and retinal nerve fibers due to a buildup of pressure within the eye; increased pressure causes a decrease of vision in the peripheral field, commonly known as *tunnel vision*

Global positioning satellite (GPS): A type of navigational system for determining one's precise geographic location based on spatial coordinates provided by satellites

Graduated guidance: System of prompts where the more intrusive physical prompts are applied initially, then faded out

Greifer: Prehensor that can be powered by a myoelectric or electronic prosthesis

H

Hand function: The ability to flex and extend the wrist and flex and extend the fingers in a coordinated manner with sufficient strength to grasp and release objects

Handling: Physical assistance provided by the therapist to the child with cerebral palsy to assist with attaining the positioning, postural stability, and voluntary movement necessary for occupational performance

Health condition: A disease, disorder, or injury as defined by medical science

Health promotion: An intervention approach that does not assume a disability is present or that any factors would interfere with performance. This approach is designed to provide enriched contextual and activity experiences that will enhance performance for all persons in the natural contexts of life

Hemianopsia: Blindness in one half the visual field of one or both eyes

Hemiparesis/Hemiplegia: Paralysis affecting only one side of the body

Heterotopic ossification: Bone formation occurring at an abnormal location in the body

Home evaluation: A step-by-step method of reviewing pertinent aspects of a person's home

Home modifications: Preventive steps to make a home safe, particularly for the persons who are elderly and/or disabled, to age comfortably in place and to live in safety

Humeral flexion: Active motion of humeral flexion which produces tension on the cable to operate terminal device and/or elbow unit

Hybrid prosthesis: Prosthesis with more than one style of component, such as a body power component and an electronic component

Hyperpigmentation: Excessive darkening of skin color due to overproduction of skin pigment, often accelerated by sun exposure

Hypertrophic scar: Excessive scar formation that rises above the level of the skin plane but does not extend beyond the original borders of the burn wound

Hypopigmentation: Lighter-than-normal skin color due to underproduction of skin pigment

I

Identity: A composite definition of the self that includes an interpersonal aspect, an aspect of possibility or potential (who we might become), and a values aspect (that suggests importance and provides a stable basis for choices and decisions). Identity can be viewed as the superordinate view of ourselves that includes both self-esteem and self-concept but also importantly reflects and is influenced by the larger social world in which humans find ourselves

Illness: An individual's actual experience of disorder or suffering, whether or not caused by an identifiable disease

Impairment: Problems in body function or structure such as a significant deviation or loss

Impairment effects: The performance consequences of impairment

Independent living movement: A philosophy in which individuals are responsible for their decision-making and performance of self-care and community activities within the limits of their capabilities

Instrumental activities of daily living (IADLs): Activities to support daily life within the home and community that often require more complex interactions than self-care used in ADLs

Intermittent catheterization: A method for bladder emptying in which a catheter is inserted into the bladder allowing urine to flow out of the catheter is removed after urine is emptied; this process is performed several times during the day on a regular timed schedule

International Classification of Functioning, Disability and Health (ICF): Provides a unified and standard language and framework for the description of health and health-related states

Intervention: The process and skilled actions taken by occupational therapy practitioners in collaboration with the client to facilitate engagement in occupation related to health and participation. The intervention process includes the plan, implementation, and review

Intervention approach: Specific strategies selected to direct the process of interventions that are based on the client's desired outcome, evaluation date, and evidence

Intervention plan: The specific plan for providing occupational therapy intervention for a client

Intervention type: The specific type of intervention used by the practitioner with the client, whether therapeutic use of self, occupation-based intervention, consultation, education, or advocacy

Intimacy: Strong feelings of attachment and closeness to another

J

Joint protection and energy conservation principles: Active strategies related to lifestyle for reducing the progressive deterioration of joints in rheumatoid arthritis; emphasis is placed on principles such as proper body alignment, adequate rest, use of assistive devices, and alternate methods of task completion

Juvenile idiopathic arthritis (JIA): A systemic joint disease characterized by three major types (systemic onset, polyarticular onset, pauciarticular onset) and seven subtypes based on symptoms after onset; all types involve fatigue, fever, and malaise. Previously referred to as *Juvenile Rheumatic Athritis (JRA)*

K

Keloid scar: Excessive scar formation that rises above the level of the skin plane and continues to extend, mushroom-like, beyond the original borders of the burn wound

L

Legal blindness: Having vision of 20/200 or less (using the Snellen Chart measurement) in the better eye with best standard eyeglass correction, or having a visual field that encompasses or subtends an angle of 20 degrees or less

Leisure: A nonobligatory activity that is intrinsically motivated and engaged in during discretionary time, that is, time not committed to obligatory occupations such as work, self-care, or sleep

Life balance: An emerging interdisciplinary concept related to the identification of lifestyle characteristics that engender health and well-being (related to the historical but unsubstantiated concept known in occupational therapy as occupational balance)

M

Macular degeneration (AMD): A condition that affects the central visual acuity, primarily in those over age 50

Maintenance: Phase where a skill is used routinely and improved under fairly stable and familiar conditions

Maintain: An intervention approach designed to provide the supports that will allow clients to preserve the performance capabilities they have regained, that continue to meet their occupational needs, or both. The assumption is that, without continued maintenance intervention, performance would decrease, occupational needs would not be met, or both, thereby affecting health and quality of life

Manual edema mobilization (MEM): A method of gentle stimulation to reduce lymphatic edema in the arms and hands following surgery, trauma, or stroke

Marginalized populations: Groups relegated to lower social standing because of poverty, race, politics, prejudice, stigma, or other factors

Microstomia: The condition of having an abnormally small mouth

Mini-Mental Status Examination (MMSE): A commonly used measure designed to evaluate the cognitive impairment of clients with dementia

Modification: An intervention approach directed at finding ways to revise the current context or activity demands to support performance in the natural setting, including compensatory techniques, such as enhancing some features to provide cues or reducing other features to reduce distractibility

Myoelectric prosthesis: The terminal device or other component of the prosthesis is operated by the electrical signal from a voluntary muscle contraction

N

Narrative: The personal story within which each individual constructs meaning through activity engagement over time

Neglect: A type of sensory perceptual loss of awareness that follows stroke. Neglect reduces a person's ability to look, listen, or make movements in one half of their environment. This can affect their ability to carry out many everyday tasks such as eating, reading, and getting dressed (also called unilateral spatial neglect)

No light perception (NLP): The designation used to mean total blindness

Norms: Performance scores or data gathered on reference groups to permit comparison with the score obtained by an individual

O

Occipital lobes: The portion of the brain at the back of the cranium that is primarily responsible for vision

Occupational deprivation: A state of prolonged preclusion from engagement in occupations of necessity or meaning due to factors outside the control of an individual

Occupational disruption: A transient or temporary condition of being restricted from participation in necessary or meaningful occupations, such as that caused by illness, temporary relocation, or temporary unemployment

Occupational performance: The act of doing and accomplishing a dynamic transaction among the client, the context, and the activity

Occupational performance problem statement: Succinctly describes the occupational status of a person, identifying the problems amenable to intervention; focuses intervention on the occupations and activities, performance skills and patterns, underlying factors, and contexts needing change in order to resolve the performance problem

Occupational profile: The initial step in the evaluation process that provides an understanding of the client's occupational history and experiences, patterns of daily living, interests, values, and needs

Osteoarthritis (OA): The most common rheumatic disease affecting both men and women equally during their middle age and beyond; it involves a progression of articular cartilage wear and bony build-up at the margins of a joint, leading to stiffness, and limited range of motion rather than pain

Osteoporosis (OP): A condition, more common in women than men, in which bones become fragile and more susceptible to fractures because the density or amount of bone decreases

Outcome: The actual result from intervention or the delivery of services

P

Paraplegia: An impairment of thoracic, lumbar, and sacral segments of the spinal cord resulting in functional impairments in the trunk, legs, and pelvic organs

Parietal lobe: A portion of the brain superior to the occipital lobe. The parietal lobe integrates sensory information from different modalities, particularly determining spatial sense and navigation

Partial participation: Ability to perform part of an activity or a somehow modified activity rather than carrying out the entire task in a typical way

Partial-thickness burn: A burn injury extending through the epidermis and into the dermis

Participation: Involvement in a life situation

Personal assistance services: Care provided by others for assistance with the requirements of daily life

Personal care attendant: A paid employee who provides in-home assistance with essential ADLs to a person with a severe disability who is functionally dependent

Personal factors: Gender, age, coping style, social background, education, profession, past and current experience, overall behavior pattern, character, and other factors that influence how disability is experienced by an individual

Photophobia: Discomfort from the abnormally increased sensitivity to bright sunlight or reflected light from water, snow, or even highly polished gems

Play: An area of occupation that provides enjoyment, entertainment, amusement, or diversion

Positioning: The placement and alignment of a body part or the entire body to prevent abnormal or unnecessary movements, allow or enhance the engagement in occupations, and/or provide safety during engagement in occupations

Post-Traumatic Amnesia Scale (PTA): A measurement obtained by estimating the duration of memory loss from the moment of the brain trauma to the time of evaluation, at which point clients are able to demonstrate the ability to communicate about memory

Postural stability: The ability to maintain a desired bodily position, such as sitting, kneeling, or propping on elbows, while engaged in a meaningful occupation

Power Mobility: Motorized devices for mobility such as wheelchairs or scooters, which use switch-activated battery power and various steering mechanisms to enable movement

Pressure ulcer: Localized area of cellular necrosis characterized by an open wound in which tissue necrosis has occurred, usually in response to externally applied pressure

Prevention: Promoting a healthy lifestyle and creating the conditions necessary for health

Probe data: Information gathered regarding a client's progress once training has begun by monitoring progress using criterion or test conditions

Problem statement: The description of a condition needing change which forms the basis for a goal

Procovery: Attaining a productive and fulfilling life regardless of the level of health assumed attainable; an approach to healing based on hope and grounded in practical everyday steps that individuals can take to move forward

Professional reasoning: Process used to design, conduct, and evaluate intervention

Psychneuroimmunology: The study of psychological influences (such as stressful situations) on the immune system

Psychoeducational approaches: Reflects an approach to teaching the basic skills of everyday living based on the goals of learning from the consumer's perspective and in the environments in which they live, work, and play

Q

Quality of life: A client's dynamic appraisal of life satisfactions (perceptions of progress toward identified goals), self-concept (the composite of beliefs and feelings about themselves), health and functioning (including health status, self-care capabilities), and socioeconomic factors (e.g., vocation, education, income)

R

Rasch Analysis: A mathematical model for calibrating measurement scales that considers the relationship between the probability of success and the difference between an individual's ability and an item's difficulty

Reliability: The consistency and precision with which an assessment measures a specific behavior or skill

Remedial: An intervention that is designed to improve or establish a skill or ability that has not yet been developed in order to meet the requirements of task demands

Remediation: Intervention designed to change a client's body functions, structures, values, skills, beliefs, performance skills, performance patterns, and overall occupational performance

Response prompts: Those cues given by the therapist to facilitate a client's performance of an activity (e.g., gestures, physical touch, modeling)

Reverse mortgages: A special type of loan used primarily by older Americans to convert the equity in their homes into cash; instead of making monthly payments to a lender, a lender makes payments to the homeowner in return for a share of the equity

Rheumatoid arthritis (RA): A systemic disease with inflammation of the synovimn (or sac), which provides lubrication for the joint, as a primary symptom, and primarily affects the extremity joints and the neck

Routines: Behaviors that are repeated over time and organized into patterns and habits

S

Scar maturation: Progressive remodeling of a scar as demonstrated by a softening and flattening of scar texture and complete resolution of erythema, usually over a 12- to 18-month period following initial burn injury or surgical reconstruction procedure

Self-care: Activities that meet basic individual or personal needs. Sometimes used as term referring to self-management, as in preventing or reducing the consequences of disease

Self-management: Client practices related to the alleviation of symptoms, prevention of complications, and the preservation of function for a chronic disease or disability

Self-management principles: Knowledge related to reducing the adverse consequences of disease on lifestyle, including understanding the disease and its causes, awareness of medications and their side effects, and recognition of practical techniques and devices that can prevent or reduce disease progression and improve function and the quality of life

Self-protection techniques: Techniques involving holding one arm (usually the nondominant one) at shoulder height, palm out, with the hand just below eye level; the dominant hand is held diagonally across the body, pulled inward, in front of the opposite upper thigh, thus protecting oneself

Sensory defensiveness (hypersensitivity): A negative reaction, motoric or emotional, to a sensory experience that most people would not consider to be harmful or unpleasant

Sensuality: The capacity for enjoying the pleasures of the senses

Serious mental illness/psychiatric disability: Typically reflects conditions such as schizophrenia, bipolar disorder, mood disorders, and personality disorders, with or without substance use disorders, which result in reduced abilities to be fully engaged in meaningful occupations of everyday life

Severe visual impairment: The inability to read standard newsprint

Sexual activity: Activities aimed toward giving or receiving sexual pleasure

Sexual counseling: Giving information to patients and clients from a functional perspective *only* related to sexuality and disability

Sexual orientation: A person's erotic, romantic, and affectional attraction to people of the same sex (homosexuality), to the opposite sex (heterosexuality), or to both sexes (bisexuality)

Sexual response stages: The physiologic responses to sexual stimulation/excitement as described by Masters and Johnson

Sexual rights: The rights of individuals to have the information, education, skills, support, and services they need to make responsible decisions about their sexuality consistent with their own values

Sexuality: How people express themselves as sexual beings, having biological, emotional, and physical aspects. It is the composite of many layers of self, including self-image, intimacy patterns, and the elements people find attractive or appealing in others especially during mate or partner selection

Sick role: A temporary excuse from normal social responsibilities (such as going to work or doing housework) due to illness; involves giving up control over one's situation and status as a competent member of society until declared well by a medical authority

Sighted guide technique: The position a blind person uses to hold the arm of a sighted guide just above the elbow; the blind person will be a half-step behind and to the side of the sighted guide. In this position, a blind person can safely follow the guide's body movements as he or she walks

Snellen chart: A test chart of lines of letters or symbols of various sizes used for assessing visual acuity

Social role: A set of behaviors that has some socially agreed-upon function and for which there is an accepted code of norms

Social suffering: The idea that many physical and mental illnesses happen to people because of conditions that affect groups (such as disasters and poverty) or as a result of social policies

Specialized amputee team/clinic: Experienced physicians, therapists, prosthetists, and other clinicians who have practiced exclusively in the field of prosthetics and amputations; the specialized team provides consultants, assessments, and treatments for individuals with amputations and meets and communicates on a scheduled basis

Spirituality: The personal quest for understanding answers to ultimate questions about life, about meaning, and about relationship with the sacred or transcendent, which may (or may not) lead to or arise from the development of religious rituals and the formation of community

Split-thickness skin graft: A skin graft containing the epidermis and the upper portion of the dermis

Stability: The consistency of a measure over time

Stages of Alzheimer's dementia: Seven progressive levels of cognitive function for persons with AD ranging from no apparent cognitive impairment to very severe impairment and the inability to respond to the environment or control movement

Stages of learning: Four specific phases in which skills are learned during intervention from acquisition through fluency, maintenance, and generalization

Standardized: Instruments that have a well-defined procedure, norms (if applicable), and standards for administration

Stigma: Prejudicial devaluing by a social group based on some characteristic or trait; negative social evaluations attached to minority ethnic and racial groups, morally disapproved behaviors, or physical differences caused by chronic illnesses or disabilities

Stimulus prompts: Graded environmental cues that provide varying levels of support for an individual's performance

Superficial burn: A brain injury that involves only the epidermis

System of least prompts: Hierarchy of 2–3 prompts that are selected to work, both for the client and the activity; they are used one at a time, starting with less assistance and moving to more assistance

Systemic lupus erythematosus (SLE): A systemic inflammation disease usually occurring in women that is characterized by a diverse clinical picture involving small vessel vasculitis

Systemic sclerosis (scleroderma, SSc): The generalized form of a group of disorders that are mainly characterized by sclerosis of the skin

T

Targeted muscle reinnervation (TMR): A surgical technique that transfers residual arm nerves to alternative muscle sites. After reinnervation, these target muscles produce EMG signals on the surface of the skin that can be measured and used to control prosthetic arms

Temporal lobe: The portion of the brain beneath the Sylvian fissure on the left and right sides of the cortex. The temporal lobe is involved in auditory processing and is home to the primary auditory cortex. It is also important for the processing of semantics in both speech and vision. The temporal lobe contains the hippocampus and plays a key role in the formation of long-term memory

Tenodesis grasp: A natural action of the wrist and hand musculature as a result of the pull of the extrinsic finger flexor and extensor muscles across the wrist; the fingers tend to flex when the wrist is extended, forming a finger pinch; fingers extend when the wrist flexes, creating a release of finger pinch

Terminal device: The end device of a prosthesis

Tetraplegia: An impairment in motor and/or sensory function in the cervical segments of the spinal cord resulting in functional impairment in the arms, trunk, legs, and pelvic organs; the term *tetraplegia* has replaced the formerly used term *quadriplegia*

Time delay: Pause or delay period added before giving a prompt on each step of an activity; the client may either wait for assistance or try the response independently during these periods

Total body surface area (TBSA): An assessment measure of burns. In adults, the "rule of nines" is used to determine the total percentage of area burned for each major section of the body. In some cases, the burns may cover more than one body part, or may not fully cover such a part; in these cases, burns are measured by using the client's palm as a reference point for 1% of the body

Training data: Performance data gathered on a client with developmental disabilities during functional skills training. This information is compared with baseline data to determine progress or improvement

Transgenerational design: The practice of making products and environments compatible with the physical and sensory impairments that limit activities and are associated with human aging

Transhumeral amputation: Amputation occurring proximal of the shoulder joint

Transradial amputation: Amputation occurring proximal of the elbow joint

Traumatic brain injury (TBI): A nonprogressive, persistent damage to the brain; usually caused by a blow to the head, either from an external object or due to internal forces caused by high-speed acceleration or deceleration

Traumatic brain injury stages: The three stages of cognitive function and/or progression described as mild, moderate, and severe; used to describe and predict behaviors that may emerge during the recovery of the brain trauma

U

Unilateral neglect: Impaired ability to attend, respond, or orient to stimuli presented unilaterally, frequently occurring across various sensory systems

Universal design: The concept of designing all products and the built environment to be aesthetic and usable to the greatest extent possible by everyone, regardless of their age, ability, or status in life

V

Validity: The extent to which one can have confidence in the results of an assessment

Visitability: The purpose of visitability is to ensure basic access for disabled people in newly constructed private homes; at least one exterior door is at ground level with no steps, and a bathroom on the main floor has a door with at least 32 inches of passage

W

Work: An area of occupation that includes activities related to remunerative employment or volunteerism

Z

Zeitgeber: Social and environmental factors that influence internal physiological clocks

Index

Boxes, figures, and tables are indicated with b, f, and t following the page number.